Current Progress in HIV Research

Current Progress in HIV Research

Edited by Chris Stinson

hayle medical

New York

Hayle Medical,
750 Third Avenue, 9th Floor,
New York, NY 10017, USA

Visit us on the World Wide Web at:
www.haylemedical.com

ISBN: 978-1-63241-442-7

The publisher's policy is to use permanent paper from mills that operate a sustainable forestry policy. Furthermore, the publisher ensures that the text paper and cover boards used have met acceptable environmental accreditation standards.

Printed in China.

Cataloging-in-Publication Data

Current progress in HIV research / edited by Chris Stinson.
p. cm.
Includes bibliographical references and index.
ISBN 978-1-63241-442-7
1. HIV infections--Research. 2. HIV infections--Prevention. 3. HIV infections--Treatment.
I. Stinson, Chris.

RC606.6 .C87 2017
616.979 2--dc23

Table of Contents

Preface ... IX

Chapter 1 **One Dose versus three Weekly Doses of Benzathine Penicillin G for Patients Co-Infected with HIV and Early Syphilis** ... 1
Chia-Jui Yang, Nan-Yao Lee, Tun-Chieh Chen, Yu-Hui Lin, Shiou-Haur Liang, Po-Liang Lu, Wen-Chi Huang, Hung-Jen Tang, Chen-Hsiang Lee, Hsi-Hsun Lin, Yen-Hsu Chen, Wen-Chien Ko, Chien-Ching Hung

Chapter 2 **Psychological Fears among Low-Paid Female Sex Workers in Southwest China and Their Implications for HIV Prevention** ... 10
Shan Qiao, Xiaoming Li, Chen Zhang, Yuejiao Zhou, Zhiyong Shen, Zhenzhu Tang, Bonita Stanton

Chapter 3 **Poor Clinical Outcomes for HIV Infected Children on Antiretroviral Therapy in Rural Mozambique: Need for Program Quality Improvement and Community Engagement** ... 2
Sten H. Vermund, Meridith Blevins, Troy D. Moon, Eurico José, Linda Moiane, José A. Tique, Mohsin Sidat, Philip J. Ciampa, Bryan E. Shepherd, Lara M. E. Vaz

Chapter 4 **Community Mobilisation and Empowerment Interventions as Part of HIV Prevention for Female Sex Workers in Southern India** ... 29
Anna Vassall, Sudhashree Chandrashekar, Michael Pickles, Tara S. Beattie, Govindraj Shetty, Parinita Bhattacharjee, Marie-Claude Boily, Peter Vickerman, Janet Bradley, Michel Alary, Stephen Moses, CHARME India Group, Charlotte Watts

Chapter 5 **Molecular Epidemiology of HIV-1 in Jilin Province, Northeastern China: Emergence of a new CRF07_BC Transmission Cluster and Intersubtype Recombinants** ... 39
Xingguang Li, Xihui Zang, Chuanyi Ning, Yi Feng, Cunxin Xie, Xiang He, Yutaka Takebe, Liuyan Sun, Qi Guo, Hui Xing, Marcia L. Kalish, Yiming Shao

Chapter 6 **Consequences of Missed Opportunities for HIV Testing during Pregnancy and Delayed Diagnosis for Mexican Women, Children and Male Partners** ... 49
Tamil Kendall

Chapter 7 **The Mpumalanga Men's Study (MPMS): Results of a Baseline Biological and Behavioral HIV Surveillance Survey in two MSM Communities in South Africa** ... 58
Tim Lane, Thomas Osmand, Alexander Marr, Starley B. Shade, Kristin Dunkle, Theodorus Sandfort, Helen Struthers, Susan Kegeles, James A. McIntyre

Chapter 8 **Suppression of Foxo1 Activity and Down-Modulation of CD62L (L-Selectin) in HIV-1 Infected Resting CD4 T Cells** ... 69
Benjamin Trinité, Chi N. Chan, Caroline S. Lee, Saurabh Mahajan, Yang Luo, Mark A. Muesing, Joy M. Folkvord, Michael Pham, Elizabeth Connick, David N. Levy

Chapter 9 **HIV-1 Conserved Elements p24CE DNA Vaccine Induces Humoral Immune Responses with Broad Epitope Recognition in Macaques** 84
Viraj Kulkarni, Antonio Valentin, Margherita Rosati, Morgane Rolland, James I. Mullins, George N. Pavlakis, Barbara K. Felber

Chapter 10 **Attrition through Multiple Stages of Pre-Treatment and ART HIV Care in South Africa** 96
Matthew P. Fox, Kate Shearer, Mhairi Maskew, Gesine Meyer-Rath, Kate Clouse, Ian Sanne,

Chapter 11 **Phosphodiesterase 8a Supports HIV-1 Replication in Macrophages at the Level of Reverse Transcription** 106
Thijs Booiman, Viviana Cobos Jiménez, Karel A. van Dort, Angélique B. van 't Wout, Neeltje A. Kootstra

Chapter 12 **Expression of the IL-7 Receptor Alpha-Chain is Down Regulated on the Surface of CD4 T-Cells by the HIV-1 Tat Protein** 115
Denny McLaughlin, Elliott Faller, Scott Sugden, Paul MacPherson

Chapter 13 **Invariant Natural Killer T (iNKT) Cells in HAART-Treated, HIV-Positive Patients with Bone and Cardiovascular Impairment** 127
Camilla Tincati, Matteo Basilissi, Elisabetta Sinigaglia, Esther Merlini, Giovanni Carpani, Antonella d'Arminio Monforte, Giulia Marchetti

Chapter 14 **HIV Testing Implementation in two Urban Cities: Practice, Policy, and Perceived Barriers** 136
Camden J. Hallmark, Jennifer Skillicorn, Thomas P. Giordano, Jessica A. Davila, Marlene McNeese, Nestor Rocha, Avemaria Smith, Stacey Cooper, Amanda D. Castel

Chapter 15 **HIV-1 Subtype C Unproductively Infects Human Cardiomyocytes *In Vitro* and Induces Apoptosis Mitigated by an Anti-Gp120 Aptamer** 146
Walter R. Lopes de Campos, Nthato Chirwa, Grace London, Lia S. Rotherham, Lynn Morris, Bongani M. Mayosi, Makobetsa Khati

Chapter 16 **Community-Based Evaluation of PMTCT uptake in Nyanza Province, Kenya** 155
Pamela K. Kohler, John Okanda, John Kinuthia, Lisa A. Mills, George Olilo, Frank Odhiambo, Kayla F. Laserson, Brenda Zierler, Joachim Voss, Grace John-Stewart

Chapter 17 **Incidence of HIV-Associated Tuberculosis among Individuals Taking Combination Antiretroviral Therapy** 165
Tendesayi Kufa, Tonderai Mabuto, Evans Muchiri, Salome Charalambous, Dominique Rosillon, Gavin Churchyard, Rebecca C. Harris

Chapter 18 **detectIR: A Novel Program for Detecting Perfect and Imperfect Inverted Repeats using Complex Numbers and Vector Calculation** 176
Congting Ye, Guoli Ji, Lei Li, Chun Liang

Chapter 19 **CD161⁺ MAIT Cells are Severely Reduced in Peripheral Blood and Lymph Nodes of HIV-Infected Individuals Independently of Disease Progression** 187
Johanna Maria Eberhard, Philip Hartjen, Silke Kummer, Reinhold E. Schmidt, Maximilian Bockhorn, Clara Lehmann, Ashwin Balagopal, Joachim Hauber, Jan van Lunzen, Julian Schulze zur Wiesch

Chapter 20 **CD8 and CD4 Epitope Predictions in RV144: No Strong Evidence of a T-Cell Driven Sieve Effect in HIV-1 Breakthrough Sequences from Trial Participants** 198
Kalpana Dommaraju, Gustavo Kijak, Jonathan M. Carlson, Brendan B. Larsen, Sodsai Tovanabutra, Dan E. Geraghty, Wenjie Deng, Brandon S. Maust, Paul T. Edlefsen, Eric Sanders-Buell, Silvia Ratto-Kim, Mark S. deSouza, Supachai Rerks-Ngarm, Sorachai Nitayaphan, Punnee Pitisuttihum, Jaranit Kaewkungwal, Robert J. O'Connell, Merlin L. Robb, Nelson L. Michael, James I. Mullins, Jerome H. Kim, Morgane Rolland

Chapter 21 **Methodological Challenges in Collecting Social and Behavioural Data Regarding the HIV Epidemic among Gay and other Men who have Sex with Men in Australia** 209
Iryna B. Zablotska, Andrew Frankland, Martin Holt, John de Wit, Graham Brown, Bruce Maycock, Christopher Fairley, Garrett Prestage

Chapter 22 **Cardiac Health Risk Stratification System (CHRiSS): A Bayesian-Based Decision Support System for Left Ventricular Assist Device (LVAD) Therapy** 220
Natasha A. Loghmanpour, Marek J. Druzdzel, James F. Antaki

Permissions

List of Contributors

Index

Preface

In my initial years as a student, I used to run to the library at every possible instance to grab a book and learn something new. Books were my primary source of knowledge and I would not have come such a long way without all that I learnt from them. Thus, when I was approached to edit this book; I became understandably nostalgic. It was an absolute honor to be considered worthy of guiding the current generation as well as those to come. I put all my knowledge and hard work into making this book most beneficial for its readers.

HIV or human immunodeficiency virus is a virus that infects the human immune system and causes AIDS. This book on HIV research discusses the ongoing research that is taking place with regard to the restoration of immunity within the human body. Early detection and treatment can greatly reduce the damage that can be caused by the HIV virus. Medication can also slow down the mutability of the virus. Through this book, we attempt to further enlighten the readers about the new concepts in this field. It presents researches and studies performed by experts across the globe. Coherent flow of topics, student-friendly language and extensive use of examples make this book an invaluable source of knowledge.

I wish to thank my publisher for supporting me at every step. I would also like to thank all the authors who have contributed their researches in this book. I hope this book will be a valuable contribution to the progress of the field.

Editor

1

One Dose versus Three Weekly Doses of Benzathine Penicillin G for Patients Co-Infected with HIV and Early Syphilis: A Multicenter, Prospective Observational Study

Chia-Jui Yang[1], Nan-Yao Lee[2], Tun-Chieh Chen[3,4], Yu-Hui Lin[5], Shiou-Haur Liang[6], Po-Liang Lu[3], Wen-Chi Huang[7], Hung-Jen Tang[8], Chen-Hsiang Lee[7], Hsi-Hsun Lin[6], Yen-Hsu Chen[3], Wen-Chien Ko[2]*, Chien-Ching Hung[9,10,11]*

1 Department of Internal Medicine, Far East Memorial Hospital, New Taipei City, Taiwan, **2** Department of Internal Medicine, National Cheng Kung University College of Medicine and Hospital, Tainan, Taiwan, **3** Department of Internal Medicine, Kaohsiung Medical University Hospital and College of Medicine, Kaohsiung Medical University, Kaohsiung, Taiwan, **4** Department of Internal Medicine, Kaohsiung Municipal Ta-Tung Hospital, Kaohsiung Medical University, Kaohsiung, Taiwan, **5** Department of Internal Medicine, Taichung Veterans General Hospital, Taichung, Taiwan, **6** Department of Internal Medicine, E-Da Hospital/I-Shou University, Kaohsiung, Taiwan, **7** Department of Internal Medicine, Kaohsiung Chang Gung Memorial Hospital, Chang Gung University College of Medicine, Kaohsiung, Taiwan, **8** Department of Internal Medicine, Chi-Mei Medical Center, Tainan, Taiwan, **9** Department of Internal Medicine, National Taiwan University Hospital and National Taiwan University College of Medicine, Taipei, Taiwan, **10** Department of Medical Research, China Medical University Hospital, Taichung, Taiwan, **11** China Medical University, Taichung, Taiwan

Abstract

Background: One dose of benzathine penicillin G (BPG) has been recommended for HIV-infected patients with early syphilis (primary, secondary, and early latent syphilis) in the sexually transmitted diseases treatment guidelines, but clinical data to support such a recommendation are limited.

Methods: We prospectively observed the serological response to 1 or 3 weekly doses of BPG in HIV-infected adults who sought treatment of early syphilis at 8 hospitals around Taiwan. Rapid plasma reagin (RPR) titers were followed every 3–6 months after treatment. The serological response was defined as a 4-fold or greater decline in RPR titers at 12 months of treatment. The missing values were treated by following the last-observed-carried-forward principle. We hypothesized that 1 dose was non-inferior to 3 weekly doses of BPG with the non-inferiority margin for the difference of serological response set to 10%.

Results: Between 2007 and 2012, 573 patients completed at least 12 months of follow-up: 295 (51.5%) receiving 1 dose of BPG (1-dose group) and 278 (48.5%) 3 doses (3-dose group). Overall, 198 patients (67.1%; 95% confidence interval [CI], 61.4–72.5%) in the 1-dose group achieved serological response at 12 months, as did 208 patients (74.8%; 95% CI, 69.3–79.8%) in the 3-dose group (one-sided 95% CI of the difference, 15.1%). In the multivariate analysis, secondary syphilis (adjusted odds ratio [AOR], 1.90; 95% CI 1.17–3.09), RPR titer ≥32 (AOR, 1.93; 95% CI, 1.38–2.69), and 3 doses of BPG (AOR, 1.68; 95% CI, 1.20–2.36) were independently associated with a serological response. The time to the first episode of treatment failure was 1184 (standard deviation [SD], 70.5) and 1436 (SD, 80.0) days for 1- and 3-dose group, respectively.

Conclusions: Single-dose BPG resulted in a higher serological failure rate and shorter time to treatment failure than 3 weekly doses of BPG in the treatment of early syphilis in HIV-infected patients.

Editor: Joseph David Tucker, UNC Project-China, China

Funding: This study was supported by grants from the Centers for Disease Control, Taiwan (grant number DOH102-DC-1401 to CCH). The funding source had no role in study design and conduct; data collection, analysis, or interpretation; or in the writing of the manuscript or the decision to submit it for publication.

Competing Interests: The authors have declared that no competing interests exist.

* Email: hcc0401@ntu.edu.tw (CCH); winston3415@gmail.com (WCK)

Introduction

Syphilis, caused by *Treponema pallidum*, is an important sexually transmitted disease. Globally, there were an estimated 36.4 million cases of syphilis in adults between the ages of 15 and 49 years in 2008 [1]. The incidence of syphilis is increasing both in developed and less developed countries, especially among men who have sex with men (MSM) [2–5]. In the United Kingdom, the newly diagnosed cases of syphilis increased from 2,650 in 2010 to 2,915 in 2011 and 75% of the cases occurred in MSM [6]. In the United States, the case numbers reported to the Centers for Disease Control and Prevention (US CDC) increased from 13,774 in 2010 to 13,970 in 2011, an increase of 1.4%, and MSM were the major risk group, accounting for 83% and 72% in 2010 and 2011, respectively [7].

Appropriate treatment of early syphilis among HIV-infected patients has been controversial because clinical studies of a sufficient sample size have been lacking. In the previous version of treatment guidelines for syphilis by the US CDC in 2006 [8], an enhanced therapy with 3 weekly doses of benzathine penicillin G (BPG) (2.4 million units [MU]) was recommended by some experts for HIV-infected patients with early syphilis. Three weekly doses of BPG had been used for treatment of neurosyphilis in 1970s and several controlled trials had concluded clinical efficacy despite report of treatment failure in a few cases [9]. Therefore, enhanced therapy was recommended to provide protective effect against neurosyphilis in immunocompromised host [9]. However, a randomized control trial conducted before the introduction of combination antiretroviral therapy (cART) demonstrated no difference in treatment response between HIV-infected and HIV-uninfected patients treated with a single dose of BPG followed by a 10-day course of oral amoxicillin plus probenecid acid, although it is unclear if the use of additional depot penicillin would have resulted in better outcomes [10]. Therefore, a single dose of BPG for early syphilis has been recommended in the most recent guidelines in the UK, US and Europe [11–13]. However, dilemmas continue to exist among infectious diseases specialists as to the appropriate dose of BPG to be administered in the management of early syphilis in HIV-infected patients in the cART era [14].

Several studies have shown that HIV-infected patients with syphilis have higher failure rates after standard treatment, while other studies have not [15–18]. The discrepant results among these studies can be attributed to limitations of the published studies, such as a small sample size, lack of stratification for different stages of syphilis, different definitions of serological failure, high rates of patients who were lost to follow up, and enrollment of patients with low non-treponemal titers. In this study, we aimed to compare the serological response rates of early syphilis to 1 dose versus 3 weekly doses of BPG therapy and to identify the factors associated with a serological response among HIV-infected patients.

Materials and Methods

Study design and participants

This multicenter, prospective observational study was conducted between January 2007 and December 2012 at 8 major hospitals around Taiwan that are designated for HIV care by the Centers for Disease Control, Taiwan, where HIV care, including cART and monitoring of CD4 count and plasma HIV RNA load, is provided free-of-charge. According to the national guidelines for HIV care in Taiwan, non-treponemal serological tests for syphilis are recommended to be performed at least once yearly and on an as-needed basis as indicated by the clinical presentations and every 3 to 6 months over a period of 2 years for those who receive

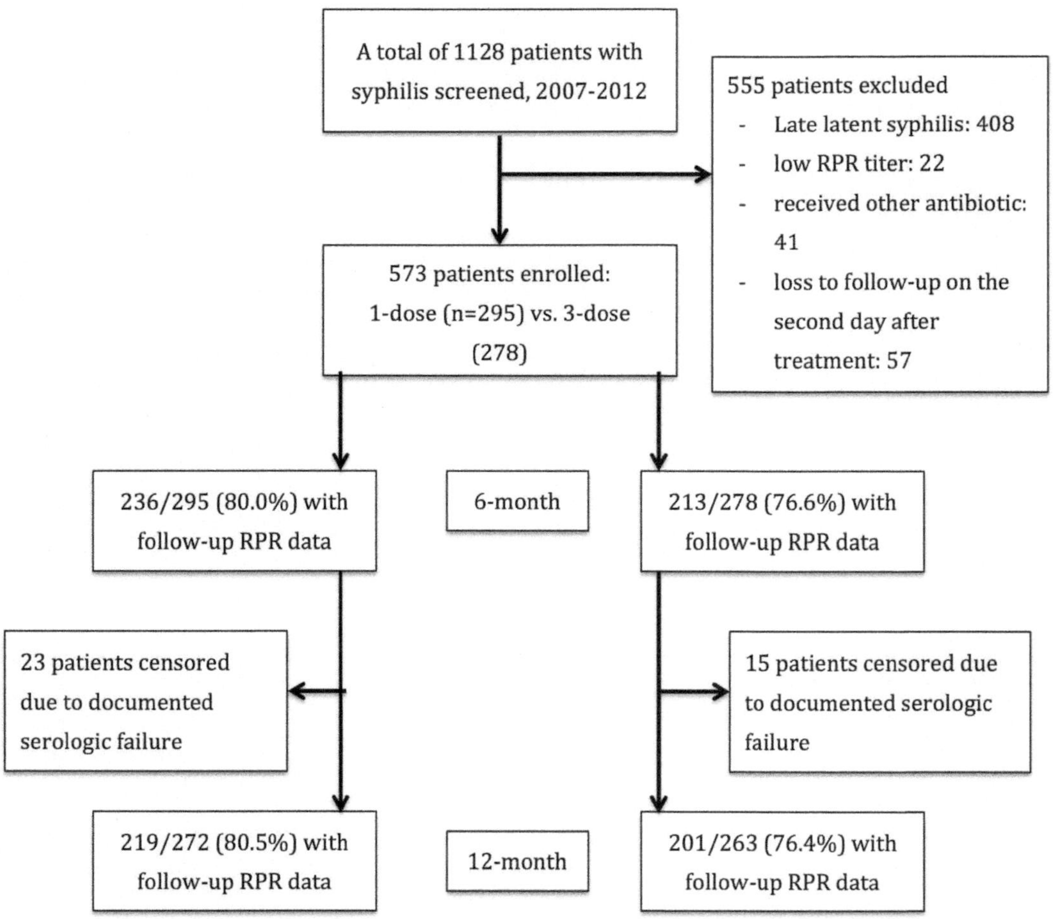

Figure 1. Study flow showing patient recruitment and patients with available rapid plasma reagin (RPR) data during the 6 and 12 months of follow-up.

Table 1. Clinical characteristics of HIV-infected patients with early syphilis receiving 1 dose or 3 weekly doses of benzathine penicillin G.

	All patients (n = 573)	1-dose (n = 295)	3-dose (n = 278)	*P*-value
Age, mean (SD), years	33.1 (7.8)	32.8 (7.9)	33.5 (7.8)	0.27
Risk for HIV transmission, n (%)				
MSM	539 (94.1)	284 (96.3)	255 (91.7)	NA
Heterosexuals	23 (4.0)	8 (2.7)	15 (5.4)	NA
Others	11 (1.9)	3 (1.0)	8 (2.9)	NA
Syphilis stage, n (%)				
Primary	51 (8.9)	28 (9.5)	23 (8.3)	0.66
Secondary	331 (57.8)	173 (58.6)	158 (56.8)	0.67
Early latent	191 (33.3)	94 (31.9)	97 (34.9)	0.48
RPR titer, median [IQR]	1:64 (32, 128)	1:64 (32, 128)	1:64 (32, 128)	0.61
CD4 count, mean (SD), cells/μl	457 (244)	462 (239)	452 (249)	0.62
CD4≤200, n (%)	71 (12.4)	33 (11.2)	38 (13.7)	0.38
CD4≤350, n (%)	207 (36.1)	103 (34.9)	104 (37.4)	0.54
PVL, mean (SD), log_{10} copies/ml	3.04 (1.49)	3.02 (1.51)	3.06 (1.48)	0.73
PVL <400 copies/ml, n (%)	305 (53.2)	156 (52.9)	149 (53.6)	0.87
Prior history of syphilis n (%)	203 (35.4)	103 (34.9)	100 (36.0)	0.79
CART, n (%)	362 (63.2)	194 (65.8)	168 (60.4)	0.26

Abbreviations: CART, combination antiretroviral therapy; IQR, interquartile range; MSM, men who have sex with men; PVL, plasma HIV RNA load; RPR, rapid plasma reagin; SD, standard deviation.

treatment for syphilis. The patients who received stable cART were usually followed as an outpatient every 3 months and monitoring of immunological and virological status was performed every 3 to 6 months.

HIV-infected patients were eligible for this observational study, if they were 20 years or older, had early syphilis (i.e. primary, secondary, or early latent), and had reactive rapid plasma reagin (RPR) titers of 1:4 or greater and a reactive result of *Treponema pallidum* particle agglutination (TPPA) test (titer ≥1:320), for which 1 or 3 weekly doses of BPG (2.4 MU, 1170 IU/mg, Biochemie Ges. M.B.H., Kundl, Australia) were administered intramuscularly. Patients with a prior history of syphilis who received treatment within 12 months before enrollment were excluded. In addition, patients were excluded if they were pregnant, received antibiotics such as penicillin, ceftriaxone, doxycycline, or macrolides for syphilis or other infections within the preceding 12 months or during follow-up, were lost to follow-up immediately after treatment, had a history of penicillin allergy, or were receiving immunosuppressants, immunomodulators, or chemotherapy. The study was approved by the Research Ethics Committee of each participating hospital and the written informed consent was waived.

Diagnosis of syphilis

Primary syphilis was diagnosed when the patients presented with reactive serologies (RPR titers >1:4 and reactive TPPA titers) and genital, anal, or oral ulceration (chancre); secondary syphilis was diagnosed when the patients presented with reactive serologies and cutaneous rashes, mucosal lesions, generalized lymphadenopathy, or other signs; and early latent syphilis was diagnosed when the patients presented with reactive serologies and documented negative RPR or 4-fold elevation of RPR titers with exposure to patients with syphilis within the preceding 12 months [11].

Laboratory investigations

Serological tests for syphilis included the RPR test (BD Macro-VueTMRPR Card tests, USA) and *T. pallidum* particle agglutination test (FTI-SERODIA-TPPA. Fujirebio Taiwan Inc., Taoyuan, Taiwan). Plasma HIV RNA loads and CD4 lymphocyte counts were quantified with the use of the Cobas Amplicor HIV-1 Monitor^{TM} Test, version 1.5, (Roche Diagnostics Corporation, Indianapolis, USA) and FACSFlow (Becton Dickinson), respectively.

Treatment and follow-up

All patients with syphilis received 1 dose or 3 weekly doses of BPG. While treatment guidelines for syphilis evolved during the 5-year study period, the decision to give 1 or 3 doses of BPG depended on the assessment of the treating physicians, which could be influenced by the characteristics of each patient. Following treatment, follow-up of RPR titers every 3 to 6 months was recommended. A standardized case record form was used to collect information on demographic characteristics, a previous history of penicillin treatment for syphilis, stage of syphilis, RPR titers at baseline and during follow-up, dose of BPG administered, receipt of cART, and CD4 count and plasma HIV RNA load.

The primary endpoint of the study was achievement of serological response that was defined as a 4-fold or greater decline in RPR titers at the 12th month follow-up visit when compared with the baseline titers. The secondary endpoint included a 4-fold or greater decline in RPR titers at the 6th month follow-up visit when compared with the baseline titers; and the time to treatment failure, which was defined as the failure to achieve a 4-fold or greater decline in RPR titers; or a 4-fold or greater increase in RPR titers after achieving serological response during the 12 months of observation; or anytime when retreatment of syphilis was given during the 12 months of follow-up.

A)

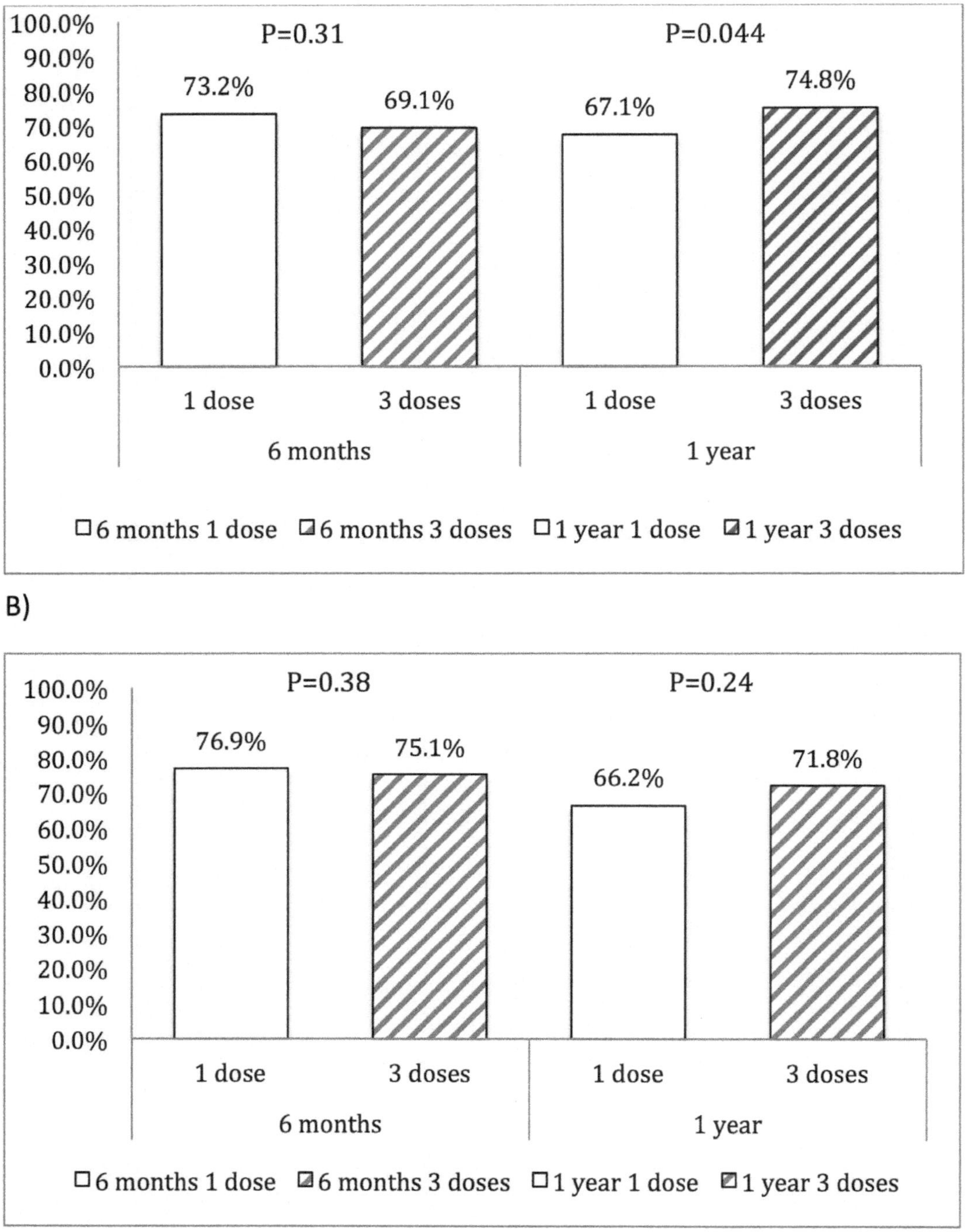

Figure 2. Serological response rates in the 1-dose and 3-dose benzathine penicillin G groups at 6 months and 12 months of follow up. A). Last-observed-carried-forward analysis; B). Per-protocol analysis.

Statistical analysis

All statistical analyses were performed using SPSS version 18.0 (SPSS, Chicago, IL) and Stata software, version 10 (StataCorp, College Station, TX, USA). All patients who received at least 1 dose of BPG were included for analyses, for which the last-observed-carried-forward principle was adopted to deal with missing data at the 6th and 12th month of follow-up. Each patient was followed at least for twice during the 12-month study period. Categorical variables were compared by Fisher's exact test or Chi-square test. Non-categorical variables were compared by Mann-Whitney U test. Factors with a P value ≤ 0.2 or biological significance were included in the multivariate analysis. Binary logistic regression analysis was used to determine the factors associated with serological responses at the time of 12 months of follow-up. We fit the data using mixed effect model in which the covariate structure of "hospitals" was considered in the model.

Table 2. Factors associated with serological response in the patients who received 1 dose or 3 doses of benzathine penicillin G at 12 months of follow-up in univariate and multivariate analysis.

	Univariate analysis			Multvariate analysis		
	Responders (n = 406)	**non-responders (n = 167)**	***P*-value**	**Adjusted odds ratio**	**95% confidence interval**	***P*-value**
Age, mean (SD), years	33.1 (8.0)	33.2 (7.3)	0.89	1.01	0.99–1.03	0.55
Risk, n (%)						
MSM	386 (95.1)	153 (91.6)	0.118	1.67	0.82–2.89	0.19
non-MSM	20 (4.9)	14 (8.4)		1	–	–
Syphilis stage, n (%)						
Primary	34 (8.4)	17 (10.2)	0.52	1	–	–
Secondary	249 (61.6)	82 (49.1)	0.005	1.90	1.17–3.09	0.01
Early latent	123 (30.3)	68 (40.7)	0.014	1.04	0.70–1.56	0.84
RPR titer, median (IQR)	1:64 (32, 128)	1:64 (32, 128)				
RPR titer ≧1:32	353 (86.9)	125 (74.9)	0.001	1.93	1.38–2.69	<0.001
CD4 count, mean (SD), cells/μl	460 (242)	449 (249)	0.61			
CD4 ≦200, n (%)	47 (11.6)	24 (14.3)	0.49	1	–	–
200<CD4 ≦350, n (%)	89 (21.9)	47 (28.1)	0.16	1.05	0.54–2.07	0.88
CD4>350, n (%)	270 (66.5)	96 (57.5)	0.084	1.51	0.69–3.51	0.30
PVL, mean (SD), log10 copies/ml	3.07 (1.51)	2.99 (1.47)	0.53			
PVL <400 copies/ml, n (%)	192 (47.3)	76 (45.5)	0.58	0.97	0.78–1.21	0.79
Prior history of syphilis, n (%)	142 (35.0)	61 (36.5)	0.77	0.98	0.79–1.21	0.82
CART, n (%)	251 (61.8)	111 (66.5)	0.29	0.75	0.47–1.20	0.23
3 doses of penicillin, n (%)	208 (51.2)	70 (41.9)	0.04	1.68	1.20–2.36	0.002

Abbreviations: CART, combination antiretroviral therapy; IQR, interquatile range; PVL, plasma HIV RNA load; RPR, rapid plasma reagin; SD, standard deviation.

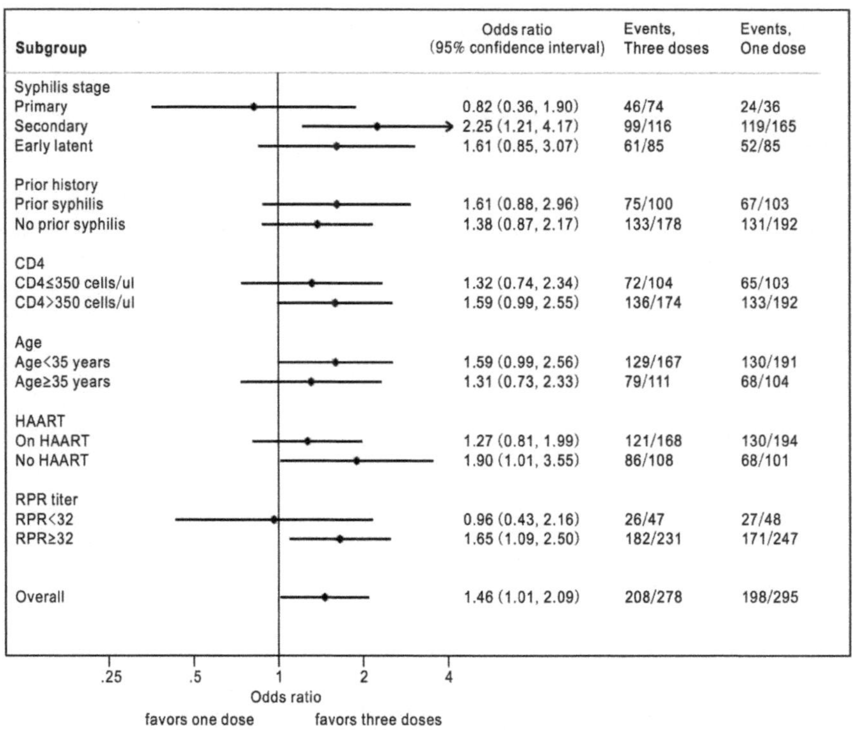

Figure 3. Forest plot showing the serological response rates in different subgroups of patients receiving 1 or 3 doses of benzathine penicillin G at 12 months of follow-up.

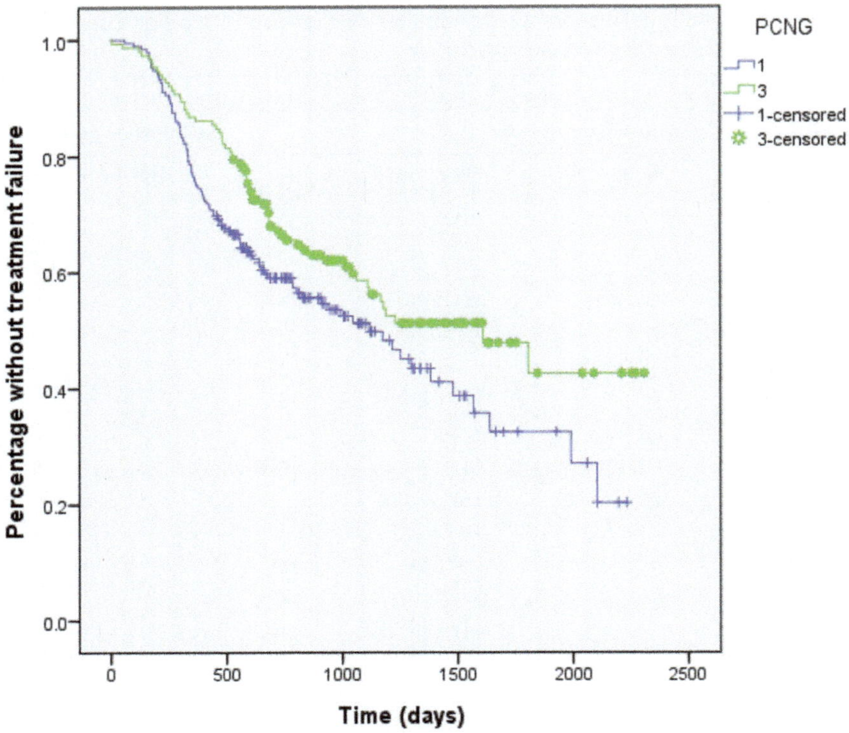

Figure 4. Kaplan-Meier plot showing the time to treatment failure to 1- or 3-dose benzathine penicillin G regimen (Log rank test, *P*=0.026).

Thus the factor "hospital" was treated as a random effect and was put into mixed effect binary logistic regression analysis. All comparisons were 2-tailed and a *P* value <0.05 was considered to be significant. We hypothesized that 1-dose BPG regimen was non-inferior to the 3-dose regimen in the HIV-infected patients with early syphilis. The non-inferiority in terms of serological response rate following 1-dose BPG therapy to 3-dose therapy would be concluded if the lower boundary of the two-sided 95% confidence interval (CI) (one-sided $\alpha = 0.025$) for the difference in the serological response rate between the two groups was at least −0·1 (that is, the non-inferiority margin was set to 10%). With the estimated serological response rate of 75% for the 3-dose BPG group, it was estimated that 232 patients were needed for each group to confirm the non-inferiority of 1-dose to 3-dose regimen with a power of 80%. Time to treatment failure was assessed by Kaplan-Meier plots and Cox proportional hazards regression analysis was used to estimate the hazard ratios (HR) for treatment failure between the two groups of patients. All patients were followed until 30 June, 2013, or the date when the patients received the diagnosis of recurrent syphilis or were lost to follow-up, or death, whichever occurred first.

Results

During the 5-year study period, 1128 HIV-infected patients with syphilis sought HIV care and treatment of syphilis at the 8 participating hospitals, and 555 (49.2%) patients were excluded due to late latent syphilis stage (n = 408), concurrent use of other antibiotics (n = 41), loss to follow-up on the second day after treatment (n = 57; 26 for 1-dose and 31 for 3-dose group), low RPR titers (<1:4) (n = 22), and without confirmed HIV infection (n = 8) (Figure 1). A total of 573 HIV-infected patients, including 295 patients receiving 1 dose and 278 patients receiving 3 doses of BPG, were enrolled. During the study period, the proportion of patients receiving 1 dose of BPG increased after 2010, when the updated treatment guidelines of US CDC in 2010 recommended 1 dose of BPG for early syphilis in HIV-infected patients (Figure S1).

Baseline characteristics of the two groups of patients are shown in Table 1. Most patients were MSM. There were no statistically significant differences between the two groups of patients in terms of age, sex, gender, the stage of syphilis, RPR titer, a prior history of syphilis, CD4 count, plasma HIV RNA load, and receipt of cART (Table 1). Of note, more than half (57.8%) of the patients had secondary syphilis at enrollment, 64% had baseline CD4 cell counts of more than 350 cells/μl, and 35.4% had a prior history of syphilis. While missing values during follow-up were dealt using the last-observed-carried-forward principle, no statistically significant differences were observed for most of the clinical characteristics assessed between the patients with missing values and those without missing values at the 6th and 12th months of follow-up (Tables S1 and S2).

The serological response rate at 12 months of BPG treatment was 67.1% (95% CI, 61.4–72.5) for the 1-dose group and 74.8% (95% CI, 69.3–79.8) for the 3-dose group ($P = 0.044$) in the last-observed-carried-forward population (Figure 2A). In the per-protocol population, the serological response rate was 66.2% (95% CI, 59.6–72.4) and 71.8% (95% CI, 64.7–78.2), respectively, for the 1-dose and 3-dose group ($P = 0.24$) (Figure 2B). The difference of serological response rates between 3-dose and 1-dose BPG group was 7.7% (95% CI, 0.3–15.1; $P = 0.041$) in the last-observed-carried-forward population, with the one-sided 95% CI of effectiveness difference between the 3-dose and 1-dose group exceeding the predefined 10% non-inferiority margin.

In the analysis of primary endpoint, the factors associated with a serological response in univariate and multivariate analysis are shown in Table 2. In univariate analysis, treatment with 3 weekly doses of BPG and secondary syphilis were associated with a higher serological response rate, while early latent syphilis was associated with a lower serological response rate. Receipt of cART, CD4 count (either <200, between 200 and 350 or >350 cells/µl), or plasma HIV RNA load was not statistically significantly associated with serological response, although a trend toward a higher serological response rate was observed in patients with CD4 counts >350 cells/µl ($P = 0.084$). In the multivariate logistic regression analysis, we found that secondary syphilis (adjusted odds ratio [AOR], 1.90; 95%CI, 1.17–3.09), RPR titers ≥32 (AOR, 1.93; 95%CI, 1.38–2.69), and 3-dose BPG (AOR, 1.68; 95%CI, 1.20–2.36) were independently associated with a serological response (Table 2).

In the two groups of patients, 88.1% and 86.0% in the 1-dose group and the 3-dose group, respectively, ever achieved a 4-fold or greater decline in RPR titers after treatment (data not shown) ($P = 0.46$). There were no statistically significant differences in the overall serological response rates before and after the change of treatment guidelines in 2010 [11]; however, a lower serological response rate to the 1-dose BPG was observed after 2011 (Figure S2).

The serological response rates in different subgroups at 12 months of follow-up are shown in the forest plot (Figure 3). The subgroup analysis demonstrated the consistency with overall serological response favoring 3 weekly doses of BPG except for the subgroups of patients who presented with primary syphilis and RPR titers <32.

We also evaluated the serologic response at 6 months of follow-up with univariate analysis and mixed effect binary logistic regression (Table S3 and Figure S4). No significant difference was observed of the serologic response rate between the 1-dose group and 3-dose group while RPR titers ≥32 and CD4 counts >350 cells/µl were found to be associated with serologic response after treatment.

During the study period, the mean observation duration was 1102 days (standard deviation [SD], 488) for the 1-dose group and 1265 days (SD, 483) for the 3-dose group. Overall, treatment failure developed in 146 (49.5%) and 120 (43.2%) patients in the 1-dose and 3-dose group ($p = 0.13$), respectively, during the follow-up; none developed clinical manifestations suggestive of neurosyphilis, however. The Kaplan-Meier survival plot to depict the time to treatment failure for the two groups of patients is illustrated in Figure 4. The mean time to treatment failure was significantly longer for the 3-dose group than the 1-dose group (1436 [SD, 80.0] vs 1184.days [SD, 70.5]; log-rank test, $P = 0.026$).

In each group of patients who developed treatment failure during the follow-up, more patients in the 1-dose group than 3-dose group experienced an increase of RPR titers by 4-fold or greater at 6 months of follow-up (16.7% [13/78] vs 3.5% [3/85], $P = 0.007$) as well as at 12 months of follow-up (70.0% [64/97] vs 47.1% [33/70], $P = 0.018$) (Figure S3). During the follow-up period, there were 5 patients with documented reinfections with primary syphilis, 17 with secondary syphilis and 6 with both primary and secondary syphilis in the 1-dose group (28.7%), while there were only 2 patients with reinfections with primary syphilis and 5 secondary syphilis in the 3-dose group (10%). In addition, 6 and 2 patients in the 1-dose and the 3-doses BPG group, respectively, received retreatment because of a delayed serological response.

Discussion

In this multicenter, prospective observational study, we demonstrated that 1-dose BPG was inferior to the 3-dose regimen in achieving a 4-fold or greater decline in RPR titers at 12 months of follow-up since a higher failure rate and a shorter time to treatment failure were noted in the 1-dose group. The better serological response was associated with higher RPR titers (RPR≥32) at baseline, secondary syphilis, and 3-dose BPG therapy. Although not statistically significant, we found a trend that a higher serologic response rate was associated with higher CD4 cell counts.

In HIV-infected patients with syphilis, the serological response rates to BPG ranged from 70.4% to 91.8% in previous retrospective studies that were conducted in the cART era [15–18]. In our study, the serological response rate at 12 months in the 1-dose and 3-dose group was 67.1% and 74.8%, respectively, while the overall serological response rate was 70.9%. In contrast to other studies that included a higher percentage of female patients or a lower proportion of MSM [15–17], our study population was mainly composed of subjects who were MSM, a population that have been reported to have a higher rate of syphilis reinfection [19], which may have contributed to the lower serological response rate observed in our study. In the retrospective study by Farhi et al, in which 95% of the population were MSM and 53% presented with secondary syphilis, the serologic response rate is higher (91.8%) than ours [18]. However, more than one fourth of the patients were excluded from the final analysis because of inadequate information; furthermore, a relatively higher preserved immune status was observed in the study population [18]. The association between lower CD4 cell counts (<200 cells/µl) and a higher serologic failure rate has been reported in a previous study [20], which was also observed in our study (Table 2).

In this study, we failed to demonstrate that the serological response of the 1-dose group was non-inferior to that of the 3-dose group during the 12-month follow-up. The subgroup analysis demonstrated the consistency with overall serological response favoring 3 weekly doses of BPG except for the subgroups of patients who presented with primary syphilis and RPR titers <32 (Figure 3). The results of a better serological response for the 3-dose group could be multifactorial, though more investigations are warranted. In our study, the interval between treatment and treatment failure for the 3-dose group was longer than that for the 1-dose group. The receipt of 3 weekly doses of BPG could theoretically maintain a longer duration of therapeutic level of BPG than a single dose, which suggests that 3-doses BPG could have a longer protective effect [21]. However, no cases of early treatment failure were noted within the first 3 months of treatment with either 1 dose or 3 doses of BPG; furthermore, the proportions of the patients ever achieving a 4-fold or greater decline of RPR titers were similar between the two groups of patients. Therefore, the difference of serological response rates between these two groups could be attributed to other reasons. One retrospective study with a large sample size concluded that no difference of serologic failure rates between 1-dose and 3-dose BPG group in treating early syphilis of HIV-infected patients [22]. However, extremely unequal sample sizes of 1-dose ($n = 47$) and 3-dose BPG ($n = 434$) groups with potential bias might make the conclusion less convincing. In addition, the follow-up of RPR titers within the study period was not mentioned in detail, which might result in underestimation of the rate of reinfection.

In our study, the patients who failed to achieve a serological response often had a 4-fold increase of RPR titer after ever achieving a serological response during the 12-month follow-up period or experienced primary or secondary syphilis suggesting reinfection with syphilis, which was more frequently observed in the patients who received 1 dose of BPG than those who received

3 weekly doses. Given the long interval between treatment administration and treatment failure, our findings of a lower response rate to 1 dose BPG therapy than to 3 weekly doses may result from higher rates of reinfection with syphilis, suggesting that more intensive safe-sex counseling is needed to be implemented in this high-risk population.

The strengths of our study include that it is a prospective observational study with a large sample size and the two groups of patients had similar baseline characteristics (Table 1), including prior syphilis; only patients with early syphilis were enrolled and those with low RPR titers (<4) were excluded; and all of the treatment responses were evaluated at 6 and 12 months of follow-up [11]. Moreover, the patients who had ever received the other antibiotics, such as doxycycline, azithromycin, amoxicillin or ceftriaxone, were excluded.

There are several limitations of our study, however. First of all, this is not a randomized clinical trial and the decision to give 1 dose or 3 doses of BPG depended on the assessment of physicians who might prefer to give the more enhanced, 3 doses of BPG to patients who were considered at a higher risk for recurrent syphilis or treatment failure such as a previous history of syphilis, higher RPR titers, early latent syphilis, or lower CD4 counts, higher plasma HIV RNA loads, a history of prior opportunistic infections and more advanced HIV disease. However, there were no statistically significant differences in the baseline characteristics when treatment for syphilis was administered between the two study groups in our study. Second, nearly one fourth of the patients had missing RPR titers at 6 and 12 months following treatment. However, if we analyze the patients with available 6-month and 12-month RPR titers, the response rate is still nearly the same between 1-dose and 3-doses BPG in 12-month (Figure 2B). Third, the validity of using serologic response as a true testament of cure remains to be investigated [23]. Because we have no clinical standard to determine bacteriologic cure, in the case of syphilis we used a 4-fold or greater decline of RPR titers as an evidence of cure as suggested by the treatment guidelines [11]. However, it's difficult to differentiate relapse from reinfection based on increased RPR titers following completion of treatment. More cases of primary and/or secondary syphilis were seen in the 1-dose group than 3-dose group during the follow-up (28.9% vs. 10%, $P = 0.004$). Therefore, we believe that more episodes of reinfection could contribute to the higher failure rate in the 1-dose group. Fourth, 94% of the patients in our study were MSM, and therefore our results may not be generalizable to other risk groups. Last, we did not perform cerebrospinal fluid study in patients with higher RPR titers or lower CD4 counts, as suggested by previous investigators [11]. However, no neurologic symptoms of all the patients had been observed during the follow-up period (data not shown).

In summary, we failed to demonstrate the non-inferiority of 1 dose of BPG to 3 weekly doses of BPG for treatment of early syphilis in HIV-infected patients. A substantial rate of treatment failure due to reinfection in both groups suggests that counseling for risk behavior modification should be integral component of management of HIV-infected patients with early syphilis.

Supporting Information

Figure S1 Trends of the proportions of the patients receiving 1 dose or 3 weekly doses of benzathine penicillin G between 2007 and 2012 before and after revision of Sexually Transmitted Diseases Treatment Guidelines by the US Centers for Disease Control and Prevention in 2010. The number inside the bar indicates the number of the patients receiving 1 dose (stippled) or 3 weekly doses (gray) of benzathine penicillin G.

Figure S2 The serological response rates of 1 or 3 doses of benzathine penicillin G therapy before and after the revision of Sexually Transmitted Diseases Treatment Guidelines in 2010.

Figure S3 The causes of treatment failure for the two groups of patients at 12 months of treatment. The numbers inside the bars indicate the cases of treatment failure.

Figure S4 Forest plot showing the serological response rates in different subgroups of patients receiving 1 or 3 doses of benzathine penicillin G at 6 months of follow-up.

Table S1 Comparisons of clinical characteristics of patients with missing rapid plasma reagin values and those without missing values at 6 months of follow-up.

Table S2 Comparisons of clinical characteristics of patients with missing rapid plasma reagin values and those without missing values at 12 months of follow-up.

Table S3 Factors associated with serological response in the patients who received 1 dose or 3 doses of benzathine penicillin G at 6 months of follow-up in univariate and multivariate analysis.

Acknowledgments

We would like to thank the Centers for Disease Control, Taiwan, for the research grant support and Professor Victor L. Yu, University of Pittsburgh, for the critical review of the manuscript.

Preliminary analyses of these data were presented as abstract no. S-119 at the 20th *Conference on Retroviruses and Opportunistic Infections*, Atlanta, Georgia, 3–6 March, 2013 and oral abstract no. 1139 at ID*Week* 2013, San Francisco, 2–6 October, 2013.

Author Contributions

Conceived and designed the experiments: CJY PLL YHL HHL YHC WCK CCH. Performed the experiments: CJY NYL TCC SHL PLL WCH HJT CHL HHL YHC CCH. Analyzed the data: CJY YHL WCK CCH. Contributed reagents/materials/analysis tools: CJY CCH. Contributed to the writing of the manuscript: CJY WCK CCH.

References

1. DoRHaR. WHO Global incidence and prevalence of selected curable sexually transmitted infections –22008. Available: http://wwwwhoint/reproductivehealth/publications/rtis/stisestimates/en/indexhtml. Accessed 2013 Jun 21.
2. Chow EP, Wilson DP, Zhang L (2011) HIV and syphilis co-infection increasing among men who have sex with men in China: a systematic review and meta-analysis. PloS one 6: e22768.

3. Simms I, Fenton KA, Ashton M, Turner KM, Crawley-Boevey EE, et al. (2005) The re-emergence of syphilis in the United Kingdom: the new epidemic phases. Sexually transmitted diseases 32: 220–226.
4. Velicko I, Unemo M (2012) Recent trends in gonorrhoea and syphilis epidemiology in Sweden: 2007 to 2011. Euro surveillance: bulletin Europeen sur les maladies transmissibles = European communicable disease bulletin 17.
5. Fenton KA, Lowndes CM (2004) Recent trends in the epidemiology of sexually transmitted infections in the European Union. Sexually transmitted infections 80: 255–263.
6. Savage EJ, Marsh K, Duffell S, Ison CA, Zaman A, et al. (2012) Rapid increase in gonorrhoea and syphilis diagnoses in England in 2011. Euro surveillance : bulletin Europeen sur les maladies transmissibles = European communicable disease bulletin 17.
7. Centers for Disease Control and Prevention (2012) Sexually Transmitted Disease Surveillance 2011. Atlanta: U.S. Department of Health and Human Services.
8. Centers for Disease Control and Prevention, Workowski KA, Berman SM (2006) Sexually transmitted diseases treatment guidelines, 2006. MMWR Recommendations and reports : Morbidity and mortality weekly report Recommendations and reports/Centers for Disease Control 55: 1–94.
9. Cuddy PG (1982) Benzathine penicillin G in the treatment of neurosyphilis. Drug intelligence & clinical pharmacy 16: 205–210.
10. Rolfs RT, Joesoef MR, Hendershot EF, Rompalo AM, Augenbraun MH, et al. (1997) A randomized trial of enhanced therapy for early syphilis in patients with and without human immunodeficiency virus infection. The Syphilis and HIV Study Group. The New England journal of medicine 337: 307–314.
11. Workowski KA, Berman S, Centers for Disease Control and Prevention (2010) Sexually transmitted diseases treatment guidelines, 2010. MMWR Recommendations and reports : Morbidity and mortality weekly report Recommendations and reports/Centers for Disease Control 59: 1–110.
12. Kingston M, French P, Goh B, Goold P, Higgins S, et al. (2008) UK National Guidelines on the Management of Syphilis 2008. International journal of STD & AIDS 19: 729–740.
13. French P, Gomberg M, Janier M, Schmidt B, van Voorst Vader P, et al. (2009) IUSTI: 2008 European Guidelines on the Management of Syphilis. International journal of STD & AIDS 20: 300–309.
14. Dowell D, Polgreen PM, Beekmann SE, Workowski KA, Berman SM, et al. (2009) Dilemmas in the management of syphilis: a survey of infectious diseases experts. Clinical infectious diseases : an official publication of the Infectious Diseases Society of America 49: 1526–1529.
15. Ghanem KG, Erbelding EJ, Wiener ZS, Rompalo AM (2007) Serological response to syphilis treatment in HIV-positive and HIV-negative patients attending sexually transmitted diseases clinics. Sexually transmitted infections 83: 97–101.
16. Gonzalez-Lopez JJ, Guerrero ML, Lujan R, Tostado SF, de Gorgolas M, et al. (2009) Factors determining serologic response to treatment in patients with syphilis. Clinical infectious diseases : an official publication of the Infectious Diseases Society of America 49: 1505–1511.
17. Manavi K, McMillan A (2007) The outcome of treatment of early latent syphilis and syphilis with undetermined duration in HIV-infected and HIV-uninfected patients. International journal of STD & AIDS 18: 814–818.
18. Farhi D, Benhaddou N, Grange P, Zizi N, Deleuze J, et al. (2009) Clinical and serologic baseline and follow-up features of syphilis according to HIV status in the post-HAART era. Medicine 88: 331–340.
19. Centers for Disease Control and Prevention (2013) Notes from the Field: Repeat Syphilis Infection and HIV Coinfection Among Men Who Have Sex With Men - Baltimore, Maryland, 2010–2011. MMWR Morbidity and mortality weekly report 62: 649–650.
20. Ghanem KG, Moore RD, Rompalo AM, Erbelding EJ, Zenilman JM, et al. (2008) Antiretroviral therapy is associated with reduced serologic failure rates for syphilis among HIV-infected patients. Clinical infectious diseases : an official publication of the Infectious Diseases Society of America 47: 258–265.
21. Currie BJ, Burt T, Kaplan EL (1994) Penicillin concentrations after increased doses of benzathine penicillin G for prevention of secondary rheumatic fever. Antimicrobial agents and chemotherapy 38: 1203–1204.
22. Jinno S, Anker B, Kaur P, Bristow CC, Klausner JD (2013) Predictors of serological failure after treatment in HIV-infected patients with early syphilis in the emerging era of universal antiretroviral therapy use. BMC infectious diseases 13: 605.
23. Lukehart SA (1991) Serologic testing after therapy for syphilis: is there a test for cure? Annals of internal medicine 114: 1057–1058.

2

Psychological Fears among Low-Paid Female Sex Workers in Southwest China and Their Implications for HIV Prevention

Shan Qiao[1]*, Xiaoming Li[1], Chen Zhang[2], Yuejiao Zhou[3], Zhiyong Shen[3], Zhenzhu Tang[3], Bonita Stanton[1]

1 Prevention Research Center, Carman and Ann Adams Department of Pediatrics, School of Medicine, Wayne State University, Detroit, Michigan, United States of America, **2** Institute of Global Health, Vanderbilt University, Nashville, Tennessee, United States of America, **3** Guangxi Center of Disease Control and Prevention, Guangxi, China

Abstract

Commercial sex plays a critical role in rapidly increasing heterosexual transmission of HIV in China. Low-paid female sex workers (FSWs) are especially vulnerable to HIV/AIDS. Because of the illegality and stigma associated with sex work, FSWs may constantly live with fears in their daily life. Based on cross-sectional study of 794 low-paid FSWs in China we described their psychological fears related to commercial sex and examined the associations between fears and HIV-related behaviors. Fear of HIV infection was significantly associated with consistent use of condoms with clients. However, fear of breaching sex worker identity significantly prevented the FSWs from consistently using condoms with clients and taking HIV tests. Fear of being arrested by the police was positively associated with consistent use of condoms but negatively associated with accessing HIV prevention services. Our findings underlined the importance of examining the triadic interaction of behavioral, psychological and environmental factors in HIV prevention interventions among low-paid FSWs.

Editor: Hong Shang, China Medical University, China

Funding: The study was supported by the National Research Grant R01AA018090 by the National Institute for Alcohol Abuse and Alcoholism (NIAAA). The funders had no role in study design, data collection and analysis, decision to publish, or preparation of the manuscript.

Competing Interests: The authors have declared that no competing interests exist.

* Email: sqiao@med.wayne.edu

Introduction

Compared with other women of reproductive age, female sex workers (FSWs) are taking a disproportionately high burden of HIV infection due to biological, behavioral and structural risk factors [1]. According to a recent meta-analysis among FSWs in low- and middle-income countries, the overall HIV prevalence is 11.8% with a pooled odds ratio of 13.5 for HIV infection [1]. Among this high-risk population, low-paid FSWs were especially vulnerable and marginalized due to their social-demographic characteristics [2], life history (e.g. child sexual abuse, adult sexual assault) [3], and working environment [4]. Low-paid FSWs refer to the FSWs who usually work on the street or lower-tier commercial sex venues and charge much less for each sex trade [5]. Struggling at the low end of the commercial sex hierarchy, they were fragile in both physical and psychological well-beings with problems of partner violence (e.g., physical or sexual abuse) [6], substance abuse (e.g., drug or alcohol dependence) [3,7], depression and posttraumatic stress disorder symptoms [8,9], and poor quality of life [10].

Existing studies also found that low-paid FSWs face a high risk of sexually transmitted infections (STIs) [11,12] and HIV infection [13]. They may be also more likely to engage in unprotected sex than their high-paid counterparts [14,15]. The HIV-related behaviors among this high-risk population may be influenced by socioeconomic factors and the contexts of their lives [16]. In Italy, some low-paid FSWs may not insist using condoms due to fear of losing clients or desire of getting extra pay for unprotected sex [17]. In Bangladesh, some low-paid FSWs spend very little money for health purposes, which may hinder their access to STI diagnosis and treatment [11]. A study among low-paid FSWs in India reported sexual coercion and forced group sex in the context of alcohol use, which made condom use negotiation difficult or even impossible [6]. In addition, drug dependence was associated with elevated rates of injection drug use and sexual risk behaviors among low-paid FSWs [18].

Commercial sex is illegal in China, but it has thrived since the economy reform in the late 1970s due to rapidly widening income disparities, increasing population mobility, and changing norms of sexuality [19]. It has also been driven by surplus rural labor and limited employment opportunities for women during the past three decades [20]. An estimated 4–10 million women are engaged in commercial sex industry with various categories [2]. According to national HIV sentinel surveillance data, the HIV prevalence rate was 0.3% among FSWs in China [21]. Although HIV prevalence rate among FSWs in China has remained relatively low in general, it is as high as 16% in some areas with dual epidemics of drug and HIV [20]. A serial cross-sectional study conducted between 2008 and 2012 suggested a decreasing trend of HIV prevalence (from 0.6% to 0.3%) but an increasing trend of syphilis prevalence (from 2.4% to 3.2%) [22]. In addition, there was a disparity between high-paid and low-paid sex workers in both disease prevalence burden in each year and the overall trends during the study period. HIV prevalence rates were higher among low-paid sex workers in both 2008 and 2012. There was a non-significant upward trend among lower-paid FSWs although syphilis prevalence rate was significantly reduced among higher-paid FSWs [22].

Low-paid FSWs in China are more likely to have higher prevalence of HIV infection and STIs, such as syphilis, HSV-2, and gonorrhea than their high-paid counterparts [23–25]. For instance, a recent systematic review reported a 2-fold increased risk of syphilis among low-paid FSWs [26]. Compared with high-paid FSWs, low-paid FSWs were older, less educated, and more often divorced or widowed [27]. Their vulnerable socio-demographic characteristics may contribute to their higher rates of unprotected sex [27], and lower utilization of HIV prevention services [27,28].

Although recent research on FSWs in China has started to pay attention to the heterogeneity of China's commercial sex industry and attempted to focus on low-paid FSWs, few studies have explored the role of psychosocial factors on HIV-related behaviors in this group [19]. Due to illegal, clandestine and discriminatory nature of commercial sex in China, FSWs may constantly live with psychological fears which can lead to a number of psychological problems such as stress, depression, hopeless, pessimism in their daily life [29]. The negative emotions were shown to be associated with high risk sexual behaviors [29]. For example, Hong and colleagues reported that depression was associated with FSWs' inconsistent use of condoms with their clients [8]. Nevertheless, empirical data are still limited regarding psychological fears in the context of commercial sex among low-paid FSWs, and the relationship between their fears and HIV-related behaviors (consistently using condoms, participating in interventions activities, and HIV-testing).

Fear is defined as "the unpleasant emotional state consisting of psychological and psychophysicological responses to a real eternal threat or danger, including agitation, alertness, tension, and mobilization of the alarm reaction" [30]. Fear is often caused by perceived threat which is composed of perceived susceptibility (likelihood of personally experiencing the threat) and perceived severity (magnitude of harm from the threat) [31]. Several meta-analysis studies have suggested that the stronger the fear, the greater the attitude, intention, and action of behavior change [32–34]. However, there is scarcity of elaboration on the role of psychological fears among low-paid FSWs. What they are afraid of may reflect their working and living contexts and interplay with their behaviors. Studies on fears therefore may demonstrate complex triadic interactions of socio- structural factors (policy, legislation and social stigma), psychological factors and HIV-related behaviors.

Utilizing data from China, the current study will explore the issue of fears among low-paid FSWs with three specific objectives: First, to delineate content of fears among low-paid FSWs; Second, to explore how the content of fears may vary along with different demographic factors, work-related factors and perceptions related to HIV/AIDS; Third, to examine associations between fears among this vulnerable population and their HIV-related behaviors. To achieve the third objective, we will test three hypotheses: 1) fear of HIV infection and fear of STIs may be positively associated with FSWs' consistent use of condoms with clients; 2) fear of police arrests and/or fear of breaching their sex worker identity may be psychological barriers for HIV testing; and 3) fear of police arrests and/or fear of identity breaching may also prevent low-paid FSWs from accessing HIV prevention services.

Methods

Study site and survey procedure

Quantitative data were collected in 2011 from a tourist city in Guangxi Zhuang Autonomous Region (Guangxi). Guangxi is ranked second at provincial level in terms of HIV prevalence and first in terms of newly reported HIV infection cases in China [35]. Based on the national sentinel surveillance data in 2010, the overall prevalence of HIV, syphilis, and HCV infections among FSWs in Guangxi were 1.0, 6.1, and 1.0%, respectively [36]. Located in the northeast of Guangxi with a population of 1.34 million, the study city is famous for tourism attracting as many as 10 million visitors each year. Commercial sex has grown rapidly along with the flourish of tourism in this city where an estimate of 2,000 FSWs worked in at least 150 commercial sex venues [28].

With the assistance of local health workers, the research team conducted ethnographic mapping for various types of low-tier commercial sex venues/locations in the city. These venues included small roadside restaurants, mini-hotels, hair salons, feet-massage salons, streets (e.g., parks, city squares, and road-side), and other small entertainment establishments (e.g., karaokes and night clubs). The research team then contacted the owners/managers or other appropriate gatekeepers of these venues for their permission to conduct survey in their premises. Once we obtained permission from the gatekeepers, trained outreach health workers from the local Center for Disease Control and Prevention (CDC) approached the FSWs in the venues to ask for their participation. The street-based FSWs were recruited by direct contact and peer referral. Around 75% of the venue owners or managers and 70% of the FSWs approached agreed to participate in the survey. A total of 794 FSWs from 131 venues/locations provided written informed consent and completed a self-administered survey on their demographic information, fears related to their work, as well as HIV/AIDS related knowledge, attitudes and behaviors.

The paper survey was conducted in separate rooms or private spaces in the venues/locations to ensure confidentiality of the responses. No one was allowed to stay with the participant during the survey except the interviewer who provided the participant with necessary assistance. The questionnaire took about 15 minutes to complete. The study protocol was approved by the Institutional Review Board at Guangxi CDC in China.

Measures

Demographic characteristics. Participants were asked about their age, ethnicity, marital status, home residence, education attainment, number of people in the family, and annual household income. For the purpose of data analysis in the current study, we dichotomized ethnicity into Han and non-Han, marital status into ever married and never married, and education attainment into less than middle school versus at least middle school.

Work-related factors. FSWs were asked to provide information on their work-related conditions and context, including length of working in commercial sex industry, types of work venues, age groups of most of their clients, number of clients per week, fees charged for each trade, income from sex work in past month, experience of police arrest, and experience of drug use. In the current study, drug use was defined to have ever used any type of illicit drugs including heroin, cocaine, marijuana, opioids, pethidine, ketamine, and ecstasy.

HIV awareness. To assess the HIV awareness, the participants were asked how much they knew about HIV/AIDS with a

4-point response ("not at all", "a little", "some", "a lot"). Participants answered "some" or "a lot" were considered as having relatively high level of HIV/AIDS awareness.

HIV susceptibility. The FSWs were asked to assess the possibility they might get HIV infection using a 4-point scale from "very impossible" to "very possible". For the purpose of data analysis in this study, responses of "very possible" and "possible" were coded as "high HIV susceptibility", while "impossible" and "very impossible" were coded as "low HIV susceptibility".

Psychological fears. To assess FSWs' fears in the context of commercial sex, we employed a multiple-response question "what are your fears when you are working in commercial sex". The potential answers included "HIV infection", "STIs", "not getting paid by clients", "being arrested by the police", "family members become aware of the nature of my job", "acquaintances become aware of the nature of my job" and "others". In data analysis, fear of family members and fear of acquaintances becoming aware of their work were combined into a single item of fear of breaching their sex worker identity.

Consistent use of condoms with clients. The participants were asked about the frequency of using condoms with clients in the past month. The potential answers were "never", "sometimes" and "every time". The respondents who answered "every time" were considered to consistently use condoms with clients in past month.

HIV testing and HIV prevention service utilization. The participants were asked whether they had tested for HIV in the past year. They were also asked in the past year if the FSWs had participated in any of the three HIV prevention activities including "condom distribution and/or voluntary counseling and testing (VCT)", "community-based methadone maintenance treatment program and/or needle exchange program", and "peer HIV/AIDS education". The FSWs who reported using at least one of these HIV prevention services were viewed as "ever used HIV prevention services", and otherwise they were considered as "never used HIV prevention services".

Data analysis

First of all, we conducted descriptive analysis to illustrate the content of fear among the FSWs. Specifically, responses to the question "what are your fears when you are working in commercial sex" were transferred into seven binary variables indicating whether or not a specific fear was reported (Yes = 1, No = 0). The frequency and proportion of each response were calculated to demonstrate the levels of various fears among the FSWs. Second, we explored the relationship between each specific fear and the FSWs' background variables (demographic characteristics, work-related factors, and HIV-related perceptions). We employed one-way ANOVA (for continuous measures) and Chi-square test (for categorical measures) to compare the differences between groups in terms of background variables. Third, univariate and multivariate logistic regression models were employed to identify background variables that were associated with each HIV-related behavior (i.e., consistent use of condoms with clients, HIV testing, and utilization of HIV prevention service). Those background variables associated with the dependent variable at the $p<0.2$ level in univariate regression models were then entered into the multivariate logistic regression models. Three multivariate logistic regression models were conducted to examine the association between fears and each of HIV-related behaviors after adjusting background variables.

In second and third steps of the analysis, the variable of venue types was dichotomized into the venues with less mobility (feet-massage salons and hair salons) and the ones with more mobility (roadside restaurants, mini-hotels, street-based and other sites). In logistic regression analysis, two income variables were transformed by taking natural logarithms of their values because of their skewed distributions. We included four most commonly reported fears (i.e., fear of HIV infection, fear of STIs, fear of identity breaching, and fear of police arrests) in final multivariate logistic regression models. VIF (i.e., Variance Inflation Factor) test in the multivariate logistics regression analysis was thus employed to test potential collinearity between the four fear variables. All statistical analyses were performed using SPSS 16.0 (SPSS Inc, Chicago, IL).

Results

Background characteristics

The background characteristics and content of fears among the FSWs is presented in Table 1. The FSWs in the current study were 31 years old on average (SD = 8.9) and 85% of them were of Han ethnicity. Nearly 71% of the participants were Guangxi residents rather than migrants from other provinces. The majority of the FSWs were ever married, 41% had not completed middle school education. There were four members in each family on average. The mean annual household income was 14,195 yuan (SD = 12,132.9).

About a half of the FSWs (51%) worked in salons (feet-massage salons and hair salons), 17% worked in roadside restaurants,15% were street-based, 9% worked in mini-hotels, and nearly 8% worked in other venues. Nearly 42% of the participants engaged in commercial sex for more than one year. About 80% of the FSWs reported that their clients were mainly aged 30–50 years, and 14% reported that the majority of their clients were older than 50 years. On average, the FSWs charged about 40 yuan for each sexual trade and had about 19 clients per week. The mean income from sex work in past month was about 1,912 yuan. Over 60% of the women reported that they knew some or a lot about HIV/AIDS, but around 80% perceived a low HIV susceptibility. Among all the respondents, 3.3% reported had ever used drug and 5.7% had ever been arrested by the police. Nearly a half of the FSWs had ever tested for HIV, and almost 73% had participated in at least one type of HIV prevention activities including condom provision/VCT, needle exchange, and peer HIV/AIDS education. However, less than 39% of the FSWs reported consistent use of condoms with clients in past month.

Psychological fears among the FSWs

Most of the FSWs feared being infected by HIV (61%) or other STIs (51%). Nearly 48% of them worried about breaching their sex worker identity (either to family members or acquaintances). About 40% of the participants feared being arrested by the police. Some of the participants (13%) expressed their fear of not getting paid by clients. Only 1.4% of the FSWs reported fears other than those listed.

Table 2 illustrated the correlations between background characteristics and each fear variable. The FSWs who expressed the fear of HIV infection had a higher proportion of ethnic minority women, higher level of education attainment, and higher annual household income. As for work-related factors, more FSWs expressing the fear of HIV infection engaged in commercial sex for at least one year, and had higher income from sex work in past month. In addition, they were less likely to work in venues with less mobility and had a higher proportion of younger clients. The respondents who feared HIV infection also showed a higher proportion of ever using drug. In addition, HIV awareness and HIV susceptibility were higher among the FSWs who feared HIV infection than those who did not.

Table 1. Summary of background characteristics among low-paid FSWs in China.

N = 794	Frequency (%)	Mean (SD)
Demographic factors		
Age in years		31.1(8.9)
Ever married*	506(64.1%)	
Guangxi residence*	558(70.6%)	
Han-Ethnicity	676(85.1%)	
Education < middle school	324(40.8%)	
No. of people in household		4.0(4.2)
Annual household income		14195.0(12132.9)
Work-related factors		
Length of working as sex workers ≥1year	336(42.3%)	
Venue types		
Feet massage salon	75(9.40%)	
Hair salon	332(41.8%)	
Roadside Restaurant	137(17.2%)	
Mini-hotel	71(9.0%)	
Other establishment-based venues	63(7.9%))	
Street-based	116(14.6%)	
Age group of clients*		
<30	47(5.9%)	
30–50	635(80.3%)	
>50	109(13.8%)	
Charge per service (Yuan)		39.6(17.8)
No. of clients per week		18.9(2.7)
Income from sex work in past month (Yuan)		1911.9(1254.2)
Ever using drug	26(3.3%)	
Eve being arrested by the police	45(5.7%)	
HIV-related perceptions		
High HIV awareness*	502(63.3%)	
Low HIV susceptibility	638(80.4%)	
Content of psychological fears		
Fear of HIV infection	482(60.7%)	
Fear of STIs	403(50.8%)	
Fear of breaching sex worker identity	356(47.7%)	
Fear of being arrested by the police	317(39.9%)	
Fear of not getting paid by clients	103(13.0%)	
Other fears	8(1.4%)	

*Missing data was not included when we calculated the proportions.

Fear of STIs had similar correlations with background characteristics. The FSWs who feared STIs had a higher proportion of being married, being ethnic minority, with lower level of education attainment, and higher annual household income. More FSWs reporting the fear of STIs engaged in commercial sex for at least one year, and had younger clients. In addition, the fear of STIs was positively correlated with HIV susceptibility.

Fear of breaching sex worker identity was correlated with demographic factors, work-related contexts and experience but not with HIV awareness or HIV susceptibility. The FSWs with the fear of breaching their identity to others were younger, from smaller size families, with higher annual household income. More FSWs in this group worked in venues with less mobility (e.g., salons), had more clients each week, charged more for each service and had higher income from sex work in past month. Both the proportions of ever using drug and ever experiencing police arrests were significantly lower among the FSWs who feared breaching their identity compared with the FSWs who did not.

The FSWs who feared police arrests had higher level of education attainment and annual household income. A higher proportion of them worked in venues with less mobility, engaged in commercial sex longer, charged more for each sex trade, had older clients, with fewer clients each week and higher income from sex work in past month. The respondents who expressed the fear of police arrests reported lower perceived HIV susceptibility.

Table 2. Correlations between fear and background characteristics among low-paid FSWs in China.

	Fear of HIV infection		Fear of STIs		Fear of breaching FSW identity		Fear of being arrested by the police	
	No	**Yes**	**No**	**Yes**	**No**	**Yes**	**No**	**Yes**
Demographic factors								
Age in years (Mean, SD)	31.5(9.0)	30.8(8.8)	31.1(9.3)	31.1(8.5)	31.7(9.5)	30.3(8.1)*	30.7(8.7)	31.9(9.2)
Ever married	62.1%	65.3%	59.7%	68.2%*	63.7%	64.4%	61.9%	67.2%
Guangxi residence	70.0%	71.0%	71.6%	69.7%	73.1%	68.0%	72.4%	68.0%
Han-Ethnicity	88.8%	82.8%*	90.3%	80.1%***	85.8%	84.4%	85.1%	85.2%
Education < middle school	62.5%	57.1%*	37.1%	44.4%*	58.6%	59.9%	63.1%	53.3%**
No. of people in household (Mean, SD)	4.2(4.1)	4.0(4.4)	3.9(3.0)	4.2(5.1)	4.6(4.9)	3.5(3.2)***	4.3(4.5)	3.6(3.9)
Annual household income(Yuan, Mean, SD)	11741.6 (9929.9)	15791.0 (13138.6)***	11421.9 (10829.3)	16843.6 (12718.6)***	12228.4 (11551.7)	16361.9 (12401.3)*	12072.7 (11339.4)	17422.8 (12598.2)*
Work-related factors								
Length of working as sex workers ≥1year	36.9%	45.9%***	37.1%	47.4%**	41.4%	43.3%	36.7%	50.8%***
Working in venues with less mobility (feet massage salons and hair salons)	62.0%	48.1%***	50.6%	53.1%	36.4%	47.0%**	55.8%	46.1%**
Age group of clients (Year)								
<30	3.2%	7.7%	4.6%	7.2%	6.6%	5.3%	6.9%	4.4%
30-50	78.3%	81.5%	78.4%	82.1%	80.8%	79.7%	82.7%	76.6%
>50	18.4%	10.8%**	17.0%	10.7%*	12.6%	15.0%	10.3%	19.0%**
Charge per service (Yuan, Mean, SD)	38.1(18.7)	40.6(17.1)	39.9(22.0)	39.4(12.3)	36.9(21.0)	42.6(12.7)*	38.1(20.4)	41.8(12.5)*
No.of clients per week (Mean, SD)	19.2(2.5)	18.7(2.8)	18.7(2.7)	19.1(2.6)	18.7(2.7)	19.1(2.6)*	19.1(2.6)	18.6(2.7)*
income from sex work past month (Yuan, Mean, SD)	1688.8 (872.7)	2056.3 (1431.0)**	1642.2 (1065.4)	2173.5 (1364.7)***	1549.2 (887.5)	2309.1 (1461.1)***	1795.1 (1001.4)	2087.6 (1544.5)**
Ever using drug	1.0%	4.8%**	2.8%	3.7%	4.8%	1.6%***	1.7%	5.7%
Eve being arrested by the police	4.5%	6.5%	6.5%	5.0%	7.6%	3.7%*	5.5%	6.0%
HIV-related perceptions								
High HIV awareness	56.0%	66.0%*	64.4%	62.3%	65.8%	60.6%	61.6%	65.8%
Low HIV susceptibility	89.4%	77.0%***	87.7%	73.2%***	79.0%	81.8%	76.1%	86.8%***

*p<.05, **p<.01, ***p<.001.

Association between psychological fears and HIV-related behaviors

Table 3 and Table 4 show results of a series of univariate and multivariate logistic regression models to identify factors associated with HIV-related behaviors, respectively. Fear of HIV infection was significantly associated with consistent use of condoms with clients in past month (aOR = 1.88, 95% CI = 1.22, 2.91) after controlling other background characteristics and other fear variables. However, fear of STIs was not significantly associated with any HIV-related behaviors. Final logistic regression model indicated that fear of breaching sex worker identity significantly prevented the FSWs from consistently using condoms with clients (aOR = .66, 95%CI = .43,.99) and taking HIV tests (aOR = .48, 95% CI = .36,.73). As we expected, fear of being arrested by the police might hamper the FSWs' accessing HIV prevention service (aOR = .39, 95% CI = .22,.68). In addition, fear of police arrests was positively associated with consistent use of condoms (aOR = 1.60, 95% CI = 1.04, 2.45).

The VIF values for all the fear variables in the final model for each dependent variable (i.e., consistent use of condoms with clients, HIV testing, utilization of HIV prevention services) were less than 1.5 which was substantially smaller than the threshold value (e.g., VIF >10) that would suggest multicollinearity among the predictors in the model [37].

Association between background characteristics and HIV-related behaviors

Some background characteristics were also independently predictive of HIV-related behaviors among the FSWs. Younger age, higher annual household income, and fewer clients each week were associated with FSWs' consistent use of condoms with their clients. Logistic regression models indicated that working in venues with less mobility, younger clientele, and high HIV awareness were positively associated with ever taking an HIV test. In addition, ever being arrested by the police was also significantly associated with having an HIV test before.

Finally, our data analysis suggested that FSWs who reported higher annual household income were more likely to participate in some HIV prevention service. Several work-related factors were also significantly associated with their utilization of HIV prevention service. The longer the FSWs engaged in commercial sex, the more likely they reported participation in HIV prevention service. Having a higher HIV awareness was positively associated with using HIV prevention service among the FSWs. The average charge for each sex trade was negatively associated with the FSWs' utilization of HIV prevention service.

Discussion

To the best of our knowledge, the current study is one of the first quantitative studies to delineate content of fears among low-paid FSWs in China. Fear of HIV infection, fear of STIs, fear of breaching their sex worker identity, and fear of being arrested by the police were the most commonly reported fears among this high-risk population. Our findings indicate complex associations between fears and background characteristics as well as unique associations between different fears and various HIV-related behaviors.

It is interesting that the FSWs who expressed various fears were not always the most disadvantageous groups in terms of socio-demographic characteristics. We noticed that these FSWs reported higher annual household income and higher income from sex work in past month. Among the FSWs who feared HIV infection and police arrest, larger proportion reported higher level of education attainment. The FSWs who feared breaching their sex worker identity reported higher fees for each service. These results suggest that psychological fears might be more relevant or become more concerning among FSWs who were relatively better off in their lives. It is also notable that ever using drug correlated with fear of HIV infection. One potential explanation is that some FSWs who had ever used drug realized their high risk behaviors and perceived high susceptibility of HIV infection and severity of the threat (fear).

The associations of psychological fears with HIV-related behaviors may depend on content of fears and may also vary by specific behaviors. The relationship between fear of HIV infection and condom use with clients is consistent with existing theoretical and empirical studies on psychological fears. The more severity of threat people have realized, the more likely they are motivated to change behaviors in order to protect themselves [34]. However, fear of STIs was not significantly associated with any of the HIV-related behavior based on our data. One possible interpretation of this result is that the perceived severity of STIs was much lower than the one of HIV infection among low-paid FSWs. STIs might have been viewed as treatable and curable, while HIV infection was generally perceived as fatal. Further studies are needed to examine the differential patterns of relationships between fear of STIs and HIV-related behaviors.

Our study indicated that FSWs' fear of breaching their identity might be an important issue that needs to be addressed in HIV prevention. Because of the stigma against sex work many FSWs conceal the nature of their work to their families, friends, and acquaintances [38]. Fear of breaching their identity was negatively associated with consistent use of condoms because FSWs might worry about potential questioning or suspicions about the nature of their work when family members or acquaintances discover their carrying condoms with themselves. Fear of breaching their sex worker identity might prevent FSWs from accessing HIV-testing, which was also evidenced in existing studies on HIV-testing behaviors among FSWs in China [28,39,40]. Visiting HIV-testing facilities may increase the risks of breaching their sex worker identity as the concern of confidentiality of testing was one of major barriers for HIV testing among FSWs [28].

Commercial sex is illegal in China. The consequences of being arrested by the police include possible jail time, a large fine, and a breach of sex worker identity [5]. Fear of police arrests reflects an individual psychological response to a structural factor. Our study suggested that the FSWs who consistently used condoms with clients were more likely to express their fear of being arrested by the police. That may be because condoms at workplace were often taken by police as material evidence of commercial sex [5]. In addition, local police may compulsorily carry out HIV-testing among arrested FSWs as part of law enforcement, which may explain why the FSWs who had ever been arrested showed a higher proportion of HIV testings or using HIV prevention service.

Findings of the current study should be interpreted with caution due to several limitations. First, our sample may not be representative of low-paid FSWs in other areas of China. Our study was conducted in a tourist city of a multi-ethnic region. Most of participants were local residents rather than rural-to-urban migrants. Second, because of cross-sectional study data, the associations between fear and HIV-related behaviors may not be interpreted as causal. For example, fear of HIV infection may stimulate motivation to practice preventive behaviors; preventive behaviors may also shape perceptions of threat and further change fear [41]. The potential reciprocal relationship between fear and behavior merits further studies with a prospective or longitudinal

Table 3. Summary of univariate logistic regression models results.

	Consistent use of condoms with clients			HIV testing			HIV prevention service		
	OR	**95% CI**	**p-value**	**OR**	**95% CI**	**p-value**	**OR**	**95% CI**	**p-value**
Demographic factors									
Age	**.933*** **	**[.914,.952]**	**.000**	1.003	[.986,1.020]	.745	1.017	[.998,1.037]	.079
Ever married	**.563*** **	**[.411,.745]**	**.000**	1.085	[.811,1.451]	.581	**1.384***	[1.005,1.908]	.047
Guangxi residence	.930	[.670,1.254]	.587	.950	[.699,1.290]	.741	.863	[.610,1.223]	.408
Han-Ethnicity	1.105	[.736,1.658]	.630	1.410	[.951,2.092]	.087	**1.582***	[1.045,2.394]	.030
Education < middle school	**1.876*** **	**[1.389,2.533]**	**.000**	1.100	[.830,1.462]	.504	.986	[.717,1.357]	.929
No. of people in household	.972	[.931,1.014]	.187	1.046	[1.000,1.095]	.049	1.026	[.978,1.077]	.297
Annual household income	**1.905*** **	**[1.562, 2.324]**	**.000**	1.085	[.912,1.290]	.356	**1.528*** **	**[1.242,1.878]**	**.000**
Work-related factors									
Length of working as sex worker ≥1 year	1.088	[.815,1.453]	.567	1.050	[.791,1.390]	.740	**1.736** **	**[1.266,2.381]**	**.001**
Working in venues with less mobility	**1.412***	**[1.056,1.884]**	**.019**	**1.800*** **	**[1.359,2.386]**	**.000**	**1.736** **	[.983,2.856]	
Age group of clients	**.606** **	**[.431,.853]**	**.004**	**.514*** **	**[.367,.718]**	**.000**	.691*	[.484,.987]	.042
Charge per service	**1.026*** **	**[1.015,1.038]**	**.000**	.998	[.990,1.006]	.561	**.989***	**[.980,.998]**	**.021**
No.of clients per week	**.821*** **	**[.768,.877]**	**.000**	.971	[.917,1.029]	.324	1.050	[.980,1.125]	.164
income from sex work past month	.915	[.776,1.079]	.290	**1.686*** **	[1.404,2.024]	.000	**2.072*** **	[1.714,2.504]	.000
Ever using drug	**2.650***	**[1.187,5.918]**	**.017**	**.424***	[.182,.987]	.047	.500	[.226,1.106]	.087
Ever being arrested by the police	.777	[.411,1.469]	.437	**3.704*** **	**[1.808,7.590]**	**.000**	**5.648*** **	[1.732,18.418]	.004
HIV-related perceptions									
High HIV awareness	**2.060*** **	**[1.509,2.813]**	**.000**	**3.636*** **	**[2.675,4.943]**	**.000**	**6.029*** **	**[4.290,8.473]**	**.000**
Low HIV susceptibility	**2.238*** **	**[1.503,3.333]**	**.000**	**1.663** **	[1.165,2.373]	.005	**2.449*** **	[1.698,3.532]	**.000**
Fear of									
HIV infection	**1.976***	**[1.458, 2.678]**	**.000**	1.250	[.940,1.663]	.125	1.194	[.870,1.640]	.273
STIs	1.125	[.844,1.498]	.421	.950	[.719,1.255]	.719	1.056	[.773,1.443]	.733
Breaching FSW identity	.994	[.746, 1.324]	.968	**.475*** **	**[.358,.631]**	**.000**	.767	[.561,1.049]	.097
Being arrested by the police	**1.952*** **	**[1.456, 2.615]**	**.000**	**.655** **	**[.492,.871]**	**.004**	**.573** **	**[.418,.786]**	**.001**

*p<.05, **p<.01, ***p<.001.

Table 4. Summary of multivariate logistic regression models results.

	Consistent use of condoms with clients			HIV testing			HIV prevention service		
	aOR	95% CI	p-value	aOR	95% CI	p-value	aOR	95% CI	p-value
Demographic factors									
Age	**.954****	**[.926,.983]**	**.002**	-	-	-	1.033	[.993,1.076]	.111
Ever married	.749	[.486,1.156]	.749	-	-	-	1.455	[.835,2.533]	.185
Guangxi residence	-	-	-	-	-	-	-	-	-
Han-Ethnicity	-	-	-	1.009	[.644,1.581]	.989	.670	[.334,1.342]	.258
Education < middle school	1.177	[.757,1.830]	.470	-	-		-	-	-
No. of people in household	.989	.925,1.056	.734	1.015	[.977,1.054]	.442	-	-	-
Annual household income	**1.771*****	**[1.333, 2.353]**	**.000**	1.120	[.902,1.390]	.307	**1.874*****	**[1.339,2.621]**	**.000**
Work-related factors									
Length of working as sex worker ≥1 year	-	-	-	-	-	-	**2.090****	**[1.218,3.585]**	**.007**
Working in venues with less mobility	.980	[.651,1.477]	.925	**1.750****	**[1.241,2.467]**	**.001**	1.676	[.983,2.856]	.058
Age group of clients	.971	[.582,1.620]	.909	**.662***	**[.441,.993]**	**.046**	.685	[.354,1.325]	.262
Charge per service	1.002	[.992,1.012]	.685	-	-	-	**.983****	**[.971,.995]**	**.007**
No. of clients per week	**.888*****	**[.813,.971]**	**.009**	-	-	-	.939	.839,1.051	.272
income from sex work past month	.922	.686,1.239	.589	.956	[.730,1.251]	.741	1.537	[.967,2.443]	.069
Ever using drug	-	-	-	.607	[.224,1.640]	.325	.908	.263,3.136	.879
Ever being arrested by the police	-	-	-	**2.748****	**[1.217,6.206]**	**.015**	4.585	.903,23.283	.066
HIV-related perceptions									
High HIV awareness	1.641*	**[1.069,2.519]**	**.023**	**2.815*****	**[1.964,4.036]**	**.000**	**6.867****	**[3.974,11.867]**	**.000**
Low HIV susceptibility	1.320	[.777,2.242]	.304	1.143	[.736,1.776]	.552	.991	[.518,1.896]	.979
Fear of									
HIV infection	**1.884****	**[1.218, 2.914]**	**.004**	1.271	[.883,1.828]	.197	1.015	[.561,1.836]	.962
STIs	.782	[.501,1.219]	.278	1.122	[.781,1.612]	.534	1.383	[.781,2.449]	.267
Breaching FSW identity	.661	[.433,.999]	.491	**.514*****	**[.363,.729]**	**.000**	.604	[.347,1.052]	.075
Being arrested by the police	**1.597***	**[1.042, 2.447]**	**.032**	.785	[.549,1.122]	.183	**.386*****	**[.219,.681]**	**.001**

*p<.05, **p<.01, ***p<.001.

design. Third, the measurement of fears was developed and used in the current study among FSWs in China. Further studies are needed to test validity and reliability of the measures. Forth, given the illegal and clandestine nature of commercial sex in China, our self-reported data are subject to socially desirable responses.

Despite of these limitations, our findings have several implications for HIV prevention and treatment service among low-paid FSWs. First, psychological fears can play an important role in HIV prevention social marketing or other public health campaigns. Strong fear may effectively motivate behavior change [34]. Many empirical studies in Africa suggest that the use of fear-based AIDS prevention campaigns often promote HIV-preventive behaviors [42]. For instance, Uganda's successful response to AIDS epidemic calls for attention to the fear appeal strategy: "Remarkably (Uganda) combined high fear approaches with openness and the capacity to rise above discrimination and to integrate prevention and care effectively" ([43], p.848).

Second, strengthening FSWs' trust in HIV-testing facilities and health care providers will be very important to promote FSWs' access to testing and other HIV prevention and treatment services. The severe stigma against both sex work and HIV/AIDS, the doubt about confidentiality of HIV clinics, and the distrust toward health care professionals or outreach workers may be sources of FSWs' fears of identity breaching and hesitation to access adequate and timely health care service [44]. In a study on utilization of VCT services among FSWs in northern China, 69% of the participants expressed their willingness to attend the VCT clinic, while only 11% were actually tested with fear of identity disclosure in the clinic being negatively related to actual HIV-testing [45]. Stigma reduction among health care professionals and secured HIV-testing results notification procedure with an emphasis on confidentiality protection are needed to decrease fear of identity breaching among FSWs. HIV education and prevention activities can be combined with other health care services that FSWs need (e.g., reproductive health, family planning and women health) to increase rapport and trust between FSWs and health care professionals [44].

Third, implementation of HIV prevention intervention needs multi-sector collaboration, including public health bureau, local authority and police. Although only a small number of FSWs had experience with law enforcement, fear of police arrests may amplify FSWs' reluctance to access HIV prevention services. It may be necessary to engage police in efforts to clarify some misunderstandings about HIV-clinics or VCT services (such as the misperception that HIV-testing records may be used by police to identify and detain FSWs) and reduce mistrust toward health care professionals.

In summary, our study has demonstrated how a psychological response among low-paid FSWs may be shaped by structural factors and how this psychological response may further influence their HIV-related behaviors. Our findings support the Social Cognitive Theory [46] which posits that socio-structural factors operate through psychological mechanism to produce behavioral effects. A growing literature has paid attention to the impact of psychological well-being on health behaviors among FSWs. For example, studies suggested that pessimism was associated with high risk sexual behaviors among FSWs [47,48]. Fear of HIV infection may motivate FSWs to employ desirable HIV-preventive behaviors with high self-efficacy of protection. However, fears related to structural factors (e.g., policy, stigma) may result in negative outcomes (stress, depression, hopelessness), which may reduce their motivation to engage in protective behaviors, and weaken their motivation to adopt a long-term perspective on avoiding the negative consequences of risk behaviors [49,50].

Fear is an emotion factor, but it may be intricately related to other cognition factors such as threat, self-efficacy, and peer norms. Further studies are needed to examine the interactions between fear and other psychological factors, and explore the mechanism of how fear affects health behaviors and mental health. Systematic studies on emotional context of FSWs will inform effective HIV prevention interventions among this high-risk population.

Author Contributions

Conceived and designed the experiments: XL. Performed the experiments: YZ ZS ZT. Analyzed the data: SQ CZ XL. Contributed reagents/materials/analysis tools: XL. Wrote the paper: SQ XL. Revised the manuscript: BS.

References

1. Baral S, Beyrer C, Muessig K, Poteat T, Wirtz AL, et al. (2012) Burden of HIV among female sex workers in low-income and middle-income countries: a systematic review and meta-analysis. Lancet Infect Dis 12: 538–549.
2. Tucker JD (2011) The social context of sexual HIV prevention among female sex workers in China. Int J Epidemiol 40: 1421–1422.
3. El-Bassel N, Witte SS, Wada T, Gilbert L, Wallace J (2001) Correlates of partner violence among female street-based sex workers: substance abuse, history of childhood abuse, and HIV risks. AIDS Patient Care STDS 15: 41–51.
4. Ling DC, Wong WC, Holroyd EA, Gray SA (2007) Silent killers of the night: an exploration of psychological health and suicidality among female street sex workers. J Sex Marital Ther 33: 281–299.
5. Zhang C, Li X, Hong Y, Zhou Y, Liu W, et al. (2013) Unprotected sex with their clients among low-paying female sex workers in southwest China. AIDS Care 25: 503–506.
6. Panchanadeswaran S, Johnson SC, Sivaram S, Srikrishnan AK, Latkin C, et al. (2008) Intimate partner violence is as important as client violence in increasing street-based female sex workers' vulnerability to HIV in India. Int J Drug Policy 19: 106–112.
7. Roxburgh A, Degenhardt L, Copeland J, Larance B (2008) Drug dependence and associated risks among female street-based sex workers in the greater Sydney area, Australia. Subst Use Misuse 43: 1202–1217.
8. Hong Y, Li X, Fang X, Zhao R (2007) Depressive symptoms and condom use with clients among female sex workers in China. Sex Health 4: 99–104.
9. Ruan Y, Cao X, Qian HZ, Zhang L, Qin G, et al. (2006) Syphilis among female sex workers in southwestern China: potential for HIV transmission. Sex Transm Dis 33: 719–723.
10. Wong WC, Holroyd EA, Gray A, Ling DC (2006) Female street sex workers in Hong Kong: moving beyond sexual health. J Womens Health (Larchmt) 15: 390–399.
11. Mondal NI, Hossain K, Islam R, Mian AB (2008) Sexual behavior and sexually transmitted diseases in street-based female sex workers in Rajshahi City, Bangladesh. Braz J Infect Dis 12: 287–292.
12. Rahman M, Alam A, Nessa K, Hossain A, Nahar S, et al. (2000) Etiology of sexually transmitted infections among street-based female sex workers in Dhaka, Bangladesh. J Clin Microbiol 38: 1244–1246.
13. Wang H, Chen RY, Ding G, Ma Y, Ma J, et al. (2009) Prevalence and predictors of HIV infection among female sex workers in Kaiyuan City, Yunnan Province, China. Int J Infect Dis 13: 162–169.
14. Fang X, Li X, Yang H, Hong Y, Stanton B, et al. (2008) Can variation in HIV/STD-related risk be explained by individual SES? Findings from female sex workers in a rural Chinese county. Health Care Women Int 29: 316–335.
15. Harcourt C, van Beek I, Heslop J, McMahon M, Donovan B (2001) The health and welfare needs of female and transgender street sex workers in New South Wales. Aust N Z J Public Health 25: 84–89.
16. Hagan JE, Dulmaa N (2007) Risk factors and prevalence of HIV and sexually transmitted infections among low-income female commercial sex workers in Mongolia. Sex Transm Dis 34: 83–87.
17. Fornasa CV, Gai F, Tarantello M, Gallina P (2005) Knowledge of sexually transmitted diseases and condom use among female street sex workers in Padua. Acta Dermatovenerol Alp Panonica Adriat 14: 107–110.
18. Roxburgh A, Degenhardt L, Copeland J (2006) Posttraumatic stress disorder among female street-based sex workers in the greater Sydney area, Australia. BMC Psychiatry 6: 24.

19. Hong Y, Li X (2008) Behavioral studies of female sex workers in China: a literature review and recommendation for future research. AIDS Behav 12: 623–636.
20. Poon AN, Li Z, Wang N, Hong Y (2011) Review of HIV and other sexually transmitted infections among female sex workers in China. AIDS Care 23 Suppl 1: 5–25.
21. China Ministry of Health (2012) 2012 China AIDS response progress report. Beijing China MInistry of Health.
22. Wang L, Tang W, Wang L, Qian S, Li YG, et al. (2014) The HIV, Syphilis, and HCV Epidemics Among Female Sex Workers in China: Results From a Serial Cross-Sectional Study Between 2008 and 2012. Clin Infect Dis.
23. Wang H, Wang N, Bi A, Wang G, Ding G, et al. (2009) Application of cumulative odds logistic model on risk factors analysis for sexually transmitted infections among female sex workers in Kaiyuan city, Yunnan province, China. Sex Transm Infect 85: 290–295.
24. Zhou Y, Li X, Zhang C, Tan G, Stanton B, et al. (2013) Rates of HIV, syphilis, and HCV infections among different demographic groups of female sex workers in Guangxi China: Evidence from 2010 national sentinel surveillance data. AIDS Care 25(11):1433–41.
25. Lu F, Jia Y, Sun X, Wang L, Liu W, et al. (2009) Prevalence of HIV infection and predictors for syphilis infection among female sex workers in southern China. Southeast Asian J Trop Med Public Health 40: 263–272.
26. Chang H, Zhi X, Chen XS, Cohen MS (2010) Systematic review and meta-analysis of syphilis seroprevalence among female sex workers in China 2010; Bethesda, MD. National Institutes of Health.
27. Li J, Chen XS, Merli MG, Weir SS, Henderson GE (2012) Systematic differences in risk behaviors and syphilis prevalence across types of female sex workers: a preliminary study in Liuzhou, China. Sex Transm Dis 39: 195-200.
28. Hong Y, Zhang C, Li X, Fang X, Lin X, et al. (2012) HIV testing behaviors among female sex workers in Southwest China. AIDS Behav 16: 44–52.
29. Gu J, Lau JT, Chen H, Chen X, Liu C, et al. (2010) Mental health and interpersonal factors associated with HIV-related risk behaviors among non-institutionalized female injection drug users who are also sex workers in China. Women Health 50: 20–36.
30. Anonymous (2007) Dorland's Medical Dictionary for Health Consumers. Saunders.
31. Witte K, Meyer G, Martell D (2001) Effective Health Risk Messages: A step-by-step guide. Newbury Park, CA: Sage.
32. Boster FJ, Mongeau P (1984) Fear-arousing persuasive messages. In: Bostrom RN, Westley BH, editors. Communication Yearbook 8. Newbury Park, CA: Sage. pp. 330–375.
33. Mongeau P (1998) Another look at fear arousing messages In: Allen M, Press R, editors. Persuation: Advances through meta-analysis. Cresskill, NJ: Hampton Press. pp. 53–68.
34. Witte K, Allen M (2000) A meta-analysis of fear appeals: implications for effective public health campaigns. Health Educ Behav 27: 591–615.
35. Guangxi Center for Disease Control and Prevention (2009) Update on HIV/AIDS epidemic in Guangxi. Paper presented at Workshop of NIAAA Venue-based HIV and Alcohol Risk Reduction among Female Sex Workers in China, July 19–21, Guilin, Guangxi, China.
36. Zhou Y, Li X, Zhang C, Tan G, Stanton B, et al. (2013) Rates of HIV, syphilis, and HCV infections among different demographic groups of female sex workers in Guangxi China: Evidence from 2010 National Sentinel Surveillance Data. AIDS Care 25: 1433–1441.
37. Kutner MH, Nachtsheim CJ, Neter J (2004) Applied linear regression models (4th ed.). New York: McGraw-Hill/Irwin.
38. Ullah AA (2005) Prostitution in Bangladesh: An Empirical Profile of Sex Workers. Journal of International Women's Studies 7: 111–122.
39. Wang Y, Li B, Zheng J, Sengupta S, Emrick CB, et al. (2009) Factors related to female sex workers' willingness to utilize VCT service: a qualitative study in Jinan city, northern China. AIDS Behav 13: 866–872.
40. Jie W, Xiaolan Z, Ciyong L, Moyer E, Hui W, et al. (2012) A qualitative exploration of barriers to condom use among female sex workers in China. PLoS One 7: e46786.
41. Gerrard M, Gibbons FX, Bushman BJ (1996) Relation between perceived vulnerability to HIV and precautionary sexual behavior. Psychol Bull 119: 390–409.
42. Green EC, Witte K (2006) Can fear arousal in public health campaigns contribute to the decline of HIV prevalence? J Health Commun 11: 245–259.
43. Wilson D (2004) Partner reduction and the prevention of HIV/AIDS. BMJ 328: 848–849.
44. Chen XS, Yin YP, Liu GG, Wei WH, Wang HC, et al. (2013) Outreach syphilis testing services by different health providers to female sex workers in southern china. PLoS One 8: e60626.
45. Wang Y, Li B, Pan J, Sengupta S, Emrick CB, et al. (2011) Factors associated with utilization of a free HIV VCT clinic by female sex workers in Jinan City, Northern China. AIDS Behav 15: 702–710.
46. Bandura A (2001) Social cognitive theory: an agentic perspective. Annu Rev Psychol 52: 1–26.
47. Silbert MH, Pines AM, Lynch T (1982) Substance abuse and prostitution. J Psychoactive Drugs 14: 193–197.
48. Paone D, Cooper H, Alperen J, Shi Q, Des Jarlais DC (1999) HIV risk behaviours of current sex workers attending syringe exchange: the experiences of women in five US cities. AIDS Care 11: 269–280.
49. Leith KP, Baumeister RF (1996) Why do bad moods increase self-defeating behavior? Emotion, risk taking, and self-regulation. J Pers Soc Psychol 71: 1250–1267.
50. Beck AT (1967) Depression: Clinical, experiemental, and theoretical aspects. New York: Hoeber.

3

Poor Clinical Outcomes for HIV Infected Children on Antiretroviral Therapy in Rural Mozambique: Need for Program Quality Improvement and Community Engagement

Sten H. Vermund[1,2,6]*, Meridith Blevins[1,3], Troy D. Moon[1,2,6], Eurico José[6], Linda Moiane[6], José A. Tique[1,6], Mohsin Sidat[7], Philip J. Ciampa[1,5], Bryan E. Shepherd[1,3], Lara M. E. Vaz[1,4,6¤]

1 Vanderbilt Institute for Global Health, Vanderbilt University School of Medicine, Nashville, Tennessee, United States of America, **2** Department of Pediatrics, Vanderbilt University School of Medicine, Nashville, Tennessee, United States of America, **3** Department of Biostatistics, Vanderbilt University School of Medicine, Nashville, Tennessee, United States of America, **4** Department of Preventive Medicine, Vanderbilt University School of Medicine, Nashville, Tennessee, United States of America, **5** Department of Medicine, Vanderbilt University School of Medicine, Nashville, Tennessee, United States of America, **6** Friends in Global Health, Quelimane and Maputo, Mozambique, **7** School of Medicine, Universidade Eduardo Mondlane, Maputo, Mozambique

Abstract

Introduction: Residents of Zambézia Province, Mozambique live from rural subsistence farming and fishing. The 2009 provincial HIV prevalence for adults 15–49 years was 12.6%, higher among women (15.3%) than men (8.9%). We reviewed clinical data to assess outcomes for HIV-infected children on combination antiretroviral therapy (cART) in a highly resource-limited setting.

Methods: We studied rates of 2-year mortality and loss to follow-up (LTFU) for children <15 years of age initiating cART between June 2006–July 2011 in 10 rural districts. National guidelines define LTFU as >60 days following last-scheduled medication pickup. Kaplan-Meier estimates to compute mortality assumed non-informative censoring. Cumulative LTFU incidence calculations treated death as a competing risk.

Results: Of 753 children, 29.0% (95% CI: 24.5, 33.2) were confirmed dead by 2 years and 39.0% (95% CI: 34.8, 42.9) were LTFU with unknown clinical outcomes. The cohort mortality rate was 8.4% (95% CI: 6.3, 10.4) after 90 days on cART and 19.2% (95% CI: 16.0, 22.3) after 365 days. Higher hemoglobin at cART initiation was associated with being alive and on cART at 2 years (alive: 9.3 g/dL vs. dead or LTFU: 8.3–8.4 g/dL, p<0.01). Cotrimoxazole use within 90 days of ART initiation was associated with improved 2-year outcomes Treatment was initiated late (WHO stage III/IV) among 48% of the children with WHO stage recorded in their records. Marked heterogeneity in outcomes by district was noted (p<0.001).

Conclusions: We found poor clinical and programmatic outcomes among children taking cART in rural Mozambique. Expanded testing, early infant diagnosis, counseling/support services, case finding, and outreach are insufficiently implemented. Our quality improvement efforts seek to better link pregnancy and HIV services, expand coverage and timeliness of infant diagnosis and treatment, and increase follow-up and adherence.

Editor: David W. Dowdy, Johns Hopkins Bloomberg School of Public Health, United States of America

Funding: This research was supported by the President's Emergency Plan for AIDS Relief (PEPFAR) through the Centers for Disease Control and Prevention (grant #U2GPS000631). The findings and conclusions in this report are those of the authors and do not necessarily represent the official position of the CDC. Dr. Tique was supported by the Fogarty AIDS International Training and Research Program, National Institutes of Health #D43TW001035. The funders had no role in study design, data collection and analysis, decision to publish, or preparation of the manuscript.

Competing Interests: Dr. Vermund is a member of the PLOS ONE editorial board. This does not alter the authors' adherence to PLOS ONE editorial policies and criteria.

* Email: sten.vermund@vanderbilt.edu

¤ Current address: Save the Children, Washington DC, United States of America

Introduction

Mozambique is one of the most HIV-affected countries with an estimated national HIV prevalence in 2009 of 11.5%, translating into approximately 1.4 million adults living with HIV. [1,2] Because of its heavy HIV burden, Mozambique is a priority nation for support from the U.S. President's Emergency Plan for AIDS Relief (PEPFAR). [3] National combination antiretroviral therapy (cART) coverage is low; only an estimated 52% of adults and 20% of children in need of cART were believed to be receiving it as of the end of 2011. [4] In 2010, an estimated 70.8% of pregnant women in their first antenatal care appointment received HIV counseling and testing and 40.2% of HIV-infected pregnant women received ARV prophylaxis for the prevention of mother-to-child transmission (PMTCT), typically single-dose nevirapine [5].

Under 5 (U5) mortality rates have been falling rapidly in Mozambique with 2011 national U5 mortality estimated at 135/1000 live births compared to 219/1000 live births in 1990, in large part because of improvements in vaccination coverage and efforts to manage childhood diarrheal and acute respiratory illnesses. [6] The most recent national estimate is 97/1000 live births, from the latest Demographic Health Survey [7], still shy of the 2015 Millennium Development Goal of 73 deaths per 1000 live births. HIV/AIDS contributes 10% to the U5 mortality nationally [6].

Zambézia Province is a very low-income region of 4.2 million persons in north-central Mozambique whose majority of residents are rural subsistence farmers and fishermen. Zambézia has the nation's second largest provincial population, representing ≈20% of Mozambique's total. [1,8] Provincial HIV prevalence among adults 15–49 years in 2009 was estimated at 12.6% overall, 15.3% among women and 8.9% among men, all higher than national averages, e.g., 13.1% for women 15–49 nationally. [1] Current U5 mortality estimates show Zambézia as having the worst U5 mortality of all provinces, with deaths estimated at 142/1000 live births. [9] Leading causes of U5 deaths in Zambézia in 2009 include neonatal deaths (26.1%), malaria (27.7%) and acute lower respiratory infection (13.7%). HIV/AIDS-related deaths account for 11.5% of U5 deaths in the province [9,10].

Children with HIV are not in care at as high a proportion as adults with HIV in Africa, and their outcomes are not as good in most programs. [11–71] To assess mortality for HIV-infected children on cART, we reviewed data from PEPFAR-supported clinics run by the Zambézia Provincial Health Directorate (Direcção Provincial de Saúde, DPS) in 10 districts where a Vanderbilt University non-governmental organization (NGO) provides technical assistance.

Methods

Both the Mozambican National Bioethics Committee for Health (*Comité Nacional de Bioética em Saúde* [CNBS]) and the Institutional Review Board of Vanderbilt University approved this analysis. Analysis was performed on routinely collected, de-identified, aggregate patient level data and no individual informed consent was obtained. The CNBS and the Vanderbilt Institutional Review Board explicitly waived the need for written informed consent from the participants.

We analyzed data from a cohort of HIV-infected children <15 years of age initiating cART between June 2006–July 2011 in 10 of 17 rural districts in Zambézia Province. Details of our Friends in Global Health NGO clinical program with the DPS and the Ministry of Health (Ministério de Saúde [MISAU]) have been reported previously. [72] Two districts for which we were responsible did not have electronic medical records at the time of analysis and so were excluded;[73] five additional districts were supported by another NGO in this time period. [74] Patients who transferred from another facility after starting cART were not included in this analysis as data on their care history was incomplete (N = 156).

Patient characteristics at treatment initiation of those alive, lost, and dead at the end of 2 years' follow-up were compared using rank sum and chi-square tests. Deaths were ascertained from both clinical records and from parental testimonials. Mozambican national guidelines define loss to follow-up (LTFU) as no effective clinical contact within 60 days after the last scheduled medication pickup. [75] Two additional definitions of LTFU from the literature were also applied for the purpose of cross-cohort comparisons. The 'universal' definition classifies patients as LTFU if there is no effective clinical contact within 180 days of database closure. [76] The 'reference' definition assigns 1 day of follow-up to any individual who does not return following treatment initiation, includes only individuals initiating ART 6 months prior to the database closure, and classifies patients as LTFU if there is no effective clinical contact within 180 days of database closure. [77] All three LTFU definitions deem the patient lost at the date of last contact as opposed to the date of missed visit. Kaplan-Meier estimates were used to compute mortality and the combined endpoint of mortality and LTFU. Cumulative incidence of LTFU was calculated by treating death as a competing risk. Mortality estimates assumed non-informative censoring, i.e., patients LTFU were assumed to have rates of death similar to patients not LTFU. This likely implies that our mortality calculations are under-estimates of true mortality.

Our study did not include children enrolled in HIV care who never initiated treatment. [78] Cotrimoxazole (CTX) data were treated as a tick box for "yes", collected each visit for the corresponding visit date. If a patient was on CTX anywhere from 0 to 365 days before ART initiation, we considered the patient as "CTX use prior to cART". If a patient was on CTX anywhere from 90 days before to 90 days after ART initiation, we considered the patient as "current CTX use".

Results

During five years of PEPFAR support, 753 HIV-infected children <15 years of age initiated cART. Of these children, 678 (90.0%) were <8 years of age at cART initiation, 397 (52.7%) were <2 years, and 191 (25.4%) were <1 years. Girls represented 57% of the pediatric cART patients. Median CD4+ T-lymphocyte cell count (CD4 counts) and percentage (CD4 percentage) at cART initiation were 497 and 15, respectively, although these quantities were missing for 62% and 70% of patients. Nearly half (48%) of children initiated cART very late in their disease progression (WHO stage III or IV), although WHO stage was missing for 58% of patients.

Two years after cART initiation, 152 patients had died and 240 were LTFU. At two years, the estimated probability of death was 29.0% (95% confidence interval [CI] 24.5–33.2), the cumulative incidence of LTFU was 38.7 (95% CI 34.8–42.9), and the probability of either death or LTFU was 62.0% (95% CI 57.6–65.9). We observed substantial heterogeneity between districts in two-year outcomes (Figure 1). Two year LTFU ranged from a district low of 25% to a high of 70% (Fig. 1A; $p<0.001$), mortality ranged from 16–34% (Fig. 1B; $p = 0.19$), and death or LTFU ranged from 51.1–88.1% (Fig. 1C; $p<0.001$). The association between treatment duration and mortality rate did not suggest a marked decline in mortality over time. At 90 days on cART, the mortality rate was 8.4% (95% CI: 6.3, 10.4). At 365 days on cART, the mortality rate was 19.2% (95% CI: 16.0, 22.3) and at 730 days (two years) on cART, the mortality rate was 29.0% (95% CI: 24.5%, 33.2%). Cumulative incidence of LTFU was lower when applying two definitions from the literature. [75] The cumulative incidence of LTFU using the 'universal' definition was 26.0% (95% CI 22.6–29.9) at 2 years. [76] The cumulative incidence of LTFU using the 'reference' definition was 26.4% (95% CI 22.9–30.2) at 2 years [77].

Table 1 compares patient characteristics at cART initiation between those who were alive, dead, and lost after two years. We did not detect any difference in CD4 counts or percentage at cART initiation in children who were alive and on treatment at 2 years compared to those who were either not alive or not in care at

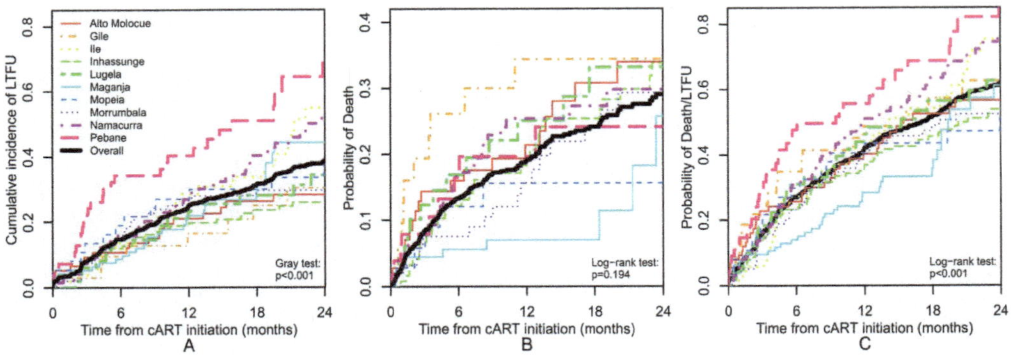

Figure 1. Variation by district in pediatric loss to follow up (LTFU), death, and death or LTFU for 2 years following combination antiretroviral therapy initiation, 10 districts of Zambézia Province, Mozambique, 2006–2011.

that time (p = 0.6), though we had high rates of missing data. We observed higher hemoglobin at the time of cART initiation among those children alive and on treatment at 2 years (alive: median 9.3 g/dL; 8.3 for dead; 8.4 g/dL for LTFU, p<0.01 for alive vs. dead or LTFU). Any cotrimoxazole use in the year prior to ART initiation was associated with improved 2-year outcomes (alive: 76%, dead: 49%, lost: 55%). Cotrimoxazole use within 90 days of ART initiation was associated with improved 2-year outcomes (alive: 69%, dead: 58%, lost: 59%).

Discussion

The experience from our PEPFAR cART program found that 29% of children initiating cART were dead within two years. It is likely that many of the 39% LTFU are at high risk of death or have already died. HIV care for children is not yet optimized in this impoverished setting with a backdrop of health workforce shortages, poor health care infrastructures, challenging transportation, poor maternal and child health outcomes, high rates of tuberculosis and malaria infections, high levels of malnutrition, low adult and pediatric cART and maternal ARV prophylaxis coverage rates, and limited formal counseling/social support programs. Similar challenges are reported elsewhere, particularly where cART is initiated late and co-infections are already extant. [20,79,80] Considerably better outcomes are reported from LMIC outside of Africa. [81–92] While a number of pediatric cART programs have reported much better success, we do not know the extent to which there is a reporting bias in the literature, i.e., overrepresentation in the literature of more favorable program outcomes. [11,44,60,64,65,68,69,85,93–110] Challenges we face have been reported from many low and middle-income nations, though we think our results are especially worrisome [25,111–117].

We observed a wide range of LTFU in different districts, suggesting possible inconsistent fidelity across sites to the active case-finding (*busca activa*) program that is in place, as well as variations in the quality of care, system infrastructure and/or community engagement. [118] In PMTCT work in Zambia and subsequently in the multinational PEARL study, similar clinic-by-clinic diversity has been seen, documenting that the specific component of the continuum of care that is "broken" in lower functioning clinics may differ by clinic [119–123].

In a poorly functioning clinic in Mozambique, we may find health providers who are able to speak only Portuguese with clients, rather than the local language. We have learned from pediatric and obstetric quality improvement work that mothers frequently do not understand complex instructions in Portuguese from health providers who often come from other provinces and may not speak one of the local languages spoken in this ethnically diverse province. [8,118,124] On aggregate, Zambézia residents have low health literacy and numeracy rates, likely contributing to patient/caregiver-provider miscommunication and, possibly to LTFU and suboptimal adherence [125].

Another common occurrence in a poorly functioning clinic generally is the failure of pyschosocial services to effectively engage caregivers fully in chronic pediatric care services, as well as HIV services for themselves. Prior to HIV services, long-term follow-up of chronic diseases was not something with which residents of Zambézia Province were familiar. It is common, especially in rural Africa, that asymptomatic or improving children, parents or guardians do not recognize the need for ongoing services. [126–132] The same applies to parents themselves; they may be LTFU once they feel better. [72,78] We have also had anecdotal reports of parents in our program avoiding care for their children (or themselves) due to stigma and fear of persons learning of the HIV infections in their children. These are daunting challenges that call for more effective counseling and trust-building between providers and clients, and potentially for earlier engagement of children in their health care. The active case-finding approach (*busca active*) of the DPS/MISAU needs serious review and improvement in the face of high mortality and LTFU data in children. It is also possible that traditional active case-finding efforts need to be tailored for special populations, such as children. Improved counseling and family-centered treatment approaches need further exploration. Any innovation in engaging HIV-infected women in their own care can be expected to improve follow-up for their children as well. [133–135] A recent review found that although there is evidence of effectiveness of interventions to improve access and adherence to cART, there is less known about major barriers and ways to address them among vulnerable groups such as women, children and adolescents [136].

There is little tradition of long-term pediatric care in rural Zambézia Province. Mothers take children for vaccines and acute illnesses, but only a tuberculosis diagnosis results in chronic care involving long-term drug administration that can reasonably be expected to be available (such medications as insulin and oncology drugs are not available in the rural clinics). In fact, loss to follow-up rates for children with HIV are high throughout southern Africa. [137] Mothers have told us that they and/or their fathers do not want the stigma of having them take the child for HIV care, that they live too far away and cannot afford the time or money for care, they do not know the health workers due to high turnover rates, and that health workers often mistreat them and violate their confidentiality and their privacy [124,138,139].

Table 1. Characteristics of children at initiation of combination antiretroviral therapy by 2 year outcome in 10 districts of Zambézia Province, Mozambique, 2006–2011 (PITC = Provider-initiated testing and counseling; PMTCT = Prevention of mother-to-child HIV transmission; BMI = Body Mass Index or weight in kg divided by height squared).

	Alive	Dead	Lost	Combined	P-value
	(n = 361)	(n = 152)	(n = 240)	(n = 753)	
Female, n(%)	204 (57%)	73 (48%)	118 (49%)	395 (52%)	0.1
Age (years), median (IQR)	2 (1, 4)	1 (0, 2)	1 (1, 3)	1 (0, 4)	<0.001
District, n(%)					0.002
Alto Molócuè	38 (11%)	19 (12%)	19 (8%)	76 (10%)	
Gilé	15 (4%)	10 (7%)	8 (3%)	33 (4%)	
Ile	23 (6%)	10 (7%)	22 (9%)	55 (7%)	
Inhassunge	69 (19%)	31 (20%)	30 (12%)	130 (17%)	
Lugela	22 (6%)	13 (9%)	15 (6%)	50 (7%)	
Maganja	58 (16%)	9 (6%)	28 (12%)	95 (13%)	
Mopeia	19 (5%)	5 (3%)	13 (5%)	37 (5%)	
Morrumbala	52 (14%)	18 (12%)	26 (11%)	96 (13%)	
Namacurra	47 (13%)	28 (18%)	50 (21%)	125 (17%)	
Pebane	18 (5%)	9 (6%)	29 (12%)	56 (7%)	
Referral site[4], n(%)					0.7
Missing	297 (83%)	134 (88%)	193 (80%)	624 (83%)	
External consultation (PITC)	10 (16%)	4 (22%)	6 (13%)	20 (16%)	
Medical inpatient (PITC)	2 (3%)	0 (0%)	4 (9%)	6 (5%)	
Tuberculosis care (PITC)	1 (2%)	0 (0%)	0 (0%)	1 (<1%)	
PMTCT site	7 (11%)	3 (17%)	8 (17%)	18 (14%)	
Voluntary counseling and testing site	44 (69%)	11 (61%)	29 (62%)	84 (65%)	
Height (cm), median (IQR)[1]	85 (67, 109)	70 (63, 84.2)	72 (66, 81.8)	75 (66, 103.5)	0.04
Missing	206 (57%)	118 (78%)	174 (72%)	498 (66%)	
Weight (kg), median (IQR)[1]	8.5 (6.3, 14)	6.7 (5, 9.5)	7 (5.8, 10)	7.5 (6, 12.4)	<0.001
Missing	4 (1%)	10 (7%)	24 (10%)	38 (5%)	
BMI (kg/m^2), median (IQR)[1]	15.2 (14.1, 16.6)	14.4 (13.8, 17.4)	14.9 (14.2, 16.6)	15.1 (14.1, 16.8)	1
Missing	274 (76%)	132 (87%)	197 (82%)	603 (80%)	
CD4+ cell count/μL, median (IQR)[2]	458 (248, 760)	595 (164, 734)	513 (314, 841)	497 (237, 774)	0.7
Missing	222 (61%)	90 (59%)	149 (62%)	461 (61%)	
CD4 percentage, median (IQR)[2]	15 (10, 21)	15 (12, 22)	15 (8, 21)	15 (10, 21)	0.6
Missing	251 (70%)	107 (70%)	171 (71%)	529 (70%)	
Hemoglobin (g/dL), median (IQR)[2]	9.3 (8, 10.4)	8.3 (7, 9.3)	8.4 (7.4, 9.4)	8.9 (7.6, 9.9)	<0.001
Missing	237 (66%)	100 (66%)	163 (68%)	500 (66%)	
WHO stage, n(%)[2]					0.1
Missing	224 (62%)	75 (49%)	130 (54%)	429 (57%)	
I	47 (34%)	18 (23%)	32 (29%)	97 (30%)	
II	30 (22%)	11 (14%)	29 (26%)	70 (22%)	
III	43 (31%)	39 (51%)	37 (34%)	119 (37%)	
IV	17 (12%)	9 (12%)	12 (11%)	38 (12%)	
Cotrimoxazole use (prior to ART), n(%)[3]	273 (76%)	75 (49%)	132 (55%)	480 (64%)	<0.001
Cotrimoxazole use (current), n(%)[3]	249 (69%)	88 (58%)	142 (59%)	479 (64%)	0.01

Percentages are computed using the number of patients with a non-missing value.
[1]Weight, height, and BMI are collected at enrollment. [2]Collected within 90 days before and 14 days after ART initiation. [3]Prior to ART means any cotrimoxazole (CTX) use recorded in 365 days prior to ART initiation. Current means any CTX use in 90 days before or 90 days after ART initiation. CTX use is recorded along with the visit date; data is not collected on non-users so we are unable to assess missing data. [4]When PITC referral sites are grouped: p = 0.9.

There is evidence from this study and elsewhere that early infant diagnosis, provider initiated testing and counseling, case finding of older children, and family support and outreach are not sufficiently developed in rural Mozambique.

[8,73,78,118,124,125,134,135,140–152] As of 2011, all HIV-infected children <2 years of age should be started on cART as per Mozambican national guidelines, based on results of the South African CHER trial. [79] As of May 2013, Mozambican guidelines changed further to mandate cART for all infected children <5 years of age, independent of clinical status or CD4+ cell count. Yet our study suggests that poor adherence by health workers to standards of screening and HIV staging and subsequent CD4 monitoring impairs pediatric outcomes by delaying recognition of children in need of cART and prophylaxis for opportunistic infections (OI). OI prophylaxis with cotrimoxazole was a protective factor for adverse outcomes in our study. We do not believe that co-trimoxazole benefits are explained by urban-rural differences, as all our sites were rural, nor by family income or assets. All HIV-related services provided by the Ministry, which includes all of the services in this study, are available free of cost, including provision of cotrimoxazole. Family income is not recorded on the clinical record, only patient (or parent) profession; we are thus unable to distinguish subsistence farmers from those who sell their crops, small merchants from larger ones. Over 80 percent of the overall population in the province subsists on less than USD 2 per day as we have documented in a baseline USAID report (Vergara, AE, Blevins M, Vaz LME, et al (2011). Baseline survey report: Improving livelihoods and health of children, women and families in the Province of Zambézia, Republic of Mozambique (available at [http://globalhealth.vanderbilt.edu/programs/scip/]).

Since many children are not diagnosed early or begun on cART early and/or fail to stay in (or adhere to) cART-based care, adverse events are high. [118] We believe that poor interpretation of the guidelines by providers and an overall reluctance to place young children on cART is playing a major role. Quality improvement efforts are essential [148] and are underway to improve infant diagnosis and treatment initiation. [124,135] Linkages across MCH services are being forged to improve treatment outcomes.

Health worker shortages contribute to poor quality of pediatric care. Given severe health care worker shortages and structural impediments to effective long-term care services, we believe that international support, such as that available from PEPFAR and the Global Fund to Fight AIDS, Tuberculosis and Malaria, will be needed for many years to come. [153–157] Whether traditional healers, far more numerous than allopathic practitioners, can be engaged in a productive way for early referral and for assistance in adherence and follow up is unknown. [158,159] More effective community engagement is essential and some success has been had with church-based outreach. [159,160] It is also unknown the extent to which efforts such as the Medical Education Partnership Initiative,[161] the Royal Society-DFID Africa Capacity Building Initiative,[162] or the Consortium of New Southern African Medical Schools [163] will make a major difference over the next 5–10 years in addressing chronic health worker shortages in rural Africa. [164–167] Task-shifting would be a reasonable approach, but nursing and medical assistants (*técnicos de medicina* in Mozambique) are also in very short supply. [8] Creative approaches to patient-to-patient adherence and retention show promise [168–170].

Our data have limitations that affect the completeness of our study. Missing data were frequent, particularly CD4 counts, CD4%, and WHO stage, limiting our ability to examine delays in initiation of treatment. Multivariable analyses were not performed to estimate independent associations with clinical outcomes due to large amounts of missing data and potential for misclassification among those LTFU. We only ask age (in years) of the child such that age subgroups are less reliable, particularly for younger ages, than if we had reliable birthdate; however, rural populations often do not know specific birthdates. Information on cotrimoxazole use was recorded; however, the nature of the documentation is to record use and thus we are unable to differentiate between non-users and missing data. If data are not missing completely at random, there would be bias in the summary statistics of non-missing data. Generalizability of findings to the whole province was limited because data were available for 10 of the total 17 districts. Our database does not collect information on risk factors for poor clinical outcomes external to the patient visit; prospective data collection on such factors (e.g., health facility staffing, drug stock-outs, family support) would permit more robust risk assessment. Nonetheless, we believe that our data clearly indicate a seriously underperforming pediatric care program in need of aggressive quality improvement; despite limitations, we have found these real-world data to be adequate to guide programmatic improvement and community engagement. These efforts are beginning to bear fruit [124,135,148].

There are many challenges not likely to be resolved soon: health care worker shortages and high turnover rates, particularly in remote rural settings, drug and supply stockouts, language barriers, gender-power distortions, literacy and numeracy challenges, poor attitudes of health care workers towards patients, lack of appreciation of the germ theory of disease, crushing rural poverty, poor transportation infrastructures, and structural barriers within the clinical care setting. [73,78,146,148,153,171–173] Co-infections prevalent in the tropics and food shortages are recurring challenges that are far less prevalent in higher income nations. [174–177] Drug resistance has not been studied widely in Mozambique [178].

Even in the face of these obstacles, we and others are having some success in pediatric care HIV quality improvement. [124,135,179–181] That our real-world findings of co-trimoxazole benefit to children in HIV care reinforces clinical trial results suggesting that HIV-infected children benefit from continued co-trimoxazole (protecting against both malaria and non-malarial disease), even when they are on cART. [182] To better retain children on cART and co-trimoxazole, more comprehensive quality improvement efforts are needed to identify staff, structural, cultural, social and policy challenges and to craft solutions for support to pediatric patients, their caregivers, and health care providers.

Acknowledgments

The authors thank Megan Pask, Wilson Silva, Tito Jequicene, Jairzinho Tereso, Carlos Castel-Branco, Ferreira Ferreira, Kulssum Faque, and Deidra Parrish for their help with this work.

Disclosures: This research was supported by the President's Emergency Plan for AIDS Relief (PEPFAR) through the Centers for Disease Control and Prevention (grant #U2GPS000631). The findings and conclusions in this report are those of the authors and do not necessarily represent the official position of the CDC. Dr. Tique was supported by the Fogarty AIDS International Training and Research Program, National Institutes of Health #D43TW001035).

Author Contributions

Conceived and designed the experiments: SHV MB TDM EJ BES LMEV. Performed the experiments: MB TDM EJ LM JAT MS LMEV. Analyzed the data: SHV MB BES LMEV. Contributed reagents/materials/analysis tools: SHV MB TDM EJ LM LMEV. Wrote the paper: SHV MB TDM BES LMEV. Edited and improved the paper: SHV MB TDM EJ LM JAT MS PJC BES LMEV.

References

1. Ministério da Saúde Instituto Nacional de Saúde (INS), Instituto Nacional de Estatística (INE), ICF Macro (2010) Inquérito Nacional de Prevalência, Riscos Comportamentais e Informação sobre o HIV e SIDA (INSIDA) em Moçambique 2009. Calverton, Maryland, EUA: INS, INE, e ICF Macro.
2. Auld AF, Mbofana F, Shiraishi RW, Sanchez M, Alfredo C, et al. (2011) Four-year treatment outcomes of adult patients enrolled in Mozambique's rapidly expanding antiretroviral therapy program. PLoS One 6: e18453.
3. U.S. State Department (2011) The United States President's Emergency Plan for AIDS Relief.
4. Republic of Mozambique, National AIDS Council, CNCS (2012) 2012 Global AIDS Response Progress Report for the Period 2010–2011. Mozambique: Ministério da Saúde Instituto Nacional de Saúde (INS).
5. National Public Health Directorate MoH, Republic of Mozambique (2011) Preliminary Report of the National Evaluation of the Prevention of Mother-to-Child Transmission Program.
6. WHO (2012) Partnership for Maternal, Newborn & Child Health, World Health Organization. Countdown to 2015: Building a Future for Women and Children, Mozambique Country Reports.
7. Instituto Nacional de Estastistica, Ministerio da Saude, US AID (2013) Moçambique Inquérito Demográfico e de Saúde 2011. Calverton, Maryland, USA.
8. Audet CM, Burlison J, Moon TD, Sidat M, Vergara AE, et al. (2010) Sociocultural and epidemiological aspects of HIV/AIDS in Mozambique. BMC Int Health Hum Rights 10: 15.
9. Institute NS (2009) Preliminary Report on the Multiple Indicator Cluster Survey, 2008. Maputo, Mozambique.
10. Republic of Mozambique, Ministry of Health, National Institute of Health (2009) Mozambique National Child Mortality Study 2009 Summary.
11. Bolton-Moore C, Mubiana-Mbewe M, Cantrell RA, Chintu N, Stringer EM, et al. (2007) Clinical outcomes and CD4 cell response in children receiving antiretroviral therapy at primary health care facilities in Zambia. JAMA 298: 1888–1899.
12. Bland RM, Ndirangu J, Newell ML (2013) Maximising opportunities for increased antiretroviral treatment in children in an existing HIV programme in rural South Africa. BMJ 346: f550.
13. Patel SD, Larson E, Mbengashe T, O'Bra H, Brown JW, et al. (2012) Increases in pediatric antiretroviral treatment, South Africa 2005–2010. PLoS One 7: e44914.
14. Munyagwa M, Baisley K, Levin J, Brian M, Grosskurth H, et al. (2012) Mortality of HIV-infected and uninfected children in a longitudinal cohort in rural south-west Uganda during 8 years of follow-up. Trop Med Int Health 17: 836–843.
15. Meyers T, Dramowski A, Schneider H, Gardiner N, Kuhn L, et al. (2012) Changes in pediatric HIV-related hospital admissions and mortality in Soweto, South Africa, 1996–2011: light at the end of the tunnel? J Acquir Immune Defic Syndr 60: 503–510.
16. Johnson LF, Davies MA, Moultrie H, Sherman GG, Bland RM, et al. (2012) The effect of early initiation of antiretroviral treatment in infants on pediatric AIDS mortality in South Africa: a model-based analysis. Pediatr Infect Dis J 31: 474–480.
17. Bland RM (2011) Management of HIV-infected children in Africa: progress and challenges. Arch Dis Child 96: 911–915.
18. Eley B (2006) Addressing the paediatric HIV epidemic: a perspective from the Western Cape Region of South Africa. Trans R Soc Trop Med Hyg 100: 19–23.
19. De Baets AJ, Bulterys M, Abrams EJ, Kankassa C, Pazvakavambwa IE (2007) Care and treatment of HIV-infected children in Africa: issues and challenges at the district hospital level. Pediatr Infect Dis J 26: 163–173.
20. Braitstein P, Nyandiko W, Vreeman R, Wools-Kaloustian K, Sang E, et al. (2009) The clinical burden of tuberculosis among human immunodeficiency virus-infected children in Western Kenya and the impact of combination antiretroviral treatment. Pediatr Infect Dis J 28: 626–632.
21. Nicoll A, Timaeus I, Kigadye RM, Walraven G, Killewo J (1994) The impact of HIV-1 infection on mortality in children under 5 years of age in sub-Saharan Africa: a demographic and epidemiologic analysis. AIDS 8: 995–1005.
22. Martinson NA, Moultrie H, van Niekerk R, Barry G, Coovadia A, et al. (2009) HAART and risk of tuberculosis in HIV-infected South African children: a multi-site retrospective cohort. Int J Tuberc Lung Dis 13: 862–867.
23. Sutcliffe CG, van Dijk JH, Bolton-Moore C, Cotham M, Tambatamba B, et al. (2010) Differences in presentation, treatment initiation, and response among children infected with human immunodeficiency virus in urban and rural Zambia. Pediatr Infect Dis J 29: 849–854.
24. Sutcliffe CG, van Dijk JH, Bolton C, Persaud D, Moss WJ (2008) Effectiveness of antiretroviral therapy among HIV-infected children in sub-Saharan Africa. Lancet Infect Dis 8: 477–489.
25. van Dijk JH, Sutcliffe CG, Munsanje B, Hamangaba F, Thuma PE, et al. (2009) Barriers to the care of HIV-infected children in rural Zambia: a cross-sectional analysis. BMC Infect Dis 9: 169.
26. Feucht UD, Kinzer M, Kruger M (2007) Reasons for delay in initiation of antiretroviral therapy in a population of HIV-infected South African children. J Trop Pediatr 53: 398–402.
27. Thomas TA, Shenoi SV, Heysell SK, Eksteen FJ, Sunkari VB, et al. (2010) Extensively drug-resistant tuberculosis in children with human immunodeficiency virus in rural South Africa. Int J Tuberc Lung Dis 14: 1244–1251.
28. Adjorlolo-Johnson G, Wahl Uheling A, Ramachandran S, Strasser S, Kouakou J, et al. (2013) Scaling up pediatric HIV care and treatment in Africa: clinical site characteristics associated with favorable service utilization. J Acquir Immune Defic Syndr 62: e7–e13.
29. Kabue MM, Buck WC, Wanless SR, Cox CM, McCollum ED, et al. (2012) Mortality and clinical outcomes in HIV-infected children on antiretroviral therapy in Malawi, Lesotho, and Swaziland. Pediatrics 130: e591–599.
30. Okomo U, Togun T, Oko F, Peterson K, Townend J, et al. (2012) Treatment outcomes among HIV-1 and HIV-2 infected children initiating antiretroviral therapy in a concentrated low prevalence setting in West Africa. BMC Pediatr 12: 95.
31. Grimwood A, Fatti G, Mothibi E, Malahlela M, Shea J, et al. (2012) Community adherence support improves programme retention in children on antiretroviral treatment: a multicentre cohort study in South Africa. J Int AIDS Soc 15: 17381.
32. Chhagan MK, Kauchali S, Van den Broeck J (2012) Clinical and contextual determinants of anthropometric failure at baseline and longitudinal improvements after starting antiretroviral treatment among South African children. Trop Med Int Health 17: 1092–1099.
33. Satti H, McLaughlin MM, Omotayo DB, Keshavjee S, Becerra MC, et al. (2012) Outcomes of comprehensive care for children empirically treated for multidrug-resistant tuberculosis in a setting of high HIV prevalence. PLoS One 7: e37114.
34. Laughton B, Cornell M, Grove D, Kidd M, Springer PE, et al. (2012) Early antiretroviral therapy improves neurodevelopmental outcomes in infants. AIDS 26: 1685–1690.
35. Haberer JE, Kiwanuka J, Nansera D, Ragland K, Mellins C, et al. (2012) Multiple measures reveal antiretroviral adherence successes and challenges in HIV-infected Ugandan children. PLoS One 7: e36737.
36. Kekitiinwa A, Asiimwe AR, Kasirye P, Korutaro V, Kitaka S, et al. (2012) Prospective long-term outcomes of a cohort of Ugandan children with laboratory monitoring during antiretroviral therapy. Pediatr Infect Dis J 31: e117–125.
37. Musiime V, Kayiwa J, Kiconco M, Tamale W, Alima H, et al. (2012) Response to antiretroviral therapy of HIV type 1-infected children in urban and rural settings of Uganda. AIDS Res Hum Retroviruses 28: 1647–1657.
38. Workneh G, Scherzer L, Kirk B, Draper HR, Anabwani G, et al. (2013) Evaluation of the effectiveness of an outreach clinical mentoring programme in support of paediatric HIV care scale-up in Botswana. AIDS Care 25: 11–19.
39. Heidari S, Mofenson LM, Hobbs CV, Cotton MF, Marlink R, et al. (2012) Unresolved antiretroviral treatment management issues in HIV-infected children. J Acquir Immune Defic Syndr 59: 161–169.
40. Kim MH, Cox C, Dave A, Draper HR, Kabue M, et al. (2012) Prompt initiation of ART With therapeutic food is associated with improved outcomes in HIV-infected Malawian children with malnutrition. J Acquir Immune Defic Syndr 59: 173–176.
41. Zyl GU, Rabie H, Nuttall JJ, Cotton MF (2011) It is time to consider third-line options in antiretroviral-experienced paediatric patients? J Int AIDS Soc 14: 55.
42. Reubenson G (2011) Pediatric drug-resistant tuberculosis: a global perspective: a global perspective. Paediatr Drugs 13: 349–355.
43. Geddes R, Giddy J, Butler LM, Van Wyk E, Crankshaw T, et al. (2011) Dual and triple therapy to prevent mother-to-child transmission of HIV in a resource-limited setting - lessons from a South African programme. S Afr Med J 101: 651–654.
44. Fatti G, Bock P, Eley B, Mothibi E, Grimwood A (2011) Temporal trends in baseline characteristics and treatment outcomes of children starting antiretroviral treatment: an analysis in four provinces in South Africa, 2004–2009. J Acquir Immune Defic Syndr 58: e60–67.
45. Ahoua L, Guenther G, Rouzioux C, Pinoges L, Anguzu P, et al. (2011) Immunovirological response to combined antiretroviral therapy and drug resistance patterns in children: 1- and 2-year outcomes in rural Uganda. BMC Pediatr 11: 67.
46. Desmonde S, Coffie P, Aka E, Amani-Bosse C, Messou E, et al. (2011) Severe morbidity and mortality in untreated HIV-infected children in a paediatric care programme in Abidjan, Cote d'Ivoire, 2004–2009. BMC Infect Dis 11: 182.
47. Ciaranello AL, Perez F, Maruva M, Chu J, Engelsmann B, et al. (2011) WHO 2010 guidelines for prevention of mother-to-child HIV transmission in Zimbabwe: modeling clinical outcomes in infants and mothers. PLoS One 6: e20224.
48. Bakanda C, Birungi J, Mwesigwa R, Nachega JB, Chan K, et al. (2011) Survival of HIV-infected adolescents on antiretroviral therapy in Uganda: findings from a nationally representative cohort in Uganda. PLoS One 6: e19261.
49. Schneider K, Puthanakit T, Kerr S, Law MG, Cooper DA, et al. (2011) Economic evaluation of monitoring virologic responses to antiretroviral therapy in HIV-infected children in resource-limited settings. AIDS 25: 1143–1151.

50. Frohoff C, Moodley M, Fairlie L, Coovadia A, Moultrie H, et al. (2011) Antiretroviral therapy outcomes in HIV-infected children after adjusting protease inhibitor dosing during tuberculosis treatment. PLoS One 6: e17273.
51. De Maayer T, Saloojee H (2011) Clinical outcomes of severe malnutrition in a high tuberculosis and HIV setting. Arch Dis Child 96: 560–564.
52. McCollum ED, Preidis GA, Golitko CL, Siwande LD, Mwansambo C, et al. (2011) Routine inpatient human immunodeficiency virus testing system increases access to pediatric human immunodeficiency virus care in sub-Saharan Africa. Pediatr Infect Dis J 30: e75–81.
53. Ndondoki C, Dabis F, Namale L, Becquet R, Ekouevi D, et al. (2011) [Survival, clinical and biological outcomes of HIV-infected children treated by antiretroviral therapy in Africa: systematic review, 2004–2009]. Presse Med 40: e338–357.
54. Peacock-Villada E, Richardson BA, John-Stewart GC (2011) Post-HAART outcomes in pediatric populations: comparison of resource-limited and developed countries. Pediatrics 127: e423–441.
55. Fatti G, Bock P, Grimwood A, Eley B (2010) Increased vulnerability of rural children on antiretroviral therapy attending public health facilities in South Africa: a retrospective cohort study. J Int AIDS Soc 13: 46.
56. Buck WC, Kabue MM, Kazembe PN, Kline MW (2010) Discontinuation of standard first-line antiretroviral therapy in a cohort of 1434 Malawian children. J Int AIDS Soc 13: 31.
57. Musoke PM, Mudiope P, Barlow-Mosha LN, Ajuna P, Bagenda D, et al. (2010) Growth, immune and viral responses in HIV infected African children receiving highly active antiretroviral therapy: a prospective cohort study. BMC Pediatr 10: 56.
58. Sutcliffe CG, Bolton-Moore C, van Dijk JH, Cotham M, Tambatamba B, et al. (2010) Secular trends in pediatric antiretroviral treatment programs in rural and urban Zambia: a retrospective cohort study. BMC Pediatr 10: 54.
59. Nyandiko WM, Mwangi A, Ayaya SO, Nabakwe EC, Tenge CN, et al. (2009) Characteristics of HIV-infected children seen in Western Kenya. East Afr Med J 86: 364–373.
60. Sauvageot D, Schaefer M, Olson D, Pujades-Rodriguez M, O'Brien DP (2010) Antiretroviral therapy outcomes in resource-limited settings for HIV-infected children <5 years of age. Pediatrics 125: e1039–1047.
61. Davies MA, Keiser O, Technau K, Eley B, Rabie H, et al. (2009) Outcomes of the South African National Antiretroviral Treatment Programme for children: the IeDEA Southern Africa collaboration. S Afr Med J 99: 730–737.
62. Leyenaar JK, Novosad PM, Ferrer KT, Thahane LK, Mohapi EQ, et al. (2010) Early clinical outcomes in children enrolled in human immunodeficiency virus infection care and treatment in lesotho. Pediatr Infect Dis J 29: 340–345.
63. Ciaranello AL, Chang Y, Margulis AV, Bernstein A, Bassett IV, et al. (2009) Effectiveness of pediatric antiretroviral therapy in resource-limited settings: a systematic review and meta-analysis. Clin Infect Dis 49: 1915–1927.
64. Janssen N, Ndirangu J, Newell ML, Bland RM (2010) Successful paediatric HIV treatment in rural primary care in Africa. Arch Dis Child 95: 414–421.
65. Memirie ST (2009) Clinical outcome of children on HAART at police referral hospital, Addis Ababa, Ethiopia. Ethiop Med J 47: 159–164.
66. Ntanda H, Olupot-Olupot P, Mugyenyi P, Kityo C, Lowes R, et al. (2009) Orphanhood predicts delayed access to care in Ugandan children. Pediatr Infect Dis J 28: 153–155.
67. Van Winghem J, Telfer B, Reid T, Ouko J, Mutunga A, et al. (2008) Implementation of a comprehensive program including psycho-social and treatment literacy activities to improve adherence to HIV care and treatment for a pediatric population in Kenya. BMC Pediatr 8: 52.
68. Kiboneka A, Wangisi J, Nabiryo C, Tembe J, Kusemererwa S, et al. (2008) Clinical and immunological outcomes of a national paediatric cohort receiving combination antiretroviral therapy in Uganda. AIDS 22: 2493–2499.
69. Jaspan HB, Berrisford AE, Boulle AM (2008) Two-year outcomes of children on non-nucleoside reverse transcriptase inhibitor and protease inhibitor regimens in a South African pediatric antiretroviral program. Pediatr Infect Dis J 27: 993–998.
70. Bock P, Boulle A, White C, Osler M, Eley B (2008) Provision of antiretroviral therapy to children within the public sector of South Africa. Trans R Soc Trop Med Hyg 102: 905–911.
71. Walker AS, Ford D, Mulenga V, Thomason MJ, Nunn A, et al. (2009) Adherence to both cotrimoxazole and placebo is associated with improved survival among HIV-infected Zambian children. AIDS Behav 13: 33–41.
72. Moon TD, Burlison JR, Sidat M, Pires P, Silva W, et al. (2010) Lessons Learned while Implementing an HIV/AIDs Care and Treatment Program in Rural Mozambique. Retrovirology: Research and Treatment 3: 1.
73. Manders EJ, Jose E, Solis M, Burlison J, Nhampossa JL, et al. (2010) Implementing OpenMRS for patient monitoring in an HIV/AIDS care and treatment program in rural Mozambique. Stud Health Technol Inform 160: 411–415.
74. Lahuerta M, Lima J, Elul B, Okamura M, Alvim MF, et al. (2011) Patients enrolled in HIV care in Mozambique: baseline characteristics and follow-up outcomes. J Acquir Immune Defic Syndr 58: e75–86.
75. Shepherd BE, Blevins M, Vaz LM, Moon TD, Kipp AM, et al. (2013) Impact of Definitions of Loss to Follow-up on Estimates of Retention, Disease Progression, and Mortality: Application to an HIV Program in Mozambique. Am J Epidemiol.
76. Chi BH, Yiannoutsos CT, Westfall AO, Newman JE, Zhou J, et al. (2011) Universal definition of loss to follow-up in HIV treatment programs: a statistical analysis of 111 facilities in Africa, Asia, and Latin America. PLoS Med 8: e1001111.
77. Grimsrud AT, Cornell M, Egger M, Boulle A, Myer L (2013) Impact of definitions of loss to follow-up (LTFU) in antiretroviral therapy program evaluation: variation in the definition can have an appreciable impact on estimated proportions of LTFU. J Clin Epidemiol.
78. Moon TD, Burlison JR, Blevins M, Shepherd BE, Baptista A, et al. (2011) Enrolment and programmatic trends and predictors of antiretroviral therapy initiation from president's emergency plan for AIDS Relief (PEPFAR)-supported public HIV care and treatment sites in rural Mozambique. Int J STD AIDS 22: 621–627.
79. Violari A, Cotton MF, Gibb DM, Babiker AG, Steyn J, et al. (2008) Early antiretroviral therapy and mortality among HIV-infected infants. N Engl J Med 359: 2233–2244.
80. Ylitalo N, Brogly S, Hughes MD, Nachman S, Dankner W, et al. (2006) Risk factors for opportunistic illnesses in children with human immunodeficiency virus in the era of highly active antiretroviral therapy. Arch Pediatr Adolesc Med 160: 778–787.
81. Rath BA, von Kleist M, Castillo ME, Kolevic L, Caballero P, et al. (2013) Antiviral resistance and correlates of virologic failure in the first cohort of HIV-infected children gaining access to structured antiretroviral therapy in Lima, Peru: a cross-sectional analysis. BMC Infect Dis 13: 1.
82. Christie CD, Pierre RB (2012) Eliminating vertically-transmitted HIV/AIDS while improving access to treatment and care for women, children and adolescents in Jamaica. West Indian Med J 61: 396–404.
83. Hansudewechakul R, Naiwatanakul T, Katana A, Faikratok W, Lolekha R, et al. (2012) Successful clinical outcomes following decentralization of tertiary paediatric HIV care to a community-based paediatric antiretroviral treatment network, Chiangrai, Thailand, 2002 to 2008. J Int AIDS Soc 15: 17358.
84. Diniz LM, Maia MM, Camargos LS, Amaral LC, Goulart EM, et al. (2011) Impact of HAART on growth and hospitalization rates among HIV-infected children. J Pediatr (Rio J) 87: 131–137.
85. Lumbiganon P, Kariminia A, Aurpibul L, Hansudewechakul R, Puthanakit T, et al. (2011) Survival of HIV-infected children: a cohort study from the Asia-Pacific region. J Acquir Immune Defic Syndr 56: 365–371.
86. Oliveira R, Krauss M, Essama-Bibi S, Hofer C, Robert Harris D, et al. (2010) Viral load predicts new world health organization stage 3 and 4 events in HIV-infected children receiving highly active antiretroviral therapy, independent of CD4 T lymphocyte value. Clin Infect Dis 51: 1325–1333.
87. Rodriguez de Schiavi MS, Scrigni A, Garcia Arrigoni P, Bologna R, Barboni G, et al. (2009) [Highly active antiretroviral therapy in HIV sero-positive children. Disease progression by baseline clinical, immunological and virological status]. Arch Argent Pediatr 107: 212–220.
88. Prasitsuebsai W, Bowen AC, Pang J, Hesp C, Kariminia A, et al. (2010) Pediatric HIV clinical care resources and management practices in Asia: a regional survey of the TREAT Asia pediatric network. AIDS Patient Care STDS 24: 127–131.
89. McConnell MS, Chasombat S, Siangphoe U, Yuktanont P, Lolekha R, et al. (2010) National program scale-up and patient outcomes in a pediatric antiretroviral treatment program, Thailand, 2000–2007. J Acquir Immune Defic Syndr 54: 423–429.
90. Souza E, Santos N, Valentini S, Silva G, Falbo A (2010) Long-term follow-up outcomes of perinatally HIV-infected adolescents: infection control but school failure. J Trop Pediatr 56: 421–426.
91. Kumarasamy N, Venkatesh KK, Devaleenol B, Poongulali S, Mothi SN, et al. (2009) Safety, tolerability and effectiveness of generic HAART in HIV-infected children in South India. J Trop Pediatr 55: 155–159.
92. Noel F, Mehta S, Zhu Y, Rouzier Pde M, Marcelin A, et al. (2008) Improving outcomes in infants of HIV-infected women in a developing country setting. PLoS One 3: e3723.
93. Reddi A, Leeper SC, Grobler AC, Geddes R, France KH, et al. (2007) Preliminary outcomes of a paediatric highly active antiretroviral therapy cohort from KwaZulu-Natal, South Africa. BMC Pediatr 7: 13.
94. Puthanakit T, Aurpibul L, Oberdorfer P, Akarathum N, Kanjananit S, et al. (2007) Hospitalization and mortality among HIV-infected children after receiving highly active antiretroviral therapy. Clin Infect Dis 44: 599–604.
95. Puthanakit T, Oberdorfer A, Akarathum N, Kanjanavanit S, Wannarit P, et al. (2005) Efficacy of highly active antiretroviral therapy in HIV-infected children participating in Thailand's National Access to Antiretroviral Program. Clin Infect Dis 41: 100–107.
96. Janssens B, Raleigh B, Soeung S, Akao K, Te V, et al. (2007) Effectiveness of highly active antiretroviral therapy in HIV-positive children: evaluation at 12 months in a routine program in Cambodia. Pediatrics 120: e1134–1140.
97. Nyandiko WM, Ayaya S, Nabakwe E, Tenge C, Sidle JE, et al. (2006) Outcomes of HIV-infected orphaned and non-orphaned children on antiretroviral therapy in western Kenya. J Acquir Immune Defic Syndr 43: 418–425.
98. Wamalwa DC, Obimbo EM, Farquhar C, Richardson BA, Mbori-Ngacha DA, et al. (2010) Predictors of mortality in HIV-1 infected children on antiretroviral therapy in Kenya: a prospective cohort. BMC Pediatr 10: 33.
99. O'Brien DP, Sauvageot D, Zachariah R, Humblet P, Medecins Sans F (2006) In resource-limited settings good early outcomes can be achieved in children

using adult fixed-dose combination antiretroviral therapy. AIDS 20: 1955–1960.
100. Adje-Toure C, Hanson DL, Talla-Nzussouo N, Borget MY, Kouadio LY, et al. (2008) Virologic and immunologic response to antiretroviral therapy and predictors of HIV type 1 drug resistance in children receiving treatment in Abidjan, Cote d'Ivoire. AIDS Res Hum Retroviruses 24: 911–917.
101. Song R, Jelagat J, Dzombo D, Mwalimu M, Mandaliya K, et al. (2007) Efficacy of highly active antiretroviral therapy in HIV-1 infected children in Kenya. Pediatrics 120: e856–861.
102. Kline MW, Matusa RF, Copaciu L, Calles NR, Kline NE, et al. (2004) Comprehensive pediatric human immunodeficiency virus care and treatment in Constanta, Romania: implementation of a program of highly active antiretroviral therapy in a resource-poor setting. Pediatr Infect Dis J 23: 695–700.
103. Kabue MM, Kekitiinwa A, Maganda A, Risser JM, Chan W, et al. (2008) Growth in HIV-infected children receiving antiretroviral therapy at a pediatric infectious diseases clinic in Uganda. AIDS Patient Care STDS 22: 245–251.
104. Kline MW, Rugina S, Ilie M, Matusa RF, Schweitzer AM, et al. (2007) Long-term follow-up of 414 HIV-infected Romanian children and adolescents receiving lopinavir/ritonavir-containing highly active antiretroviral therapy. Pediatrics 119: e1116–1120.
105. Evans-Gilbert T, Pierre R, Steel-Duncan JC, Rodriguez B, Whorms S, et al. (2004) Antiretroviral drug therapy in HIV-infected Jamaican children. West Indian Med J 53: 322–326.
106. Pierre RB, Steel-Duncan JC, Evans-Gilbert T, Rodriguez B, Moore J, et al. (2008) Effectiveness of antiretroviral therapy in treating paediatric HIV/AIDS in Jamaica. West Indian Med J 57: 223–230.
107. Eley B, Davies MA, Apolles P, Cowburn C, Buys H, et al. (2006) Antiretroviral treatment for children. S Afr Med J 96: 988–993.
108. Collins IJ, Jourdain G, Hansudewechakul R, Kanjanavanit S, Hongsiriwon S, et al. (2010) Long-term survival of HIV-infected children receiving antiretroviral therapy in Thailand: a 5-year observational cohort study. Clin Infect Dis 51: 1449–1457.
109. Meyers TM, Yotebieng M, Kuhn L, Moultrie H (2011) Antiretroviral therapy responses among children attending a large public clinic in Soweto, South Africa. Pediatr Infect Dis J 30: 974–979.
110. van Kooten Niekerk NK, Knies MM, Howard J, Rabie H, Zeier M, et al. (2006) The first 5 years of the family clinic for HIV at Tygerberg Hospital: family demographics, survival of children and early impact of antiretroviral therapy. J Trop Pediatr 52: 3–11.
111. Kamya MR, Mayanja-Kizza H, Kambugu A, Bakeera-Kitaka S, Semitala F, et al. (2007) Predictors of long-term viral failure among ugandan children and adults treated with antiretroviral therapy. J Acquir Immune Defic Syndr 46: 187–193.
112. Zanoni BC, Phungula T, Zanoni HM, France H, Feeney ME (2011) Risk factors associated with increased mortality among HIV infected children initiating antiretroviral therapy (ART) in South Africa. PLoS One 6: e22706.
113. Bong CN, Yu JK, Chiang HC, Huang WL, Hsieh TC, et al. (2007) Risk factors for early mortality in children on adult fixed-dose combination antiretroviral treatment in a central hospital in Malawi. AIDS 21: 1805–1810.
114. Callens SF, Shabani N, Lusiama J, Lelo P, Kitetele F, et al. (2009) Mortality and associated factors after initiation of pediatric antiretroviral treatment in the Democratic Republic of the Congo. Pediatr Infect Dis J 28: 35–40.
115. Raguenaud ME, Isaakidis P, Zachariah R, Te V, Soeung S, et al. (2009) Excellent outcomes among HIV+ children on ART, but unacceptably high pre-ART mortality and losses to follow-up: a cohort study from Cambodia. BMC Pediatr 9: 54.
116. Taye B, Shiferaw S, Enquselassie F (2010) The impact of malnutrition in survival of HIV infected children after initiation of antiretroviral treatment (ART). Ethiop Med J 48: 1–10.
117. Anaky MF, Duvignac J, Wemin L, Kouakoussui A, Karcher S, et al. (2010) Scaling up antiretroviral therapy for HIV-infected children in Cote d'Ivoire: determinants of survival and loss to programme. Bull World Health Organ 88: 490–499.
118. Groh K, Audet CM, Baptista A, Sidat M, Vergara A, et al. (2011) Barriers to antiretroviral therapy adherence in rural Mozambique. BMC Public Health 11: 650.
119. Stringer EM, Sinkala M, Stringer JS, Mzyece E, Makuka I, et al. (2003) Prevention of mother-to-child transmission of HIV in Africa: successes and challenges in scaling-up a nevirapine-based program in Lusaka, Zambia. AIDS 17: 1377–1382.
120. Stringer JS, Sinkala M, Maclean CC, Levy J, Kankasa C, et al. (2005) Effectiveness of a city-wide program to prevent mother-to-child HIV transmission in Lusaka, Zambia. AIDS 19: 1309–1315.
121. Reithinger R, Megazzini K, Durako SJ, Harris DR, Vermund SH (2007) Monitoring and evaluation of programmes to prevent mother to child transmission of HIV in Africa. BMJ 334: 1143–1146.
122. Stringer EM, Ekouevi DK, Coetzee D, Tih PM, Creek TL, et al. (2010) Coverage of nevirapine-based services to prevent mother-to-child HIV transmission in 4 African countries. JAMA 304: 293–302.
123. Stringer EM, Chintu NT, Levy JW, Sinkala M, Chi BH, et al. (2008) Declining HIV prevalence among young pregnant women in Lusaka, Zambia. Bull World Health Organ 86: 697–702.
124. Ciampa PJ, Burlison JR, Blevins M, Sidat M, Moon TD, et al. (2011) Improving retention in the early infant diagnosis of HIV program in rural Mozambique by better service integration. J Acquir Immune Defic Syndr 58: 115–119.
125. Ciampa PJ, Vaz LM, Blevins M, Sidat M, Rothman RL, et al. (2012) The association among literacy, numeracy, HIV knowledge and health-seeking behavior: a population-based survey of women in rural Mozambique. PLoS One 7: e39391.
126. Nyandiko W, Vreeman R, Liu H, Shangani S, Sang E, et al. (2013) Nonadherence to clinic appointments among HIV-infected children in an ambulatory care program in western Kenya. J Acquir Immune Defic Syndr 63: e49–55.
127. Sengayi M, Dwane N, Marinda E, Sipambo N, Fairlie L, et al. (2013) Predictors of loss to follow-up among children in the first and second years of antiretroviral treatment in Johannesburg, South Africa. Glob Health Action 6: 19248.
128. Wachira J, Middlestadt SE, Vreeman R, Braitstein P (2012) Factors underlying taking a child to HIV care: implications for reducing loss to follow-up among HIV-infected and -exposed children. SAHARA J 9: 20–29.
129. Langat NT, Odero W, Gatongi P (2012) Antiretroviral drug adherence by HIV infected children attending Kericho District Hospital, Kenya. East Afr J Public Health 9: 101–104.
130. McNairy ML, Lamb MR, Carter RJ, Fayorsey R, Tene G, et al. (2012) Retention of HIV-infected children on antiretroviral treatment in HIV care and treatment programs in Kenya, Mozambique, Rwanda and Tanzania. J Acquir Immune Defic Syndr.
131. Okomo U, Togun T, Oko F, Peterson K, Jaye A (2012) Mortality and loss to programme before antiretroviral therapy among HIV-infected children eligible for treatment in The Gambia, West Africa. AIDS Res Ther 9: 28.
132. Chetty T, Knight S, Giddy J, Crankshaw TL, Butler LM, et al. (2012) A retrospective study of Human Immunodeficiency Virus transmission, mortality and loss to follow-up among infants in the first 18 months of life in a prevention of mother-to-child transmission programme in an urban hospital in KwaZulu-Natal, South Africa. BMC Pediatr 12: 146.
133. Audet CM, Silva Matos C, Blevins M, Cardoso A, Moon TD, et al. (2012) Acceptability of cervical cancer screening in rural Mozambique. Health Educ Res 27: 544–551.
134. Moon TD, Silva-Matos C, Cordoso A, Baptista AJ, Sidat M, et al. (2012) Implementation of cervical cancer screening using visual inspection with acetic acid in rural Mozambique: successes and challenges using HIV care and treatment programme investments in Zambezia Province. J Int AIDS Soc 15: 17406.
135. Ciampa PJ, Tique JA, Juma N, Sidat M, Moon TD, et al. (2012) Addressing poor retention of infants exposed to HIV: a quality improvement study in rural Mozambique. J Acquir Immune Defic Syndr 60: e46–52.
136. Scanlon ML, Vreeman RC (2013) Current strategies for improving access and adherence to antiretroviral therapies in resource-limited settings. HIV AIDS (Auckl) 5: 1–17.
137. Fenner L, Brinkhof MW, Keiser O, Weigel R, Cornell M, et al. (2010) Early mortality and loss to follow-up in HIV-infected children starting antiretroviral therapy in Southern Africa. Journal of acquired immune deficiency syndromes (1999) 54: 524.
138. Groh K, Audet C, Baptista A, Sidat M, Vergara A, et al. (2011) Barriers to antiretroviral therapy adherence in rural Mozambique. BMC public health 11: 650.
139. Audet CM, Groh K, Moon TD, Vermund SH, Sidat M (2012) Poor-quality health services and lack of programme support leads to low uptake of HIV testing in rural Mozambique. African Journal of AIDS Research 11: 327–335.
140. Geelhoed D, Lafort Y, Chissale E, Candrinho B, Degomme O (2013) Integrated maternal and child health services in Mozambique: structural health system limitations overshadow its effect on follow-up of HIV-exposed infants. BMC Health Serv Res 13: 207.
141. Lambdin BH, Micek MA, Sherr K, Gimbel S, Karagianis M, et al. (2013) Integration of HIV care and treatment in primary health care centers and patient retention in central Mozambique: a retrospective cohort study. J Acquir Immune Defic Syndr 62: e146–152.
142. Audet CM, Sidat M, Blevins M, Moon TD, Vergara A, et al. (2012) HIV knowledge and health-seeking behavior in Zambezia Province, Mozambique. SAHARA J 9: 41–46.
143. Ciampa PJ, Skinner SL, Patricio SR, Rothman RL, Vermund SH, et al. (2012) Comprehensive knowledge of HIV among women in rural Mozambique: development and validation of the HIV knowledge 27 scale. PLoS One 7: e48676.
144. Lehe JD, Sitoe NE, Tobaiwa O, Loquiha O, Quevedo JI, et al. (2012) Evaluating operational specifications of point-of-care diagnostic tests: a standardized scorecard. PLoS One 7: e47459.
145. Bandali S (2013) HIV Risk Assessment and Risk Reduction Strategies in the Context of Prevailing Gender Norms in Rural Areas of Cabo Delgado, Mozambique. J Int Assoc Provid AIDS Care 12: 50–54.
146. Yao J, Murray AT, Agadjanian V, Hayford SR (2012) Geographic influences on sexual and reproductive health service utilization in rural Mozambique. Appl Geogr 32: 601–607.

147. Wandeler G, Keiser O, Pfeiffer K, Pestilli S, Fritz C, et al. (2012) Outcomes of antiretroviral treatment programs in rural Southern Africa. J Acquir Immune Defic Syndr 59: e9–16.
148. Cook RE, Ciampa PJ, Sidat M, Blevins M, Burlison J, et al. (2011) Predictors of successful early infant diagnosis of HIV in a rural district hospital in Zambezia, Mozambique. J Acquir Immune Defic Syndr 56: e104–109.
149. Noden BH, Gomes A, Ferreira A (2010) Influence of religious affiliation and education on HIV knowledge and HIV-related sexual behaviors among unmarried youth in rural central Mozambique. AIDS Care 22: 1285–1294.
150. Posse M, Baltussen R (2009) Barriers to access to antiretroviral treatment in Mozambique, as perceived by patients and health workers in urban and rural settings. AIDS Patient Care STDS 23: 867–875.
151. Agadjanian V, Sen S (2007) Promises and challenges of faith-based AIDS care and support in Mozambique. Am J Public Health 97: 362–366.
152. Vuylsteke B, Bastos R, Barreto J, Crucitti T, Folgosa E, et al. (1993) High prevalence of sexually transmitted diseases in a rural area in Mozambique. Genitourin Med 69: 427–430.
153. Vermund SH, Sidat M, Weil LF, Tique JA, Moon TD, et al. (2012) Transitioning HIV care and treatment programs in southern Africa to full local management. AIDS 26: 1303–1310.
154. Gormley W, McCaffery J, Quain EE (2011) Moving forward on human resources for health: next steps for scaling up toward universal access to HIV/AIDS prevention, treatment, and care. J Acquir Immune Defic Syndr 57 Suppl 2: S113–115.
155. Lambdin BH, Micek MA, Koepsell TD, Hughes JP, Sherr K, et al. (2011) Patient volume, human resource levels, and attrition from HIV treatment programs in central Mozambique. J Acquir Immune Defic Syndr 57: e33–39.
156. Fulton BD, Scheffler RM, Sparkes SP, Auh EY, Vujicic M, et al. (2011) Health workforce skill mix and task shifting in low income countries: a review of recent evidence. Hum Resour Health 9: 1.
157. Adjorlolo-Johnson G, Wahl A, Ramachandran S, Strasser S, Kouakou J, et al. (2012) Scaling up Pediatric HIV Care and Treatment in Africa: Clinical Site Characteristics Associated with Favorable Service Utilization. J Acquir Immune Defic Syndr.
158. Audet CM, Blevins M, Moon TD, Shepherd BE, Vergara A, et al. (2012) Knowledge and Treatment of HIV/AIDS by traditional healers in central Mozambique. J Altern Comlement Med [In Press].
159. Audet CM, Blevins M, Moon TD, Sidat M, Shepherd BE, et al. (2012) Traditional healers in rural Mozambique: Qualitative survey of HIV/AIDS-related attitudes and practices. Journal of Social Aspects of HIV/AIDS [In Press].
160. Agadjanian V, Menjivar C (2011) Fighting down the scourge, building up the church: organisational constraints in religious involvement with HIV/AIDS in Mozambique. Glob Public Health 6 Suppl 2: S148–162.
161. MEPI (Medical Education Partnership Initiative) (2010)Medical Education Partnership Initiative.
162. The Africa Capacity Building Initiative (1991) The Africa Capacity Building Initiative.
163. CONSAMS (Consortium of New Southern African Medical Schools) (2011) Consortium of New Southern African Medical Schools.
164. Eichbaum Q, Nyarango P, Bowa K, Odonkor P, Ferrao J, et al. (2012) "Global networks, alliances and consortia" in global health education - The case for south-to-south partnerships. J Acquir Immune Defic Syndr.
165. Chen C, Buch E, Wassermann T, Frehywot S, Mullan F, et al. (2012) A survey of Sub-Saharan African medical schools. Hum Resour Health 10: 4.
166. Mullan F, Frehywot S, Omaswa F, Sewankambo N, Talib Z, et al. (2012) The Medical Education Partnership Initiative: PEPFAR's effort to boost health worker education to strengthen health systems. Health Aff (Millwood) 31: 1561–1572.
167. Mullan F, Frehywot S, Omaswa F, Buch E, Chen C, et al. (2011) Medical schools in sub-Saharan Africa. Lancet 377: 1113–1121.
168. Decroo T, Telfer B, Biot M, Maikere J, Dezembro S, et al. (2011) Distribution of antiretroviral treatment through self-forming groups of patients in Tete Province, Mozambique. J Acquir Immune Defic Syndr 56: e39–44.
169. Decroo T, Panunzi I, das Dores C, Maldonado F, Biot M, et al. (2009) Lessons learned during down referral of antiretroviral treatment in Tete, Mozambique. J Int AIDS Soc 12: 6.
170. Decroo T, Van Damme W, Kegels G, Remartinez D, Rasschaert F (2012) Are Expert Patients an Untapped Resource for ART Provision in Sub-Saharan Africa? AIDS Res Treat 2012: 749718.
171. Bandali S (2012) HIV Risk Assessment and Risk Reduction Strategies in the Context of Prevailing Gender Norms in Rural Areas of Cabo Delgado, Mozambique. J Int Assoc Physicians AIDS Care (Chic).
172. Bandali S (2011) Norms and practices within marriage which shape gender roles, HIV/AIDS risk and risk reduction strategies in Cabo Delgado, Mozambique. AIDS Care 23: 1171–1176.
173. Lahuerta M, Lima J, Nuwagaba-Biribonwoha H, Okamura M, Alvim MF, et al. (2012) Factors associated with late antiretroviral therapy initiation among adults in Mozambique. PLoS One 7: e37125.
174. Hendriksen IC, Ferro J, Montoya P, Chhaganlal KD, Seni A, et al. (2012) Diagnosis, Clinical Presentation, and In-Hospital Mortality of Severe Malaria in HIV-Coinfected Children and Adults in Mozambique. Clin Infect Dis 55: 1144–1153.
175. Naniche D, Letang E, Nhampossa T, David C, Menendez C, et al. (2011) Alterations in T cell subsets in human immunodeficiency virus-infected adults with co-infections in southern Mozambique. Am J Trop Med Hyg 85: 776–781.
176. Modjarrad K, Vermund SH (2010) Effect of treating co-infections on HIV-1 viral load: a systematic review. Lancet Infect Dis 10: 455–463.
177. Modjarrad K, Vermund SH (2011) An addition to the effect of treating co-infections on HIV-1 viral load. Lancet Infect Dis 11: 81.
178. Vaz P, Augusto O, Bila D, Macassa E, Vubil A, et al. (2012) Surveillance of HIV drug resistance in children receiving antiretroviral therapy: a pilot study of the World Health Organization's generic protocol in Maputo, Mozambique. Clin Infect Dis 54 Suppl 4: S369–374.
179. Holmes CB, Blandford JM, Sangrujee N, Stewart SR, DuBois A, et al. (2012) PEPFAR's past and future efforts to cut costs, improve efficiency, and increase the impact of global HIV programs. Health Aff (Millwood) 31: 1553–1560.
180. Jani IV, Sabatier J, Vubil A, Subbarao S, Bila D, et al. (2012) Evaluation of a high-throughput diagnostic system for detection of HIV-1 in dried blood spot samples from infants in Mozambique. J Clin Microbiol 50: 1458–1460.
181. Jani IV, Sitoe NE, Alfai ER, Chongo PL, Quevedo JI, et al. (2011) Effect of point-of-care CD4 cell count tests on retention of patients and rates of antiretroviral therapy initiation in primary health clinics: an observational cohort study. Lancet 378: 1572–1579.
182. Bwakura-Dangarembizi M, Kendall L, Bakeera-Kitaka S, Nahirya-Ntege P, Keishanyu R, et al. (2014) A Randomized Trial of Prolonged Co-trimoxazole in HIV-Infected Children in Africa. New England Journal of Medicine 370: 41–53.

4

Community Mobilisation and Empowerment Interventions as Part of HIV Prevention for Female Sex Workers in Southern India: A Cost-Effectiveness Analysis

Anna Vassall[1]*, Sudhashree Chandrashekar[1,2], Michael Pickles[1,3], Tara S. Beattie[1], Govindraj Shetty[4], Parinita Bhattacharjee[2], Marie-Claude Boily[3], Peter Vickerman[1], Janet Bradley[5], Michel Alary[5,6], Stephen Moses[4], CHARME India Group¶, Charlotte Watts[1]

1 London School of Hygiene and Tropical Medicine, London, United Kingdom, 2 St John's Research Institute, Bangalore, India, 3 Imperial College, London, United Kingdom, 4 Karnataka Health Promotion Trust, Bangalore, India, 5 URESP, Centre de recherche du CHU de Québec, Québec, Canada, 6 Département de médecine sociale et préventive, Université Laval, Québec, Canada

Abstract

Background: Most HIV prevention for female sex workers (FSWs) focuses on individual behaviour change involving peer educators, condom promotion and the provision of sexual health services. However, there is a growing recognition of the need to address broader societal, contextual and structural factors contributing to FSW risk behaviour. We assess the cost-effectiveness of adding community mobilisation (CM) and empowerment interventions (eg. community mobilisation, community involvement in programme management and services, violence reduction, and addressing legal policies and police practices), to core HIV prevention services delivered as part of *Avahan* in two districts (Bellary and Belgaum) of Karnataka state, Southern India.

Methods: An ingredients approach was used to estimate economic costs in US$ 2011 from an HIV programme perspective of CM and empowerment interventions over a seven year period (2004–2011). Incremental impact, in terms of HIV infections averted, was estimated using a two-stage process. An 'exposure analysis' explored whether exposure to CM was associated with FSW's empowerment, risk behaviours and HIV/STI prevalence. Pathway analyses were then used to estimate the extent to which behaviour change may be attributable to CM and to inform a dynamic HIV transmission model.

Findings: The incremental costs of CM and empowerment were US$ 307,711 in Belgaum and US$ 592,903 in Bellary over seven years (2004–2011). Over a 7-year period (2004–2011) the mean (standard deviation, sd.) number of HIV infections averted through CM and empowerment is estimated to be 1257 (308) in Belgaum and 2775 (1260) in Bellary. This translates in a mean (sd.) incremental cost per disability adjusted life year (DALY) averted of US$ 14.12 (3.68) in Belgaum and US$ 13.48 (6.80) for Bellary - well below the World Health Organisation recommended willingness to pay threshold for India. When savings from ART are taken into account, investments in CM and empowerment are cost saving.

Conclusions: Our findings suggest that CM and empowerment is, at worst, highly cost-effective and, at best, a cost-saving investment from an HIV programme perspective. CM and empowerment interventions should therefore be considered as core components of HIV prevention programmes for FSWs.

Editor: Eduard J. Beck, UNAIDS, Trinidad And Tobago

Funding: The funder of this work was the Bill and Melinda Gates Foundation. The funder had no role in study design, data collection and analysis, decision to publish, or preparation of the manuscript.

Competing Interests: The authors have declared that no competing interests exist.

* Email: Anna.Vassall@lshtm.ac.uk

¶ Membership of the CHARME India Group is provided in the Acknowledgments.

Introduction

The UNAIDS strategic investment approach for an effective response to HIV/AIDS proposes a package of basic programme interventions, including HIV prevention for key populations [1,2]. Traditionally, core HIV prevention interventions for female sex workers (FSWs) are individual behaviour change involving peer educators, condom promotion and the provision of sexual health services [3,4]. However, there is a growing recognition that wider social and community level factors influence an individual's ability to adopt safer sexual behaviours [5]. As a result, many actors working in HIV prevention argue it is necessary to simultaneously address the broader societal and contextual factors that may contribute to HIV-related risk behaviour [6–12] as an essential element in achieving and sustaining the impact and efficiency of HIV prevention services targeted at FSWs [2].

Within the UNAIDS investment framework, 'critical enablers' are defined as activities that are necessary to support the effectiveness and efficiency of basic programme activities [13]. For FSW-targeted HIV prevention these community mobilisation (CM) and empowerment interventions may include: community mobilisation, community involvement in programme management and services, violence reduction, and addressing legal policies and police practices. These interventions are argued to improve programme effectiveness through the 'empowerment' of FSWs, with empowerment defined as 'the *process* by which those who have been denied the ability to makes choices (the disempowered) acquire such an ability'[14] - in this case the aim being to empower individual FSWs to negotiate safer sex and access services, as well as address other issues affecting their lives (such as violence or poverty), supported by the social solidarity of the broader community of FSWs [15].

There are a number of studies on the cost-effectiveness of HIV prevention targeted at FSWs [16–18]. For example, a recent study, modelling the potential cost-effectiveness of FSW-targeted HIV prevention in India (including impact on the general population), found an incremental cost per disability adjusted life year (DALY) averted of US$ 10 [19] for a basic package of services. Several further studies also suggest that cost-effectiveness can be achieved in practice and at a scale [20–22]. However, despite this clear evidence that investment in HIV prevention for FSWs is highly cost-effective in concentrated epidemic settings, the 'added value' of investing in the mobilisation and empowerment of FSWs as part of the HIV prevention package for key populations remains unclear. This lack of evidence can provide a substantial constraint to those seeking funding to implement comprehensive approaches to supporting FSWs, when funders are seeking 'value for money' and are scrutinising any cost that may be seen as 'non-essential'. Given the growing evidence that CM and empowerment improve programme impact [23–27], without sound evidence of cost-effectiveness there is a risk that the gains that have been made to date by more comprehensive HIV prevention programmes for FSWs [28,29] will be jeopardised.

We therefore present here a cost-effectiveness analysis of CM and empowerment interventions, when added to the core package of HIV prevention for FSWs, as part of the *Avahan* Programme in two districts of Karnataka state, South India, in order to inform funders, policy makers and programme managers designing HIV prevention for FSWs globally.

Methods

Study setting and population studied

It is estimated that 2.27 million people are living with HIV in India [30]. The epidemic is concentrated, and predominately driven by marginalised groups, particularly FSWs, men who have sex with men (MSM), and in some contexts injecting drug users [31,32]. The *Avahan* programme, the India AIDS Initiative of the Bill & Melinda Gates Foundation (BMGF), is one of the largest HIV prevention programmes targeted at high risk groups in the world. The programme operates across six Indian states and had a funding commitment of US$ 258 million between 2004 and 2009 [33], and thereafter was transitioned to national ownership. *Avahan* is implemented through contracted state lead partners (SLPs), who in turn contract a plethora of local non-governmental organisations (NGOs) at the district level.

The state of Karnataka is one of the four southern states in India supported by *Avahan*, with an estimated HIV adult prevalence of 0.9% (2008), and it contributes 11% of the HIV burden in the country [30]. Unprotected heterosexual sex is a key factor in the spread of the epidemic, with overall prevalence among FSWs in the state being 16.4% [32]. The *Avahan* SLP in HIV prevention efforts is the Karnataka Health Promotion Trust (KHPT), supported by the University of Manitoba - and has worked with 17 NGOs across 19 districts since 2004. Our cost-effectiveness analysis focuses on two districts in Karnataka, Belgaum and Bellary. These two districts were chosen purposively, based on Karnataka's socio-cultural regions, the size of the high-risk population and the availability of detailed behavioural, biological and costing data. Table 1 shows the number of FSWs reached at least once a year. For Belgaum this ranges from 806 in 2004 to 3072 in 2011; and in Bellary from 2741 in 2004 to 5743 in 2011.

Intervention description

The package of core HIV prevention services provided by the Avahan NGOs in both districts includes outreach through peers, behaviour change communication, condom distribution, and clinical services for sexually transmitted infections (STIs). Peer educators provided services to about 25–50 people each, sharing prevention information, distributing supplies (condoms and lubricants) and providing referral for STI management. Referral clinics followed standard protocols for STI management. There was active referral of individuals for HIV testing and positive key populations were referred to government anti-retroviral treatment (ART) centres for care and support. This core package has been demonstrated as cost-effective [34].

CM services and actions to create an 'enabling environment' were added to these core services in order to empower FSWs. Full details of the intervention are also publically available [35,36]. In the initial stages, activities concentrated on drop-in centres (DICs) as a focal point for community mobilization (2004–6). DICs provided a platform to motivate FSWs to use HIV prevention, but also drew in FSWs by holding special events. In rural areas, at the village level, FSW peer groups were established as a platform for FSWs to share and discuss issues and develop income generation activities (2006–07). FSW peer groups aimed to create awareness on HIV/AIDS, but also address non-health needs such as helping to access government welfare schemes including ration cards, education for the children of FSWs, etc. From 2008 onwards, FSW peer groups were strengthened through the formation of district-level collectives; and over time these provided the basis to form community-based organizations that could take on an active role in programme implementation and management. Similarly, building on the connections made in the DICs, FSWs were further encouraged to be involved in the planning of HIV prevention services through the formation of various programme committees.

In addition to the formation of communal structures, broader efforts to create an 'enabling environment' were taken to improve the FSWs' interaction with the wider community, further contributing towards their empowerment. This included conventions to encourage community members to interact with other FSWs in different villages and the provision of legal empowerment sessions [12]. There were also sensitization sessions for local leaders, youth organizations and secondary stakeholders like pimps, brothel owners, police and others – particularly focused on violence reduction [11]. All the activities were supported through capacity building from the SLP and its supporting partners. Table 1 shows the numbers of DICs, FSW peer groups and FSW membership and attendances to committee meetings in each district.

Intervention effectiveness

We have recently conducted a study [37,38] examining the impact of CM on FSW empowerment, risk behaviours and HIV/STI prevalence in four districts in Karnataka. This study used data from serial cross-sectional bio-behavioural surveys, termed inte-

Table 1. HIV prevention core and community mobilisation and empowerment services provided by year (US$ 2011).

	2004/5	2005/6	2006/7	2007/8	2008/9	2009/10	2010/11
Belgaum							
FSW population contacted at least once a year	806	2,776	3,143	4,237	2,294	2,679	3,072
Drop-in Centres	1	8	15	17	17	16	16
FSW peer groups			18	186	233	163	117
FSW members of peer groups			250	2,328	2,609	2,155	1,607
FSWs attendances to committee meetings			582	4,597	19,481	20,712	13,697
Bellary							
FSW population contacted at least once a year	2,741	3,066	4,464	4,157	4,341	5,055	5,743
Drop-in Centres	0	7	14	14	13	14	14
FSW peer groups				158	168	168	168
FSW members of peer groups				2,364	2,568	2,568	2,568
FSWs attendances to committee meetings				25,529	25,264	34,541	38,450

Data from routine management data sources (Avahan Comprehensive Management Information System).

grated behavioural and biological assessments (IBBAs), that were carried out amongst FSWs and clients in districts in Karnataka state in 2008 (3 years after programme initiation) and in 2011 (further details below). Detailed results of this exposure analysis are presented elsewhere [37,38], and a summary of the methods and results used can be found in Appendix S1 (Tables S1 and S2).

We used a conceptual hierarchical framework of protective factors for HIV and STI infection to explore the possible pathways through which CM may impact key HIV related outcomes, over and above peer education activities alone [37]. By 2011, for all measures of power, HIV/STI service uptake and condom use, adjusting for CM, caused the adjusted odds ratio (AOR) (for peer education and these HIV related outcome variables) to shift substantially closer to 1.0, suggesting CM was having a key mediating effect on the pathway between peer education and these HIV related outcomes (Table S2 in Appendix S1). When peer education was significantly associated with an outcome variable, we then calculated the proportion difference in the adjusted ORs between peer education and the HIV related outcome variable, and the adjusted ORs with the adjustment for CM (OR adjusted for confounders – OR adjusted for confounders and CM)/OR adjusted for confounders) (last column of tables S1–S2). In particular, and for the purposes of this study, the AOR for peer education and reported condom use at last sex with occasional clients changed from 10.96 (5.00, 24.01) ($p<0.001$), to 6.78 (1.96, 23.44) ($p=0.003$), when we included CM in the model, representing a proportional reduction in the AOR of 38.1% in 2010/11. Similar results were also seen in baseline (Table S1 in Appendix S1), where the proportional reduction in the AOR was found to be 46.2%.

Framework for cost-effectiveness analysis

Drawing upon these findings, we estimate the incremental (additional) costs and impact of CM and empowerment activities described above compared to a base case of providing just the core HIV prevention activities for FSWs from an HIV programme [39] (provider) perspective for a seven year period (2004–2011). We estimate two measures of incremental cost-effectiveness, incremental cost per HIV infection averted (within the seven year period), and incremental cost per DALY averted, (DALYs averted from HIV infections averted within the seven year period over the potential lifetime of FSWs). The latter is compared to a World Health Organisation (WHO) defined willingness to pay (WTP) threshold of Gross National Income (GNI) per capita (US$ 1410) for India in 2011 [40,41] to assess cost-effectiveness. A discount rate of 3% is used in our primary estimates for both costs and DALYS.

Incremental cost estimation. An ingredients approach was used to estimate incremental economic costs prospectively from the perspective of the HIV programme. The UNAIDS 'Costing Guidelines for HIV Prevention Strategies' were taken as the basis for the costing methodology [42]. Costs were collected from every organizational level that was involved in the provision of services: NGO, SLP, the BMGF office in Delhi (including pan-*Avahan* capacity building costs).

Cost data were obtained from routine financial and management reporting, as well as from staff records and interviews with staff. Details of donated goods and services were collected from each district. The economic costs of donated items were valued at market prices. Capital costs were annualised using a standard discount rate of 3% [43,44]. Start-up and training costs were annualised over the first five years. The start-up period was defined as district-level inception until the start of service delivery to the target population.

Personnel costs covered the salaries and expenses of all staff, including peer educators, volunteers and shared resource personnel. Peer educator time was valued at the honorarium paid, except when not paid. In the latter case, and for other volunteers, time costs were valued using self-reported average earnings or, if unemployed, the payment made to peers in interventions undertaken by the National Aids Control Organisation (NACO), Government of India. Condom costs were estimated using the lowest-priced market alternative.

All costs that were not spent on a specific use were allocated to different programme activities on the basis of time sheets (personnel-related costs) or interviews with staff (use of capital items), supported by programme activity reports. BMGF and pan-*Avahan* capacity building costs were allocated to SLPs according to the size of the grant during the year of analysis. SLP costs that could not be allocated for a specific use were broadly allocated according to either interviews with staff, on an equal basis for costs associated with programme management, or using estimated population for activities directly related to service provision.

Incremental costs for CM and empowerment activities were calculated for the numbers of FSWs reached per year. The number of people contacted at least once in a year reflects programme reach and was measured using programme management information system (MIS) data. All data were entered into a specifically designed MS Excel workbook and converted to US$ 2011 prices using the GDP deflator index [45] and the mid-year exchange rate for 2011 [43].

Incremental impact estimation. Incremental impact, in terms of HIV infections averted, was estimated using a two-stage process drawing on the exposure analysis. The exposure analysis, described above was used to estimate the incremental changes in HIV-related sexual risk behaviour related to exposure to the CM and empowerment intervention in Bellary and Belgaum. In the second stage, the results of this exposure analysis were then inputted into a dynamic transmission model that estimated the number of HIV infections averted from the incremental changes in HIV-related sexual risk behaviour relative to a simulated control scenario where no CM and empowerment activities were present.

Survey data used

As part of the evaluation of *Avahan,* IBBAs surveys were carried out amongst FSWs and clients in districts in Karnataka state. Programmes were initiated between April 2004 and July 2005, with the IBBA surveys in FSWs conducted in 2005/6, 2008 and 2011. Client IBBA surveys were carried out in October 2007 in Belgaum and Bellary. Sample size calculations and the sampling methodology have been described in detail previously [46], with approximately 400 respondents randomly sampled at each round in most districts, using a probability-based sampling method. Appropriate weights were used to account for the differential non-response rates and differential probabilities of selection across districts, as well as the differential recruitment of FSW by typology within districts.

In addition to questions on sexual behaviour and risk factors for HIV, blood samples were taken to test for HIV, HSV-2 and syphilis [47]. IBBA survey data were subsequently used in the exposure analysis and to calibrate the dynamic HIV transmission model.

Exposure analysis

Following discussions with project staff, we used the following data from the IBBAs as proxy measures to define exposure to CM activities: "high" if a woman reported being a member of a FSW peer group or FSW collective; "medium" if she had ever attended a drop-in center or a nongovernmental organization (NGO) meeting; and "low" if she had not done any of the preceding. Measures of collective power (power with) were explored using the following questions: "I feel a strong sense of unity with FSWs I do not know"; "In the last 1 year, have you negotiated with or stood up against a powerbroker to help a fellow FSW?"; and "In the last 6 months, have you attended any public events, such as a rally or a gathering of sex workers, where you could be identified as a sex worker?". A measure of individual power (power to) was developed by looking at whether respondents had answered "no" to "In the past 1 month, was there a time when you wanted to use a condom during sexual intercourse but did not use it?" or "In the past 1 month, was there a time when you wanted to use a condom during sexual intercourse with a client but did not use it?"

For the exposure analysis, we used the results from this analysis [37] derived from data from the 2005/6 and 2011 IBBA surveys for FSWs pooled across four districts (Bangalore and Shimoga in addition to Belgaum and Bellary) and applied them to Belgaum and Bellary. This was justified because the implementation of CM and empowerment was standardized across *Avahan* districts, and the district-pooled analysis was necessary to have sufficient unexposed individuals to CM and empowerment activities (incremental to the broad HIV programme). The effect size (proportional AOR) derived from the exposure analysis was assumed to vary over time, starting at the 2005/6 value (46.2%) and then increasing linearly over time to the value at 2011 (38.1%), after which it was taken to be constant. This effect size was then incorporated in the dynamic HIV transmission model described below.

It should be noted that the examination of effect did include controls for socio-demographic variables. District, duration in sex work, sex work typology (place where solicit clients or place where have sex with clients), relationship status (marital status or regular partner), and socio-economic status (literacy or additional income to sex work) were added a priori. The adjusted Wald test was used to test for effect modification for the following socio-demographic variables: age, duration in sex work, place where solicit clients, place where have sex with clients, charge per sex act, and regular partner.

Impact model

A purpose-built dynamic compartmental model of HIV/STI transmission was then used to calculate HIV infections averted in FSWs and their clients, as well as their partners in the general population, over the first seven years of the *Avahan* programme [48]. Further details of the model are publically available [29,49]. Within the model, the basic package of services is assumed to have two effects: increasing FSW condom use with clients, and enhancing STI treatment in clinics. Other intervention components such as structural interventions, and CM and empowerment, are considered to act indirectly on HIV transmission through increasing condom use. The effect estimates from the causal pathway model for condom use at last sex with occasional clients (see Tables S1 and S2 in Appendix S1) were used to parameterise the fraction of increases in FSW condom use with clients associated with the CM and empowerment component of the intervention, and thus explore the impact of CM and empowerment activities on HIV infections averted using the simulated matched control groups described below. Unlike most previous exercises in modelling impact for cost-effectiveness analyses at scale in India [19,21,22], the model used is dynamic (incorporating indirect population-level effects not captured in cohort models) and is employed within a Bayesian framework [1,29] to allow a better quantification of uncertainty.

Each district was parameterized separately, using behavioural parameters derived from the relevant district FSW and client IBBA surveys. For each parameter a range was defined using the 95% confidence interval of the survey data. Ranges for biological parameters such as per-act HIV transmission probabilities were obtained from extensive reviews of published literature, and the same parameter ranges were used for both districts (see Table S3 in Appendix S1 which summarises the key model parameter ranges and references). A full list of parameters, along with a detailed description of the model equations and structure, is also publically available [29,49]. All parameter ranges were sampled extensively through Latin hypercube sampling (LHS) to generate combinations of parameters for each district. Enough combinations of parameters were generated through LHS to fully account for parametric uncertainty in each district, with one million and 100,000 parameter sets sampled for Belgaum and Bellary districts respectively.

In a previous evaluation of the overall HIV impact of *Avahan* [29,49] the *intervention* scenario in which condom use increased as given by trends in IBBA survey data was compared against a control scenario describing how condom use might have changed without the intervention (i.e. a first matched simulated control group). For the intervention scenario, condom use over time in each district was estimated using a historical cohort method [50]. Condom use increased at a slower rate before *Avahan*, and then increased sequentially up to the level of each FSW IBBA survey, remaining constant after the last round. The model was then run under the *intervention* scenario with each parameter set as an input to obtain "fits" to the confidence intervals of the first round of local HIV/STI prevalence derived from IBBA survey data for FSWs and clients, as well as the FSW HIV prevalence ratio between Round 1 and subsequent rounds.

In the *control* scenario, condom use was assumed to have increased during *Avahan* at the pre-intervention rate, while STI treatment was assumed to continue at pre-intervention levels. The difference between the *intervention* scenario and evaluation *control* scenario thus gives the increase in condom use due to *Avahan* over time. This incremental effect is used to generate our primary estimates for the impact and cost-effectiveness analysis of the entire *Avahan* package of services.

The effect size of CM and empowerment on FSW condom use, which was taken to be the same in both districts, was used in a similar way to define a second simulated control group. This second simulated control group, with no exposure to CM and empowerment activities, was created by assuming that a fraction of the total increase in condom use due to *Avahan*, as defined above, was due to CM and empowerment activities, as estimated through the exposure analysis. Removing this fraction created a *no-CM and empowerment (no-CME) control* group scenario. The multiple parameter combinations which were found to be "fits" to survey prevalence data under the intervention scenario were re-run for the *no-CME control scenario* to obtain the number of new HIV infections without the CM and empowerment component of the intervention. By comparison with the number of HIV infections occurring in each of the corresponding original "fits" from the intervention scenario, estimates for the incremental infections averted over 7 years by CM and empowerment were obtained, with the multiple "fits" producing an uncertainty range. DALYs averted were estimated from incremental infections averted generated by the impact model, using standard formulae and disability weights [41], a 3% discount rate and no age weighting. Table S4 also includes the parameters used to estimate DALYS.

Sensitivity Analyses

We conducted a probabilistic sensitivity analysis randomly sampling cost parameters with 5,000 iterations to estimate mean incremental costs per DALY averted. The parameters sampled at this stage were annual NGO, SLP and BMGF costs, age at HIV infection (based on IBBA data), and DALY weights (see Table S4 in Appendix S1 for details). In addition, the impact model "fits" were also sampled uniformly at the same time, corresponding to different impacts of CM and empowerment.

We also conducted a one-way analysis to examine how our results may change if antiretroviral therapy (ART) was available. We did not include prevention effects from ART, as ART was not provided in a widespread manner during the time of intervention, but rather explored the likely impact in terms of the future cost savings associated with reductions in the need for ART from infections averted. This was done using the dynamic HIV transmission model to predict the number of individuals who would have started ART by 2011 assuming future coverage rates of 21–40% of people meeting the eligibility criterion CD4< 350 cells/mm^3. For the sensitivity analysis, coverage of ART, the incremental increase in life expectancy from ART, and the annual unit cost of ART were all sampled as well. We also conducted a further sensitivity analysis using discount rates of 0%, 5% and examined the probability that any incremental cost-effectiveness ratios were below the WTP threshold using an acceptability curve, which shows the probability of the incremental cost effectiveness being below the WTP taking into account the parameter uncertainty.

Ethical approval

The estimates of the effect of CM and empowerment come from the secondary analysis of IBBA data in Karnataka. Participation in the IBBAs was by witnessed, verbal, informed consent. Only women aged 18 years or more were recruited in the study. The surveys were conducted anonymously, with no names or personal identifiers recorded. A detailed and standardized consent process was implemented for each respondent, and consent was obtained separately for the interview and for giving biological samples. Participants' consent was provided in writing, either by themselves, or for illiterate participants, by an independent witness who confirmed that verbal consent was provided. Statutory approval for the conduct of the IBBAs and their protocols was obtained from the Government of India's Health Ministry Screening Committee (HMSC). The study was approved by the Institutional Ethical Review Board of St. John's Medical College, Bangalore, India, and the Health Research Ethics Board of the University of Manitoba, Winnipeg, Canada.

Results

Costs

Community mobilisation and empowerment activities cost between US$ 31,690–US$ 64,304 in Belgaum and US$ 53,349–US$ 135,572 in Bellary per year (Table 2). Total costs rise initially then fall after the first four to five years of the intervention, broadly in line with the pattern of total HIV prevention costs. Overall HIV prevention costs increased until 2007/8 as the programme reached out to more people (also see Table 3). In 2008 the programme began to transition to national ownership and fell back dramatically. Total CM and empowerment costs increased from the first to second year, due to the increased ability of NGOs to expand CM and empowerment once the rapport with the community was built. In the later years, post 2008, as with overall prevention costs, CM and empowerment costs start to decrease

Table 2. Incremental community mobilisation (CM) and empowerment costs by organisational level and year (US$ 2011) and CM and empowerment as a percentage of total HIV prevention costs.

	2004/5	2005/6	2006/7	2007/8	2008/9	2009/10	2010/11	Total	%
Belgaum									
NGO Level	16,309	23,053	35,518	20,296	17,508	10,584	8,071	131,339	42.7
SLP Level	0	19,081	4,218	1,895	10,008	12,078	9,595	56,874	18.5
Programme Level	15,381	22,169	17,857	32,860	4,427	10,482	16,321	119,498	38.8
Total CM & empowerment costs	**31,690**	**64,304**	**57,593**	**55,051**	**31,942**	**33,144**	**33,986**	**307,711**	100.0
Total HIV prevention costs	256,407	361,204	530,550	1,015,644	763,946	619,066	562,240	4,109,056	
CM & empowerment costs/HIV prevention costs (%)	**12.4%**	**17.8%**	**10.9%**	**5.4%**	**4.2%**	**5.4%**	**6.0%**	**8.9%**	
Bellary									
NGO Level	8,188	21,807	66,240	51,380	41,548	26,818	22,085	238,065	40.2
SLP Level	-	27,263	5,877	8,960	3,929	6,343	6,071	58,416	9.9
Programme Level	48,397	63,640	63,455	57,239	8,526	20,188	34,975	296,422	50.0
Total CM & empowerment costs	**56,585**	**112,711**	**135,572**	**117,578**	**54,004**	**53,349**	**63,131**	**592,903**	**100.0**
Total HIV prevention costs	415,796	502,869	635,771	628,652	297,274	298,942	302,835	3,082,140	
CM & empowerment costs/HIV prevention costs (%)	**13.6%**	**22.4%**	**21.3%**	**18.7%**	**18.2%**	**17.8%**	**20.8%**	**19.0%**	

due to preparation for transition in funding to local state HIV programmes. Reductions in costs may also reflect improvements in efficiency with programme maturity and scale [51].

Community mobilisation and empowerment costs contribute between 4.2% to 17.8% in Belgaum and 13.6% to 22.4% in Bellary of total annual programme costs. Bellary shows a more sustained resource commitment for this overall compared to Belgaum; this in parts reflects NGO priorities and also the larger target population of brothel-based workers, which meant that it was feasible to achieve a high attendance at community mobilisation events. In addition Belgaum expanded its more general activities to new areas during the period, which also meant that less attention was able to be placed on supporting community mobilisation. As with the basic HIV prevention package of services, most cost was incurred above the NGO service level for activities such as capacity building, programme management, and support and supervision [52].

The allocation of costs between different activities (Table 4) shows that the majority of the cost was allocated to DICs and events, although this decreased over time. Activities that did not require fixed centres (advocacy and & enabling environment, self-help groups and capacity building for FSWs) required relatively low proportions of total cost, compared to funding for the DICs. The relatively high costs of DICs, was not due to expenditure on buildings, but was due to the costs of holding events in the early years of community mobilisation and empowerment activities. Personnel costs also accounted for a high proportion of the total costs of community mobilisation and empowerment (44% in Belgaum and 32% in Bellary) (Table S4 in Appendix S1).

The numbers of persons reached at least once a year increases between 2004 and 2011. However in Belgaum it falls in 2008 when the programme is taken over by national authorities in 2008, and also at a time when the programme was beginning to expand to new key populations (high risk men who have sex with men/ transgenders); thereafter the numbers of FSWs increases again, but does not rebound to the levels achieved in 2008. The unit cost per FSW reached ranges from US$ 11 to US$ 39 for Belgaum and US$ 11 to US$ 37 in Bellary (Table 4). As with total costs, the highest costs are observed in the first 2–4 years of the intervention – and thereafter costs stabilise at lower levels.

HIV impact and cost-effectiveness

We estimate that the incremental mean (standard deviation, sd.) impact of community mobilisation and empowerment is 1,256 (308) infections averted in Belgaum, and 2,775 (1,260) infections averted in Bellary in the first seven years of the intervention (Table 5) compared to a situation where no CM and empowerment activities were present. This represents 31% and 39% respectively of the total impact of *Avahan* over this period [29]. Assuming no ART is available to prolong the lives of those in these groups with HIV, we estimate a mean of 20,837 DALYs averted in Belgaum and 46,932 DALYs averted in Bellary as a consequence of the HIV infections averted during the seven year period. In the univariate sensitivity analysis, where ART is available (at a coverage rate of 21–40%) [53], we predict that CM and empowerment would prevent around 383 persons in Belgaum starting treatment and 846 persons in Bellary during this period.

Bringing together this incremental impact with incremental cost we estimate a mean (sd.) incremental cost per infection averted of US$ 234 (61) in Belgaum and US$ 228 (114) in Bellary. Assuming no ART this results in a mean (sd.) incremental cost per DALY averted of US$ 14.12 (3.68) in Belgaum and US$ 13.48 (6.80) in Bellary. Exploring the inclusion of ART in a sensitivity analysis we find that if ART cost savings are included, the intervention becomes cost saving. The sensitivity analysis around discount rates did not increase the incremental cost per DALY above the WTP threshold (Figure S1 in Appendix S1).

Discussion

Our findings suggest that investment in CM and empowerment, as a critical enabler of basic HIV prevention services aimed at

Table 3. Unit costs of community mobilisation per person reached by district and year (US$ 2011).

	2004/5	2005/6	2006/7	2007/8	2008/9	2009/10	2010/11	Mean 2004/11
Belgaum								
Total CM & empowerment costs	31,690	64,304	57,593	55,051	31,942	33,144	33,986	
NGO CM & empowerment costs	16,309	23,053	35,518	20,296	17,508	10,584	8,071	
Number of persons reached at least once a year	806	2,776	3,143	4,237	2,294	2,679	3,072	
Unit cost per person reached at least once a year	**39**	**23**	**18**	**13**	**14**	**12**	**11**	**19**
NGO level unit cost per person reached at least once a year	**20**	**8**	**11**	**5**	**8**	**4**	**3**	**8**
Bellary								
Total CM & empowerment costs	56,585	1,12,711	1,35,572	1,17,552	54,004	53,349	63,131	
NGO CM & empowerment costs	8,188	21,807	66,240	51,380	41,548	26,818	22,085	
Number of persons reached at least once a year	2,741	3,066	4,464	4,157	4,341	5,055	5,743	
Unit costs per person reached at least once a year	**21**	**37**	**30**	**28**	**12**	**11**	**11**	**21**
NGO level costs per person reached at least once a year	**3**	**7**	**15**	**12.4**	**10**	**5**	**4**	**8**

FSWs, is cost-effective; may even be cost saving if future ART savings are taken into account and therefore are good 'value for money'. While some may be concerned that additional expenditure on CM and empowerment has an opportunity cost in terms of other HIV prevention and treatment activities forgone (given current resource constraints on HIV programmes), the very low incremental cost-effectiveness ratio of CM and empowerment suggests that this is unlikely - and that CM and empowerment should be considered as an integral component of HIV prevention programming for FSWs [16,18]. In this sense, CM and empowerment can be argued to be as much of an essential HIV prevention activity for FSWs as many other HIV interventions labeled as 'core' HIV prevention services.

Moreover our findings are likely to be conservative from a broader economic welfare perspective as our analysis focuses on outcomes in terms of the HIV prevention benefits alone. We have excluded other health benefits that may arise from this type of intervention, such as reductions in violence and alcohol use [11]. We have also not examined possible impact on ART uptake or adherence. Beyond these health benefits, there may be broader benefits derived in terms of economic welfare (access to income generation schemes) and poverty reduction objectives (access of this very vulnerable group to social entitlements and education for their children) [12]. Therefore, while our results suggest that investment in community mobilization and empowerment is justifiable from the HIV perspective alone, exploring wider economic and health benefits further may also justify funding from those with a broader development perspective – at a time when HIV funding is increasingly required to find its place in the broader post-Millennium Development Goals context.

For those interested in broader social welfare as their primary funding objective, it is important to consider the added value of making the most efficient use of the infrastructure developed by HIV prevention programmes such as *Avahan* to reach many vulnerable population groups who may not have previously been reached at this scale by other development efforts. From a poverty reduction perspective, the potential of incurring relatively low incremental costs to expand development efforts to improve the welfare of FSWs more generally may be an opportunity not to be missed – and thus greater synergies between traditional HIV funders and development funders need to be explored.

The high cost-effectiveness of community mobilization and empowerment found is likely to be primarily due to the underlying cost-effectiveness of HIV prevention in India [20,22,54]. The low cost of HIV prevention in India [55], together with a sizeable impact on the HIV epidemic [29], means that community mobilization and empowerment, as an intertwined intervention that enhances the effectiveness of the HIV prevention, has a sound basis on which to yield substantial returns from an HIV perspective. However, in environments where HIV prevention targeted at key populations is less cost-effective, it remains to be seen whether the same results as we find here could be achieved. In India the costs of CM and empowerment range between 10–20% of the total HIV prevention cost; and the incremental unit cost per person reached a year is around US$ 11, which may be considered affordable within the current National Aids Control Organisation expenditures of around US$ 50 per person reached. But this may not be the case in other settings. There are a number of key contextual factors that are likely to impact on the likely transferability of our findings to other settings. These include the legal context of sex work – for example, where sex work is highly criminalised, it may be far more difficult to implement sex worker mobilisation interventions, or they may require a different combination of intervention inputs. Other contextual issues

Table 4. Community mobilisation and empowerment costs by activity and year (US$ 2011).

	2004/5	2005/6	2006/7	2007/8	2008/9	2009/10	2010/11	Total	%
Belgaum									
Advocacy & Enabling Environment	5,810	11,789	10,559	10,093	55,856	6,076	6,231	56,414	18.3
Drop-in centres and events	17,165	34,831	31,196	29,819	17,302	17,953	18,409	166,677	54.2
Self-help groups and community based organisations	3,169	6,430	5,759	5,505	3,194	3,314	3,399	30,771	10.0
Capacity building and training for FSWs	5,546	11,253	10,079	9,634	5,590	5,800	5,948	53,849	17.5
Total	**31,690**	**64,304**	**57,593**	**55,051**	**31,942**	**33,144**	**33,986**	**307,711**	100.0
Bellary									
Advocacy & Enabling Environment	9,313	18,550	22,313	19,347	8,888	8,780	10,390	97,582	16.5
Drop-in centres and events	26,053	51,894	62,420	54,123	24,864	24,563	29,067	272,982	46.0
Self-help groups and community based organisations	6,955	13,854	16,664	14,449	6,638	6,557	7,760	72,878	12.3
Capacity building and training for FSWs	14,264	28,412	34,175	29,633	13,613	13,448	15,914	149,461	25.2
Total	**56,585**	**112,711**	**135,572**	**117,552**	**54,004**	**53,349**	**63,131**	**592,903**	100.0

Table 5. Mean and standard deviation (sd.)infections averted, cost per infection, DALYs averted, Cost per DALY averted, persons on ART and ART savings, by district and year (U$S2011).

	Infections averted		Cost per infection averted (no ART)		DALYs averted (no ART)		Cost per DALY averted (no ART)		NGO cost per DALY averted (no ART)		Persons on ART averted		ART savings		Cost per DALY averted (including ART savings)	
	Over first 4 years	Over 7 years	Over first 4 years	Over 7 years	Over first 4 years	Over 7 years	Over first 4 years	Over 7 years	Over first 4 years	Over 7 years	Over first 4 years	Over 7 years	Over first 4 years	Over 7 years	Over first 4 years	Over 7 years
Belgaum																
Mean	**719**	**1257**	**273**	**234**	**11916**	**20837**	**16.48**	**14.12**	**8.44**	**6.70**	**219**	**383**	424249	741989	Cost Saving	Cost Saving
mean-1.96sd	391	653	137	114	6333	10557	8.28	6.90	4.51	3.44	92	153	29781	41046	Cost Saving	Cost Saving
mean+1.96sd	1046	1860	408	353	17499	31118	24.67	21.33	12.38	9.96	346	613	818718	1442933	9.42	Cost Saving
Bellary																
Mean	**1332**	**2775**	**323**	**228**	**22533**	**46932**	**19.12**	**13.48**	**7.80**	**6.22**	**406**	**846**	787793	1642173	Cost Saving	Cost Saving
mean-1.96sd	247	305	27	3	4035	4843	1.53	0.15	0.87	0.21	43	28	-163829	-449356	Cost Saving	Cost Saving
mean+1.96sd	2417	5246	619	452	41031	89021	36.71	26.82	14.73	12.22	769	1664	1739414	3733701	18.88	10.97

include the acceptability to the community of the specific intervention models evaluated here, existing levels of sex worker empowerment and organisation, socio-cultural norms and the characteristics of sex work in different settings.

Our results may also be viewed by some as limited, even with the setting studied, as the analysis of the causal pathway relies on a conceptual framework, observational data and model-based evidence of effectiveness, rather than on experimental evidence. This approach provides plausible evidence of effect [29]; and is feasible in settings where experimental designs are not appropriate [56]. However, while we adjusted for socio-demographic confounders in our exposure analysis, and carefully constructed our control group in the modelling, our results may still be limited by some selection bias, in that we may not have entirely removed endogeneity in the relationship between FSW behaviour related to HIV prevention and their involvement in community mobilisation. In addition, our approach allows estimation of the impact of CM and empowerment activities including reduced onwards transmission from FSWs who were infected prior to engaging with CM and empowerment. Through the combination of Bayesian methods and a probabilistic sensitivity analysis around the incremental cost-effectiveness ratio we also attempt to provide a realistic and transparent presentation of the uncertainty inherent in this type of analysis. In particular, our estimates of infections averted have high standard deviations, primarily due to uncertainty around the estimated population size studied [29]. But nevertheless we find our results to be robust.

As an economic evaluation, our study is also limited in that the strength of much of our evidence is based on data from costs and effects which are derived from a single study setting. We chose this approach due to the dearth of data on costs and effects of community mobilisation and empowerment (from the same setting) globally. However, our findings on effects are supported by a recent meta-analysis of CM and empowerment interventions [57]. Finally, our study is limited in the fact that it takes a provider rather than a societal perspective, and thus excludes the costs that FSWs and other providers may incur and contribute towards any intervention effect. This may mean we over-estimate cost-effectiveness. However, given the very low incremental cost-effectiveness ratio, this is highly unlikely to impact our main findings and inference above. Nevertheless, given the local nature of our study, and these limitations, we strongly suggest that further research across a number of settings is conducted to bring added precision and confirmation to our findings.

Overall, our findings provide strong evidence of the value of investment in sex worker community mobilization, and lead us to recommend the sustained funding of community mobilisation and empowerment activities as part of HIV prevention for FSWs in India, and the consideration of funding for scaling up similar interventions in other contexts, (accompanied with a careful evaluation of impact and cost-effectiveness during scale-up). The potential for multiple HIV, development and poverty reduction benefits for a low cost are an important element of such investments, meriting further research, as part of a broader, developmental perspective on future investments. Finally, our findings suggest that community mobilisation for especially at risk and vulnerable populations play a central role in the HIV response, and merit consideration by HIV programme managers and their funders, as central components of the core package of HIV prevention for FSWs.

Supporting Information

Appendix S1 Text S1, Summary of Exposure Analysis. **Table S1,** Peer education and service uptake, risk and HIV/STI prevalence, adjusted for socio-demographic characteristics and community mobilisation (IBBA Round 1 (2005), pooled data from 4 districts). **Table S2,** Peer education and power, service uptake, risk and HIV/STI prevalence, adjusted for socio-demographic characteristics and community mobilisation (IBBA 2011 and STI data 2008, pooled data from 4 districts). **Table S3,** Impact and cost-effectiveness model parameters. **Table S4,** NGO* and SLP** community mobilisation economic costs by input and year (US$ 2011). **Figure S1,** Acceptability Curves. **Figure S2,** FSW HIV prevalence (%) by year in four districts used in the exposure analysis. **Figure S3,** Condom use by year in four districts used in the exposure analysis.

Acknowledgments

This research was funded by the Bill & Melinda Gates Foundation and UK Aid from the Department for International Development (Dfid), through the STRIVE research programme consortium. The views expressed herein are those of the authors and do not necessarily reflect the official policy or position of the Bill & Melinda Gates Foundation or Dfid. The authors are grateful for all the staff at the Karnataka Health Promotion Trust and the *Avahan* supported NGO sites in Belgaum, Bellary, Shimoga and Bangalore Urban who supported the study. The authors would like to thank Professor Judith Glynn for useful discussions on causal pathway analyses and James Moore and Tisha Wheeler from the Bill and Melinda Gates Foundation for helpful contributions during the study design. The authors are also grateful to Annie Tangri for her work providing us with programme data. Finally, the authors are grateful to the members of the *Avahan* Evaluation Advisory Group, convened by WHO, for their valuable advice and guidance on the design and implementation of the evaluation of the *Avahan* programme: Ties Boerma, Amy Tsui, Basia Zaba, Charles Gilks, David Evans, Geoff Garnett, Isabelle de Zoysa, Laith Abu-Raddad, Michael Merson, Peter Ghys, Bernhard Schwartlander, Shiva Halli, Swarup Sarkar.

CHARME India Group

In alphabetical order: James Blanchard[8], Shajy Isac[4], Catherine M. Lowndes[7], Banadakoppa M Ramesh[4,8],Sushena Reza-Paul[5,8], Reynold Washington[2,4]

1. London School of Hygiene and Tropical Medicine, London, UK;
2. St John's Research Institute, Bangalore India;
3. Imperial College, London, UK;
4. Karnataka Health Promotion Trust, Bangalore, India
5. URESP, Centre de recherche du CHU de Québec, Québec, Canada
6. Département de médecine sociale et préventive, Université Laval, Québec, Canada
7. Public Health England, London, UK;
8. University of Manitoba, Winnipeg, Canada

Author Contributions

Conceived and designed the experiments: AV SC MP TB GS PB MB PV JB MA SM CW CHARME India Group. Performed the experiments: AV SC MP TB GS PB MB PV JB MA SM CW. Analyzed the data: AV SC MP TB GS PB MB PV JB MA SM CW. Wrote the paper: AV SC MP TB GS PB MB PV JB MA SM CW.

References

1. Boily MC, Lowndes CM, Vickerman P, Kumaranayake L, Blanchard J, et al. (2007) Evaluating large-scale HIV prevention interventions: study design for an integrated mathematical modelling approach. Sex Transm Infect 83: 582–589.
2. Schwartlander B, Stover J, Hallett T, Atun R, Avila C, et al. (2011) Towards an improved investment approach for an effective response to HIV/AIDS. Lancet 377: 2031–2041.

3. Foss AM, Hossain M, Vickerman PT, Watts CH (2007) A systematic review of published evidence on intervention impact on condom use in sub-Saharan Africa and Asia. Sex Transm Infect 83: 510–516.
4. Shahmanesh M, Patel V, Mabey D, Cowan F (2008) Effectiveness of interventions for the prevention of HIV and other sexually transmitted infections in female sex workers in resource poor setting: a systematic review. Trop Med Int Health 13: 659–679.
5. Rhodes T, Singer M, Bourgois P, Friedman SR, Strathdee SA (2005) The social structural production of HIV risk among injecting drug users. Soc Sci Med 61: 1026–1044.
6. Auerbach JD, Parkhurst JO, Caceres CF (2011) Addressing social drivers of HIV/AIDS for the long-term response: conceptual and methodological considerations. Glob Public Health 6 Suppl 3: S293–309.
7. Blankenship KM, Bray SJ, Merson MH (2000) Structural interventions in public health. AIDS 14 Suppl 1: S11–21.
8. Evans C, Jana S, Lambert H (2009) What makes a structural intervention? Reducing vulnerability to HIV in community settings, with particular reference to sex work. Glob Public Health: 1–13.
9. Parkhurst JO (2012) HIV prevention, structural change and social values: the need for an explicit normative approach. J Int AIDS Soc 15 Suppl 1: 1–10.
10. Kerrigan D, Baral S, Decker M, Murray L, Poteat T, et al. (2013) The Global HIV Epidemics among Sex Workers International Bank for Reconstruction and Development/The World Bank.
11. Beattie TS, Bhattacharjee P, Ramesh BM, Gurnani V, Anthony J, et al. (2010) Violence against female sex workers in Karnataka state, south India: impact on health, and reductions in violence following an intervention program. BMC Public Health 10: 476.
12. Gurnani V, Beattie TS, Bhattacharjee P, Mohan HL, Maddur S, et al. (2011) An integrated structural intervention to reduce vulnerability to HIV and sexually transmitted infections among female sex workers in Karnataka state, south India. BMC Public Health 11: 755.
13. Schwartlander B, Stover J, Hallett T, Atun R, Avila C, et al. (2011) Towards an improved investment approach for an effective response to HIV/AIDS. Lancet 377: 2031–2041.
14. Kerrigan D, Moreno L, Rosario S, Gomez B, Jerez H, et al. (2006) Environmental-structural interventions to reduce HIV/STI risk among female sex workers in the Dominican Republic. American Journal of Public Health 96: 120–125.
15. Kabeer N (1999) Resources, Agency, Achievements: Refections on the Measurement of Women's Empowerment. Development and Change 30: 435–464.
16. Creese A, Floyd K, Alban A, Guinness L (2002) Cost-effectiveness of HIV/AIDS interventions in Africa: a systematic review of the evidence. Lancet 359: 1635–1643.
17. Bertozzi S, Wegbreit J, DeMaria LM, Feldman B, Gayle H, et al. Disease control prioirities in developing countries New York; Washington: Oxford Univeristy Press; World Bank. 331–370.
18. Galarraga O, Colchero MA, Wamai RG, Bertozzi SM (2009) HIV prevention cost-effectiveness: a systematic review. BMC Public Health 9 Suppl 1: S5.
19. Prinja S, Bahuguna P, Rudra S, Gupta I, Kaur M, et al. (2011) Cost effectiveness of targeted HIV prevention interventions for female sex workers in India. Sex Transm Infect.
20. Fung IC, Guinness L, Vickerman P, Watts C, Vannela G, et al. (2007) Modelling the impact and cost-effectiveness of the HIV intervention programme amongst commercial sex workers in Ahmedabad, Gujarat, India. BMC Public Health 7: 195.
21. Dandona L, Kumar SG, Kumar GA, Dandona R (2009) Economic analysis of HIV prevention interventions in Andhra Pradesh state of India to inform resource allocation. AIDS 23: 233–242.
22. Dandona L, Kumar SG, Kumar GA, Dandona R (2010) Cost-effectiveness of HIV prevention interventions in Andhra Pradesh state of India. BMC Health Serv Res 10: 117.
23. Blankenship KM, West BS, Kershaw TS, Biradavolu MR (2008) Power, community mobilization, and condom use practices among female sex workers in Andhra Pradesh, India. AIDS 22 Suppl 5: S109–116.
24. Erausquin JT, Biradavolu M, Reed E, Burroway R, Blankenship KM (2012) Trends in condom use among female sex workers in Andhra Pradesh, India: the impact of a community mobilisation intervention. J Epidemiol Community Health 66 Suppl 2: ii49–54.
25. Parimi P, Mishra RM, Tucker S, Saggurti N (2012) Mobilising community collectivisation among female sex workers to promote STI service utilisation from the government healthcare system in Andhra Pradesh, India. J Epidemiol Community Health 66 Suppl 2: ii62–68.
26. Lippman SA, Chinaglia M, Donini AA, Diaz J, Reingold A, et al. (2012) Findings from Encontros: a multilevel STI/HIV intervention to increase condom use, reduce STI, and change the social environment among sex workers in Brazil. Sexually Transmitted Diseases 39: 209–216.
27. Halli SS, Ramesh BM, O'Neil J, Moses S, Blanchard JF (2006) The role of collectives in STI and HIV/AIDS prevention among female sex workers in Karnataka, India. Aids Care-Psychological and Socio-Medical Aspects of Aids/Hiv 18: 739–749.
28. Ghose T, Swendeman D, George S, Chowdhury D (2008) Mobilizing collective identity to reduce HIV risk among sex workers in Sonagachi, India: the boundaries, consciousness, negotiation framework. Soc Sci Med 67: 311–320.
29. Boily MC, Pickles M, Lowndes CM, Ramesh BM, Washington R, et al. (2013) Positive impact of a large-scale HIV prevention program among female sex workers and clients in Karnataka state, India. AIDS.
30. National AIDS Control Organsation, Ministry of Health and Family Welfare, Government of India (2010) Annual Report 2009–10
31. Chandrasekaran P, Dallabetta G, Loo V, Mills S, Saidel T, et al. (2008) Evaluation design for large-scale HIV prevention programmes: the case of Avahan, the India AIDS initiative. AIDS 22 Suppl 5: S1–15.
32. Vickerman P, Foss AM, Pickles M, Deering K, Verma S, et al. (2010) To what extent is the HIV epidemic in southern India driven by commercial sex? A modelling analysis. AIDS 24: 2563–2572.
33. Bill and Melinda Gates Foundation (2008) Avahan - The India AIDS initiative: The Business of HIV prevention and scale. New Delhi: Bill and Melinda Gates Foundation
34. Vassall A PM, Chandrashekar S, Boily MC, Shetty G, Guinness L, et al. (2014) The cost-effectiveness of HIV prevention for high-risk groups at scale: an economic evaluation of the Avahan programme in South India. Lancet Global Health *In press*.
35. Bill and Melinda Gates Foundation (2013) Community Led Crisis Response Systems–A Handbook.
36. Bill and Melinda Gates Foundation (2013) Micro-Planning in Peer Led Outreach Programs–A Handbook.
37. Beattie TS, Mohan HL, Bhattacharjee P, Chandrashekar S, Isac S, et al. (2014) Community mobilization and empowerment of female sex workers in Karnataka State, South India: associations with HIV and sexually transmitted infection risk. Am J Public Health. Aug; 104(8): 1516–25.
38. Beattie TS, Bhattacharjee P, Mohan HL, Chandrashekar S, Suresh M, et al. Exposure to community mobilisation is associated with increased power, increased service use, increased condom use and lower HIV and STI prevalence among female sex workers in Bellary district, South India. 19th International AIDS Conference. Abstract no. THPE275
39. Bill and Melinda Gates Foundation (2010) Avahan Common Minimum Program for HIV Prevention in India. New Delhi.
40. World Bank (2011) Available: www.databank.worldbank.org.
41. World Health Organisation (2004) Global Burden of Disease Update. Geneva: World Health Organisation.
42. UNAIDS (2000) Costing guidelines for HIV prevention strategies. Geneva: UNAIDS.
43. Reserve Bank of India (2009) Selected Economic Indicators. Reserve Bank of India Bulletin Jun 11 2009.
44. Drummond M, Stoddart GL, Torrance GW (1997) Methods for the Economic Evaluation of Health Care Programmes. Oxford: Oxford Medical Publications.
45. International Monetary Fund (2011) imf.stat.
46. Ramesh BM, Beattie TS, Shajy I, Washington R, Jagannathan L, et al. (2010) Changes in risk behaviours and prevalence of sexually transmitted infections following HIV preventive interventions among female sex workers in five districts in Karnataka state, south India. Sexually Transmitted Infections 86 Suppl 1: i17–24.
47. B S, Hegde AH, K CR, J S (2012) Exploring the binding mechanism of ondansetron hydrochloride to serum albumins: spectroscopic approach. Spectrochim Acta A Mol Biomol Spectrosc 86: 410–416.
48. Pickles M, Foss AM, Vickerman P, Deering K, Verma S, et al. (2010) Interim modelling analysis to validate reported increases in condom use and assess HIV infections averted among female sex workers and clients in southern India following a targeted HIV prevention programme. Sex Transm Infect 86 Suppl 1: i33–43.
49. Pickles M, Boily MC, Vickerman P, Lowndes CM, Moses S, et al. (2013) HIV prevention at scale: has it worked? Evaluation of the impact of the Avahan programme in South India. Lancet Global Health. 2013 Nov; 1(5): e289–99
50. Lowndes CM, Alary M, Verma S, Demers E, Bradley J, et al. (2010) Assessment of intervention outcome in the absence of baseline data: 'reconstruction' of condom use time trends using retrospective analysis of survey data. Sexually Transmitted Infections 86 Suppl 1: i49–55.
51. Chandrashekar S, Guinness L, Kumaranayake L, Reddy B, Govindraj Y, et al. (2010) The effects of scale on the costs of targeted HIV prevention interventions among female and male sex workers, men who have sex with men and transgenders in India. Sexually Transmitted Infections 86 Suppl 1: i89–94.
52. Chandrashekar S, Vassall A, Reddy B, Shetty G, Vickerman P, et al. (2011) The costs of HIV prevention for different target populations in Mumbai, Thane and Bangalore. BMC Public Health 11 Suppl 6: S7.
53. UNAIDS (2011) AIDS at 30: Nations at the Crossroads.
54. Prinja S, Bahuguna P, Rudra S, Gupta I, Kaur M, et al. (2011) Cost effectiveness of targeted HIV prevention interventions for female sex workers in India. Sex Transm Infect 87: 354–361.
55. Chandrashekar S, Guinness L, Kumaranayake L, Reddy B, Govindraj Y, et al. (2010) The effects of scale on the costs of targeted HIV prevention interventions among female and male sex workers, men who have sex with men and transgenders in India. Sex Transm Infect 86 Suppl 1: i89–94.
56. Laga M, Moodie R (2012) Avahan and impact assessment. Lancet 379: 1003–1004.
57. Kerrigan DL, Fonner V, Stromdahl S, Kennedy CE (2013) Community Empowerment Among Female Sex Workers is an Effective HIV Prevention Intervention: A Systematic Review of the Peer-Reviewed Evidence from Low- and Middle-Income Countries. AIDS Behav 17: 1926–1940.

5

Molecular Epidemiology of HIV-1 in Jilin Province, Northeastern China: Emergence of a New CRF07_BC Transmission Cluster and Intersubtype Recombinants

Xingguang Li[1,2]☯, Xihui Zang[3]☯, Chuanyi Ning[1,6], Yi Feng[1], Cunxin Xie[1], Xiang He[1], Yutaka Takebe[1,4], Liuyan Sun[3], Qi Guo[3], Hui Xing[1], Marcia L. Kalish[5], Yiming Shao[1]*

1 State Key Laboratory for Infectious Disease Prevention and Control, National Center for AIDS/STD Control and Prevention, Chinese Center for Disease Control and Prevention, Beijing, China, and Collaborative Innovation Center for Diagnosis and Treatment of Infectious Diseases, Hangzhou, Zhejiang, China, **2** HIV Molecular Epidemiology and Virology Research Group, The State Key Laboratory of Virology, Wuhan Institute of Virology, University of Chinese Academy of Sciences, Wuhan, Hubei, China, **3** Jilin Provincial Center for Disease Control and Prevention, Changchun, Jilin, China, **4** AIDS Research Center, National Institute of Infectious Diseases, Tokyo, Japan, **5** Vanderbilt Institute for Global Health, Vanderbilt University School of Medicine, Nashville, Tennessee, United States of America, **6** Guangxi Key Laboratory of AIDS Prevention and Treatment & School of Public Health, Guangxi Medical University, Nanning, Guangxi, China

Abstract

Objective: To investigate the HIV-1 molecular epidemiology among newly diagnosed HIV-1 infected persons living in the Jilin province of northeastern China.

Methods: Plasma samples from 189 newly diagnosed HIV-1 infected patients were collected between June 2010 and August 2011 from all nine cities of Jilin province. HIV-1 nucleotide sequences of *gag* P17–P24 and *env* C2–C4 gene regions were amplified using a multiplex RT-PCR method and sequenced. Phylogenetic and recombination analyses were used to determine the HIV-1 genotypes.

Results: Based on all sequences generated, the subtype/CFR distribution was as follows: CRF01_AE (58.1%), CRF07_BC (13.2%), subtype B′ (13.2%), recombinant viruses (8.1%), subtype B (3.7%), CRF02_AG (2.9%), subtype C (0.7%). In addition to finding CRF01_AE strains from previously reported transmission clusters 1, 4 and 5, a new transmission cluster was described within the CRF07_BC radiation. Among 11 different recombinants identified, 10 contained portions of gene regions from the CRF01_AE lineage. CRF02_AG was found to form a transmission cluster of 4 in local Jilin residents.

Conclusions: Our study presents a molecular epidemiologic investigation describing the complex structure of HIV-1 strains co-circulating in Jilin province. The results highlight the critical importance of continuous monitoring of HIV-infections, along with detailed socio-demographic data, in order to design appropriate prevention measures to limit the spread of new HIV infections.

Editor: Chiyu Zhang, Institut Pasteur of Shanghai, Chinese Academy of Sciences, China

Funding: This study was supported by the National Science and Technology Major Project for Infectious Diseases Control and Prevention (2008ZX10001-004, 2012ZX10001-002, and 2012ZX10001-008), National Natural Science Foundation of China (81261120379), NIH Foundation (1R01AI094562-01), International Cooperative Grant (2009DFB30420) and SKLID Development Grant (2012SKLID103). This work was also supported by U.S. National Institute of Health grants R01AI094562. The funders had no role in study design, data collection and analysis, decision to publish, or preparation of the manuscript.

Competing Interests: The authors have declared that no competing interests exist.

* Email: yshao08@gmail.com

☯ These authors contributed equally to this work.

Introduction

In China, it is estimated that 780,000 people were living with HIV by the end of 2011, according to the "China AIDS Response Progress Report" [1]. China is experiencing a dynamic and complex HIV/AIDS epidemic. The reported predominant co-circulating HIV-1 genotypes are: subtype B', circulating recombinant form (CRF) CRF01_AE, CRF07_BC, and CRF08_BC [2,3]. These three CRFs and the B' subtype constituted 92.8% of reported HIV-1 infections in China in 2006 based on our nationwide molecular epidemiology survey, and were detected in all high-risk groups including former plasma donors (FPDs), injecting drug users (IDUs), men having sex with men (MSM) and heterosexual transmissions [2]. Co-circulation with strains from different HIV-1 subtypes, CRFs, and unique recombinant forms (URFs) in these risk groups can create opportunities for the emergence of new, hybrid recombinants [4–7].

Jilin province is located in the center of northeast China, bordering with Russia to the east, the Democratic People's Republic of Korea (DPRK, also referred to as North Korea) across the rivers of Yalu and Tumen to the southeast, Liaoning province to the southwest, Inner Mongolia Autonomous Region to the west, and Heilongjiang province to the north. Jilin province encompasses an area of 187,400 square kilometers, and is divided into nine regions: Changchun (the capital of Jilin province), Jilin (located in the center of Jilin province), Siping, Tonghua, Baishan, Liaoyuan, Baicheng, Songyuan and Yanbian Korean Autonomous Prefecture. According to the sixth nationwide population census of 2010 [8], Jilin province had a population of 27,462,297, with a total of 44 ethnicities, including Han, Manchu, Mongol and Hui. Jilin's central location contributes to a persistent influx and outflow of people, mainly due to trade, labor, tourism, and education; this increasingly mobile population provides an increased opportunity for importing new HIV-1 strains and increasing transmissions.

The first known AIDS case in Jilin province was in a laborer infected through heterosexual contact with a female commercial sex worker (CSW) in Mombasa, Kenya in 1993, however, the HIV genotype of the infected patient was unknown. Jilin province experienced a low level of new HIV infections between 1993 and 1994, and then the number of reported HIV infections increased yearly [8]. A total of 1,477 HIV infections had been reported by the end of 2010 among all risk groups [9].

Between 2004 and 2010, the major risk for HIV-1 infections changed from FPDs (2.09% in 2010 compared with 42.19% in 2004) to those infected through sexual transmission (93.4% in 2010 compared with 35.9% in 2004) [10]. In addition, the proportion of HIV-1 infections among MSM surged approximately 28-fold: from 1.8% (2/114) in 2005 to 48.6% (139/286) in 2010 [10]. However, the most heavily affected regions in Jilin province were still concentrated in several big regions, including Changchun, Jilin and Yanbian Korean Autonomous Prefecture [9,10].

The current distribution of HIV-1 subtypes, CRFs, and recombinants in Jilin province is largely unknown. Therefore, a detailed HIV-1 molecular epidemiologic investigation to determine the genotypic distribution and the emergence and spread of new subtypes and CRFs is of great importance for understanding the dynamics of the HIV-1 epidemic in this region. In the present study, we performed an HIV-1 molecular epidemiological investigation of 189 newly diagnosed HIV-infections in Jilin province.

Methods

Study subjects and dataset information

A total of 189 newly diagnosed HIV-infected persons identified between January 2008 and December 2010 at local voluntary counseling and testing sites (VCT), sentinel surveillance sites, and medical institutions in Jilin province were agreed to be enrolled in this study. All newly diagnosed HIV-infected people were identified from various cities and risk groups. Whole blood samples were collected in 2010 (n = 93) and 2011 (n = 96); plasma was separated and stored at −80°C. The study was approved by the institutional review board of the National Center for AIDS/STD Control and Prevention, China CDC. A written informed consent, as well as a socio-demographic questionnaire, was obtained from each participant in this study.

The socio-demographic data that was collected included sex, age, ethnicity, marital status, education background, year of diagnosis, year of sampling, site of sampling, CD4+ T Cell Count and risk group.

HIV-1 RNA extraction, amplification and sequencing

Plasma samples from 189 newly diagnosed HIV infected participants were collected and submitted for RT-PCR and sequencing. Viral RNA was extracted from 280 μl of plasma using the QIAamp Viral RNA Mini kit (Qiagen, Valencia, California, USA) following the manufacturer's instructions [11,12]. The extracted viral RNA was subjected to a multiplex reverse transcription, polymerase chain reaction (RT-PCR) to obtain the nucleotide sequences of HIV-1 *gag* P17–P24 (HXB2: position 781-1836 for 1056 base pairs (bp)) and *env* C2–C4 (HXB2: positions 7002-754 for 540 bp) gene regions as previously described [13].

The positive PCR products were purified using QIAquick Gel Extraction Kit (Qiagen, Valencia, California, USA) and sequenced directly on an ABI 3730XL automated sequencer using BigDye terminators (Applied Biosystems, Foster City, California, USA) by Beijing Biomed Technology Development CO., Ltd (Beijing, China).

Phylogenetic tree and recombination analysis

The nucleotide sequences of the 134 HIV-1 *gag* P17–P24 and 121 *env* C2–C4 gene regions were aligned separately using the Gene Cutter software (http://www.hiv.lanl.gov/cotent/sequence/.html) with HIV-1 group M subtype reference sequences [Los Alamos National Laboratory (LANL) HIV Sequence Database (http://www.hiv.lanl.gov/cotent/sequence/NEWALIGN/align.html, accessed in April 2013)] as follows: A1 (3), A2 (3), B (4), C (4), D (4), F1 (4), F2 (4), G (4), H (4), J (3), K (2), CRF01_AE (2), CRF02_AG (3), CRF08_BC (1) and group N (3). In addition to these 48 reference strains, we used 62 reference sequences from viruses that represent subtypes/CRFs commonly identified in China as follows: subtypes A1 (1), B (6), B' (7), C (2), CRF07_BC (5) and CRF01_AE (39), CRF08_BC (2). Both *gag* and *env* sequences from these 110 reference strains were available. Following alignment, manual adjustments were made taking into consideration protein coding sequences using BioEdit software [14,15]. Neighbor-joining phylogenetic trees were constructed using the Kimura 2-parameter model of evolution, including both transitions and transversions [16], implemented in the MEGA 5.0 software package [17]. The reliability of the tree structure or branching order was evaluated by bootstrap analysis with 1000 replicates [18]. In order to better display the phylogenetic trees of the HIV-1 *gag* P17–P24 and *env* C2–C4 regions, the sequences were separated into two different Neighbor-joining trees, one containing only the subtype A, CRF01_AE, CRF02_AG-related sequences and the other representing the B/B', C, CRF07_BC related sequences. If there was evidence of recombination in any of the sequences (i.e., discordant gene regions or outlier position in a tree), they were further analyzed using the jumping profile Hidden Markov Model program (jpHMM; http://jphmm.gobics.de/) [19]. In order to confirm the possible recombinant structures and identify recombinant breakpoints of the potential HIV-1 recombinants, Bootscanning analysis was performed using Simplot 3.5.1 software package with window size of 300 bp, step size of 20 bp) [20].

Nucleotide sequence accession numbers

All the nucleotide sequences obtained in this study were submitted to GenBank under accession numbers of KF818784–KF818917 for the HIV-1 *gag* P17–P24 gene region and

Table 1. Demograpic and epidemiologic information of the study subjects and the distribution of HIV-1 genotypes.

					HIV-1 Genotypes[d]									
Characteristics	Total	B (n=5)	B′ (n=18)	C (n=1)	CRF01_AE (n=79)					CRF07_BC (n=18)			CRF02_AG (n=4)	URFs (n=11)
					CRF01-1	CRF01-4	CRF01-5	JL.DG[e]	CRF01-NG[f]	CRF07-1	CRF07-2	CRF07-NG[g]		
Sex[a]														
M	111	5	6	1	0	20	53	1	0	5	8	2	1	9
F	25	0	12	0	1	2	1	0	1	1	0	2	3	2
Ethnicity														
Han	120	5	16	1	1	21	52	1	0	5	6	3	0	9
Korean	7	0	1	0	0	0	1	0	0	1	0	0	4	0
Manchu	3	0	0	0	0	1	0	0	0	0	2	0	0	0
Others[b]	5	0	1	0	0	0	1	0	1	0	0	1	0	1
Unknown	1	0	0	0	0	0	0	0	0	0	0	0	0	1
Site of sampling														
Changchun	92	3	5	0	1	21	45	1	0	4	7	0	1	4
Jilin	19	0	8	0	0	1	3	0	0	0	0	3	0	4
Yanbian	11	0	3	0	0	0	1	0	1	1	0	0	3	2
Tonghua	3	0	0	0	0	0	2	0	0	0	0	0	0	1
Baishan	4	0	2	0	0	0	2	0	0	0	0	0	0	0
Baicheng	3	1	0	0	0	0	0	0	0	1	0	1	0	0
Liaoyuan	2	1	0	1	0	0	0	0	0	0	0	0	0	0
Songyuan	2	0	0	0	0	0	1	0	0	0	1	0	0	0
Risk group[c]														
MSM	83	5	0	0	0	18	46	1	0	3	8	0	0	2
Hetero	43	0	13	0	1	4	8	0	1	3	0	3	3	7
FPD	5	0	4	0	0	0	0	0	0	0	0	0	0	1
IDU	3	0	0	1	0	0	0	0	0	0	0	1	1	0
MTCT	1	0	1	0	0	0	0	0	0	0	0	0	0	0
Unknown	1	0	0	0	0	0	0	0	0	0	0	0	0	1
Total	136	5	18	1	1	22	54	1	1	6	8	4	4	11

[a]Sex: M, male; F, female.
[b]Other: other ethnic minority including Yi, Dai, Lisu and Mongol.
[c]Risk Groups: MSM, men who have sex with men; Hetero, heterosexual; FPD, former plasma donor; IDU, injecting drug user; MTCT, mother-to-child transmission.
[d]HIV-1 Genotypes: genotypes were determined based on all sequences available.
[e]JL.DG: samples with different genotypic identification assigned to the *gag* P17–P24 and *env* C2–C4 regions were designated as discordant genotype and were abbreviated as JL.DG.
[f]CRF01-NG: ungrouped CRF01_AE lineage.
[g]CRF07-NG: ungrouped CRF07_BC lineage.

Table 2. HIV-1 genotype information of 12 subjects of Jilin province with new recombinants.

Sequence ID	Site of sampling	Year of sampling	Sex[a]	Age	Risk group	*p17–p24* (HXB2: 781-1836 nt)	*C2–C4* (HXB2: 7002-7541 nt)	Genotype[b]
JL.RF01	Tonghua	2010	M	38	Hetero	CRF01/B'/C	NA[d]	CRF01/B'/C
JL.RF02	Changchun	2010	M	23	MSM	CRF01-4	B	CRF01-4//B
JL.RF03	Changchun	2010	M	51	Hetero	CRF01-5/CRF07-2	CRF07-2	CRF01-5/CRF07-2
JL.RF04	[c]YKAP	2010	M	27	Hetero	CRF01/C	CRF01	CRF01/C//CRF01
JL.RF05	Jilin	2010	M	34	Hetero	CRF01/C	C	CRF01/C//C
JL.RF06	Jilin	2010	F	23	Hetero	CRF01/C	C	CRF01/C//C
JL.RF07	Jilin	2010	M	49	MSM	B	CRF01-5	B/CRF01-5
JL.RF08	Changchun	2011	M	68	Hetero	CRF07-2	CRF01-4	CRF07-2//CRF01-4
JL.RF09	Changchun	2011	M	21	Hetero	CRF07-2	CRF01-4	CRF07-2/CRF01-4
JL.RF10	Jilin	2011	F	41	FPD	A1/G	H	A1/G//H
JL.RF11	[c]YKAP	2011	M	unknown	unknown	CRF07-1	CRF01-5	CRF07-1//CRF01-5
JL.DG01	Changchun	2011	M	24	MSM	CRF01-5	CRF01-4	CRF01-5//CRF01-4

[a]Sex: M, male; F, female.
[b]Genotype was determined based on both *gag* and *env* gene region sequences.
[c]YKAP: Yanbian Korean Autonomous Prefecture.
[d]NA: not available.

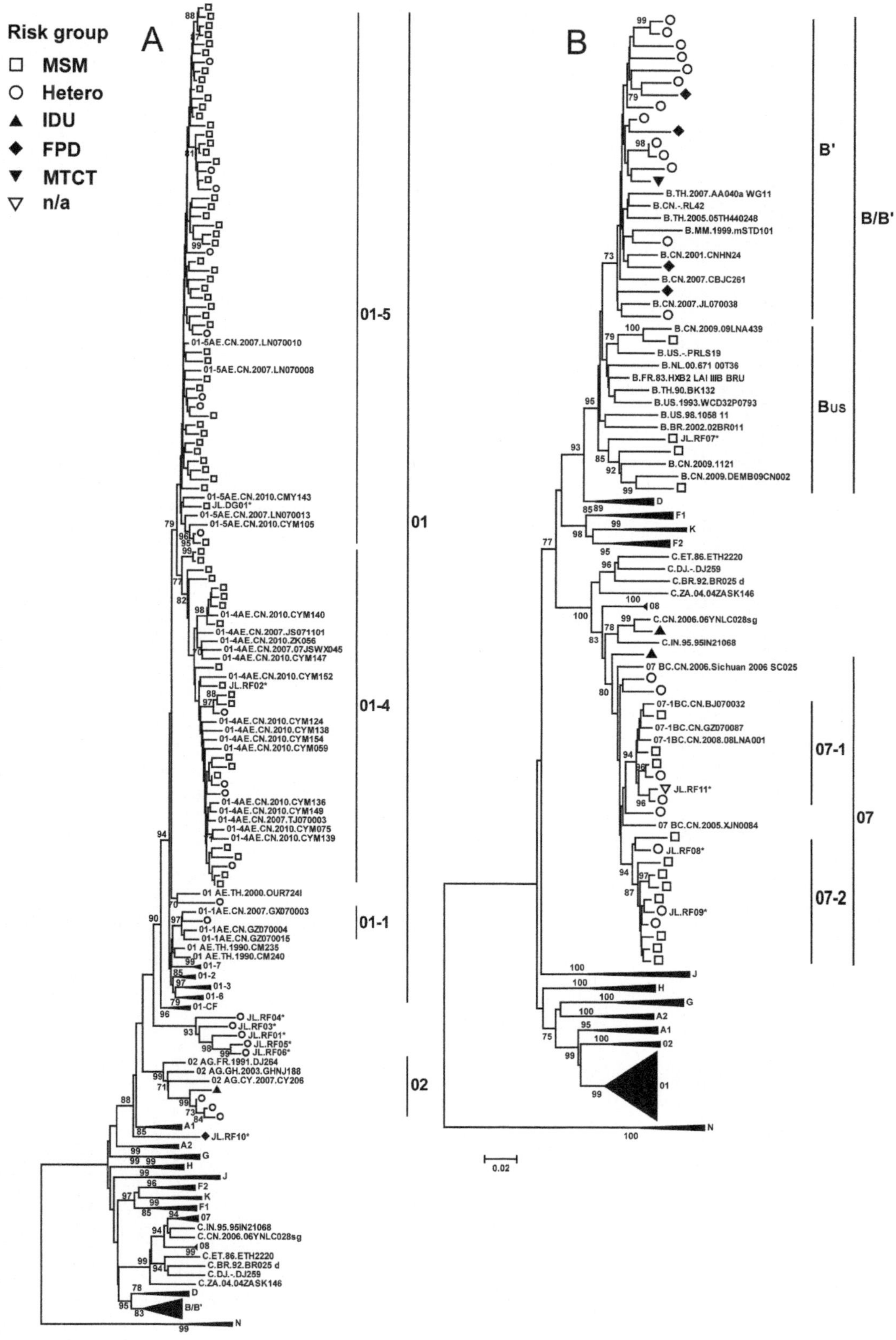

Figure 1. Neighbor-joining phylogenetic tree of HIV-1 *gag* P17–P24 gene of study samples from the Jilin province of northeastern China. Neighbor-joining phylogenetic trees were constructed for 134 DNA sequences of HIV-1 *gag* P17–P24 and reference sequences. The 134 *gag* P17–P24 gene sequences were separated into two different neighbor-joining trees, Fig. 1A containing only the subtype A, CRF01_AE, CRF02_AG-related sequences and Fig. 1B representing the B/B′, C, CRF07_BC related sequences. The stability of each node was assessed by bootstrap analyses with 1000 replicates and only bootstrap values ≥70 are shown at the corresponding nodes. CRF01_AE, CRF02_AG, CRF07_BC and CRF08_BC are labeled CRF01, CRF02, CRF07 and CRF08, respectively, for simplicity. The seven unique CRF01_AE lineages detected in China are labeled CRF01-1

through CRF01-7 and the Central African CRF01_AE sequences are labeled CRF01-CF. The two distinct CRF07_BC lineages identified among MSM are labeled CRRF07-1 and CRF07-2. The asterisk (*) next to sequence name indicates the identified recombinant or discordant genotype in the study. The symbols representing the risk groups are shown at the top-left corner of the figure.

KF818661–KF818713, KF818715–KF818772, KF818774–KF818783 for the HIV-1 *env* C2–C4 gene region.

Results

Demographic and epidemiologic information on the study participants

A total of 189 newly diagnosed HIV-1 infected samples were collected from local voluntary counseling and testing sites (VCT), sentinel surveillance sites and medical institutions in Jilin province and were used for the HIV-1 genetic analysis. For each sample, *gag* P17–P24 and *env* C2–C4 genes were amplified and sequenced. From the 189 plasma samples, 134 *gag* P17–P24 and 121 *env* C2–C4 gene sequences were obtained; 119 samples had both *gag* P17–P24 and *env* C2–C4 sequences; a total of 136 samples were genotyped with a success rate of 72.0% (136/189). The failure of PCR amplification or sequencing was likely related to factors such as poor transportation and storage conditions, low plasma volumes, low viral load, repeated freezing and thawing, and poor amplification and/or sequencing primer specificity.

The demographic and epidemiologic data are summarized in Table S1. Among the 189 participants, 81.5% were males. The mean age of the participants was 37.3±12.9 years. 88.4% (167/189) of participants were of Han nationality and 11.6% (22/189) of participants were minority nationalities, including Korean, Manchu, Dai, Yi, Hui, Lisu, and Mongol. The median CD4+ T Cell Count was 380 cells/μl, suggesting that most of these newly diagnosed participants had chronic infections. The following risk groups were identified: MSM (107/189, 56.6%); heterosexuals (65/189, 34.4%); FPDs (9/189, 94.8%); IDUs (3/189, 1.6%); blood transfusion recipients (2/189, 1.1%); mother-to-child transmission (1/189, 0.5%); unknown (2/189, 1.1%) and geographical regions in Jilin province: Changchun (125/189, 66.1%); Jilin (20/189, 10.6%); Yanbian Korean Autonomous Prefecture (15/189, 7.9%); Tonghua (10/189, 5.3%); Liaoyuan (4/189, 2.1%); Baishan (4/189, 2.1%); Baicheng (4/189, 2.1%); Songyuan (4/189, 2.1%); and Siping (3/189, 1.6%).

HIV-1 genotype distribution of the study participants

Phylogenetic analyses of the nucleotide sequences of 134 *gag* P17–P24 and 121 *env* C2–C4 gene regions are shown in Fig. 1 and Fig. 2, respectively. A total of 136 HIV-1 samples were successfully amplified and genotyped for at least one gene region, and most for both gene regions (Table 1 and Table S2). The classifications for the 119 samples having both *gag* and *env* sequences (*gag/env*) were as follows: CRF01/CRF01 (69/119, 58.0%), subtype B'/B' (17/119, 14.3%), CRF07/CRF07 (16/119, 13.4%), CRF02/CRF02 (4/119, 3.4%), subtype B/B (2/119, 1.7%), and subtype C/C (1/119, 0.8%). Furthermore, there were 10 (8.4%) samples with discordant *gag//env* phylogenies, and 2 of these showed complex levels of recombination involving gene regions from at least 3 different subtypes/CRFs: CRF07//CRF01 (3/119, 2.5%), CRF01//B (1/119, 0.8%), B//CRF01 (1/119, 0.8%), CRF01/C//C (2/119, 1.7%), CRF01/CRF07//CRF07 (1/119, 0.8%), CRF01/C//CRF01 (1/119, 0.8%) and A1/G//H (1/119, 0.8%) (Table 2 and Table S2). The distribution of genotypes for the samples having only *gag* sequences were as follows: CRF01_AE (10/17, 58.8%), subtype B (2/17, 11.8%), CRF07_BC (2/17, 11.8%), CRF01/B'/C (1/17, 5.9%) and the two with only *env* sequences were both subtype B (2/17, 11.8%) (Table S2). Six *gag* sequences were located outside of the subtype/CRF clusters, suggesting that they might be intersubtype recombinants. Bootscanning analyses of the 6 *gag* sequences showed the following recombinant structures: 3 CRF01_AE/C, 1 CRF01_AE/B'/C, 1 CRF01_AE/CRF07_BC and 1 A1/G (Fig.S1). The demographic and genotypic characteristics of the 136 participants with available nucleotide sequences are summarized in Table 1.

Our previous national-wide study [21] identified 7 major, distinct lineages among China's CRF01_AE epidemic. We found that some Jilin province CRF01_AE strains sub-clustered with CRF01-4 (22/79, 27.8%) and CRF01-5 (54/79, 68.4%) lineages, predominantly found among MSM in both this and our previous study (Fig. 1A and Fig. 2A) [21], and just one strain of CRF01-1 (1/79, 1.3%), commonly found among heterosexuals and IDUs in the previous study, but in a heterosexual transmission in this study. In addition, one sequence did not group with other known transmission clusters (1/79, 1.3%) (designated as CRF01-NG). In the present study, we found 1 CRF01_AE recombinant consisting of CRF01-5 in *gag* and CRF01-4 regions in *env*.

We also identified two strongly supported monophyletic transmission sub-clusters of CRF07_BC among sexual transmissions based on both *gag* and *env* sequences; CRF07_BC-1 was previously identified [24–26]. However, in the current study, a new lineage, designated CRF07_BC-2, was identified only in MSM from Jilin and Songyuan. Among 18 CRF07_BC strains identified in the present study, 6 (33.3%) and 8 (44.4%) belonged to CRF07-1 and CRF07-2 respectively, and 4 (22.2%) CRF07_BC strains were located outside of these two clusters (Fig. 1B and Fig. 2B and Table 1).

HIV-1 genotype distribution by risk group

As summarized in Table 1, a socio-demographic study was performed to better characterize the distribution of HIV-1 genotypes. We found intermixing of HIV-1 subtypes/CRFs in sexual transmissions (MSM and heterosexual) accounting for 92.6% of the genotyped infections. Based on HIV-1 *gag* P17–P24 and/or *env* C2–C4, among the MSM population, CRF01_AE, CRF07_BC, subtype B and recombinants accounted for 78.3%, 13.3%, 6.0% and 2.4% of HIV-infections, respectively. The greatest diversity of HIV subtypes and recombinant viruses was observed among the heterosexual population with CRF01_AE, subtype B', recombinants, CRF07_BC and CRF02_AG accounting for 32.6%, 30.2%, 16.3%, 14.0% and 7.0% of the infections, respectively. Recombinants were primarily found among the heterosexual transmissions compared to other risk groups, accounting for 63.6% (7/11) of all recombinants (Table 1 and Table 2). Subtype B' (13/18, 72.2%) and CRF02_AG (3/4, 75.0%) were most frequently identified among the heterosexual population; none were found in our 83 MSM. CRF01_AE was the primary HIV-1 genotype found among the MSM and heterosexual populations, while no CRF01_AE strains were identified in our 3 IDUs. Three different genotypes were detected among our 3 IDUs: subtype C (33.3%), CRF02_AG (33.3%) and CRF07_BC (33.3%).

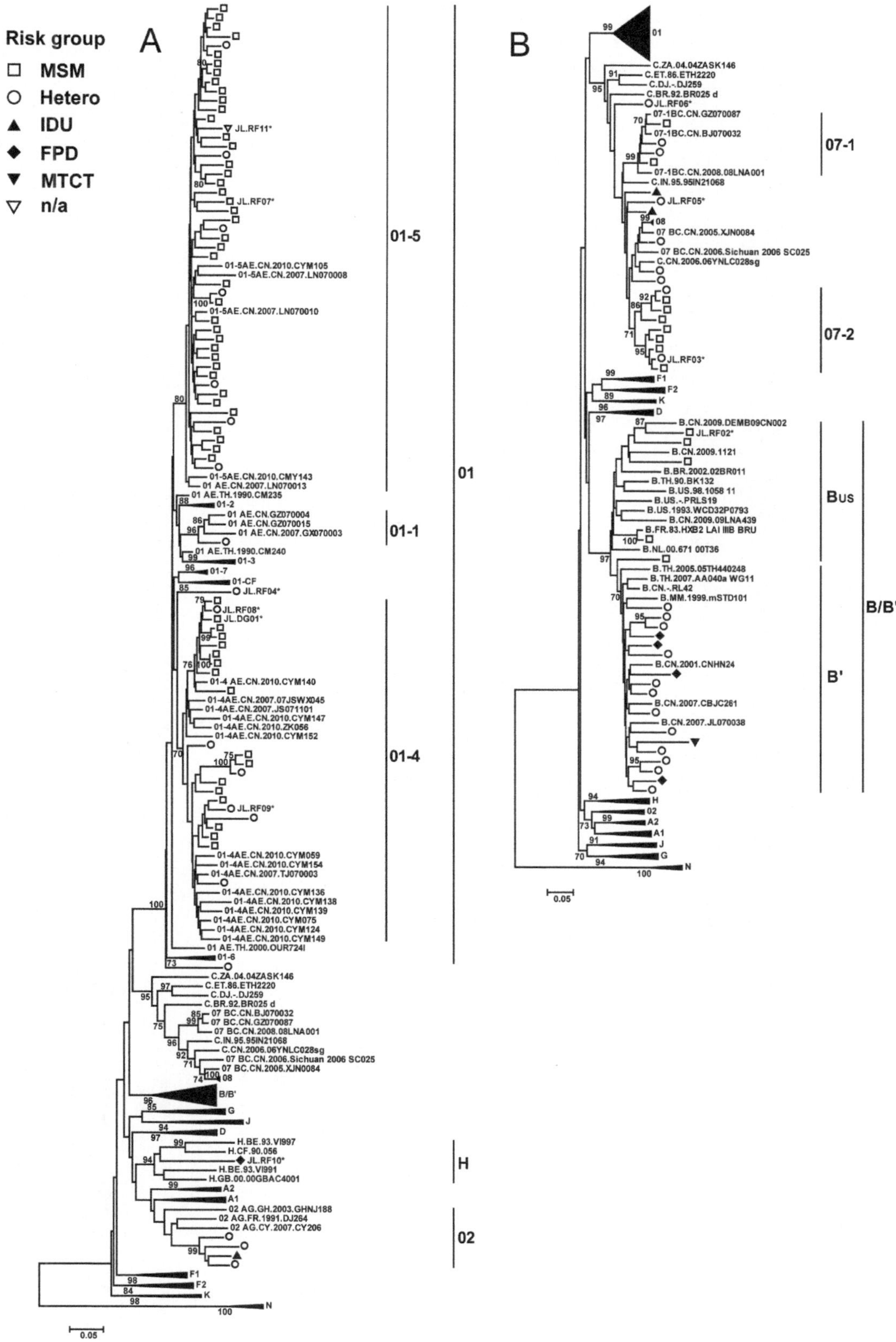

Figure 2. Neighbor-joining phylogenetic tree of HIV-1 *env* C2–C4 gene of study samples from the Jilin province of northeastern China. Neighbor-joining phylogenetic trees were constructed for 121 nucleotide sequences of HIV-1 *env* C2–C4 and reference sequences. The phylogenetic trees were constructed using methods described in Figure 1.

HIV-1 genotype distribution by geographic region

As shown in Table 1 and Figure 2, most HIV sequences were collected in Changchun (92/136, 67.6%), Jilin (19/136, 14.0%) and Yanbian Korean Autonomous Prefecture (11/136, 8.1%). Six out of the 7 identified subtypes/CRFs of HIV-1 were found in Changchun. Most of these HIV-infections were found in MSM (72/92, 78.3%) and heterosexuals (19/92, 20.7%), and the two predominant genotypes were CRF01_AE (68/92, 73.9%) and CRF07_BC (11/92, 12.0%). Seven out of 8 (87.5%) of the newly identified CRF07-2 strains were identified in Changchun, and the other CRF07-2 infection was found in the neighboring city of Songyuan. Of note, 95.5% of CRF01-4 and 83.3% of CRF01-5 co-circulated in Changchun, therefore, it was not surprising that we discovered a recombinant genotype (designated JL.DG01) comprised of gene regions from both CRF01-4 and CRF01-5. However, it should be noted that 68% of all our sequences were from Changchun.

In the city of Jilin, heterosexual (9/19, 47.4%) and FPD (5/19, 26.3%) were the two major risk groups for HIV-infections with subtype B' (8/19, 42.1%), followed by CRF01_AE (4/19, 21.1%), URFs (4/19, 21.1%) and CRF07_BC (3/19, 15.8%). In Yanbian Korean Autonomous Prefecture, the major risk group was heterosexual transmission (10/11, 90.9%), which was comprised of subtype B' (3/11, 27.3%), CRF02_AG (3/11, 27.3%), CRF01_AE (2/11, 18.2%), recombinant viruses (2/11, 18.2%) and CRF07-1 (1/11, 9.1%). The sampling size in the remaining cities was very small (Table 1, Fig. 3).

Discussion

Here we describe the most comprehensive HIV-1 molecular epidemiologic investigation, to date, on the characteristics and trends of the HIV/AIDS epidemic in the Jilin province of northeastern China between 2010 and 2011. Jilin province, as well as most of China, is experiencing an increasingly complex HIV epidemic. We identified subtypes B, B', and C, CRF01_AE (including lineages CRF01-1, CRF01-4 and CRF01-5), CRF02_AG, CRF07_BC (CRF07-1 and the newly identified lineage CRF07-2), and recombinant viruses; CRF01_AE was the predominant genotype in both heterosexual and MSM sequences.

In a previous nation-wide study [21], we identified 7 unique, strongly supported, phylogenetic sub-clusters or lineages among the CRF01_AE radiation nation-wide. These lineages were partially segregated by geographic regions of China and different risk groups. The first three lineages (CRF01-1through CRF01-3) were prevalent among IDUs and heterosexuals from the south and southwest, lineages CRF01-4 and CRF01-5 were primarily found in MSM from northern cities, and sub-clusters CRF01-6 and CRF01-7 were found in heterosexuals from southern China. In the current study, we identified three of these CRF01_AE lineages. CRF01-4 and CRF01-5 were found among sexual transmissions, both heterosexual and MSM, while the one CRF01-1 virus was identified in a heterosexual male.

Previous studies have found that there was a large and strongly supported transmission sub-cluster of CRF07_BC strains among MSM in Beijing, Liaoning, and Shijiazhuang within the CRF07 radiation [22–24], we designated this CRF07_BC sub-cluster as CRF07-1. In this current study, we found the route of transmissions

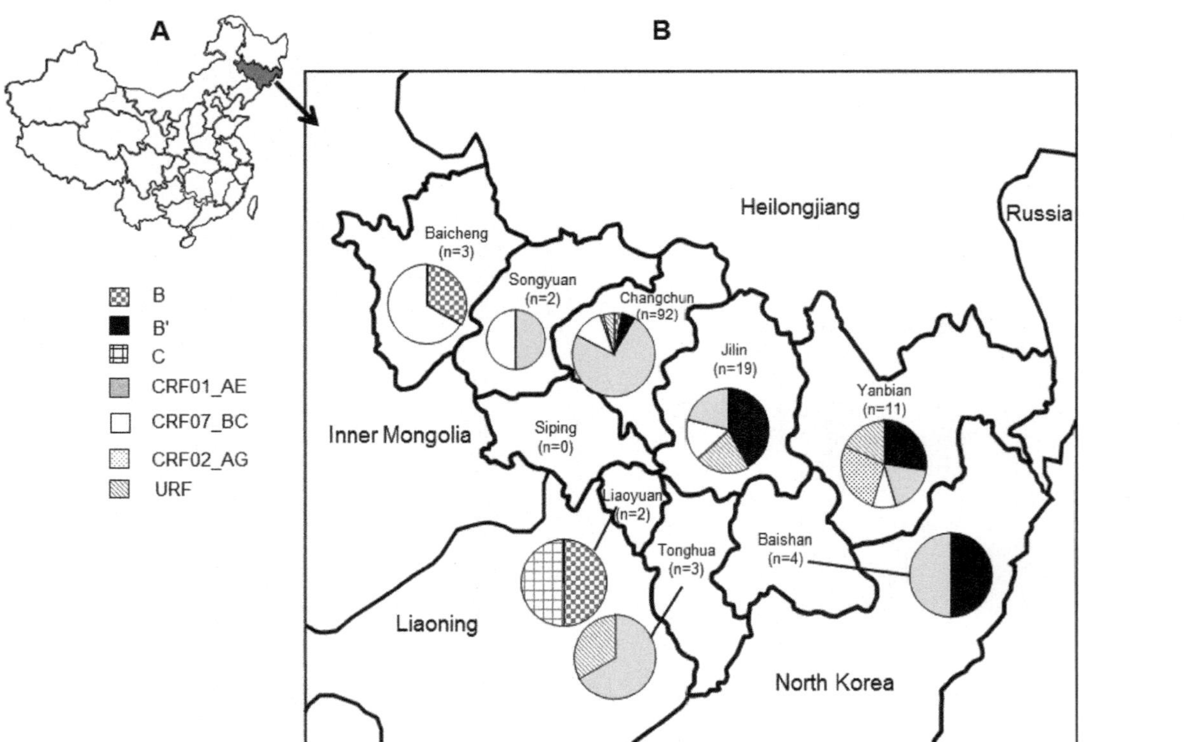

Figure 3. Maps of the study regions and HIV-1 genotype distribution of each geographical region in Jilin province of northeastern China. At the top-left corner of the figure is map of China (A), Jilin province of northeastern China is marked in gray. The map on the right of the figure represents Jilin province of northeastern China (B), the geographical location of the nine regions within Jilin province and the numbers of samples with genotypes from each region are shown. Pie charts show the distribution of HIV-1 genotypes in each region of Jilin province of northeastern China. The symbols representing different HIV-1 genotypes are shown at the left of the figure.

for CRF07-1 had expanded to include heterosexuals as well as MSM in Jilin province. Furthermore, a new statistically supported, monophyletic transmission cluster of CRF07_BC (designated CRF07-2) was identified among seven MSM from Changchun and one MSM from Songyuan, which is geographically adjacent to the northwestern portion of Changchun. Although the sample sizes are still fairly small relative to the epidemic, CRF07-1 has spread throughout much of Jilin province and is transmitted by both heterosexuals and MSM, while CRF07-2 has only been found among MSM in Changchun and neighboring Songyuan.

Originally subtype B' infections in China were identified primarily among IDU in Yunnan province and subsequently among FPD and heterosexual in inland China, due to unhygienic commercial plasma collections during the early to mid-1990s, after which the practice was banned [25]. The majority of subtype B' infections are now found in the heterosexual population [2]. This shift in risk groups is most likely the result of national policies in China that strictly regulated blood donations, which began in the late 1990s [26] and the fact that the HIV-infected FPD were spreading subtype B' viruses through heterosexual transmissions to their sex partners. Indeed, we found no subtype B' infections among our 83 MSM from Jilin province. While these comparisons of genotypes and risk groups are interesting, and appear to indicate certain trends, it must be highlighted that the samples were collected by convenience and do not represent a random sampling. An unknown degree of sampling bias is likely.

In the present study, we also detected a new statistically supported monophyletic cluster of 4 CRF02_AG uniquely associated with Korean ethnicity and heterosexuals near the Jilin-North Korean border (Yanbian Korean Autonomous Prefecture). The exception was an IDU in Changchun, who was also a citizen of Yanbian Korean Autonomous Prefecture but was imprisoned in Changchun. In a previous study, it was also showed that CRF02_AG predominated among heterosexuals in Cina, accounting for at least 68.8% of all detected CRF02_AG in a nationwide cross-sectional study of HIV-1 epidemic in China. In light of the fact that the four study participants were all of Korean ethnicity, it is tempting to speculate that the CRF02_AG cluster detected in the present study originated in Yanbian Korean Autonomous Prefecture. It is the first report of CRF02_AG forming a transmission cluster in a local resident population in China. In the past, CRF02_AG had only been found in migrating workers from West Africa [27,28].

Among the complex mix of subtypes and CRFs that co-circulate in China, it was not surprising to find the emergence of *gag* and *gag/env* recombinants. All but 1 (90.9%) of the 11 recombinants we found contained at least a portion of CRF01_AE, which is consistent with CRF01_AE being the predominant genotype among both heterosexual and MSM transmissions. Overall, the highest HIV-1 genotype diversity was observed among the heterosexual population, however, we only had three IDU samples. If we had a larger sampling of IDUs, we may have found a larger genotype diversity in this risk group too, due to the presence of both needle sharing and sexual routes of infection. In fact, from the three Jilin IDU sequences, we found three different genotypes, subtype C, CRF07_BC, and CRF02_AG, supporting the hypothesis that if more samples were available from IDUs, we might have found a genotype diversity at lease as high as that seen in heterosexual transmissions.

China's HIV epidemic is very heterogeneous, composed of a series of overlapping local sub-epidemics defined by risk groups, as well as temporal and/or spatial variation [29–34]. Detecting these sub-epidemics can be challenging because HIV diagnosis may take place many years after infection, and because of reliance on risk group self-reporting. IDU, MSM, and heterosexual risk factors are complicated by frequent 'bridging' between risk groups, caused by concurrent risk behaviours. IDUs constitute a high-risk group, which can facilitate HIV spread to lower risk populations through sexual risk factors [35–43]. While MSM has become the predominant route of HIV transmission [40,44,45], it is common for MSM in China to be bisexual [41–43], because of traditional values and family expectations; 17–35% of MSM are married [46–49] and more than 70% will be married in their lifetime [48,50]. Furthermore, an estimated 8.3% of MSM used drugs in the past 6 months and 5–25% sold sex to other men [50–56].

In conclusion, our study indicates that the HIV epidemic in Jilin province is very complex; effective control will require an understanding of the dynamics that drives the spread of HIV through social/sexual transmission networks [57,58]. Future molecular epidemiologic studies need to focus on collecting detailed behavioral and socio-demographic information that will allow the characterization of common behavioral risk factors for each of the identified social/sexual transmission clusters. Since transmission clusters significantly drive the HIV-1 epidemic in China, characterizing the specific, common risk behaviors for these networks will help target intervention strategies.

Supporting Information

Figure S1 Bootscanning analyses of 6 *gag* sequences of HIV-1 URFs strains isolated from Jilin province of northeastern China. The conditions used for bootscanning analyses are described in Methods. The representative subtypes/CRFs reference sequences with corresponding colors are shown at the bottom right of the figure.

Author Contributions

Conceived and designed the experiments: XGL. Performed the experiments: XHZ QG LYS XGL CXX. Analyzed the data: XGL CYN YF YT MLK. Contributed reagents/materials/analysis tools: XGL XH HX YMS. Contributed to the writing of the manuscript: XGL MLK YMS.

References

1. Health CMo, (WHO) WHO (2011) 2011 Estimates for the HIV/AIDS Epidemic in China. China Ministry of Health. Beijing.
2. He X, Xing H, Ruan Y, Hong K, Cheng C, et al. (2012) A comprehensive mapping of HIV-1 genotypes in various risk groups and regions across China based on a nationwide molecular epidemiologic survey. PLoS One 7: e47289.
3. Chen M, Yang L, Ma Y, Su Y, Yang C, et al. (2013) Emerging variability in HIV-1 genetics among recently infected individuals in Yunnan, China. PLoS One 8: e60101.
4. Guo H, Guo D, Wei JF, Yang H, Huan X, et al. (2009) First detection of a novel HIV Type 1 CRF01_AE/07_BC recombinant among an epidemiologically linked cohort of IDUs in Jiangsu, China. AIDS Res Hum Retroviruses 25: 463–467.
5. Chen L, Yang S, Li J, Li J, Liu Y, et al. (2011) Near full-length genomic characterization of a novel HIV type 1 CRF07_ BC/CRF08_ BC recombinant strain from Yunnan, China. AIDS Res Hum Retroviruses 27: 693–699.

6. Li X, Ning C, He X, Yang Y, Li F, et al. (2013) Genome Sequences of a Novel HIV-1 Circulating Recombinant Form (CRF61_BC) Identified among Heterosexuals in China. Genome Announc 1.
7. Yang Y, Lei-ming Z, Yi-le X, Qi-chao P, Lai-yi K, et al. (2008) Near full-length sequence analysis of a unique CRF01_AE/B' recombinant existed in Shanghai. JOURNAL OF DIAGNOSTICS CONCEPTS & PRACTICE 7: 511–516.
8. Council PCOutS, Statistics DoPaE, Statistics NBo (2010) Tabulation on the 2010 population census of people's republic of china: China Statistics Press.
9. Wang L, Meng X, Guo W, Meng X, Guo W, et al. (2010) Estimation and projection for HIV epidemic trend in Jilin province. Inter J Epidemiol Infect Dis 37: 361–364.
10. Huang L, Meng X, Qiu B, Sun L, Li Z (2011) Status and analysis of network direct reporting of HIV/AIDS epidemic in Jilin Province. Chinese Journal of Public Health Engineering 10: 515–516.
11. Rousseau CM, Birditt BA, McKay AR, Stoddard JN, Lee TC, et al. (2006) Large-scale amplification, cloning and sequencing of near full-length HIV-1 subtype C genomes. J Virol Methods 136: 118–125.
12. Li Z, He X, Wang Z, Xing H, Li F, et al. (2012) Tracing the origin and history of HIV-1 subtype B' epidemic by near full-length genome analyses. AIDS 26: 877–884.
13. Cham F, Heyndrickx L, Janssens W, Van der Auwera G, Vereecken K, et al. (2000) Study of HIV type 1 gag/env variability in The Gambia, using a multiplex DNA polymerase chain reaction. AIDS Res Hum Retroviruses 16: 1915–1919.
14. Hall TA (1999) BioEdit: a user-friendly biological sequence alignment editor and analysis program for Windows 95/98/NT. Nucleic Acids Symposium Series 41: 95–98.
15. Thompson JD, Gibson TJ, Plewniak F, Jeanmougin F, Higgins DG (1997) The CLUSTAL_X windows interface: flexible strategies for multiple sequence alignment aided by quality analysis tools. Nucleic Acids Res 25: 4876–4882.
16. Kimura M (1980) A simple method for estimating evolutionary rates of base substitutions through comparative studies of nucleotide sequences. J Mol Evol 16: 111–120.
17. Tamura K, Peterson D, Peterson N, Stecher G, Nei M, et al. (2011) MEGA5: molecular evolutionary genetics analysis using maximum likelihood, evolutionary distance, and maximum parsimony methods. Mol Biol Evol 28: 2731–2739.
18. Sanderson MJ, Wojciechowski MF (2000) Improved bootstrap confidence limits in large-scale phylogenies, with an example from Neo-Astragalus (Leguminosae). Syst Biol 49: 671–685.
19. Zhang M, Schultz AK, Calef C, Kuiken C, Leitner T, et al. (2006) jpHMM at GOBICS: a web server to detect genomic recombinations in HIV-1. Nucleic Acids Res 34: W463–465.
20. Lole KS, Bollinger RC, Paranjape RS, Gadkari D, Kulkarni SS, et al. (1999) Full-length human immunodeficiency virus type 1 genomes from subtype C-infected seroconverters in India, with evidence of intersubtype recombination. J Virol 73: 152–160.
21. Feng Y, He X, Hsi JH, Li F, Li X, et al. (2013) The rapidly expanding CRF01_AE epidemic in China is driven by multiple lineages of HIV-1 viruses introduced in the 1990s. AIDS 27: 1793–1802.
22. Wang W, Xu J, Jiang S, Yang K, Meng Z, et al. (2011) The dynamic face of HIV-1 subtypes among men who have sex with men in Beijing, China. Curr HIV Res 9: 136–139.
23. Li L, Lu X, Li H, Chen L, Wang Z, et al. (2011) High genetic diversity of HIV-1 was found in men who have sex with men in Shijiazhuang, China. Infect Genet Evol 11: 1487–1492.
24. Han X, Dai D, Zhao B, Liu J, Ding H, et al. (2010) Genetic and epidemiologic characterization of HIV-1 infection In Liaoning Province, China. J Acquir Immune Defic Syndr 53 Suppl 1: S27–33.
25. Mastro TD, Yip R (2006) The legacy of unhygienic plasma collection in China. AIDS 20: 1451–1452.
26. Wu Z, Sullivan SG, Wang Y, Rotheram-Borus MJ, Detels R (2007) Evolution of China's response to HIV/AIDS. Lancet 369: 679–690.
27. Zhu J, Tian Z, Xing H, Fang Y, Zhang X, et al. (2008) Subtype study and sequence analysis of HIV-1 strains in *env* C2–V3 region isolated from passengers entering or exiting the Shanghai port. Chin J AIDS STD 14: 111–114.
28. Tian Z, Fang Y, Zhang Q, Yan J, Zhang X, et al. (2009) Study of Molecular Epidemiology on Infected with Human Immunodeficiency Virus-1 in 2001~2005 at Shanghai Frontier Port. Chinese Frontier Health Quarantine 32: 339–345.
29. Young AM, Jonas AB, Mullins UL, Halgin DS, Havens JR (2013) Network structure and the risk for HIV transmission among rural drug users. AIDS Behav 17: 2341–2351.
30. Klovdahl AS, Potterat JJ, Woodhouse DE, Muth JB, Muth SQ, et al. (1994) Social networks and infectious disease: the Colorado Springs Study. Soc Sci Med 38: 79–88.
31. Rothenberg RB, Potterat JJ, Woodhouse DE, Muth SQ, Darrow WW, et al. (1998) Social network dynamics and HIV transmission. AIDS 12: 1529–1536.
32. Rothenberg RB, Sterk C, Toomey KE, Potterat JJ, Johnson D, et al. (1998) Using social network and ethnographic tools to evaluate syphilis transmission. Sex Transm Dis 25: 154–160.
33. Potterat JJ, Rothenberg RB, Muth SQ (1999) Network structural dynamics and infectious disease propagation. Int J STD AIDS 10: 182–185.
34. Helleringer S, Kohler HP, Chimbiri A, Chatonda P, Mkandawire J (2009) The Likoma Network Study: Context, data collection, and initial results. Demogr Res 21: 427–468.
35. Kral AH, Bluthenthal RN, Lorvick J, Gee L, Bacchetti P, et al. (2001) Sexual transmission of HIV-1 among injection drug users in San Francisco, USA: risk-factor analysis. Lancet 357: 1397–1401.
36. Pisani E, Dadun, Sucahya PK, Kamil O, Jazan S (2003) Sexual behavior among injection drug users in 3 indonesian cities carries a high potential for HIV spread to noninjectors. J Acquir Immune Defic Syndr 34: 403–406.
37. Howard DL, Latkin CA (2006) A bridge over troubled waters: factors associated with non-injection drug users having injection drug-using sex partners. J Acquir Immune Defic Syndr 42: 325–330.
38. Lindenburg CE, Krol A, Smit C, Buster MC, Coutinho RA, et al. (2006) Decline in HIV incidence and injecting, but not in sexual risk behaviour, seen in drug users in Amsterdam: a 19-year prospective cohort study. AIDS 20: 1771–1775.
39. Kretzschmar M, Wiessing L (2008) New challenges for mathematical and statistical modeling of HIV and hepatitis C virus in injecting drug users. AIDS 22: 1527–1537.
40. Beyrer C, Trapence G, Motimedi F, Umar E, Iipinge S, et al. (2010) Bisexual concurrency, bisexual partnerships, and HIV among Southern African men who have sex with men. Sex Transm Infect 86: 323–327.
41. Chow EP, Iu KI, Fu X, Wilson DP, Zhang L (2012) HIV and sexually transmissible infections among money boys in China: a data synthesis and meta-analysis. PLoS One 7: e48025.
42. Chow EP, Wilson DP, Zhang L (2011) HIV and syphilis co-infection increasing among men who have sex with men in China: a systematic review and meta-analysis. PLoS One 6: e22768.
43. Liao M, Kang D, Jiang B, Tao X, Qian Y, et al. (2011) Bisexual behavior and infection with HIV and syphilis among men who have sex with men along the east coast of China. AIDS Patient Care STDS 25: 683–691.
44. Zhang L, Chow EP, Jing J, Zhuang X, Li X, et al. (2013) HIV prevalence in China: integration of surveillance data and a systematic review. Lancet Infect Dis 13: 955–963.
45. Beyrer C, Baral SD, van Griensven F, Goodreau SM, Chariyalertsak S, et al. (2012) Global epidemiology of HIV infection in men who have sex with men. Lancet 380: 367–377.
46. Feng L, Ding X, Lu R, Liu J, Sy A, et al. (2009) High HIV prevalence detected in 2006 and 2007 among men who have sex with men in China's largest municipality: an alarming epidemic in Chongqing, China. J Acquir Immune Defic Syndr 52: 79–85.
47. Xiao Y, Ding X, Li C, Liu J, Sun J, et al. (2009) Prevalence and correlates of HIV and syphilis infections among men who have sex with men in Chongqing Municipality, China. Sex Transm Dis 36: 647–656.
48. Zhang B, Li X, Chu Q, Wang N, Wang Z, et al. (2008) A survey of HIV/AIDS related behaviors among 2250 MSM in nine major cities of China. Chinese Journal of AIDS & STD 14: 541–547.
49. Qu S, Zhang D, Wu Y, Zhu H, Zheng X (2002) Seroprevalence of HIV and risk behaviors among men who have sex with men in a northeast city of China. Chinese JSTD & AIDS Prevention Control 8: 145–147.
50. Zhang B, Li X, Hu T, Liu D, Shi T (2000) HIV/AIDS interventions targeting men who have sex with men (MSM): theory and practice. Chinese JSTD & AIDS Prevention Control 6.
51. Choi KH, Gibson DR, Han L, Guo Y (2004) High levels of unprotected sex with men and women among men who have sex with men: a potential bridge of HIV transmission in Beijing, China. AIDS Educ Prev 16: 19–30.
52. Zhang D, Bi P, Lv F, Zhang J, Hiller JE (2007) Changes in HIV prevalence and sexual behavior among men who have sex with men in a northern Chinese city: 2002–2006. J Infect 55: 456–463.
53. Liu H, Wang N, Zhang Q, Shao Y, Wu T, et al. (2007) Study of HIV and syphilis infection situation and sexual behavioral characteristics among 416 MSM. Chin J AIDS STD 13: 230–232.
54. Ruan Y, Li D, Li X, Qian HZ, Shi W, et al. (2007) Relationship between syphilis and HIV infections among men who have sex with men in Beijing, China. Sex Transm Dis 34: 592–597.
55. Liu H, Yang H, Li X, Wang N, Liu H, et al. (2006) Men who have sex with men and human immunodeficiency virus/sexually transmitted disease control in China. Sex Transm Dis 33: 68–76.
56. Choi KH, Liu H, Guo Y, Han L, Mandel JS, et al. (2003) Emerging HIV-1 epidemic in China in men who have sex with men. Lancet 361: 2125–2126.
57. Anderson RM, May RM, Boily MC, Garnett GP, Rowley JT (1991) The spread of HIV-1 in Africa: sexual contact patterns and the predicted demographic impact of AIDS. Nature 352: 581–589.
58. Doherty IA, Padian NS, Marlow C, Aral SO (2005) Determinants and consequences of sexual networks as they affect the spread of sexually transmitted infections. J Infect Dis 191 Suppl 1: S42–54.

6

Consequences of Missed Opportunities for HIV Testing during Pregnancy and Delayed Diagnosis for Mexican Women, Children and Male Partners

Tamil Kendall*

Women and Health Initiative and Takemi Program in International Health, Department of Global Health and Population, Harvard School of Public Health, Boston, Massachusetts, United States of America

Abstract

Introduction: HIV testing during pregnancy permits prevention of vertical (mother-to-child) transmission and provides an opportunity for women living with HIV to access treatment for their own health. In 2001, Mexico's National HIV Action Plan committed to universal offer of HIV testing to pregnant women, but in 2011, only 45.6% of women who attended antenatal care (ANC) were tested for HIV. The study objective was to document the consequences of missed opportunities for HIV testing and counseling during pregnancy and late HIV diagnosis for Mexican women living with HIV and their families.

Methods: Semi-structured-interviews with 55 women living with HIV who had had a pregnancy since 2001 were completed between 2009 and 2011. Interviews were analyzed thematically using *a priori* and inductive codes.

Results: Consistent with national statistics, less than half of the women living with HIV (42%) were offered HIV testing and counseling during ANC. When not diagnosed during ANC, women had multiple contacts with the health-care system due to their own and other family members' AIDS-related complications before being diagnosed. Missed opportunities for HIV testing and counseling during antenatal care and health-care providers failure to recognize AIDS-related complications resulted in pediatric HIV infections, AIDS-related deaths of children and male partners, and HIV disease progression among women and other family members. In contrast, HIV diagnosis permitted timely access to interventions to prevent vertical HIV transmission and long-term care and treatment for women living with HIV.

Conclusions: Omissions of the offer of HIV testing and counseling in ANC and health-care providers' failure to recognize AIDS-related complications had negative health, economic and emotional consequences. Scaling-up provider-initiated HIV testing and counseling within and beyond antenatal care and pre-service and in-service trainings on HIV and AIDS for health-care providers can hasten timely HIV diagnosis and contribute to improved individual and public health in Mexico.

Editor: Claire Thorne, UCL Institute of Child Health, University College London, United Kingdom

Funding: This research was supported by a Canadian Institutes of Health Research Postdoctoral Fellowship (http://www.cihr-irsc.gc.ca/e/193.html), a Pierre Elliott Trudeau Foundation Doctoral and Post-Doctoral Scholarship (http://www.trudeaufoundation.ca/en), a Social Sciences and Humanities Research Council Canada Vanier Canada Graduate Scholarship (http://www.vanier.gc.ca/eng/home-accueil.aspx), and a grant from UNIFEM (now UNWOMEN) sub-regional office for Mexico, Central America, Cuba and the Dominican Republic (http://www.unwomen.org/). The funders had no role in study design, data collection and analysis, decision to publish, or preparation of the manuscript.

Competing Interests: The author declares that no competing interests exist.

* Email: tkendall@hsph.harvard.edu

Introduction

Prevention of vertical (mother-to-child) transmission of HIV is recognized as an important action to achieve the Millennium Development Goals, particularly the health-related goals of reducing child and maternal mortality and turning the tide of the HIV epidemic [1,2]. Antenatal HIV testing is necessary to prevent vertical HIV transmission and also offers an opportunity for women and other family members to learn their HIV status and access treatment for their own health [3]. In 2012 only 38% of pregnant women in low and middle-income countries were tested for HIV; in the Americas the proportion was 62% [4]. This is despite the fact that in 2001, member countries of the United Nations committed to providing antiretroviral prophylaxis to prevent vertical HIV transmission to 80% of women who needed it by 2011 [5].

After endorsing the United Nations Political Declaration on HIV and AIDS in 2001, Mexico, like many other countries around the world, strengthened domestic policies to prevent vertical HIV transmission. The 2001 Mexican National Action Plan on HIV and AIDS established the universal offer of HIV testing to pregnant women; the 2007–2012 National Action Plan on HIV and AIDS reaffirmed this objective [6,7]. The most important operational intervention to promote HIV testing during antenatal care (ANC) after 2001 was the national distribution of 800,000 rapid HIV tests to primary care clinics that serve the population without employer-provided health insurance at the end of 2006 and beginning of 2007 with the instruction to offer HIV testing to all pregnant women [8]. However, Mexican HIV legislation was not modified to include the obligation of health-care services to offer HIV testing to all pregnant women until 2010 [9] and, as of June 2014, the national ANC legislation still stated that antenatal HIV testing should only be offered to "high risk women–those who have received blood transfusions, drug addicts, and prostitutes" [10]. This disjuncture between the commitment to offer of HIV testing to all pregnant women in the HIV National Action Plan and the legislative frameworks for HIV and reproductive health care, combined with the vertical organization of HIV and reproductive health services, assignation of the responsibility for prevention of vertical HIV transmission to the HIV program, and competing priorities in both HIV and reproductive health have been identified as policy and political barriers to the scale-up of HIV testing among pregnant women in Mexico, as well as other Latin American countries [11,12]. Additional operational barriers to antenatal HIV testing identified in Mexico between 2001 and 2011 included a limited number of health workers trained in HIV testing and counseling in reproductive health services and insufficient availability of commodities [12].

Mexico's national prenatal care legislation has recommended a minimum of five ANC visits since 1993 and the national HIV action plan introduced universal offer of HIV testing in 2001 [6,10]. Since 2006, 81.5% of women have begun ANC during the first trimester and beginning in 2009 national guidelines for antiretroviral management recommended HIV testing during the first trimester of pregnancy or as soon as possible thereafter [13,14]. However, when the current study began in 2009, despite 95.8% of Mexican women attending at least one ANC visit and 86.3% of women attending four or more ANC visits [15], only 42.1% of Mexican women who attended ANC were tested for HIV [16]. In 2011 when the study concluded, only 45.6% of women who attended ANC were tested for HIV [16]. The objective of this analysis is to describe missed opportunities for HIV diagnosis during pregnancy and document the consequences for the health and well-being of women living with HIV and their families.

Methods

Ethics statement

The design and conduct of this study was reviewed and approved annually by the University of British Columbia-Okanagan Behavioural Research Ethics Board and the Mexican National AIDS Program (CENSIDA) Ethics Board. To ensure confidentiality, pseudonyms were assigned to all women living with HIV who participated in the research, and physicians and decision-makers are identified only by their professional role.

Data collection and analysis

The analysis draws on semi-structured interviews with 55 Mexican women of reproductive age living with HIV conducted between July 2009 and January 2011. The criteria for women's inclusion in the study were: living with HIV, speaking Spanish, being at least 18 and of reproductive age (18–49 years of age), and having had a pregnancy since 2001 when universal offer of HIV testing during ANC was first included in the Mexican National Action Plan on HIV and AIDS. Women living with HIV were recruited from eight ambulatory HIV clinics in Central Mexico (Mexico State, Morelos, and Mexico City) that serve the population without employer-provided health insurance. The population attending these health services is generally economically disadvantaged. Reported monthly family incomes of the women living with HIV ranged from 200 pesos (USD 16) to 10,000 pesos (USD 777) per month, with a median family income of 3000 pesos per month (USD 233) and a mean income of 3500 pesos per month (USD 272). All of the women living with HIV reported monthly household incomes below the Mexican national mean of USD 950 a month [17]. The exchange rate of 12.86 Mexican pesos for a US Dollar was calculated using the Federal Reserve Rate on the first day of each month between July 2009 and December 2010 (http://www.federalreserve.gov). Based on the cost of the basic monthly food basket in urban areas in 2008, which Mexico uses to estimate poverty, two-thirds of the women faced food insufficiency at the household level even before taking into account the cost of rent and other living expenses [18].

Women of reproductive age living with HIV were given a written invitation to participate by clinic staff. If they met the selection criteria and wished to participate, clinic staff made an appointment to conduct an interview. Interviews were conducted in Spanish by the author, who has been doing qualitative research with Mexican women living with HIV for more than a decade, or a female Mexican anthropologist experienced in reproductive health research who was trained by the author about HIV and in the use of the interview guide. A site which afforded sufficient privacy was chosen by the woman living with HIV; most interviews were conducted in a private office at the HIV clinic. Research participants were given 100 pesos (approximately eight dollars) to pay for their travel and childcare. All research participants signed written informed consent prior to the interview. As one of the study objectives was to analyze implementation of the Mexican program to prevent vertical HIV transmission, and consequences of successful or failed implementation for women and their families, this was a purposive sample of women living with HIV diagnosed during ANC as well as women who were diagnosed in other settings. Sample size was determined by the principle of saturation, which refers to the point at which additional interviews do not provide novel information about the primary areas of interest [19]. Interviews were continued until saturation was reached with respect to women's narratives about the offer of HIV testing during antenatal care, the circumstances of their HIV diagnosis, and referral to services to prevent vertical HIV transmission. Numerical balance between women living with HIV diagnosed during ANC and those diagnosed in other settings was not sought.

Interviews with women living with HIV ranged from one to two hours in length and included questions about the circumstances of the HIV diagnosis, pregnancy history, sexual and reproductive practices and desires before and after the HIV diagnosis, experience of and management of HIV disease, prevention of vertical HIV transmission, interactions with the health-care system and health-care providers, and social and economic situation. This analysis focuses on the experiences of women living with HIV however data from 60 additional interviews with health-care providers, policymakers and other experts about prevention of vertical HIV transmission in Mexico between 2001 and 2011 are drawn upon to contextualize women's experiences.

All interviews were audiotaped and transcribed verbatim. The author conducted analysis during fieldwork and modified the interview guide to explore emerging issues. Interviews were coded thematically by the author, using a combination of predefined codes related to areas of interest and codes which were generated inductively from the interviews. Examples of *a priori codes* were HIV diagnosis during ANC and circumstances of the HIV diagnosis; examples of inductive codes include diagnosis because of AIDS-related morbidity or mortality of a child or a male partner, diagnosis when women developed AIDS-related complications, or through provider-initiative testing and counseling outside of ANC. Data were managed using the qualitative analysis package Atlas-ti 6.0.

Results

In total, 48 of the 55 women living with HIV attended ANC without knowledge of their diagnosis between 2001 and 2009. Figure 1 describes two routes to HIV diagnosis for these 48 women who attended ANC after 2001 and were diagnosed subsequently with HIV: 1) provider initiated testing and counseling (PITC) as part of ANC or intrapartum care, or 2) missed opportunities for HIV diagnosis during ANC/intrapartum care and subsequent HIV testing in another setting, usually when the woman, her child(ren), or the male partner developed AIDS-related complications.

As shown in Figure 1, all 14 pregnant women who were offered PITC and tested positive during ANC or intrapartum care received interventions to prevent vertical HIV transmission, as did another seven women who were diagnosed with HIV during pregnancy outside of ANC (21/48). Of the 34 women who were not diagnosed in ANC/intrapartum care, 27 were diagnosed after delivery and did not receive any interventions to prevent vertical HIV transmission (27/48). Four women who were offered and accepted PITC during ANC or intrapartum care had an initial negative test result. These four women, two women who refused HIV testing during ANC, and twenty-four women not offered PITC in ANC were subsequently diagnosed when the woman, her child(ren), or the male partner became ill with AIDS-related complications (30/48).

Seven women living with HIV were excluded from Figure 1 because they were already aware of their HIV diagnosis before becoming pregnant and accessing ANC post-2001. Their routes to HIV diagnosis were similar to other women who were not diagnosed during ANC: the woman becoming ill with AIDS-related complications, the male partner becoming ill or dying of AIDS-related complications, or PITC of asymptomatic women in other settings e.g. at work or prior to surgery.

HIV diagnosis during pregnancy

On average, women went to 6.5 ANC visits in the pregnancy prior to HIV-diagnosis or the pregnancy during which they were diagnosed [range 1–10], providing ample opportunities for health workers to offer HIV testing. Nevertheless, of the 48 women who attended ANC after 2001 but before being diagnosed with HIV, only 20 (42%) were offered HIV testing during ANC or labor and delivery (Figure 1). Many of the women who reported antenatal HIV testing were pregnant during 2007 and 2008 (after the national distribution of rapid tests to public primary care clinics), however other women who attended ANC in those years were not offered testing. The haphazard offer of HIV testing and counseling during ANC is exemplified by Nancy's experience. In 2008, she attended ANC at the public primary health care center "in my neighborhood, where my mother lives" and was not offered HIV testing and counseling. Nancy only learned she was living with HIV during pregnancy because, by chance, she went to an ANC visit at a different public primary health care center in the same city and was offered an HIV test.

Of the 20 women who received PITC during ANC, two refused testing, for an acceptance rate similar to the 85–90% identified in other Mexican studies [20,21]. Women who refused testing said they had not received specific information about preventing vertical HIV transmission as part of counseling. The perception among a few women that HIV testing was compulsory during pregnancy also suggests that the quality of counseling was sub-optimal. For instance, Jacinta wanted to be tested but understood HIV testing to be "a requirement of the health center to receive prenatal care".

Four of the women tested during ANC received negative test results (Figure 1). While one woman reported that she acquired HIV from a partner who she met after the index pregnancy, the other three women had the same male partner at the time of diagnosis as during the index pregnancy and were diagnosed shortly after delivery. This finding indicates that repeat HIV testing in the third trimester of pregnancy could provide additional benefit for identifying women living with HIV, preventing vertical HIV transmission, and enabling women's timely referral to long-term care.

Another group of women (n = 7) were not offered HIV testing as a routine part of ANC but were diagnosed during pregnancy. Among these women, four were diagnosed because their male partner became ill with AIDS-related complications during the pregnancy, one male partner disclosed his HIV status after his female partner became pregnant, one woman's husband received PITC as part of his application for work, and one woman happened to test at a street testing fair held in her neighbourhood.

Provision of interventions to prevent vertical HIV transmission and linkage to long-term HIV care and treatment

Once women had an HIV-positive test result, health-care providers and administrators reported that they expedited confirmation of pregnant women's HIV test results and access to interventions to prevent vertical HIV transmission, including antiretroviral prophylaxis. The head of a state HIV Program, explained "we consider a pregnant woman an emergency so we don't wait to have the viral load and CD4, we start the [prophylactic antiretroviral] regimen immediately." These efforts were reflected in women's reported experiences. Of the 21 women who learned their HIV status during pregnancy, all took steps to prevent vertical HIV transmission: 17/21 received antiretroviral prophylaxis; one woman diagnosed at 38 weeks gestation delivered by cesarean section and her child was given antiretroviral prophylaxis; none of the three women diagnosed during labor received antiretroviral prophylaxis for themselves or their children but two delivered by caesarean section; and none of the women breastfed. Of the 21 women who learned their diagnosis during ANC or intrapartum, 16 had children with an HIV-negative diagnosis, three children were too young to have a confirmed diagnosis, and two women were pregnant at the time of the interview.

With respect to linkage to and uptake of long-term HIV care, whether they were diagnosed during prenatal care or in another context, most women reported a relatively smooth and speedy transition from initial diagnosis to being referred to a public HIV clinic, confirmatory testing of HIV status and receiving the first CD4 and viral load count. At the time of the interview, all of the participants were enrolled in long-term HIV care and treatment for their own health. Sara's experience was typical of that reported by most participants, in that during the month after her child was born she "started to go to the [HIV] clinic with the doctor, my medical visits, my medications, and did everything to take care of myself." However, 7 of 55 women (12.7%) reported delaying seeking care and treatment after their diagnosis (from a few months up to several years), suspending HIV care for a period before they were treatment eligible, and temporarily stopping treatment during the postpartum period; only one of these women was diagnosed during pregnancy. Reasons given by women for

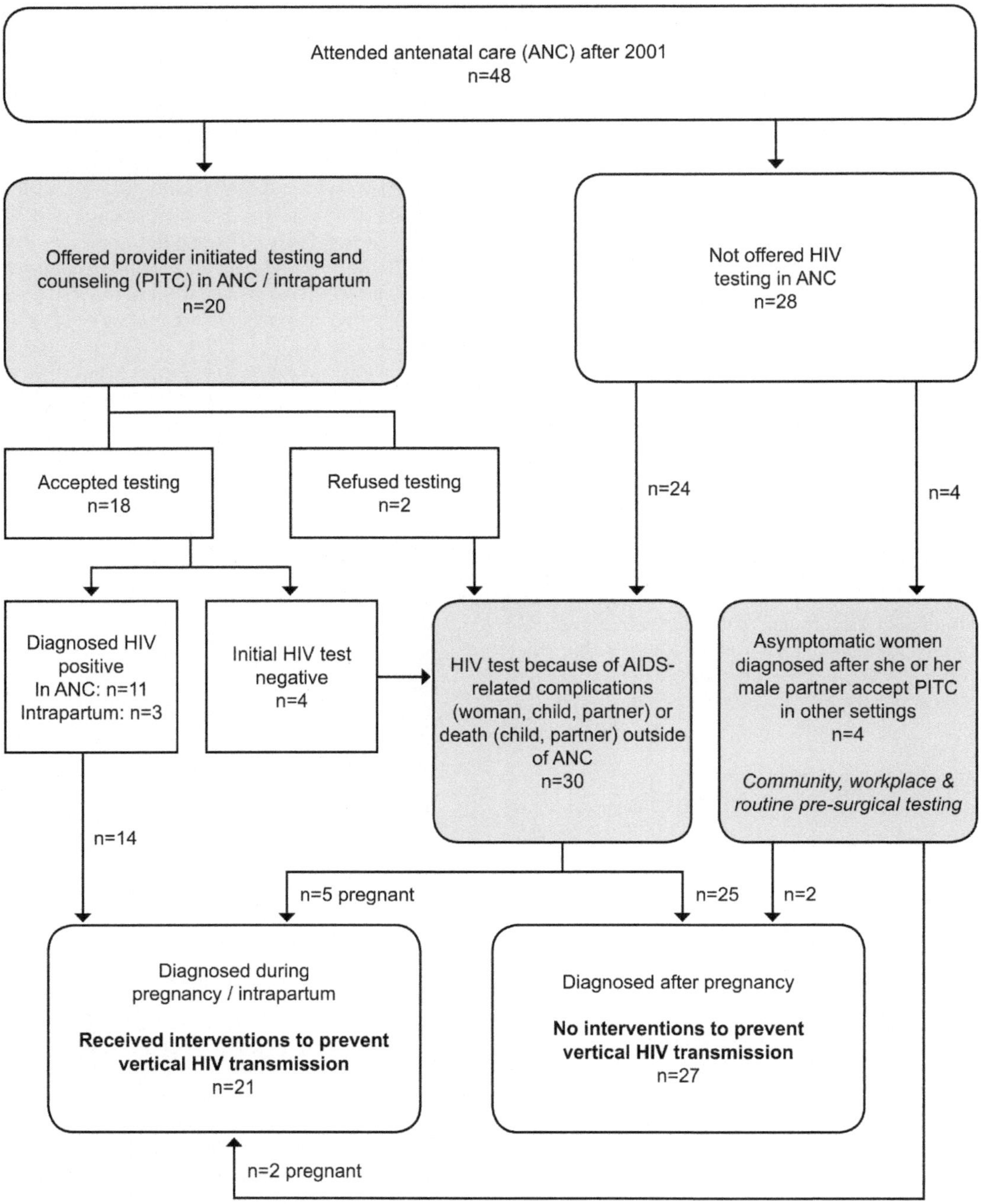

Figure 1. Routes to HIV diagnosis for Mexican women who attended antenatal care (ANC) after 2001.

delaying or suspending HIV care and treatment included lack of knowledge about HIV disease and treatment, perceived lack of empathy from health-care providers, antiretroviral side effects, prioritizing a child's treatment over their own health, and the cost of transportation. For example, Amparo said that before she was eligible for treatment she "stopped coming for about a year. I thought 'I'm fine, the doctor doesn't even give me a check-up, so why I am paying for transport and leaving my little kid."

Health, economic and emotional consequences of missed opportunities for HIV testing and delayed diagnosis

When the opportunity to offer HIV testing during ANC was missed, the most common route to the HIV diagnosis was when women or their family members experienced AIDS-related complications (Figure 1). As discussed in more detail below, the health, economic and emotional consequences of missing the opportunity to diagnose HIV during pregnancy were frequently exacerbated by health-care providers' failure to recognize HIV and AIDS-related complications among children, male partners, and women.

AIDS-related morbidity and mortality among children

In this sample, only women who were not diagnosed with HIV during pregnancy had children who were known to be living with HIV, or who had died from complications that were known or suspected to be AIDS-related. Four of the women interviewed experienced the death of a child who tested positive for HIV, three lost a child who had symptoms that could be due to AIDS without a diagnosis, and ten were mothers of children living with HIV. Children's AIDS-related illness or death was a common way for women to learn their HIV diagnosis. The tragedy of the preventable child death due to vertical HIV transmission is compounded by the fact that the parents invariably sought medical care for their children without receiving a timely HIV diagnosis. Itzel and her husband were typical in this respect. Despite their limited income (she is a maid and he is a day labourer), they sought specialized medical care in the public and private sectors for their son, and became deeply indebted. Itzel said:

> Test after test, they pricked him wherever they wanted and they never did this one [HIV], until the very last days when he had a convulsion and then, according to them, they wanted to do a more advanced test. By then we had gone through everything. Paediatricians and paediatricians, private ones, and the best–we spent so much money. [...] And we got deeply into debt. And for what? Nothing. Doctors and doctors and nothing. Why did it not occur to them to think just for a minute about [HIV]? And we did not either because, well, we never could have imagined it.

By the time of her son's death from AIDS-related complications at two years of age in 2008, Itzel had also progressed to AIDS. Mother and child had the same clinical symptoms: extreme weight loss (wasting), vomiting, and diarrhoea. Itzel explained that it "seemed strange to me that I had the same symptoms as him, you understand? I had totally lost weight, a lot of diarrhoea, and everything that we ate, I threw up, and that was how he was." If Itzel's husband had not taken the initiative to track down the physician who had ordered the HIV test for their son because he wanted to know what his son had died of, even their son's death would not have resulted in them learning their HIV diagnosis.

Similar to Itzel, Karen sought health-care for her son but did not learn he was living with HIV until shortly before he died. Karen's son died of AIDS-related complications at three years of age, and her younger daughter is HIV-positive. The history of Karen's pregnancies and the AIDS-defining illnesses experienced by the family illustrate that health-care providers had multiple opportunities and indications for recommending HIV testing. During her first pregnancy in 2004, Karen and her husband were both public sector employees with health insurance. Yet despite attending eight ANC visits and doing "eight ultrasounds with my son, every month I did one," Karen was not offered HIV testing and counseling. Her son was born vaginally and she breastfed exclusively for three months after which time she fed him with formula and breast milk. He was a sickly child and was being hospitalized regularly for infections and respiratory problems when she became pregnant with her daughter. During her second pregnancy in 2006 Karen attended six ANC visits but was not offered HIV testing. Her son's repeated illnesses, her husband's AIDS-defining illness (oesophageal candidiasis) and both of them being hospitalized did not result in health-care providers recommending HIV testing. Karen said she feels "impotent about my son because we knew that my husband got sick a lot from this. He was hospitalized several times and they never, ever diagnosed anything". Just as her husband's symptoms did not provoke suspicion of HIV, her son was also misdiagnosed. Karen was told her son "had adenoiditis, and that was why he was always getting sick in his throat. So we finally got together enough money, and my father also lent us [money], so that he could have an operation." After the operation, Karen's son became acutely ill and remained hospitalized. At the same time, his younger sister became ill and was hospitalized. Karen related that "when they saw the two little siblings hospitalized, they asked why. It seemed strange to them, and they started to do tests". The simultaneous hospitalization of Karen's two children led to Karen, her husband and their two children learning that they were living with HIV.

Three other women living with HIV had lost children due to symptoms that could be AIDS-related but who died without a diagnosis. For example, Lilia miscarried and then, "in 2005, I had another baby who died at twenty-seven days old. He got pneumonia in one of his little lungs." Antonina's daughter died, but "even now, three years later, I don't know what killed her. She was sick to her throat. We took her to the doctor, but never found out what was wrong with her."

AIDS-related morbidity and mortality among male partners

Another route to the HIV diagnosis for women was when a male partner became ill with AIDS-related complications. In Carmen's case, health-care services missed the opportunity to diagnose her in 2003 while she was pregnant, but when her husband became ill with AIDS-related complications in 2009, they were both diagnosed. Similarly, Luisa was not offered HIV testing and counseling though she attended ANC during three pregnancies between 2002 and 2006. She learned she was HIV-positive in 2008 when her husband "started to get sick with fever, his whole body hurt, his bones, and when we came to the hospital for a vaccine, because he felt sick, the doctor told me that he did not have anemia, that probably he had AIDS." She and her husband both tested positive for HIV, and he died shortly afterwards. Very late diagnosis and deaths from AIDS-related complications were a hallmark of the family medical histories of women who participated in the research.

Women's HIV disease progression

The other common route to diagnosis was when a woman presented symptoms of HIV disease or AIDS-related complications. However, these diagnoses were frequently delayed. Over and over again, women reported that they had sought health care for a variety of HIV-related ailments without physicians ever suggesting an HIV test. Paola's story exemplifies the difficulty that women have receiving an HIV diagnosis despite being symptomatic. She said that

> for almost a year I was doing tests. I was going to urologists and other specialists because it seemed that I had a urinary tract infection. I had pain that wouldn't go away. I went to several different physicians but none sent me to do the [HIV] test. It was only when I felt really sick, I had a lot of diarrhoea and fever, I went to a doctor who knows my father, a family doctor. And because I trusted him, and based on the symptoms, the medicines [I had taken], and that I hadn't gotten better, he sent me to do an ELISA [Enzyme-linked immunosorbent assay].

Research has shown a close relationship between gynaecological disorders and HIV among women, yet despite her symptomology and determined health seeking, Paola progressed to the third clinical stage of HIV disease before she received her diagnosis [22]. Noemi had different symptoms than Paola, but she also experienced a long period of health-care seeking and became very ill before she was diagnosed.

> They told me that it was pneumonia. They controlled it, I was okay, and then I got sick again. After that, they did tests but they never did one of these [HIV] tests. Because they did not think that it could be this [HIV]. They said that no, well it was just pneumonia, it was pneumonia, and they prescribed medicine, and I got better, and then again.

Noemi presented with recurrent pneumonia, an AIDS-defining illness, for years without an HIV test being suggested. When Noemi was finally tested for HIV, she was extremely ill:

> They put me in intensive care because I had third grade dehydration; they said I arrived weighing thirty kilos (66 lbs.). By then I had pneumonia, dehydration, I was in the third stage of HIV. And as well, I had genital herpes, and also in the mouth. I was at the end. In fact, they [the physicians] told my family to come and say goodbye because they couldn't do anything for me.

Women living with HIV repeatedly narrated becoming very ill–losing weight, having fevers and diarrhoea, a chronic chest infection or pneumonia, or on-going gynaecological complications, and consulting a variety of physicians without receiving the recommendation of an HIV test.

Economic consequences

Futile health-care seeking that included consultations with specialists who ordered numerous laboratory tests but never recommended HIV testing, prescribed medicines and performed surgical interventions to treat AIDS-related symptoms and disease progression that limited women and men's ability to work had negative economic consequences for families. In many cases, the families of these women living with HIV simply could not afford their odyssey through the health system, and became indebted in order to pay their medical bills. Itzel explains that when seeking a diagnosis for her now deceased son, "sometimes my husband said, or I said: 'Well, now there is no money.' And then he'd say: 'well, we'll get it from wherever we can, what's important is that he's healthy and well.'" When men and women experienced AIDS-related complications, they became unable to work, digging their families into an ever deeper economic hole. For instance, Pamela was not diagnosed with HIV during her first pregnancy. While she was pregnant with their second child, her husband became ill with AIDS-related complications. The family was forced to migrate from another state to live with her male partner's family, increasing the economic precariousness of two households. Pamela said her greatest fear was her husband getting

> sick again, right now he is in bed, and he cannot do almost anything .... He will not be able to work until I don't know when. We rely on my father-in-law. And it's not the same as before. Before, my husband gave me my money, and I could buy what I wanted–things for my daughter. And now it is very different. We are dependent on my father-in-law, and with him it's only food, and hospital bills.

Death or abandonment by the male partner also left women and children in difficult economic situations. For example, at the time of the interview in March 2010, Anel was the only economic support for her family. She described being the sole breadwinner and the primacy of her job as a burden and a barrier to her HIV treatment: "I arrive too early for my appointments, and I apologize a million times, because at work they don't give me time off. And if I lose [my job] how do I eat? It is the only thing I have to support my kids."

Emotional consequences

The emotional costs of the failure to prevent vertical HIV transmission were also high, both for those women who had children living with HIV and those whose children had died of AIDS-related complications. A psychologist working in an ambulatory HIV clinic called the transmission of HIV to a child a "double grief" for their mothers.

> I am speaking about part of the Mexican culture in which the value of maternity is channelled into moral questions, questions of values, of virtues, right? A good woman is a good mother, a good mother gives everything for her child, and a good mother who gives everything for her child would not forgive herself for an irresponsible act or let herself be, let herself be-I don't know how I can express this–to not provide protection to avoid that the child be born infected. Based on my work experience, this is how I could sum it up: when children are born infected because they did not realize in time, the mothers experience a double grief and they have to work doubly hard to accept [the diagnosis]. First, to accept that they are the ones who are alive. And afterwards to work out the guilt that they were the ones who infected their children.

Women's guilt because they had, unknowingly, transmitted HIV to their children was a recurrent theme of the interviews. Gisela said that having a child who is living with HIV "isn't nice, because they are going to suffer. Right now my daughter is little and everything, but when she is bigger, she is going to say that it is my fault." Karen, who was inconsolable about the AIDS-related death of her son and wept for most of the two hour long interview, said that "it hurts me because he was a child and he wasn't guilty of anything. I feel that I am [guilty] because I did not take care of myself, and I never realized that he was sick [with AIDS-related complications]." Karen never suspected she could be living with HIV, assiduously sought health-care services during pregnancy and to promote her son's health, and still blames herself for his death. The cultural construction of motherhood that condemns women for their children's ill health, irrespective of women's circumstances and efforts to promote their children's well-being, is made clear by Lourdes' experiences with health-care providers when seeking care for her son before either of them were diagnosed with HIV. Lourdes went to the regional hospital with

> a bag of [his] medicines and prescriptions and I don't know what all. And even then the doctors who were there hit me with everything they had. They said, 'What an irresponsible mother. How is it possible that she is just letting this child die? Can you believe it?' 'No Miss, [Lourdes responded], I

am not letting him die. Here are all of his prescriptions, all of his medicines, everything that I am giving him, and he just doesn't get better.' 'Why?' I also wanted to know what was wrong with my child.

Vertical HIV transmission, disability and death among children is mainly attributable to health-care providers' failure to offer HIV testing and counseling during pregnancy and failure to recognize AIDS-related complications among children, yet women living with HIV experienced guilt and were blamed by health-care providers for their children's ill-health.

Discussion

One of the central findings of this study is that these women were in regular contact with the health-care system for ANC and on multiple other occasions while seeking a diagnosis for AIDS-related complications for themselves or other family members and that often HIV counseling and testing was not offered. For more than half of the women living with HIV, the first failure to offer HIV testing and counselling occurred when they attended ANC during pregnancy. This omission of the offer of HIV testing and counselling was then frequently repeated when women and their families subsequently sought health-care for HIV and AIDS-related complications. Consequences of the omission of the offer of HIV testing and counseling during ANC and then during repeated contacts with the health care system included: new pediatric HIV infections, including younger siblings becoming infected with HIV because the woman wasn't diagnosed during the earlier pregnancy, disease progression of women, children and male partners, and deaths due to AIDS-related causes among children and male partners. The women living with HIV who participated in the research had survived these omissions. Beyond negative health consequences, futile health-care seeking and delayed diagnoses had negative economic and emotional consequences for women living with HIV and their families.

The serious health, economic and emotional consequences of the failure to offer HIV testing and counseling during ANC and delayed HIV diagnoses for women and their families could be averted by: 1) routine PITC in ANC and 2) improved recognition of AIDS-related complications by health-care providers.

To address low levels of HIV testing during ANC internationally, both the Centers for Disease Control and Prevention in the United States and the World Health Organization have advocated routine PITC [23,24]. Studies in both high- and low-income countries have demonstrated that antenatal PITC results in significantly higher HIV screening rates and increased implementation of programs to prevent vertical HIV transmission without a corresponding drop in clinic attendance because of fears of HIV testing [25–28]. The high uptake of PITC described in this study reiterates other Mexican studies that have found that PITC in ANC is acceptable to a large proportion of pregnant women with HIV (85–90%) and emphasizes the importance of counseling that informs pregnant women that vertical HIV transmission exists, that it can be prevented, and that there is effective and free treatment for HIV disease available for women's own health [20,21]. The need to improve and monitor the quality of counseling is also highlighted by the finding that a few women understood testing during pregnancy to be compulsory, substantiating concerns that PITC can contravene principles of informed consent; it is crucial to monitor PITC to ensure informed consent and confidentiality [24,29,30].

This research also suggests that the failure to offer HIV testing and counseling in Mexico is not simply an issue of financial constraints-either for the health-care system or for individual families. Frequently ANC included many tests and procedures which are more expensive than an HIV test. In fact, some of the care provided could be considered superfluous. The most dramatic example of this was reported by Karen who underwent eight ultrasounds during ANC but was not offered an HIV test–this omission resulted in the death of her son from AIDS, the subsequent transmission of HIV to her younger daughter, and delayed her and her husband's HIV diagnosis until he was experiencing AIDS-related complications. In response to AIDS-related complications, these low-income families actively sought health-care in both the for-profit and not-for-profit sectors, and paid for physician visits, laboratory tests, medications, and surgery.

Late HIV diagnosis is a serious individual and public health problem in Mexico and around the globe. For individuals living with HIV, late diagnosis (lower CD4 count, higher viral load, or an AIDS-defining illness) has been associated with a greater probability of progression to AIDS and death [31]. In Mexico, half of those people newly diagnosed with HIV in 2011 were categorized as having AIDS [32]. Similarly, a study from a tertiary level Mexico City hospital categorized 61% of people as late-testers because within six months of diagnosis, they had CD4 counts below 200 and/or they had experienced an AIDS-defining illness [27]. Free lifelong antiretroviral treatment for people living with HIV has been available to beneficiaries of the Social Security Institutes for private and public sector workers since the late 1990 s and those without employer-provided health insurance since 2003 [33]. However, many of the women living with HIV who participated in this study and their family members weren't able to take advantage of freely available antiretroviral treatment in a timely fashion because of delayed HIV diagnosis. This study makes a novel contribution to the literature by documenting how missed opportunities to offer HIV testing and counseling to women when they attend ANC during pregnancy and to recognize the symptoms of HIV and AIDS when women and other family members seek health-care resulted in late diagnosis.

After the HIV diagnosis, women's experiences of linkage to and uptake of health-care services suggest both the existence of a relatively strong referral system within the public health-care system and women's strong motivation to prevent vertical HIV transmission and access long-term HIV care and treatment for themselves and other family members. At the time of the interview, all of the women living with HIV were participating in long-term HIV care and treatment. A small proportion of women (7 of 55, 12.7%) reported that they had delayed or interrupted HIV care and treatment for their own health. Reasons given, such as lack of knowledge about HIV disease and treatment, not having symptoms, negative interactions with health-care providers, and transportation costs have also been identified in other settings and should be addressed [34,35]. Research from sub-Saharan Africa has raised concerns about the large proportion of women (ranging from 38% to 88% depending on the study) who do not enroll in care and treatment for their own health after being diagnosed with HIV during pregnancy [35,36].

Study limitations

The experiences of women attending public HIV clinics located in three Central Mexican States may not be relevant for women of different socioeconomic status, or those who live in other areas of the country. Despite increasing coverage of HIV testing during the period under study, omission of HIV testing in ANC remains a significant problem in Mexico. The most recently published national statistics indicate that in 2012 only 59.8% of pregnant women who attended ANC were tested for HIV [16]. In addition, as women were reporting on events that could have occurred up to a decade prior to the interview, recall bias may have influenced their responses. Finally, as this study recruited women living with HIV from care and treatment clinics, it cannot provide insight into the linkage to and uptake of long-term HIV care and treatment by all women testing for HIV during ANC. Studies to explore this issue should be considered a priority for HIV research in Mexico and other Latin American countries.

Conclusions

A decade after universal HIV testing for pregnant women was included in Mexico's National Action Plan on HIV and AIDS, less than half of Mexican women attending ANC were tested for HIV [6,16]. The seriousness of the negative health, economic and emotional consequences of this omission for women and their families and the high acceptance rate of HIV testing by pregnant Mexican women are compelling arguments firstly to create a favorable policy environment by harmonizing ANC legislation with existing HIV legislation and secondly to make the necessary investments in health-care provider training, commodities, supervision and monitoring to rapidly accelerate scale-up of routine provider-initiated HIV testing and counseling during ANC. This research also documents the need to undertake national education campaigns for health-care workers about the HIV epidemic and the symptoms of AIDS in collaboration with medical and nursing schools, health-care institutions, and professional associations. There is an urgent need for both pre-service and in-service training to increase health-care providers' awareness of HIV as well as their abilities to provide HIV testing and counseling, identify HIV and AIDS-related complications, and appropriately refer people to HIV care and treatment. PITC within and beyond ANC and more pre-service and in-service medical education about HIV will not only prevent vertical HIV transmission but will reduce extremely late HIV diagnosis and facilitate timely access to free, lifesaving antiretroviral treatment for women and other family members.

Acknowledgments

This research was only possible thanks to the generosity of all of those who gave of their time and knowledge to participate, particularly the women living with HIV who shared their stories. The author received institutional support during the research and preparation of the manuscript from the Mexican non-governmental organization Balance, as well as from the Takemi Program in International Health and the Women and Health Initiative at the Harvard School of Public Health. Thanks are also due to Lauren Ng and Rebecca Hope for their helpful comments.

Author Contributions

Conceived and designed the experiments: TK. Analyzed the data: TK. Contributed reagents/materials/analysis tools: TK. Wrote the paper: TK.

References

1. UNAIDS (2011) Countdown to Zero: Global Plan Towards the Elimination of New HIV Infections Among Children by 2015 and Keeping Their Mothers Alive, 2011–2015. Geneva.
2. WHO (2010) Towards Universal Access: Scaling up priority HIV/AIDS intervention in the health sector. Progress Report 2010. Geneva.
3. UNAIDS (2012) UNAIDS World AIDS Day Report 2012. Geneva.
4. WHO UNICEF, UNAIDS (2013) Global update on HIV treatment 2013: results, impact and opportunities, June 2013 Brief summary. Geneva. WHO/HIV/2013.9 WHO/HIV/2013.9.
5. UN (2001) Declaration of Commitment on HIV/AIDS: United Nations General Assembly Special Session on HIV/AIDS, 25–27 June 2001, UNAIDS/02.31E. Geneva: UNAIDS. 92-9173-190-0 92-9173-190-0.
6. Secretaría de Salud (2002) Programa de Acción: VIH/SIDA e Infecciones de Transmisión Sexual (ITS) (2001–2006). Mexico City.
7. Secretaría de Salud (2008) Programa de Acción Especifico 2007–2012 en respuesta al VIH/SIDA e ITS. Mexico City: Secretaría de Salud.
8. Godinez Leal L (2007) Tiene Censida pruebas rápidas de VIH para embarazadas. CIMAC Noticias. Mexico City, Mexico: CIMAC.
9. Secretaría de Salud (2010) Norma Oficial Mexicana NOM-010-SSA2-2010, Para la prevención y control de la infección por de Inmunodeficiencia Humana. Mexico City: Secretaría de Salud.
10. Secretaría de Salud (1993) Norma Oficial Mexicana NOM-007-SSA2-1993, Atención de la mujer durante el embarazo, parto y puerperio y del recién nacido. Criterios y procedimientos para la prestación del servicio. Mexico City: Secretaría de Salud: Secretaría de Salud.
11. Kendall T, López-Uribe E (2010) Improving the HIV Response for Women in Latin America: Barriers to Integrated Advocacy for Sexual and Reproductive Health and Rights. Global Health Governance 4.
12. Kendall TR (2012) Prevention of Vertical HIV Transmission and the HIV Response for Women in Latin America [PhD]. Kelowna, British Columbia: University of British Columbia. 242 p.
13. Guttierez J, Rivera-Donmarco J, Shamah-Levy T, Villalpando-Hernandez S, Franco A, et al. (2013) Encuesta Nacional de Salud y Nutrición Resultados Nacionales 2012; Oropeza-Abundez C, editor. Cuernavaca: Instituto Nacional de Salud Pública.
14. CENSIDA (2009) Guía de manejo de antirretroviral de las personas con VIH, cuarta edición Mexico City: Secretaría de Salud.
15. United Nations Statisctics Division (2011) Millenium Development Goals Indicators: The official United Nations site for the MDG Indicators. In: United Nations Statisctics Division, editor.
16. CONASIDA (2013) Boletin del Grupo de Informacion Sectorial en VIH/SIDA No. 10. Mexico City: Secretaria de Salud.
17. INEGI (2009) El INEGI da a conocer los resultados de la Encuesta Nacional de Ingresos y Gastos de los Hogares (ENIGH) 2008. Comunicado numero 191/09.
18. CONEVAL (2011) Measurement: Frequently Asked Questions. Mexico City: CONEVAL.
19. Charmaz K (2005) Grounded Theory in the 21st Century: Applications for Advancing Social Justice Studies. In: Denizen NK, Lincoln YS, editors. The Sage Handbook of Qualitative Research. 3 ed. Thousand Oaks, CA: Sage Publications. 507–535.
20. Romero-Gutierrez G, Delgado-Macias AA, Mora-Escobar Y, Ponce-Ponce de Leon AL, Amador N (2007) Mexican women's reasons for accepting or declining HIV antibody testing in pregnancy. Midwifery 23: 23–27.
21. Vera Gamboa L, Gongora Biachi RA, Pavia Ruz N, Gaber Osorno J, Lara Perera D, et al. (2005) Aceptabilidad para la detección de anticuerpos contra el VIH en un grupo de mujeres embarazadas de Yucatán, México. Ginecol Obstet Mex 73: 355–359.
22. Squires KE (2007) Gender differences in the diagnosis and treatment of HIV. Gend Med 4: 294–307.
23. Branson BM, Handsfield HH, Lampe MA, Janssen RS, Taylor AW, et al. (2006) Revised Recommendations for HIV Testing of Adults, Adolescents, and Pregnant Women in Health-Care Settings. Atlanta: Centers for Disease Control and Prevention. 1–17 p.
24. WHO UNAIDS (2007) Guidance on Provider-Initiated HIV Testing and Counselling in Health Facilities. Geneva.
25. Creek TL, Ntumy R, Seipone K, Smith M, Mogodi M, et al. (2007) Successful introduction of routine opt-out HIV testing in antenatal care in Botswana. J Acquir Immune Defic Syndr 45: 102–107.
26. Manzi M, Zachariah R, Teck R, Buhendwa L, Kazima J, et al. (2005) High acceptability of voluntary counselling and HIV-testing but unacceptable loss to follow up in a prevention of mother-to-child HIV transmission programme in rural Malawi: scaling-up requires a different way of acting. Trop Med Int Health 10: 1242–1250.
27. Moses A, Zimba C, Kamanga E, Nkhoma J, Maida A, et al. (2008) Prevention of mother-to-child transmission: program changes and the effect on uptake of the HIVNET 012 regimen in Malawi. Aids 22: 83–87.
28. Walmsley S (2003) Opt in or opt out: what is optimal for prenatal screening for HIV infection? CMAJ 168: 707–708.
29. Rennie S, Behets F (2006) Desperately seeking targets: the ethics of routine HIV testing in low-income countries. Bull World Health Organ 84: 52–57.
30. Maman S, King E (2008) Changes in HIV testing policies and the implications for women. J Midwifery Womens Health 53: 195–201.
31. Egger M, May M, Chene G, Phillips AN, Ledergerber B, et al. (2002) Prognosis of HIV-1-infected patients starting highly active antiretroviral therapy: a collaborative analysis of prospective studies. Lancet 360: 119–129.
32. CENSIDA (2012) El VIH/SIDA en México 2012. Mexico City, Mexico: Secretaria de Salud.
33. Saavedra-Lopez J, Bravo-Garcia E (2006) Panorama del VIH/SIDA en el 2006. In: Rodríguez CM, Bárcenas HB, Kenefick SB, editors. SIDA: Aspectos de Salud Pública. Cuernavaca: Instituto Nacional de Salud Pública. 3–14.
34. Ferguson L, Grant AD, Lewis J, Kielman K, Watson-Jones D, et al. (2014) Linking women who test HIV-positive in pregnancy-related services to HIV care

and treatment services in Kenya: A mixed methods prospective cohort study. PLoS One 9: e89764.

35. Ferguson L, Grant AD, Watson-Jones D, Kahawita T, Ong'ech JO, et al. (2012) Linking women who test HIV-positive in pregnancy-related services to long-term HIV care and treatment services: a systematic review. Tropical Medicine & International Health 17: 564–580.

36. Watson-Jones D, Balira R, Ross DA, Weiss HA, Mabey D (2012) Missed opportunities: poor linkage to ongoing care for HIV-positive pregnant women in Mwanza, Tanzania. PLoS One 7: e40091.

7

The Mpumalanga Men's Study (MPMS): Results of a Baseline Biological and Behavioral HIV Surveillance Survey in Two MSM Communities in South Africa

Tim Lane[1]*, Thomas Osmand[1], Alexander Marr[1], Starley B. Shade[1], Kristin Dunkle[2], Theodorus Sandfort[3], Helen Struthers[4,5], Susan Kegeles[1], James A. McIntyre[4,6]

1 Center for AIDS Prevention Studies, University of California San Francisco, San Francisco, California, United States of America, **2** Rollins School of Public Health, Emory University, Atlanta, Georgia, United States of America, **3** HIV Center for Clinical and Behavioral Studies, Columbia University, New York, New York, United States of America, **4** Anova Health Institute, Johannesburg, South Africa, **5** Division of Infectious Diseases & HIV Medicine, Department of Medicine, University of Cape Town, Cape Town, South Africa, **6** School of Public Health & Family Medicine, University of Cape Town, Cape Town, South Africa

Abstract

The Mpumalanga Men's Study (MPMS) is the assessment of the Project *Boithato* HIV prevention intervention for South African MSM. *Boithato* aims to increase consistent condom use, regular testing for HIV-negative MSM, and linkage to care for HIV-positive MSM. The MPMS baseline examined HIV prevalence and associated risk behaviors, and testing, care, and treatment behaviors among MSM in Gert Sibande and Ehlanzeni districts in Mpumalanga province, South Africa in order to effectively target intervention activities. We recruited 307 MSM in Gert Sibande and 298 in Ehlanzeni through respondent-driven sampling (RDS) between September 2012-March 2013. RDS-adjusted HIV prevalence estimates are 28.3% (95% CI 21.1%–35.3%) in Gert Sibande, and 13.7% (95% CI 9.1%–19.6%) in Ehlanzeni. Prevalence is significantly higher among MSM over age 25 [57.8% (95% CI 43.1%–72.9%) vs. 17.9% (95% CI 10.6%–23.9%), $P<0.001$ in Gert Sibande; 34.5% (95%CI 20.5%–56.0%) vs. 9.1% (95% CI 4.6%–13.9%), $P<0.001$ in Ehlanzeni]. In Gert Sibande, prevalence is higher among self-identified gay and transgender MSM vs. other MSM [39.3% (95%CI, 28.3%–47.9%), $P<0.01$], inconsistent condom users [38.1% (18.1%–64.2%), $P<0.05$], those with a current regular male partner [35.0% (27.1%–46.4%), $P<0.05$], and those with lifetime experience of intimate partner violence with men [40.4%, (95%CI 28.9%–50.9%), $P<0.05$]. Prevalence of previous HIV testing was 65.8% (95%CI 58.8%–74.0%) in Gert Sibande, and 69.3% (95%CI 61.9%–76.8%) in Ehlanzeni. Regular HIV testing was uncommon [(34.6%, (95%CI 27.9%–41.4%) in Gert Sibande; 31.0% (95%CI 24.9%–37.8%) in Ehlanzeni]. Among HIV-positive participants, few knew their status (28.1% in Gert Sibande and 14.5% in Ehlanzeni), or were appropriately linked to care (18.2% and 11.3%, respectively), or taking antiretroviral therapy (13.6% and 9.6% respectively). MPMS results demonstrate the importance of implementing interventions for MSM to increase consistent condom use, regular HIV testing, and linkage and engagement in care for HIV-infected MSM.

Editor: Susan Marie Graham, University of Washington, United States of America

Funding: This research was supported by the National Institute of Allergy and Infectious Disease (NIAID) R01AI089292. The funder had no role in the study design, data collection and analysis, decision to publish, or preparation of the manuscript.

Competing Interests: The authors have declared that no competing interests exist.

* Email: Tim.Lane@ucsf.edu

Introduction

Multiple studies have confirmed the severity of the HIV epidemic among men who have sex with men (MSM) in sub-Saharan African countries. [1–8] In South Africa, surveys of the MSM population have found prevalence of 13.2% in Soweto, [9] 25.5% in Cape Town, [10] 27.5% in Durban, and 49.5% in greater Johannesburg. [11] HIV incidence among MSM in the region is also high. One cohort study in Kenya estimated incidence at 5.8 per 100 person-years for men who have sex with both men and women, and 35.2 per 100 person-years for men who have sex with men exclusively; [12] another found 6.8 per 100 person-years in its MSM cohort. [13] Behavioral factors may not by themselves provide a compelling explanation of high HIV prevalence and incidence of infection among MSM. [14,15] Sexual transmission between men in the region is likely facilitated by a combination of biological, structural, and social factors, including high per-act transmission risks of anal intercourse; criminalization of homosexuality in most countries, which has been used to exclude many MSM from receiving HIV services [16]; and experiences of stigma and discrimination, particularly in the health sector, which discourage MSM from accessing available prevention and treatment services [2,6,11,17–19].

The Republic of South Africa's explicit constitutional prohibition of discrimination on the basis of sexual orientation is unique in Africa; there are no legal barriers to providing HIV services to MSM in RSA. The World Health Organization recommends "regular" HIV testing for key affected populations, including

MSM. [20] The United States Centers for Disease Control and Prevention (CDC) recommends MSM test regularly at least every six months. [21] Although there has been a dramatic expansion of treatment and prevention programming since 2009, [22] it is not known whether South African MSM currently access testing and treatment services in proportion to their need, or in sufficient numbers to check the further spread of the epidemic. In particular, critical data gaps exist for this key population on regular HIV testing, timely diagnosis of HIV infection, and timely linkage to HIV care.

To address the unmet need for targeted MSM interventions in South Africa, we established the Project Boithato HIV prevention intervention for South African MSM. Boithato is adapted from Mpowerment, a multilevel HIV prevention intervention that is effective at increasing consistent condom use among MSM. [23–25] As adapted, Boithato is designed to encourage greater uptake of prevention and treatment behaviors, including consistent condom use, regular HIV testing (following the CDC recommendation of every 6 months) among HIV-negative MSM, and linkage to HIV care among HIV-positive MSM.

The Mpumalanga Men's Study is intended to evaluate the effectiveness of Boithato. MPMS is a set of serial cross-sectional, integrated biological and behavioral HIV surveillance surveys of the MSM population in the Boithato intervention community in Gert Sibande district municipality, and the comparison community in Ehlanzeni district municipality. Gert Sibande is a primarily rural district whose primary industries include agriculture, coal mining, and electricity production. Its Census 2011 population was 1.04 million. The seat of District government is Msukaligwa (Ermelo) local municipality. Ehlanzeni is also a largely rural district of 1.69 million, whose primary industries include agriculture and tourism. The seat of District government is Mbombela (Nelspruit), which is also the seat of Mpumalanga's provincial government. [26] The two districts share a border. Each is well connected to Johannesburg (roughly 200 km from Msukaligwa and 400 km from Mbombela) by well-maintained national highways. The main population centers of each district are roughly 200 km apart over relatively poorly maintained rural roads (See Figure 1 for a map of Mpumalanga).

The baseline assessment was completed between September 2012 and March 2013, prior to the Boithato intervention launch in April 2013, with follow-up assessments at 12-months and 18-months post-intervention. MSM are recruited into each wave of the assessment through respondent-driven sampling (RDS). Independent samples are recruited in each district, and each RDS recruitment wave is independent of the preceding wave. Each follow-up wave will track recapture of participants from the previous wave; staff will initiate targeted recruitment of those participants not recaptured through RDS.

In this paper, we describe the results of the MPMS baseline assessment survey of the two MSM communities. We report findings on HIV prevalence, associated risk behaviors, and health-seeking behaviors as they relate to the Boithato efficacy assessment's primary endpoints: consistent condom use, regular uptake of HIV testing, and regular uptake of care among HIV-positive MSM.

Methods

Recruitment and Study Procedures

Recruitment into the MPMS baseline assessment wave began simultaneously in each district and continued over 24 weeks of recruitment between September 2012 and March 2013. Following RDS recruitment procedures described by Heckathorn, [27,28] seed participants were identified at each MPMS site based on a matrix of criteria designed to encourage the recruitment of a diverse sample of MSM from each district. These criteria included age, self-described sexual identity (e.g., gay, bisexual), educational attainment, and place of residence within the district. Each site launched recruitment with two seed participants recruited by MPMS staff, who then recruited non-seed participants, by means of study-issued coupons; these non-seed participants in turn recruited other non-seed participants via coupons, and so on. Coupons were pre-printed with an alphanumeric code consisting of a letter to identify recruitment site, a four-digit number (2000–2999) to facilitate tracking of recruitment chains, and a study phone number for recruits to call or text the local MPMS office for additional information and schedule an interview appointment. The study issued up to three recruitment coupons sequentially to each participant who completed the required study procedures, with instructions to recruit three other MSM from within their social network within the following four weeks by giving them a coupon. Monitoring of recruitment and sample characteristics at each site occurred on a weekly basis. Staff purposefully recruited two seeds to launch recruitment at each site, and additional seeds as needed based on weekly assessments of sample diversity with respect to the demographic variables of interest listed above. In total, 8 seeds were recruited in Gert Sibande, and 11 in Ehlanzeni. Participants received their choice of a mobile phone air-time voucher or a supermarket gift voucher valued at ZAR30 (US$3.00) for each participant successfully recruited and enrolled.

MSM over the age of 18 in possession of a valid study coupon, who lived, worked, or socialized with other MSM in the district where he received the coupon, and who reported anal or oral sexual activity with a man in the previous six months were eligible to enroll in the study. Recruits were screened for eligibility by MPMS staff through verification that the potential participant was in possession of a valid study coupon received from someone he knew, and by asking ten standardized screening questions about sexual activity designed to elicit answers indicative of specialized knowledge of the local MSM population and its social and sexual behaviors. To prevent the possibility that ineligible individuals could be coached into providing acceptable answers, no more than four questions were asked on any given day, and the order of questions was rotated. Individuals were deemed ineligible if they were not in possession of a coupon given to them by someone they knew, if they did not report sexual activity with another man within the specified time period, or if their replies to screening questions suggested the recruit was not likely a member of the target MSM population.

Eligible recruits who wished to enroll in the study were then asked to provide their fingerprint through the use of a commercially available digital fingerprint scanner (360 Biometrics, San Jose, CA). The scanner worked with software to generate a unique, anonymous, numeric study code for each participant, which was then linked to their coupon recruitment code. This fingerprint-generated personal identification number (PID) was used both for registration and identification purposes for future study visits to collect HIV test results or secondary study incentives, and to link a participant's behavioral data to his HIV testing results.

Participants' behavioral data were collected via an interviewer-administered computer-assisted interview on an ASUS Eee PC 1011CX N2600 netbook programmed with a QDS survey (NOVA Research, Bethesda, MD). Interviews took approximately 45–60 minutes. Interviews took place primarily in English, with interviewers offering simultaneous translation into isiZulu, Siswati, or Sesotho as requested. Data was collected over ten domains

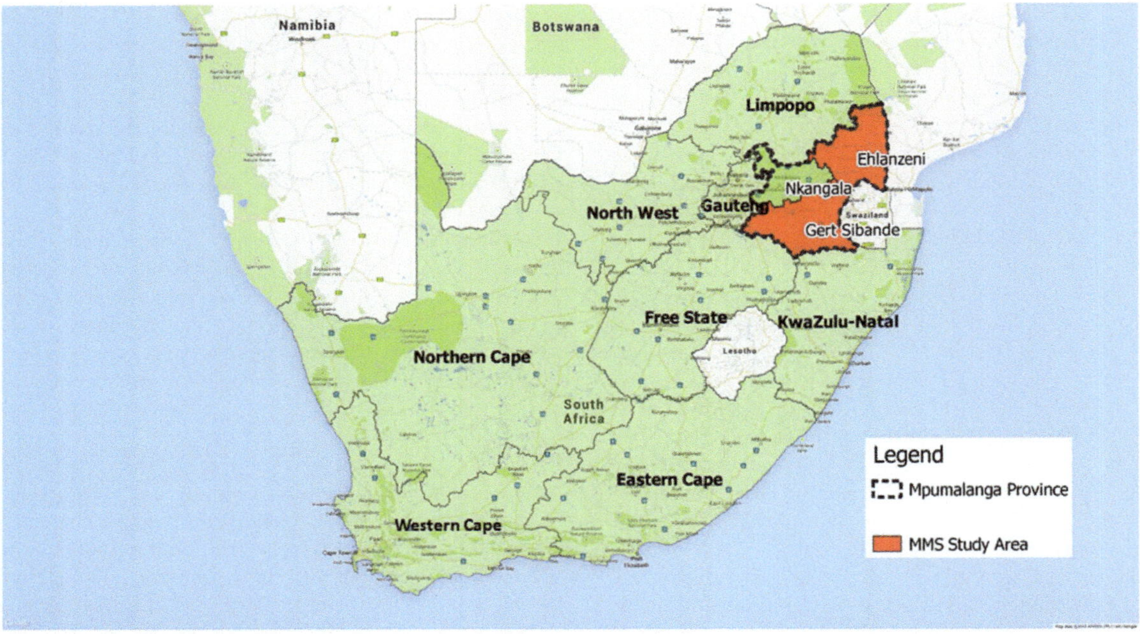

Figure 1. Location of Gert Sibande and Ehlanzeni District Municipalities, Mpumalanga Province, South Africa.

including: demographic characteristics and RDS-specific network size questions; condom use self-efficacy and safer sex social norms; perceived community cohesion and collective power; alcohol and other drug use; sexual behaviors with up to 5 of their most recent female or male sexual partners in the prior six months; knowledge of HIV transmission and prevention; knowledge and recent history of STI symptoms; experiences of MSM- or HIV-related stigma and discrimination; intimate partner violence (IPV) with regular and non-regular sexual partners; and HIV testing and treatment history and behaviors. Participants were compensated ZAR100 (~US$10) for their time and effort in completing the survey. Participants were then offered rapid HIV testing and the option of receiving results. Participants provided separate informed consent for HIV testing per South African law. Study staff followed South African national HIV guidelines for HIV counseling, testing, and referral services.

Return of HIV results to participants was strongly encouraged but not mandatory for purposes of survey compensation of receiving recruitment coupons. For HIV-positive participants who opted to receive their results, results disclosure, post-test counseling, and appropriate referral to care and treatment were provided immediately following the rapid tests for HIV. Anova Health Institute's "Health4Men" program (www.health4men.co.za) provided training to clinical staff at four Mpumalanga Provincial Department of Health (MPDOH) referral clinics (2 per district) on providing culturally competent HIV and STI care for MSM. All participants received information packs that included condoms, water-based lubricant packets, and contact information for local referral clinics. All participants who received HIV-positive results or who reported currently experiencing STI symptoms (e.g., urethral discharge, genital ulcer) were provided with a referral letter from the study addressed to the clinics and describing their clinical needs.

Participants received up to three study coupons to recruit members of their social network after their fingerprick for HIV rapid results, but before results disclosure for those who opted to receive their results. For those who opted not to test, recruitment coupons were issued at the conclusion of the survey.

Measurement

The behavioral survey was based on a standardized behavioral surveillance survey for MSM which had been adapted [9,29] and used previously with South African MSM. For this assessment, we included psychosocial measures adapted by Kegeles and colleagues for the Mpowerment assessment instrument, [23] as well as additional behavioral and community measurements appropriate to the risk behavior, HIV testing, and HIV treatment behavioral outcomes of the efficacy assessment. Measurements described below pertain only to results presented in the current analysis.

Demographic indicators: Participants reported their age, highest level of educational attainment (secondary/post-secondary education), and employment in the prior six months. Participants were asked how frequently they ran out of money for basic needs in the prior six months (never/rarely/sometimes/often/always). Participants self-identified their sexual orientation as gay, bisexual, heterosexual, transgender or woman, or other.

Behavioral and HIV indicators: Participants reported the number and types of sexual partnerships with female and male partners in the prior six months. Partner types were dichotomized as "regular" and "non-regular". Regular partnerships with men and women were defined as "someone whom you lived with, saw a lot, or felt a special emotional connection to," and assessed as ever had and currently has a regular partner. Transactional sex was assessed by asking whether participants had ever received from or provided to a partner any of the following in exchange for sex: money or valuable goods or services, food or shelter, or drugs or alcohol. Consistent condom use was assessed by self-report on a per-partner basis. Participants were first asked to list up to 5 partners (male or female) in the prior six months, the number of vaginal, insertive anal, or receptive anal sex acts with each partner, and the number of those acts where a condom was used (protected acts). Those reporting an equal number of sex acts and protected acts were classified as consistent condom users, those with fewer protected acts than sex acts as inconsistent condom users. Alcohol consumption was assessed by the AUDIT-C screening measure, a 3-item screen asking about alcohol use in the last year, number of alcoholic drinks consumed in a typical day of drinking, and frequency of drinking six or more drinks in one day. A score of 4 or more in males is interpreted as indicative of alcohol misuse. [30] For the current analysis, because the vast majority of participants had scores indicating misuse, we separately classified those reporting drinking six or more drinks on a typical day of drinking more than one time per month in the last year as "heavy drinkers"; those who drank less were classified as "non-heavy drinkers". Marijuana and other substance use was assessed by asking if participants had ever used marijuana, cocaine, methamphetamine ("tik"), ecstasy, or methcathinone ("khat") and whether they had used these in the previous six months. IPV victimization was assessed by asking whether participants had ever been physically assaulted (hit, beaten, or kicked) or sexually assaulted (coercion or rape) by male partners in the prior six months. Those who reported either experience were classified as having experienced IPV.

HIV testing history and behaviors were assessed by asking whether participants had ever tested, how many times they had tested, when they last tested, and the result of their last test. MSM who had tested more than once and who reported an HIV-negative test result at their last test, were asked to describe the frequency of HIV testing as at least once every six months, at least once annually, or less than annually. Those who reported testing at least once every six months were classified as regular testers.

Knowledge of HIV infection, recency of HIV infection and linkage to HIV care are composite measures of multiple survey items. Individuals whose rapid HIV test result was positive and who self-reported their HIV-positive status were classified as aware of their HIV infection; those whose rapid test result was positive and who self-reported never having tested or having received a result of HIV-negative or indeterminate on their last HIV test were classified as newly diagnosed HIV infection (also presented as undiagnosed HIV infection in Figure 2). Those individuals whose rapid test result was positive and who self-reported an HIV-negative result within the prior 12 months were classified as a recent HIV infection. Those who self-reported their last HIV test result prior to the survey as HIV-positive were classified as linked to care if they self-reported seeking medical attention for HIV within 30 days of their HIV diagnosis. Current use of antiretroviral therapy was established by self-report.

Laboratory procedures

HIV infection was established by interpreting results of fingerprick blood samples on approved commercial rapid HIV testing kits using a parallel testing algorithm. Consenting participants were tested using EZ Trust Rapid Anti-HIV (1 &2) (CS Innovation, Singapore) [hereafter A1] and First Response HIV 1–2.0 Rapid test kits (Premier Medical Corporation, Ltd., India) [hereafter A2]. A1 and A2 non-reactive samples were interpreted as negative. A1 and A2 reactive samples were interpreted as positive. The protocol called for A1 reactive and A2 non-reactive samples to be interpreted as indeterminate and to refer participants to a local accredited laboratory for confirmatory testing following the laboratory's approved protocols for ELISA using blood collected via venipuncture.

Statistical methods

Population prevalence estimates of demographic characteristics, HIV infection, and associated risk and health-seeking behaviors

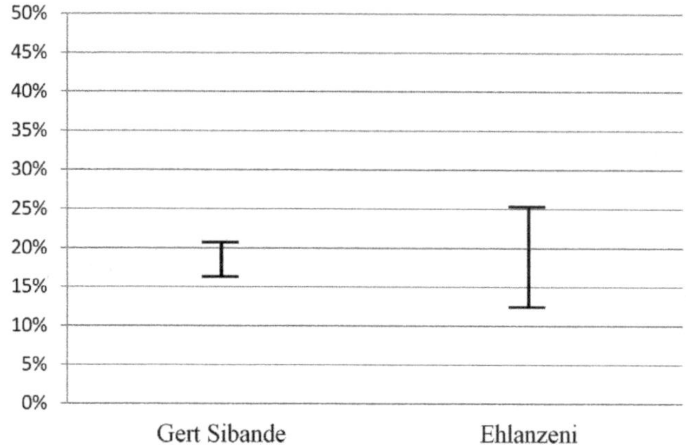

Figure 2. Plausibility Bounds of Undiagnosed HIV Infection. The graph indicates the upper and lower plausibility bounds of undiagnosed infection in Mpumalanga MSM. We estimate that between 16.3% and 20.6% of MSM in Gert Sibande, and 12.5% and 25.2% in Ehlanzeni, currently have an undiagnosed HIV infection. This range between lower and upper plausibility boundaries accounts for the small number of participants at each site who declined testing. The upper plausibility bound assumes all untested participants are HIV-positive, and the lower assumes all untested participants are HIV-negative.

were calculated using RDSAT software version 7.1 (www.respondentdrivesampling.org). Because a small number of participants declined HIV rapid testing, undiagnosed HIV infection is presented as a range of upper and lower RDS-adjusted proportions where all non-testers were classified as HIV-positive and HIV-negative, respectively. We employed weighted logistic regression to describe the relationship between demographic and behavioral variables and HIV infection using individualized HIV outcome weights calculated in RDSAT [31,32]. Bivariable analyses were conducted in SAS, version 9.2 (Cary, NC). Statistical associations were determined by chi-square tests at $P<0.05$ significance level. Small cell sizes prevented calculation of RDS adjusted estimates and/or 95% confidence intervals for some variables: these are noted in Tables 1–3 as "NC." In addition, small cell sizes prevented meaningful RDS-adjusted estimates of linkage and utilization of care variables in Table 4: these results are presented as unadjusted proportions of the crude sample at each site. In our presentation of results below, we describe RDS-adjusted results in the present tense under the RDS assumption that these estimates apply to the entire population at present, and unadjusted (crude) sample results in the past tense as these refer specifically to the properties of the sample at the time it was recruited.

Ethics Statement

This study was approved by the University of Witwatersrand Human Research Ethic Committee (Medical) (FWA00000715) and the University of California, San Francisco Committee on Human Research (FWA00000068). All participants in this study were requested to provide written informed consent to both the behavioral questionnaire and voluntary counseling and testing (VCT). Participants who wished to remain anonymous were encouraged to use a pseudonym. All participants were able to opt out of any portion of the study.

Table 1. Demographic Indicators for Mpumalanga Men's Study.

Measure	Gert Sibande (N = 307)				Ehlanzeni (N = 298)			
	Crude		Adjusted		Crude		Adjusted	
	N	%	%	95% CI	N	%	%	95% CI
Age								
18–24	199	64.8	70.4	62.8–77.5	206	69.6	72	63.1–77.4
25+	108	35.2	29.6	22.5–37.2	90	30.4	28	22.6–36.9
Highest Education Attained								
Secondary or less	199	65.5	64.2	55.1–71.4	121	41.2	47.3	38.2–54.3
Tertiary	105	34.5	35.8	28.6–45.0	173	58.8	52.7	45.7–61.8
Employment in Last 6 Months								
Had paid work	122	39.7	35.7	28.9–44.1	129	43.3	40.7	34.4–49.7
No paid work	185	60.3	64.3	55.9–71.1	169	56.7	59.3	50.3–65.6
Ran out of Money for Basic Needs in Last 6 Months								
Never/Rarely	148	48.2	45	37.6–53.1	169	56.7	45.6	38.7–54.0
Sometimes/Often/Always	159	51.8	55	46.9–62.4	129	43.3	54.4	46.0–61.3
Sexual Orientation								
Gay/Homosexual	163	53.1	46.6	38.3–55.5	151	50.7	44.5	26.6–44.1
Bisexual	128	41.7	45.4	37.3–53.7	92	30.9	35.3	36.0–51.7
Heterosexual	13	4.2	7.3	NC	7	2.4	4.5	NC
Trans/Woman	1	0.3	0.1	NC	5	1.7	0.6	NC
Other	0	0	0	NC	4	1.3	2	NC
None Reported	2	0.7	0.6	NC	39	13.1	13.1	7.7–20.3

NC = Not calculated due to small cell size.

Table 2. Behavioural and HIV Indicators in Mpumalanga Men's Study.

Measure	Gert Sibande (N = 307)				Ehlanzeni (N = 298)			
	Crude		Adjusted		Crude		Adjusted	
	N	%	%	95% CI	N	%	%	95% CI
Female Partners								
Current regular female partner	113	38.6	40.6	32.2–48.9	67	22.7	25.7	18.05–33.2
Past female partners	85	27.7	32.3	24.9–40.2	67	22.7	23.2	17.5–29.9
Never had a female partner	109	35.5	27.1	19.4–35.7	161	54.6	51.1	43.4–58.2
Male Partners								
Current regular male partner	215	70.5	66.0	58.2–73.7	224	75.7	74.2	65.9–79.9
Past regular male partner	63	20.7	21.7	7.3–18.5	21	7.1	5.7	2.4–11.5
Never had a male partner	27	8.9	12.2	7.3–18.5	51	17.2	20.1	14.2–27.5
Number of Female Partners in Last 6 Months								
None	286	93.2	91.9	88.5–95.3	292	98.0	97.7	95.7–99.3
>=1 Partner	21	6.8	8.1	4.7–11.5	6	2.0	2.3	NC
Number of Male Partners in Last 6 Months								
=1 Partner	188	61.2	70.3	62.8–76.4	172	57.7	62.2	53.5–69.0
>=2 Partners	119	38.8	29.7	23.6–37.2	126	42.3	37.8	31.0–46.5
Transactional Sex								
Received money, other goods	57	18.6	21.1	14.8–28.5	34	11.4	13.2	81.9–92.0
Gave money, other goods	35	11.4	12.7	8.0–19.0	22	7.4	9.0	4.2–14.0
Condom Use with Last 5 Male Partners								
Consistent	244	83.3	85.1	78.2–90.7	169	58.9	63.7	55.9–70.1
Inconsistent	49	16.7	14.9	9.3–21.8	118	41.1	36.3	29.9–44.1
Drink>=6 Drinks in One Sitting								
Never	49	16	17.4	11.4–23.4	127	42.6	41.3	34.9–49.3
<1/month	114	37.1	42.7	34.2–50.9	68	22.8	23.9	16.3–28.8
2–4 times/month	141	45.9	39.9	32.5–48.5	79	26.5	26.5	20.8–33.8
2–3 times/week	0	0	0	NC	17	5.7	6.6	3.4–10.8
More than 4 times/week	3	1	0	NC	7	2.3	1.6	NC
Marijuana								
Used in past 6 months	35	11.4	8.2	4.6–11.6	7	2.3	0.4	NC
Partner Violence								
Any victimization in past 6 months	142	46.3	38.4	29.8–46.1	37	12.4	12.8	7.8–19.1
HIV Testing Behavior								
Ever Tested in Lifetime								
Yes	223	72.6	65.8	58.8–74.0	213	71.5	69.3	61.9–76.8

Table 2. Cont.

Measure	Gert Sibande (N = 307)				Ehlanzeni (N = 298)			
	Crude		Adjusted		Crude		Adjusted	
	N	%	%	95% CI	N	%	%	95% CI
No	84	27.4	34.2	26.0–41.2	85	28.5	30.7	23.2–38.1
Regular Tester[1]	115	37.5	34.6	27.9–41.4	97	32.6	31.0	24.9–37.8
HIV Rapid Test Result								
Positive	110	35.8	28.3	21.1–35.3	62	20.8	13.7	9.1–19.6
Negative	185	60.3	67.8	61.0–75.4	197	66.1	72.4	65.2–78.5
Not Tested	12	3.9	3.9	1.4–6.5	39	13.1	13.9	8.8–19.8

NC = Not calculated due to small cell size.
[1]"Regular tester":>1 lifetime HIV test & tests every 6 months.

Results

Demographic characteristics of the two communities are presented in Table 1. The MSM population in these two Mpumalanga districts is young, largely under the age of 25. Each MSM community is characterized by relatively low levels of post-secondary education and regular employment, and nearly half of MSM in each community run short of money to meet their basic needs. The overwhelming majority of MSM describe themselves as either "gay" or "bisexual," with similar proportions of MSM in each community self-describing their sexual identity as "gay." Bisexual identity is more common among Gert Sibande MSM than among Ehlanzeni MSM. Few participants identify as transgender women. A sizeable proportion of MSM in Ehlanzeni do not identify as "gay," "bisexual," "heterosexual," or "transgender" categories.

Key behavioral indicators are described In Table 2. Sizeable proportions of MSM have ever had a regular female partner, and most have ever had a regular male partner. Around a third of MSM had only one male partner in the prior six months, with large majorities reporting using condoms consistently with their male partners. Transactional sex is relatively common among MSM in Mpumalanga, and particularly in the Gert Sibande district where more than 1 in 5 MSM have received money, goods or services in exchange for sex. IPV is also common, particularly in Gert Sibande where nearly 2 in 5 MSM have been physically or sexually assaulted by a male partner. Substance use in the Mpumalanga MSM population is limited primarily to heavy alcohol use, where more than one-third of Ehlanzeni MSM and one-half of Gert Sibande MSM drank 6 or more alcoholic drinks in one sitting at least twice per month. Marijuana (known locally as "dagga") is much less common. Less than one percent use stimulants including methamphetamine ("tik"), methcathinone ("khat"), cocaine, and ecstasy (data not shown).

Previous HIV testing is common among Mpumalanga MSM: around two-thirds of MSM in the two districts had tested for HIV at least once. Regular HIV testing, however, was not common, with only a third of MSM in each district reporting testing at least once every six months (See Table 2). Fifty-one MSM declined to test in the study; consequently, we estimate that at least 3.9% of MSM in Gert Sibande and 13.9% in Ehlanzeni are reluctant to test, despite a culturally competent testing environment.

We estimate HIV prevalence at 28.3% (95% CI 21.1%–35.3%) among Gert Sibande MSM, and 13.7% (95% CI 9.1–19.6%) among Ehlanzeni MSM (Table 2). HIV-positive men were disproportionately gay-identified, and 25 years of age or older—in each district, prevalence was 3 times greater in the older age group. In bivariable analysis (Table 3), HIV infection among Gert Sibande MSM was significantly associated with age 25 years or older, having a regular male partner, inconsistent condom use, and experiencing IPV from a male partner. In Ehlanzeni, age 25 years or older and consistent condom use were associated with HIV infection.

We estimate that 16.3% to 20.6% of MSM in Gert Sibande, and 12.5% to 25.2% in Ehlanzeni, currently have an undiagnosed HIV infection (Figure 2). Included in this measure were all MSM who tested positive in the survey, and those who had either never tested, or who self-reported the result of their last test as negative. (*N.B.* All participants who had self-reported the result of their last HIV test as positive provided a rapid-test sample that confirmed their HIV-positive serostatus for the study.) We present these estimates as a range between lower and upper plausibility boundaries due to the small number of participants at each site (12 and 39, respectively) who declined testing. The upper

Table 3. Associations between HIV infection and demographic and behavioural indicators in Mpumalanga Men's Study.

Measure	Gert Sibande (N = 307)	Ehlanzeni (N = 298)
	Adj % (95% CI)	Adj % (95% CI)
Age		
18–24	17.9 (10.6–23.9)	9.1 (4.6–13.9)
25+	57.8 (43.1–72.9)***	34.5 (20.5–56.0)***
Sexual Identity		
Gay/Trans/Woman	39.3 (26.1–48.2)	13.8 (8.3–21.7)
Bisexual	20.2 (11.4–28.8)	21.3 (10.5–31.2)
None Reported	NC	14.4 (0.0–34.9)
Current Regular Female Partner	20.7 (8.3–28.1)	13.4 (1.0–14.6)
Male Partners		
Current regular male partner	35.0 (27.1–46.4)**	15.0 (8.8–23.3)
Past regular male partners	16.1 (7.2–30.5)	6.8 (0.0–21.1)
Never had a regular male partner	7.6 (0.5–20.2)	24.5 (8.6–40.2)
Transactional Sex		
Received money, goods, services	29.50 (15.2–49.5)	13.5 (2.9–39.6)
Provided money, goods, services	42.70 (16.8–70.4)	NC
Condom Use with Male Partner (6 months)		
Consistent	26.6 (19.2–35.3)	26.7 (17.2–34.3)*
Inconsistent	38.1 (18.1–64.2)*	11.6 (6.0–19.9)
Alcohol Consumption		
"Heavy drinkers"	30.8 (18.2–39.7)	18.2 (8.–27.5)
Never drank heavily	22.4 (9.8–35.4)	18.7 (10.2–31.3)
Marijuana Use (6 Months)	14.4 (2.7–30.3)	NC
IPV with Male Partners	40.4 (28.9–50.9)*	NC
Negative Result on Last HIV Test	16.2 (8.8–22.9)	14.3 (3.5–17.0)

*p<0.05, **p<0.01, ***p<0.001 NC = Not calculated due to small cell size.

plausibility bound assumes all untested participants are HIV-positive, and the lower assumes all untested participants are HIV-negative.

We present unadjusted analysis of HIV testing utilization, linkage, and treatment among the subset of HIV-positive MSM in each sample in Table 4. No indeterminate results were observed through rapid testing. Roughly 1 in 4 HIV-positive Gert Sibande participants and 1 in 7 Ehlanzeni participants were aware of their HIV infection. Fewer than 1 in 5 HIV-positive participants were linked to care, and roughly 1 in 10 were taking antiretroviral therapy. We observed that 1 in 5 MSM in Gert Sibande, and 2 in 5 in Ehlanzeni, who had received an HIV-negative test result within the 12 months prior to the survey, were diagnosed with HIV through rapid HIV testing in the MPMS and referred to care.

Table 4. Utilization of Testing and Care Among HIV+ MSM in Mpumalanga Men's Study.

Measure	Gert Sibande (N = 307)	Ehlanzeni (N = 298)
	% (n)	% (n)
HIV Rapid Test Result Positive	35.8 (110)	20.8 (62)
Previously aware of HIV positive status	28.1 (31)	14.5 (9)
Linked to care	18.2 (20)	11.3 (7)
Currently taking ART	13.6 (15)	9.6 (6)
Newly diagnosed HIV+	71.8 (79)	85.4 (53)
Never tested for HIV	31.6 (25)	37.7 (20)
Recent HIV infection (12 months)	22.1 (30)	39.6 (21)

NB: Figures are not RDS-adjusted estimates; all variables other than rapid results are self-reported.

Discussion

These results demonstrate Mpumalanga MSM do not currently access HIV testing, care and treatment services in proportion to what is needed to substantially impact the course of the epidemic in this population. We observed high HIV prevalence in these communities, low uptake of regular HIV testing, and consequently a high burden of undiagnosed HIV infection. If unaddressed, this high burden of undiagnosed HIV infection will lead to increased morbidity and mortality and continued transmission of HIV within these communities of MSM. That we observed a third of the MSM in our sample who had tested negative within the last twelve moths had been infected by the time of their enrolment suggests high incidence in this population and the urgent need for expanding prevention, testing, care, and treatment programming for MSM.

HIV prevalence is markedly higher among Gert Sibande MSM than among Ehlanzeni MSM. We speculate that lower prevalence in Ehlanzeni may be attributable to the higher level of tertiary education observed in this MSM community compared to that of Gert Sibande. We further speculate that higher background HIV prevalence in Gert Sibande among the general population, (estimated at 40.5% among women from antenatal surveillance), may also contribute to higher prevalence among MSM in this district. [33] (The severity of the HIV epidemic in Gert Sibande district had not been documented at the time the sites were selected for the trial in 2010.) Nonetheless, distribution of HIV by age is markedly similar between districts: we observed prevalence roughly 3 times higher among men aged 25 and older compared to men 18–24. Additionally, in both districts HIV disproportionately affects MSM who self-identify either as gay, transsexual, or bisexual. This finding corroborates others where elevated prevalence among MSM who are gay or bisexually identified was observed. [9] It also indicates that those MSM most affected by HIV in South Africa are also those most open about their sexuality, and potentially most easily reached by existing MSM intervention models' focus on the specialized prevention needs of gay and bisexually identified MSM. Moreover, the lower observed prevalence among MSM under the age of 25 indicates that reaching younger MSM with interventions to reinforce HIV prevention behaviors including consistent condom use may yield significant results in checking the spread of HIV as MSM progress through their adult lives. Like Mpowerment, the Boithato intervention focuses explicitly on mobilizing gay- and bisexual-identified MSM to support each other in risk reduction, and has been adapted to provide a structured way of informing MSM about clinical HIV services, and for MSM to support each other to access those services they need. These would include pre- and post-exposure chemoprophylaxis and other HIV treatment services that are currently available or may soon be made available to them.

We observed significantly higher HIV prevalence among MSM in current regular partnerships than among those with non-regular partners. Other data from South Africa show that risk behavior is more likely to take place in partnerships perceived as regular versus non-regular, and that regular partnerships are often not long-lasting. [34,35] In light of MPMS findings of low prevalence of regular testing and high prevalence of undiagnosed HIV, coupled with previous studies showing that MSM in regular partnerships are not likely to communicate about HIV status, [36] it is unlikely that unprotected sex between partners reflects negotiated safety based on individuals' accurate knowledge of their HIV status and disclosure of that status to a partner. Rather, given the low utilization of regular HIV testing, higher prevalence among those in regular partnerships is more likely indicative of a high probability of HIV transmission within these partnerships. This suggests that interventions focused on communication between sexual partners about condom use and testing for HIV, including testing for HIV as a couple, may potentially be of great benefit to MSM. Increasing efficacy for communication between partners about condom use and HIV testing, including couples testing, are among the prevention behaviors that the adapted Boithato intervention aims to encourage. MSM couples-based testing has been shown to be acceptable to South African MSM, [37,38] and is available in Mpumalanga, but does not appear currently to be well-utilized by MSM.

The number of MSM in the MPMS baseline who were aware of their HIV-positive status and had linked to care, while well below optimum levels, was comparable to what has been observed generally in the Sub-Saharan Africa region. [39] Among men who were already aware of their HIV infection, the proportion reporting being linked to care was similar to what has been observed among MSM in comparatively higher-income settings in the USA. [40] However, it is unknown whether these participants' post-diagnosis health-seeking behavior is typical for South African MSM. On the basis of other data, we hypothesize that this is not likely to be typical behavior for Mpumalanga MSM; rather, these HIV-positive participants may be relatively empowered individuals who previously sought HIV testing and attended clinics despite social vulnerabilities that are highly prevalent in this population, including low socioeconomic status and limited educational attainment, associated with low uptake of testing, [41] and clinical environments perceived to be unwelcoming to MSM. [18,19] These MSM have therefore found their way into care despite the lack of social interventions to encourage and support testing and treatment behaviors among MSM, or structural interventions in clinical settings. The baseline assessment provided the initial HIV diagnosis for nearly three-quarters of HIV-infected MSM in this sample. There is a high likelihood that most of these participants will be recaptured in subsequent analysis waves, which will provide a more accurate understanding of post-diagnosis health seeking behaviors, as well as an assessment of whether the social support provided by the Boithato intervention offers additional impetus to successful linkage and engagement in care.

The Boithato intervention aims in part to encourage greater uptake of both regular HIV testing and treatment. In conjunction with the MPMS and Project Boithato, the Anova Health Institute has established a culturally competent standard of care in Mpumalanga for MSM though its Health4Men program (www.health4men.co.za). Follow-up assessments of Project Boithato will consequently measure whether direct exposures to and community diffusion of the Boithato intervention provides additional impetus towards regular utilization of HIV testing, diagnosis of HIV, and linkage and engagement in care in a culturally competent clinical setting.

Limitations of the MPMS include those that pertain to the assumptions of RDS methodology: specifically, that unbiased RDS estimates depend on fulfilling several related assumptions, namely that MSM in each district form a single, networked population; that individuals can accurately assess their personal network size; and that the crude samples were sufficiently representative of the underlying characteristics of the population. The disproportionate number of young men in these crude samples may have biased RDS-adjusted estimates towards characteristics of this subpopulation; in this case, HIV prevalence could be underestimated, and HIV risk behavior and testing behavior overestimated. Moreover, the MPMS offered HIV counseling and testing in a culturally competent setting, and those MSM more motivated to test for HIV may have been overrepresented in the crude sample. [42] In addition, due to structural and operational constraints, the survey measured several key variables normally associated with HIV infection, risk behavior, or health seeking behavior outcomes through self-report that are subject to social desirability bias. It is possible that previous HIV diagnosis, number of partners, and receptive anal intercourse were underreported, and that regular partnerships, consistent condom use, and regular recent HIV testing were over-reported. In addition, our findings on linkage to care are limited by the small numbers of men who self-reported an HIV-positive status and having sought care after their diagnosis prior to MPMS enrolment. The MPMS was not able to independently verify whether any of its HIV-positive participants were previously in care, nor if those diagnosed in the study sought care in the public health service.

The MPMS is, to our knowledge, the first study to report on HIV prevalence, associated risk behaviors, and HIV testing, care and treatment behaviors in an MSM population outside of South Africa's largest urban centers of Cape Town, eThekwini/Durban, Johannesburg, and Tshwane/Pretoria. As such, it may be representative of the state of the HIV epidemic among MSM in more resource-challenged rural provinces, [43] as well as an indication of the state of the national response to the epidemic among MSM outside of these major metropolitan centers. South Africa's current HIV/AIDS National Strategic Plan has set ambitious benchmarks for the HIV response with key affected populations, including MSM, that include halving HIV prevalence, ensuring at least 90% are reached by a social and behavioral change communication strategy to increase demand for testing and treatment, and ensuring at least 80% are engaged in care that includes early ART initiation, all by 2017. [44] The MPMS findings demonstrate a critical need for a comprehensive intervention to bring more MSM into timely, regular, and meaningful contact with HIV prevention, testing, and treatment services. Follow up MPMS waves in 2014 and 2015 will show if Project Boithato's approach to building a healthy, supportive MSM community can add value to government and non-governmental organizations' current efforts to engage MSM in HIV prevention and treatment with culturally competent HIV prevention and care services in Mpumalanga, and potentially elsewhere in South Africa.

Author Contributions

Conceived and designed the experiments: TL TO TS. Performed the experiments: TL TO. Analyzed the data: TL TO AM SBS. Contributed reagents/materials/analysis tools: TL TS KD SK. Wrote the paper: TL TO AM SBS TS HS SK JAM.

References

1. Baral SD, Ketende S, Mnisi Z, Mabuza X, Grosso A, et al. (2013) A cross-sectional assessment of the burden of HIV and associated individual- and structural-level characteristics among men who have sex with men in Swaziland. J Int AIDS Soc 16 Suppl 3: 18768.
2. Beyrer C, Baral SD, van Griensven F, Goodreau SM, Chariyalertsak S, et al. (2012) Global epidemiology of HIV infection in men who have sex with men. Lancet 380: 367–377.
3. Baral S, Sifakis F, Cleghorn F, Beyrer C (2007) Elevated risk for HIV infection among men who have sex with men in low- and middle-income countries 2000–2006: a systematic review. PLoS Med 4: e339.
4. Dahoma M, Johnston LG, Holman A, Miller LA, Mussa M, et al. (2011) HIV and related risk behavior among men who have sex with men in Zanzibar, Tanzania: results of a behavioral surveillance survey. AIDS Behav 15: 186–192.
5. Merrigan M, Azeez A, Afolabi B, Chabikuli ON, Onyekwena O, et al. (2011) HIV prevalence and risk behaviours among men having sex with men in Nigeria. Sex Transm Infect 87: 65–70.
6. Baral S, Trapence G, Motimedi F, Umar E, Iipinge S, et al. (2009) HIV prevalence, risks for HIV infection, and human rights among men who have sex with men (MSM) in Malawi, Namibia, and Botswana. PLoS ONE 4: e4997.
7. Park JN, Papworth E, Kassegne S, Moukam L, Billong SC, et al. (2013) HIV prevalence and factors associated with HIV infection among men who have sex with men in Cameroon. J Int AIDS Soc 16 Suppl 3: 18752.
8. Vu L, Adebajo S, Tun W, Sheehy M, Karlyn A, et al. (2013) High HIV prevalence among men who have sex with men in Nigeria: implications for combination prevention. J Acquir Immune Defic Syndr 63: 221–227.
9. Lane T, Raymond HF, Dladla S, Rasethe J, Struthers H, et al. (2011) High HIV prevalence among men who have sex with men in Soweto, South Africa: results from the Soweto Men's Study. AIDS Behav 15: 626–634.
10. Baral S, Burrell E, Scheibe A, Brown B, Beyrer C, et al. (2011) HIV risk and associations of HIV infection among men who have sex with men in peri-urban Cape Town, South Africa. BMC Public Health 11: 766.
11. Rispel LC, Metcalf CA, Cloete A, Reddy V, Lombard C (2011) HIV prevalence and risk practices among men who have sex with men in two South African cities. J Acquir Immune Defic Syndr 57: 69–76.
12. Sanders EJ, Okuku H, Smith AD, Mwangome M, Wahome E, et al. (2013) High HIV-1 incidence, correlates of HIV-1 acquisition, and high viral loads following seroconversion among men who have sex with men in Coastal Kenya. AIDS 27: 437–446.
13. Price MA, Rida W, Mwangome M, Mutua G, Middelkoop K, et al. (2012) Identifying at-risk populations in Kenya and South Africa: HIV incidence in cohorts of men who report sex with men, sex workers, and youth. J Acquir Immune Defic Syndr 59: 185–193.
14. Millett GA, Jeffries WLt, Peterson JL, Malebranche DJ, Lane T, et al. (2012) Common roots: a contextual review of HIV epidemics in black men who have sex with men across the African diaspora. Lancet 380: 411–423.
15. Millett GA, Peterson JL, Wolitski RJ, Stall R (2006) Greater Risk for HIV Infection of Black Men Who Have Sex With Men: A Critical Literature Review. Am J Public Health 96: 1007–1019.
16. Johnson C (2007) Off the Map: How HIV/AIDS Programming is Failing Same-Sex Practicing People in Africa. New York: International Gay and Lesbian Human Rights Commission.
17. Beyrer C (2006) HIV Epidemiology Update and Transmission Factors: Risks and Risk Contexts; Toronto.
18. Rispel LC, Metcalf CA, Cloete A, Moorman J, Reddy V (2011) You become afraid to tell them that you are gay: health service utilization by men who have sex with men in South African cities. J Public Health Policy 32 Suppl 1: S137–151.
19. Lane T, Mogale T, Struthers H, McIntyre J, Kegeles SM (2008) "They see you as a different thing": the experiences of men who have sex with men with healthcare workers in South African township communities. Sex Transm Infect 84: 430–433.
20. WHO (2014) Consolidated Guidelines on HIV Prevention, Diagnosis, Treatment and Care for Key Populations. Geneva.
21. CDC (2011) HIV Testing Among Men Who Have Sex with Men — 21 Cities, United States, 2008. Morbidity and Mortaility Weekly Report 60: 694–699.
22. UNAIDS (2013) Global Report: UNAIDS report on the global AIDS epidemic 2013.
23. Kegeles SM, Hays RB, Coates TJ (1996) The Mpowerment Project: a community-level HIV prevention intervention for young gay men. Am J Public Health 86: 1129–1136.
24. Kegeles SM, Hays RB, Pollack LM, Coates TJ (1999) Mobilizing young gay and bisexual men for HIV prevention: a two-community study. Aids 13: 1753–1762.
25. Hays RB, Rebchook GM, Kegeles SM (2003) The Mpowerment Project: community-building with young gay and bisexual men to prevent HIV1. Am J Community Psychol 31: 301–312.
26. Statistics South Africa (2011) Statistics by place.
27. Heckathorn D (1997) Respondent-Driven Sampling: A New Approach to the Study of Hidden Populations. Social Problems 44: 174–199.
28. Heckathorn D (2002) Respondent-Driven Sampling II: Deriving Valid Population Estimates from Chain-Referral Samples of Hidden Populations. Social Problems 49: 11–34.
29. Lane T, Shade SB, McIntyre J, Morin SF (2008) Alcohol and sexual risk behavior among men who have sex with men in South african township communities. AIDS Behav 12: S78–85.
30. Bush K, Kivlahan DR, McDonell MB, Fihn SD, Bradley KA (1998) The AUDIT alcohol consumption questions (AUDIT-C): an effective brief screening test for problem drinking. Ambulatory Care Quality Improvement Project (ACQUIP). Alcohol Use Disorders Identification Test. Arch Intern Med 158: 1789–1795.
31. Heckathorn D (2007) Extensions of respondent driven sampling: Analyzing continuous variables and controlling for differential recruitment. Sociological Methodology 37: 151–207.
32. Salganik M, Heckathorn D (2004) Sampling and Estimation in Hidden Populations Using Respondent-Driven Sampling. Sociological Methodology forthcoming.

33. South African National Department of Health (2011) The 2011 National Antenatal Sentinel HIV & Syphilis Prevalence Survey in South Africa. In: Epidemiology & Surveillance, editor. Pretoria: National Department of Health.
34. Knox J, Yi H, Reddy V, Maimane S, Sandfort T (2010) The fallacy of intimacy: sexual risk behaviour and beliefs about trust and condom use among men who have sex with men in South Africa. Psychol Health Med 15: 660–671.
35. Arnold MP, Struthers H, McIntyre J, Lane T (2012) Contextual Correlates of Per Partner Unprotected Anal Intercourse Rates Among MSM in Soweto, South Africa. AIDS Behav.
36. Knox J, Reddy V, Kaighobadi F, Nel D, Sandfort T (2013) Communicating HIV status in sexual interactions: assessing social cognitive constructs, situational factors, and individual characteristics among South African MSM. AIDS Behav 17: 350–359.
37. Stephenson R, Rentsch C, Sullivan P (2012) High levels of acceptability of couples-based HIV testing among MSM in South Africa. AIDS Care 24: 529–535.
38. Stephenson R, Rentsch C, Sullivan P, McAdams-Mahmoud A, Jobson G, et al. (2013) Attitudes toward couples-based HIV counseling and testing among MSM in Cape Town, South Africa. AIDS Behav 17 Suppl 1: S43–50.
39. Kranzer K, Govindasamy D, Ford N, Johnston V, Lawn SD (2012) Quantifying and addressing losses along the continuum of care for people living with HIV infection in sub-Saharan Africa: a systematic review. J Int AIDS Soc 15: 17383.
40. Mugavero MJ, Amico KR, Horn T, Thompson MA (2013) The state of engagement in HIV care in the United States: from cascade to continuum to control. Clin Infect Dis 57: 1164–1171.
41. Knox J, Sandfort T, Yi H, Reddy V, Maimane S (2011) Social vulnerability and HIV testing among South African men who have sex with men. Int J STD AIDS 22: 709–713.
42. Johnston LG, Khanam R, Reza M, Khan SI, Banu S, et al. (2008) The effectiveness of respondent driven sampling for recruiting males who have sex with males in Dhaka, Bangladesh. AIDS Behav 12: 294–304.
43. Imrie J, Hoddinott G, Fuller S, Oliver S, Newell ML (2013) Why MSM in rural South African communities should be an HIV prevention research priority. AIDS Behav 17 Suppl 1: S70–76.
44. South Africa. Department of Health (2011) National Strategic Plan on HIV, STIs, and TB, 2012–2016.

8

Suppression of Foxo1 Activity and Down-Modulation of CD62L (L-Selectin) in HIV-1 Infected Resting CD4 T Cells

Benjamin Trinité[1], Chi N. Chan[1], Caroline S. Lee[1], Saurabh Mahajan[1], Yang Luo[2], Mark A. Muesing[2], Joy M. Folkvord[3], Michael Pham[3¤], Elizabeth Connick[3], David N. Levy[1]*

1 Department of Basic Science, New York University College of Dentistry, New York, New York, United States of America, **2** Aaron Diamond AIDS Research Center, New York, New York, United States of America, **3** Department of Medicine, University of Colorado Denver, Aurora, Colorado, United States of America

Abstract

HIV-1 hijacks and disrupts many processes in the cells it infects in order to suppress antiviral immunity and to facilitate its replication. Resting CD4 T cells are important early targets of HIV-1 infection in which HIV-1 must overcome intrinsic barriers to viral replication. Although resting CD4 T cells are refractory to infection *in vitro*, local environmental factors within lymphoid and mucosal tissues such as cytokines facilitate viral replication while maintaining the resting state. These factors can be utilized *in vitro* to study HIV-1 replication in resting CD4 T cells. *In vivo*, the migration of resting naïve and central memory T cells into lymphoid tissues is dependent upon expression of CD62L (L-selectin), a receptor that is subsequently down-modulated following T cell activation. CD62L gene transcription is maintained in resting T cells by Foxo1 and KLF2, transcription factors that maintain T cell quiescence and which regulate additional cellular processes including survival, migration, and differentiation. Here we report that HIV-1 down-modulates CD62L in productively infected naïve and memory resting CD4 T cells while suppressing Foxo1 activity and the expression of KLF2 mRNA. Partial T cell activation was further evident as an increase in CD69 expression. Several other Foxo1- and KLF2-regulated mRNA were increased or decreased in productively infected CD4 T cells, including IL-7rα, Myc, CCR5, Fam65b, $S1P_1$ (EDG1), CD52, Cyclin D2 and $p21^{CIP1}$, indicating a profound reprogramming of these cells. The Foxo1 inhibitor AS1842856 accelerated *de novo* viral gene expression and the sequella of infection, supporting the notion that HIV-1 suppression of Foxo1 activity may be a strategy to promote replication in resting CD4 T cells. As Foxo1 is an investigative cancer therapy target, the development of Foxo1 interventions may assist the quest to specifically suppress or activate HIV-1 replication *in vivo*.

Editor: Yuntao Wu, George Mason University, United States of America

Funding: This work was supported by R01 AI078783, National Institute of Allergy and Infectious Diseases, National Institutes of Health to DNL; R01 AI081615, National Institute of Allergy and Infectious Diseases, National Institutes of Health to MAM; and R01 AI096966, National Institute of Allergy and Infectious Diseases, National Institutes of Health to EC. The funders had no role in study design, data collection and analysis, decision to publish, or preparation of the manuscript.

Competing Interests: The authors have declared that no competing interests exist.

* Email: dnlevy@nyu.edu

¤ Current address: School of Medicine, University of Virginia, Charlottesville, Virginia, United States of America

Introduction

Resting CD4+ T cells in lymphoid tissues and mucosa constitute at least 90% of HIV/SIV RNA+ cells [1–5] and are massively depleted during acute infection, [2–6], a period in which antiviral immunity is established and the outcome of infection determined [7]. Although peripheral blood CD4+ T cells are resistant to infection *in vitro* [8–10], viral replication occurs predominantly in lymphoid and mucosal tissues, where microenvironmental factors, including cytokines such as IL-4 and IL-7 maintain resting T cell viability [11–17], and fortuitously (for the virus), facilitate their productive infection [18–22]. IL-7 is the primary cytokine maintaining the survival and homeostasis of mature T cells [17,23,24]. In addition, HIV-1 can itself manipulate infected cells in order to enhance viral replication; for example, binding of viral envelope proteins to CD4 and coreceptors CXCR4 and CCR5 can stimulate actin remodeling to facilitate early replication steps in resting T cells [25]. Viral proteins such as Env, Tat and Nef interact with cell signaling pathways and can stimulate partial T cell activation that enhances virus expression in resting T cells [26–29].

An important revelation of the past decade has been that T cell quiescence results not merely from an absence of antigenic stimulation, but is actively maintained by constitutive expression of certain transcription factors [30–32]. Chief among these is Foxo1, a member of the Forkhead box protein family of proteins, (the other members being Foxo3a, Foxo4 and Foxo6) that respond to environmental stimuli (growth factors, oxidative stress, nutritional availability) and regulate the expression of many genes involved in cell growth, proliferation, differentiation, and survival [33–37]. Foxo3a has been implicated in HIV-1 neuropathology [38] and disease progression [39,40]. Foxo1 is specifically upregulated during T cell maturation [41] and is constitutively active in resting T cells [35,42] and many other tissues [43]. Deletion of Foxo1 leads to spontaneous T cell activation and differentiation [44], while ectopic expression of constitutively active Foxo1 suppresses T cell proliferation [36,45]. Foxo1 binds directly to a consensus

DNA sequence on promoters that it regulates [35,46] and it also associates with many binding partners [47] to regulate gene expression. Foxo1 transactivates and maintains expression of CD62L, CCR7, KLF2 (LKLF) [45] and the IL-7 receptor alpha chain (IL-7rα) in resting T cells. Transcriptional repression of these genes is an indicator of Foxo1 inactivation and early T cell activation [45,48–50]. Thus, by controlling these genes, Foxo1 regulates both T cell quiescence and T cell trafficking [33,48,51].

CD62L is expressed on resting naïve, central memory and some effector memory T cells and regulates their migration into lymph nodes [52]. Disruption of CD62L expression has detrimental effects on T cell migration and immune responses [35,53,54]. Antigenic activation in the LN leads first to rapid CD62L shedding by protease cleavage and then to transcriptional suppression [55] as a result of Foxo1 inactivation [33]. CD62L down-modulation functions to prevent activated and CD62L-negative effector memory T cells from re-entering LN. KLF2, often cooperatively with Foxo1, also transactivates CD62L [56] as well as a further set of genes involved in cell growth, differentiation, and migration [57–61].

In this study we examine the consequences of HIV-1 infection to naïve and memory resting CD4+ T cells, finding that CD62L was specifically down-modulated, the early activation marker CD69 was upregulated, and that these occurred concomitantly with HIV-1 suppression of Foxo1 activity. Several genes that are known targets of Foxo1 and KLF2 were activated or repressed in infected resting T cells [34,45,62–64], including IL-7 receptor (IL-7rα), Myc, $S1P_1$ (EGD1), CD52, CCR5, Fam65b, Cyclin D2 and $p21^{CIP1}$. Each of these genes regulates cell survival, differentiation, activation and/or migration. Application of the Foxo1 inhibitor AS1842856 resulted in an acceleration of HIV-1 replication in resting CD4+ T cells, suggesting that targeting Foxo1 may be a viral tactic to promote its own replication.

Results

HIV-1 infection of resting CD4+ T cells leads to down-modulation of CD62L and upregulation of CD69

We first tested whether common gamma chain cytokines alter CD62L expression on resting naïve and memory peripheral blood CD4 T cells, finding that each maintained high CD62L expression at concentrations which enhance HIV-1 infection (Figure S1 in File S1). Because of the demonstrated importance for IL-7 in maintaining T cell homeostasis *in vivo* [23], we chose this cytokine for the majority of the following studies. Maintenance of CD62L expression in IL-7 culture is consistent with the finding that submitogenic levels of IL-7 do not activate PI3K [65].

We next examined the influence of HIV-1 infection on expression of CD4, CD69 and CD62L on resting CD4+ T cells (Figure 1). We activated a subset of cells with anti-CD3/CD28 beads 2 days after infection in order to compare receptor expression on infected resting vs. activated cells. CD4 was efficiently down-modulated by the virus, as expected, whether the cells were activated or not after infection (Figure 1A). Interestingly, the early activation marker CD69 was modestly upregulated in both memory (CD4+CD45RA+) and naïve (CD4+CD45RA−) resting GFP+ cells, (Figure 1B). There was variability in the effect of infection on both receptors among cell donors, but with a single exception, all infections produced significant CD62L down modulation and CD69 upregulation. Late activation markers such as CD25, CD38 and HLA Class II were unaffected (not shown). Mock infected cells remained uniformly CD69-negative (not shown), thus HIV-1 is actively inducing CD69 expression.

CD62L was strongly down-modulated in both the naïve (T_N) and memory subsets (Figure 1A–B), becoming progressively lower as GFP intensity increased past an apparent threshold level of gene expression. After 48 hours of activation with anti-CD3/CD28 beads, which down-modulates CD62L, the GFP+ cells expressed even less CD62L than GFP-negative activated cells. A prior study of pre-activated cells reported HIV-1-induced CD62L down-modulation [66], which these data confirm, despite the natural down-modulation provided by stimulation through the T cell receptor. We further observed that CD62L was down-modulated by HIV-1 on both T_{CM} and T_{EM} subsets identified by CCR7 expression (Figure S2A in File S1). While TN are uniformly CD62L+, a subset of T_{EM} naturally do not express CD62L, complicating interpretation of the data. However, the overall shape of the relationship between GFP levels and CD62L levels provides evidence that HIV-1 is indeed down-modulating CD62L on those cells which did express this receptor prior to infection. CCR7 was modestly down-modulated in GFP+ resting naïve and memory cells (Figure S2B in File S1). This is consistent with a recent study in activated T cells, where CCR7 was down-modulated by HIV-1 Vpu [67]. Interestingly, HIV-1 expression was considerably higher in T_{EM} than in either T_N or T_{CM} (Figure S2C in File S1). To test whether a pre-existing CD62L-negative subpopulation was being preferentially expanded after infection, as opposed to HIV-1 actively down-modulating CD62L, we examined cell replication by dilution of the intracellular dye eFluor670 (Figure 1C). Whether left resting or when activated with beads, the population of GFP+ cells did not expand, held in check by Vpr [68] in this post-infection activation scenario [22]. Therefore, CD62L down-modulation appears to be driven by *de novo* HIV-1 expression in these cells.

IL-4 is a product of activated T cells present in lymphoid tissues, including tonsils, where it enhances HIV-1 infection [69]. We have utilized this cytokine to provide a convenient *in vitro* model for HIV-1 infection and latency after direct infection of resting CD4+ T cells [22]. Because of its favorable characteristic of inducing little homeostatic proliferation while efficiently enhancing HIV-1 infection [22], IL-4 is a useful alternative to IL-7 in such studies. We examined CD62L in IL-4 treated resting peripheral blood CD4+ T cells, finding similar down-modulation as in IL-7 treated cells (Figure 1D). Next, we examined infection of tonsil cells cultured with IL-4, finding that CD62L was reduced in these cells as well, though not as strongly as in peripheral blood cells. The difference may be that in our infection of tonsil cells the virus was not held to a single round of infection but was allowed to spread within the target cell population. In this expanding infection, many cells are likely to have been infected too recently to fully down-modulate CD62L.

CD62L down-modulation is reduced by PI3K inhibition

To explore the mechanism(s) responsible for HIV-1-induced CD62L down-modulation, we first tested whether apoptosis of GFP+ cells was inducing CD62L shedding [70,71]. However, Annexin V and 7-AAD staining were very low (0.9%) on GFP+ cells that were down-modulating or had down-modulated CD62L (Figure 2A). Prior studies have reported that HIV-1 binding to cells can induce ADAM17-dependent shedding of CD62L through the interaction between envelope protein and CD4 or CXCR4 [72,73], while another study reported upregulation [74]. To test whether virus binding influenced CD62L expression in our system, we stained cells soon after spinoculation of virus onto cells. Infection was performed in the presence of the reverse transcriptase inhibitor efavirenz (EFV) in order to block events downstream of virus binding and entry. No effect on CD62L expression was

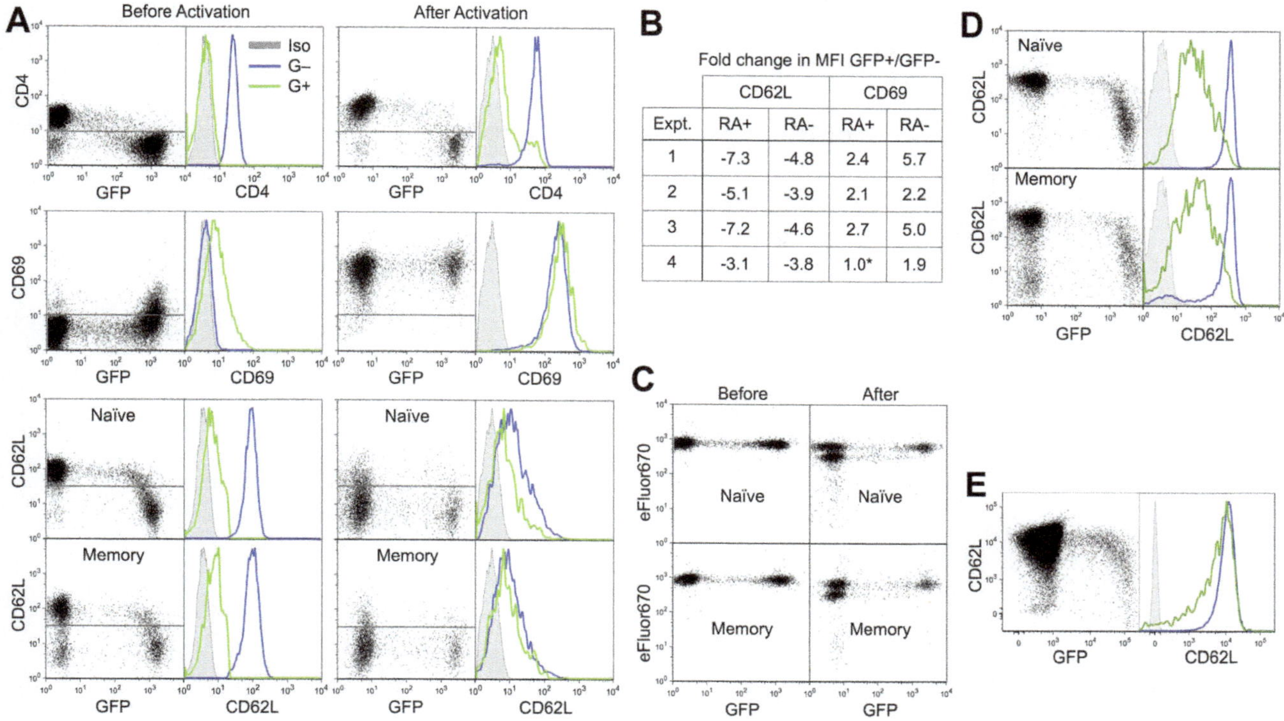

Expt.	CD62L RA+	CD62L RA-	CD69 RA+	CD69 RA-
1	-7.3	-4.8	2.4	5.7
2	-5.1	-3.9	2.1	2.2
3	-7.2	-4.6	2.7	5.0
4	-3.1	-3.8	1.0*	1.9

Figure 1. Down-modulation of CD62L and upregulation of CD69 and on productively infected naïve and memory resting CD4 T cells. A. Resting IL-7 treated CD4+ T cells were infected with the GFP reporter virus NLENG1, restricted to a single round of infection by treatment with the protease inhibitor indinavir (2 μM). Flow analysis was carried out on day 5 post infection on cells with and without activation by αCD3/CD28 beads on day 3 p.i. Grey: isotype-matched IgG control antibody staining. Blue: GFP-negative cells. Green: GFP+ cells. Data are representative of 4 independent experiments. **B.** Fold change in CD62L and CD69 expression on naïve and memory CD4+ resting T cells in A. With on exception (*) all values were statistically different ($p<0.01$) from the negative control by a T(x) population comparison test [134]. **C.** Failure of GFP+ cells proliferate demonstrates that CD62L-low cells are not produced by preferential expansion of an existing CD62L-low population. Experiment shown is representative of >5 similar experiments. **D.** IL-4 supports HIV-1-induced down-modulation of CD62L on both naïve and memory resting CD4+ T cells. Experiment shown is representative of >3 similar experiments. **E.** CD62L down-modulation on HIV-1 infected naïve tonsil T cells 7 days after infection. Similar results were observed on CD45R0+cells (not shown). Experiment shown is representative of 2 similar experiments.

observed at any time from 4 hours to 5 days after infection in the presence of EFV (Figure 2B). It has also been reported that contact between Jurkat T cells infected with an Envelope wild type virus and uninfected primary cells led to CD62L shedding [72], but in a separate test we observed no CD62L loss by this method either (data not shown). Failure of coculture of infected and uninfected cells to affect CD62L expression is consistent with the results in Figure 1A that CD62L down-modulation was restricted to the productively infected GFP+ cells and was not observed on GFP-negative bystander cells.

CD62L shedding and transcriptional repression can be triggered by a PI3K/Akt-dependent pathway, and this can be inhibited by the PI3K inhibitors LY294002 or PI-103. These inhibitors reduced the HIV-1-induced down-modulation of CD62L (Figure 2C), confirming that at least part of HIV-1's effect on CD62L expression is through activation of PI3K/Akt pathway. PI3K inhibition can block HIV-1 infection when added early [75,76], so we added them after the appearance of GFP+ cells but before CD62L down modulation was evident. The timing of addiction to culture may have been too late to completely block CD62L down modulation by HIV-1. We next directly tested whether a metalloprotease was responsible for CD62L loss by applying the metalloprotease inhibitor (MTPI) TAPI-1 to cells. A control experiment utilizing PMA-induced CD62L shedding demonstrated the effectiveness of MTPI to block this strong stimulus (Figure 2D left panel). On the other hand, MTPI had no effect on HIV-1-induced CD62L down-modulation, indicating that in these cells CD62L is being lost from the cell surface by a mechanism other than MTP cleavage.

Foxo1- and KLF2-regulated mRNA levels in HIV-1 infected resting CD4+ T cells

We hypothesized that CD62L transcription was being suppressed in the productively infected cells and that we would observe alterations in the transcription of this and other Foxo1 and KLF2 regulated genes. To test this, we sorted naïve CD4+ T cells with varying degrees of GFP and CD62L expression (Figure 3A) and performed qRT-PCR on their RNA (Figure 3B–C, Table S2 in File S1). We chose to purify naïve cells because they uniformly express CD62L and thus would provide a more consistent test of CD62L mRNA regulation. The comparison between GFP+ and GFP− cells allows us to specifically isolate the effects of HIV-1 gene expression within these cells. We first confirmed that HIV-1 RNA levels corresponded to GFP intensity [22,77]. Consistent with our hypothesis, CD62L RNA decreased in concordance with increasing HIV-1 expression and decreasing CD62L surface expression. KLF2 mRNA was strongly reduced in progression with HIV-1 and CD62L expression, as were several other Foxo1-regulated mRNA, including IL-7rα, and Fam65B. The KLF2- and Foxo1-regulated $S1P_1$, Myc, and CD52 mRNA [62] were all suppressed, and the KLF2-regulated CCR5 mRNA [61] was lower in GFP+ bright cells. Interestingly, CCR5 RNA was

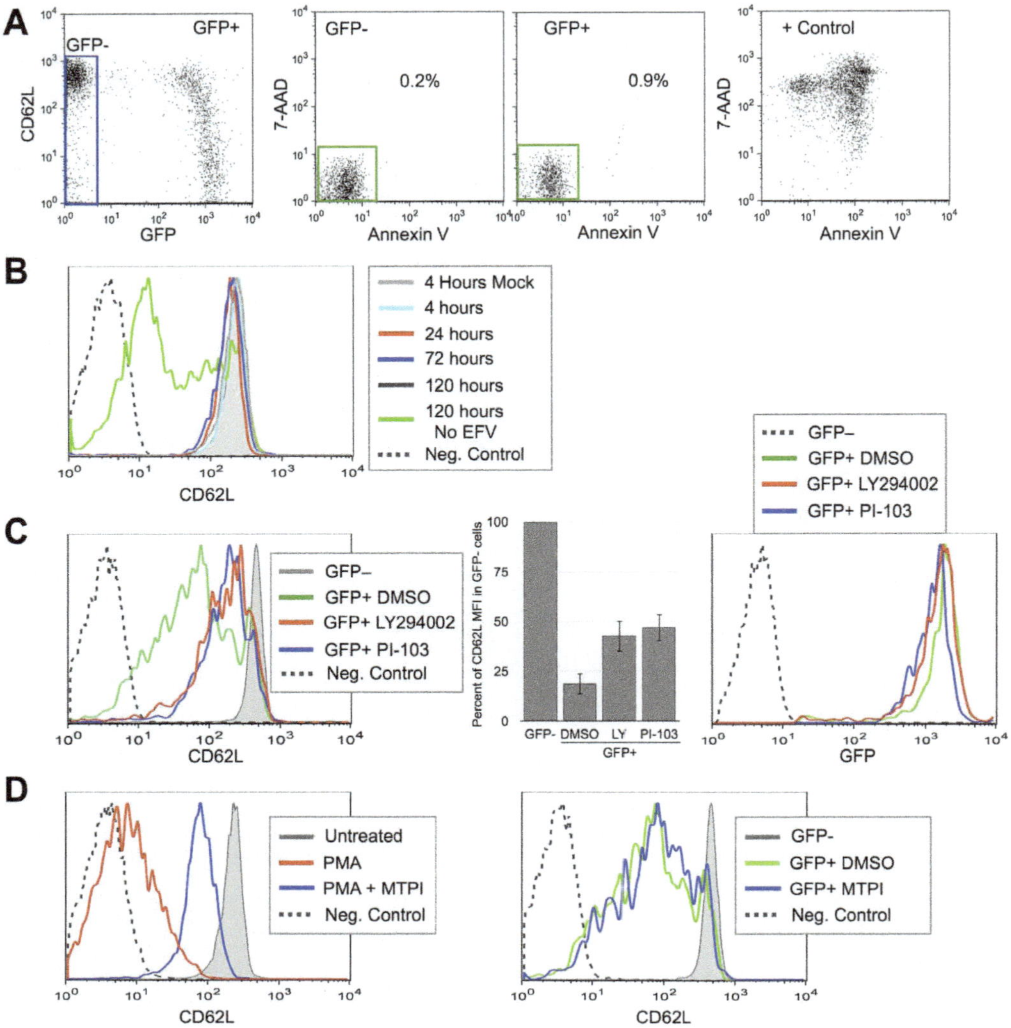

Figure 2. CD62L down-modulation is not the result of apoptosis, virus contact or protease cleavage, but is influenced by PI3K. A. Cells infected with for 5 days, then were analyzed for GFP, CD62L and Annexin V surface expression, and permeability to 7-AAD. Data are representative of >5 independent experiments. **B.** Contact with HIV-1 virions does not affect CD62L surface expression. Cells were treated with the reverse transcriptase inhibitor efavirenz (EFV) (2 μg/ml) and infected by spinoculation or spinoculated without virus (Mock). Surface CD62L expression was analyzed at the indicated times after infection. A positive control infection was performed without EFV as indicated. EFV completely prevented the appearance of GFP+ cells (not shown). **C.** The PI3K and mTORC2 inhibitors LY294002 and PI-103 suppress HIV-1-induced CD62L down-modulation. Infected cells were treated with LY294002 (5 μM), PI-103 (5 μM) or a carrier control (DMSO) 1 day and again 4 hours prior to staining for CD62L. Middle graph: Data from 3 independent experiments with different cell donors. Y axis = the mean fluorescence intensity of CD62L staining (MFI) for each condition expressed as a percentage of the CD62L MFI of the GFP-negative cells. Right: GFP expression is modestly suppressed by LY294002 and PI-103 (MFI = 1761 and 1471 respectively, vs.1981 for DMSO control). LY294002 and PI-103 treatments were statistically different ($p < 0.01$) from their respective DMSO controls by a T(x) population comparison test [134]. **D.** Metalloprotease inhibitor (MTPI) TAPI-1 (50 μM) does not inhibit HIV-1-induced CD62L surface down-modulation. Left: Control experiment demonstrating inhibition of PMA-induced CD62L downmodulation by MTPI. Cells were treated with PMA with and without MTPI and analyzed one hour later. Right: Cells infected with HIV-1 GFP reporter virus were treated with MTPI 1 day and again 3 hours prior to staining. Data are representative of 2 independent experiments.

modestly increased in the GFP+ dim cells in 2 independent experiments for reasons that are not clear. $p21^{CIP1}$ mRNA was also increased in all productively infected cells. CD69 and Cyclin D2 are negatively regulated by Foxo1, and their RNA increased in progression with HIV-1 expression. Interestingly, some other known targets of Foxo1 transcriptional regulation were not altered in productively infected cells, including CCR7, Foxo3a and Foxo1 itself. The abundances of these mRNA were similar to the starting abundances of the other genes examined (CD62L, etc.) (not shown), so the absence of regulation was genuine and not the result being transcriptionally inactivated prior to infection. Transcriptional regulation is highly complex and cell-type dependent, and since much prior work on these genes has been performed in transgenic mice and in transformed cells *in vitro*. It may not be surprising that some known Foxo1/KLF2 targets genes do not fit the expected pattern in this primary human cell system. Finally, CD4 and HLA-A, genes that are not thought to be Foxo1 or KLF2 targets but which are upregulated in activated T cells, remained unaltered in productively infected cells. This demonstrates that the effect of HIV-1 on T cell activation phenotype is selective and apparently restricted to early activation markers such as CD69.

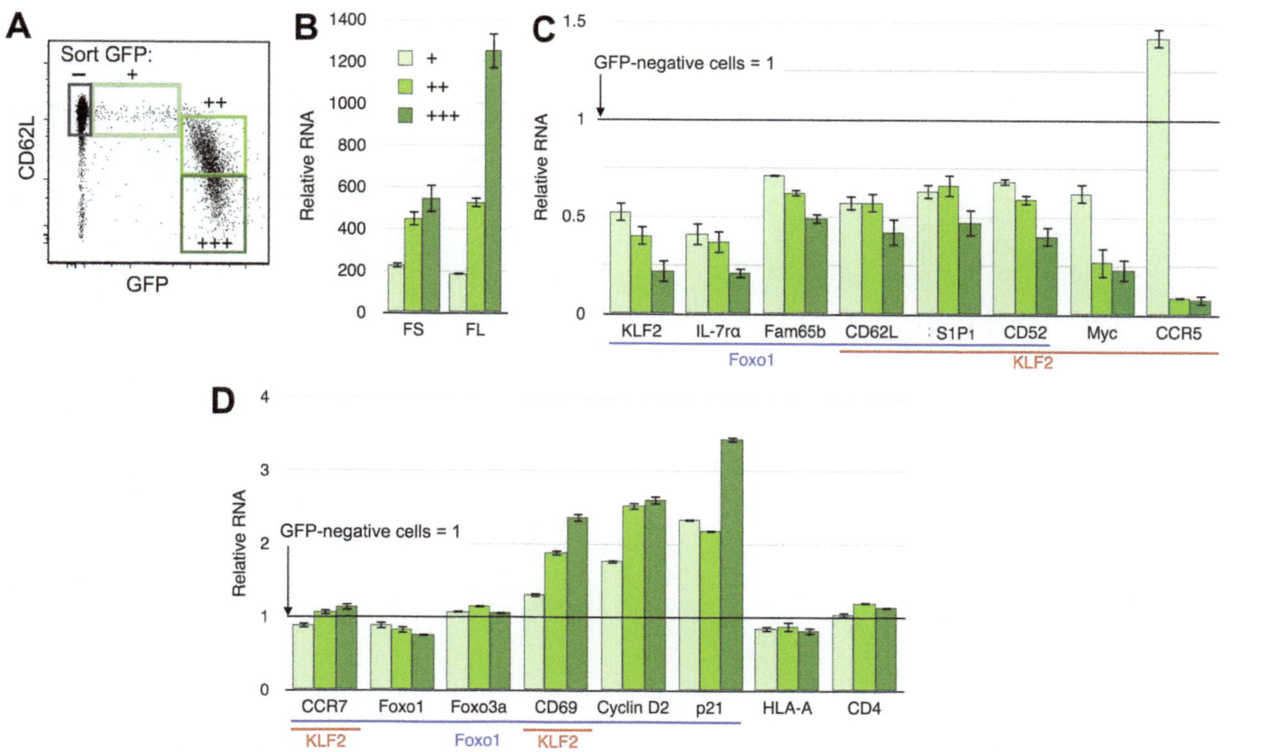

Figure 3. mRNA levels of several known Foxo1- and KLF2-regulated genes in HIV-1 infected naïve CD4+ T cells. Data are representative of 3 independent experiments. Error bars represent SD of triplicate PCR reactions. **A.** CD45RO-CD4+ T cells were infected with sing-round GFP reporter virus for 7 days then sorted by FACS into 4 populations of GFP- and GFP+ cells according to GFP and CD62L expression. **B.** HIV-1 early fully spliced RNA (FS) and late full length RNA (FL) in each group of sorted cells. Data are normalized to a value of 1 for the FS RNA in GFP- cells. GFP- FL RNA was 1.5. A synthetic RNA standard containing both the FS and FL targets was used in order to allow the FS and FL values to be directly compared. Values are presented in Table S2 in File S1. **C.** mRNA of genes that were suppressed in GFP+ cells. Values are normalized to the GFP- cells set to a value of 1 for each gene. Genes regulated by Foxo1 or KLF2 are indicated by color-matched under lines. All $p<0.01$ (paired T-test). **D.** mRNA of genes that were changed <2 fold or were increased in GFP+ cells. mRNA in GFP-negative cells is set to a relative value of 1 for each gene as in C.

Foxo1 relocalizes to the cytoplasm in naïve and memory HIV-1 infected resting CD4+ T cells

Freed from DNA binding, inactivated Foxo1 relocalizes to the cytoplasm; thus cytoplasmic translocation is a direct indication of Foxo1 inactivation. We next examined Foxo1 localization by ImageStream analysis, a technique that combines flow cytometry with cell imaging to provide spatial and intensity information within individual cells (Figure 4). We first observed that total Foxo1 levels were not altered in the productively infected naïve CD4 T cells, and slightly increased in memory cells (Figure 4A). When nuclear and cytoplasmic expression were analyzed, translocation of Foxo1 from nucleus to the (very thin) cytoplasm, was observed in both the naïve and memory resting T cells (Figure 4B). This translocation was clearly evident in images of individual cells (Figure 4C). By contrast with Foxo1, NF-κB remained almost completely cytoplasmic (Figure 4D–F). However, similar to Foxo1, NF-κB total levels were increased in the GFP+ memory cells (Figure 4D), though no nuclear translocation was observed. GFP+ cells tended to be more elongated and irregular in shape, resembling polarized T cells, a further indication of partial activation (see the middle cells in memory GFP+ cells stained for Foxo1 in Figure 4C).

Foxo1 DNA binding activity is suppressed in HIV-1 infected resting CD4+ T cells

We next directly examined nuclear Foxo1 activity using the TransAM transcription factor ELISA (Active Motif), which measures ability of Foxo1 to bind an oligonucleotide containing a Foxo1 target consensus sequence. We first performed a timecourse control experiment to examine the kinetics of Foxo1 inactivation following activation of resting T cells with anti-CD3/CD28 beads, observing that Foxo1 activity was progressively reduced in the first 24 hours after activation (Figure 5A). We then tested Foxo1 activity in HSA+ and HSA− cells, comparing them to mock infected or 24 hour beads-activated cells (Figure 5B). HSA− cells contained slightly less Foxo1 activity than mock control. Most importantly, in productively infected cells, Foxo1 activity was reduced to the low level observed in cells activated through the T cell receptor/coreceptor complex for 24 hours.

A Foxo1 inhibitor accelerates HIV-1 replication

The question arises whether inactivation of Foxo1 confers a replicative advantage to HIV-1. The capacity of a cell to support viral replication is closely linked to its activation status, and Foxo1 is a primary suppressor of T cell activation. Therefore, we hypothesized that direct inhibition of Foxo1 might increase or accelerate HIV-1 replication. The Foxo1 inhibitor AS1842856 binds to Foxo1 and disables its ability to transactivate [78]. We first observed that AS1842856 did not interfere with nuclear Foxo1 binding to its DNA target sequence in the TransAM assay (not shown), consistent with a proposed mechanism of action in which AS1842856 does not interfere with DNA attachment but instead block unphosphorylated Foxo1 from binding to the its co-activator cAMP response element-binding protein [78].

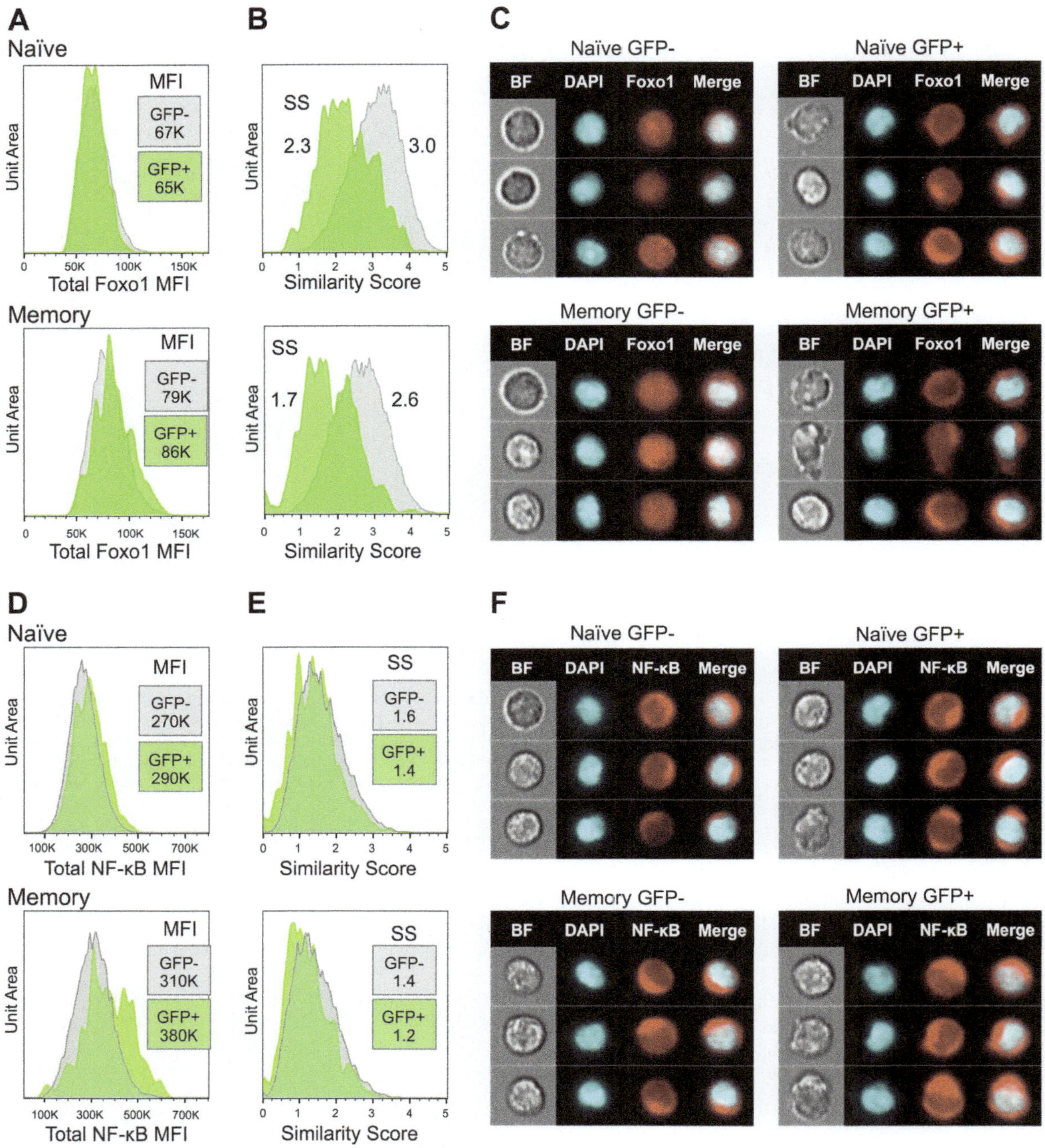

Figure 4. ImageStream analysis of Foxo1 and NF-κB in HIV-1 infected cells. HIV-1 GFP-reporter virus-infected resting CD4+ T cells were stained for CD45RA, intracellular Foxo1 or NF-κB and for DNA (DAPI) 7 days after infection, then analyzed by ImageStream. One representative experiment of two is shown. **A.** Total Foxo1 expression in naïve and memory GFP+ and GFP- cells. MFI = Mean Fluorescence Intensity. **B.** Nuclear localization was analyzed in IDEAS software by comparison of Foxo1 distribution to nuclear DAPI staining using the Similarity Score (see materials and methods). **C.** Representative ImageStream pictures of individual cells stained for Foxo1. **D.** Total NF-κB expression in naïve and memory GFP+ and GFP- cells. **E.** NF-κB nuclear Similarity Scores. **F.** Representative ImageStream pictures of individual cells stained for NF-κB.

We applied AS1842856 to cells from two donors prior to and one day after infection with a single round pseudotyped virus. We then measured GFP, CD62L and CD69 expression, viral cDNA and RNA within the cells, and *de novo* virus output (Figure 6). GFP+ cells emerged earlier in the AS1842856 treated cultures, and at two days after infection, the total GFP fluorescence in the culture was enhanced by an order of magnitude, consistent with the interpretation that Foxo1 suppression assists the establishment of infection in cells (Figure 6A–D). Reverse transcription was unaffected by AS1842856 (Figure 6E), but the production of HIV-1 RNA was accelerated (Figure 6F). Interestingly, AS1842856 did not increase the maximum RNA production from the cells but only accelerated the achievement of this peak. Application of AS1842856 to sorted GFP+ cells that had reached their maximum expression had little effect, increasing GFP fluorescence 16% after 3 days (Figure S3 in File S1). CD62L was modestly down-modulated in the GFP-negative (Figure 6A, 6H) and control uninfected cells by a single AS1842856 dosing on day 0 (not

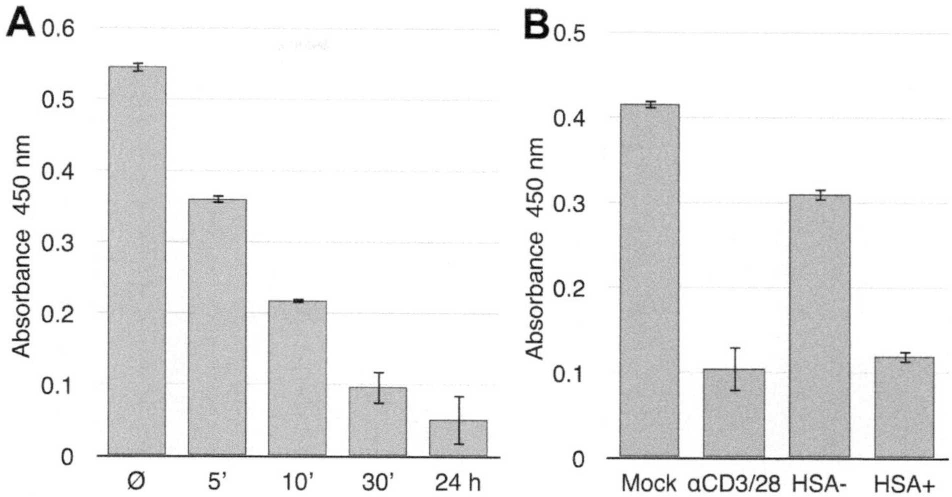

Figure 5. Foxo1 activity by TransAM ELISA. A. Time course of Foxo1 inactivation following T cell activation with anti-CD3/CD28 beads. The ability of nuclear Foxo1 to bind a target DNA oligonucleotide was analyzed using a TransAM Foxo1 kit (Active Motif). SD of triplicate analysis of each condition are shown from one representative experiment of 3. Specificity was demonstrated by successful competition with a free Foxo1 binding oligonucleotide but not with a negative control oligonucleotide (not shown). Error bars are SD of triplicate wells. **B.** Foxo1 activity in HIV-1 infected resting CD4 T cells, mock infected and beads activated cells. Cells were infected with HIV-1 HSA reporter virus for 7 days, then separated into HSA+ and HSA-negative subsets using an antibody to HSA and magnetic beads. Data are from one representative experiment of three independent experiments. Error bars are SD of triplicate wells.

shown), which when left untreated increased their CD62L expression over time. GFP+ AS1842856 treated cells down-modulated CD62L more rapidly than untreated cells in parallel with accelerated HIV-1 expression. Repeated dosing with AS1842856 over 9 days resulted in down modulation similar to HIV-1 infection (not shown). AS1842856 synergized with HIV-1 in productively infected cells to increase CD69 expression (Figure 6I), especially in memory cells, indicating early T cell activation. There are no Foxo1 or KLF2 consensus binding sequences in this HIV-1 strain, so these transcription factors are unlikely to be enhancing virus expression through direct binding to the viral promoter.

Discussion

The suppression of Foxo1 activity of both infected resting naïve and memory CD4 T cells is a hitherto unknown dysregulation of cells by HIV-1. Foxo1 regulates fundamental properties of T cells, including their activation state and expression of a series of receptors controlling T cell migration such as CD62L; consequently the implications of this finding are wide ranging. The activation state of productively infected resting CD4 T cells was elevated, as they displayed increased CD69 and cyclin D2 expression and down-modulation of CD62L, all of which are Foxo1 target genes. A primary implication of this finding is that by raising the activation state of the infected cell, Foxo1 inactivation might enhance virus replication. Indeed, application of the Foxo1 inhibitor AS1842856 accelerated virus expression. Interestingly, the herpesvirus Epstein-Barr Virus also suppresses Foxo1 activity [79], suggesting that Foxo1 inactivation might not be an unusual viral strategy. Foxo1 is dysregulated in many cancers and the possibility of its therapeutic manipulation is avidly investigated [80]. Control of Foxo1 activity might also provide a means to activate or suppress HIV-1 expression in resting T cells.

We demonstrated Foxo1 inactivation in productively infected cells by both functional assays (DNA binding) and by Image-Stream analysis showing that Foxo1 relocated to the cytoplasm in productively infected naïve and memory CD4 T cells. We confirmed this result by Western blot (unpublished data). Cytoplasmic Foxo1 can be degraded in a ubiquitin-dependent pathway [35,50,81], however we found that the total Foxo1 protein staining as well as its mRNA were nearly equal in cells with and without HIV-1 gene expression, indicating that Foxo1 inactivation by HIV-1 did not entail a reduction in Foxo1 protein or necessarily its transcription. The best characterized mechanism for Foxo1 inactivation is through phosphorylation, primarily by Akt (protein kinase B) that is activated in a PI3K dependent pathway following T cell receptor ligation, though phosphorylation by SGK (serum and glucocorticoid-induced kinase), casein kinase 1 and Cdk2 as well as acetylation and ubiquitinization can inhibit Foxo1 activity [82]. The ability of PI3K inhibitors to partially inhibit CD62L down-modulation in infected cells, plus the relocalization of Foxo1 to the cytoplasm both implicate phosphorylation in HIV-1-induced Foxo1 inactivation. HIV-1 is known to activate PI3K and Akt by the interaction of envelope with resting T cells [83] and through the activities of Tat and Nef [26,84]. Each of these proteins has long been known to enhance both T cell activation [85–89] and infection of resting T cells [25,29]. Our findings likely add another consequence of HIV-1-induced Akt activation; however, Foxo1 phosphorylation has been difficult to document in our system. Studies are underway to define the kinetics of Foxo1 inactivation and the HIV-1 gene(s) and signaling pathway(s) responsible.

PI3K is an upstream activator of Akt, which phosphorylates and inactivates Foxo1. Akt activation is an important mechanism to promote cell survival [90,91], in part by reducing activity of Foxo1 and the related Foxo3a transcription factors. Inhibitors of PI3K and Akt are under development to treat cancers and certain inflammatory and infectious diseases [91–95]. HIV-1 Tat protein activates Akt in infected macrophages, providing a cytoprotective function; thus it has been proposed that Akt inhibition could provide a way to specifically target infected macrophages for death [96–98]. It may be that Foxo1 links HIV-1 infection and Akt

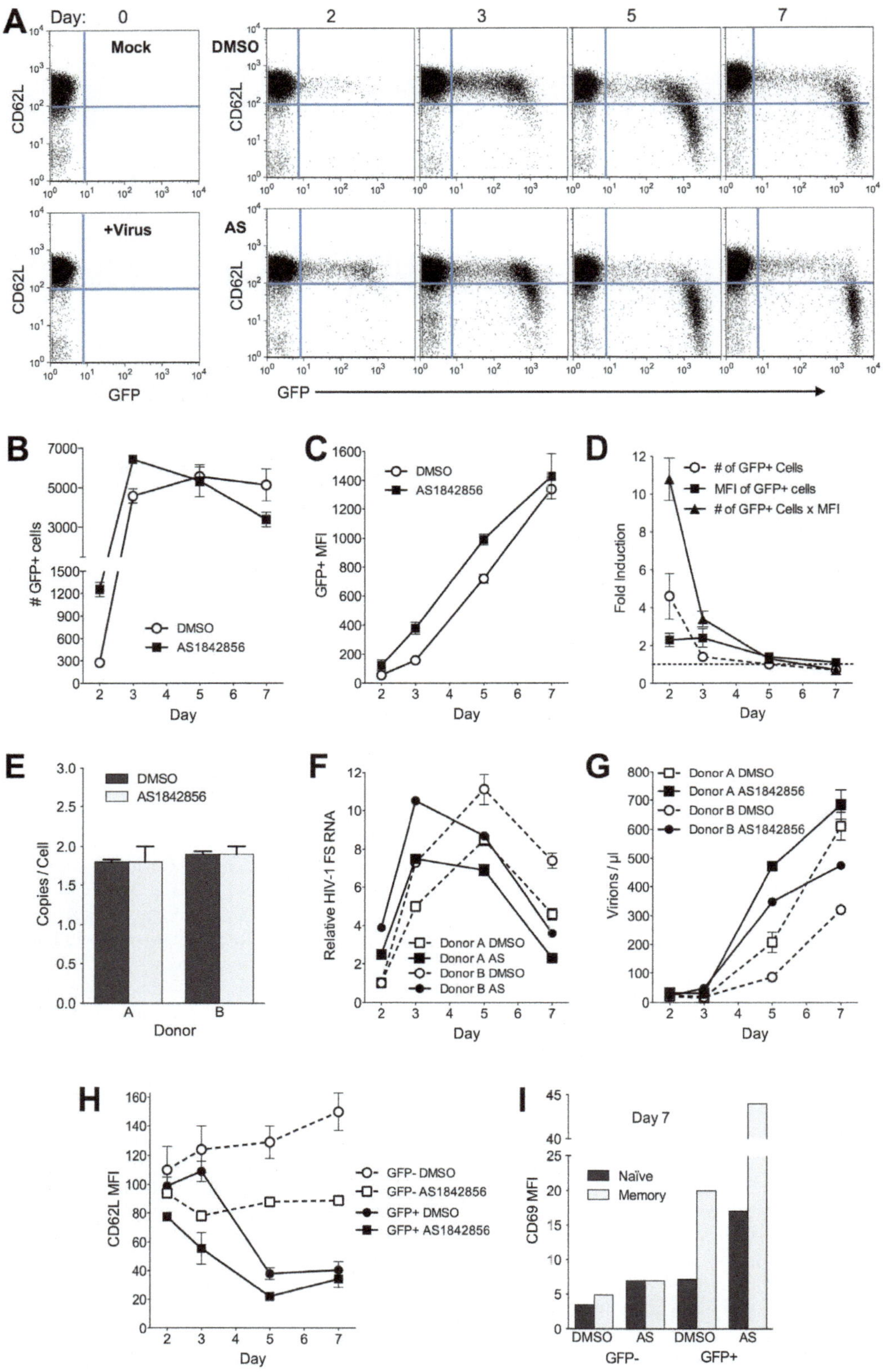

Figure 6. Foxo1 inhibitor AS1842856 accelerates HIV-1 expression. AS1842856 (AS) was applied to cells 1 day before and 1 day after infection with single round GFP reporter virus. CD45RO- naïve T cells are shown. **A.** GFP and CD62L expression in infected naïve CD4+ T cells on the indicated day after infection. Donor A is shown. **B.** The number of GFP+ cells on the indicated day after infection. Data are average and SD of the two donors. **C.** Mean fluorescence intensity (MFI) of GFP in the GFP+ cells. Data are average and SD of the two donors. **D.** Fold increase in the number and the MFI of GFP+ cells, and total GFP fluorescence in the cells calculated as the product of the number of GFP+ cells multiplied by their MFI. Data are average and SD of the two donors. **E.** Near-full length reverse transcripts on day 2 after infection for one representative cell donor. Data are averages and SD for replicate PCR reactions for each donor. **F.** HIV-1 fully spliced RNA presented relative to day 1 DMSO condition. Data are averages and SD for replicate PCR reactions for each donor. **G.** Virus production measured by genomic RNA in culture medium. Data are averages and SD for replicate

PCR reactions for each donor. **H.** CD62L MFI on the indicated day. Data are MFI of GFP+ cells divided by background staining. Data are average and SD of the two donors. **I.** CD69 MFI on day 7 post infection on naïve and memory resting CD4+ T cells for donor A.

activity with various sequella of infection to provide a therapeutically useful target for pharmacologic development.

CD62L down-modulation did not occur rapidly, but instead required several days of HIV-1 gene expression (Figure 6H) or treatment with Foxo1 inhibitor (unpublished data). These kinetics are similar to the genetic down-modulation that occurs following T cell activation, except that we did not observe the initial protease cleavage step following infection that has been reported by others [72,73]. The half-life of CD62L mRNA is long [33,55] and our unpublished data indicate that CD62L persists on the resting T cell surface for several days, so further studies will be required to reveal the kinetics of Foxo1, KLF2 and CD62L mRNA suppression after infection. Since *de novo* HIV-1 expression was required for these effects, there will of necessity be some delay between infection and Foxo1 suppression.

We hypothesized that the inhibition of Foxo1 activity with AS1842856 would increase or accelerate viral replication, and indeed, AS1842856 accelerated HIV-1 RNA transcription, but not reverse transcription. It was interesting that the peak of RNA production was similar between AS1842856 treated and control infections, consistent with the notion that Foxo1 inhibition mainly accelerates the establishment of infection. Also consistent with this interpretation was the observation that AS1842856 only modestly increased GFP fluorescence of cells that had been infected several days prior to treatment. As stated above, we find that daily dosing of uninfected CD4 T cells with AS1842856 results in much more complete CD62L down-modulation than the single dose we employed to assist HIV-1 infection (unpublished findings), consistent with the long half-life of CD62L mRNA and with the proposed mechanism of AS1842856 action [78].

Besides enhancing virus output, what are likely consequences of the reprogramming of infected naïve and memory resting T cells via Foxo1 suppression? Each of the genes that were up or down regulated can have a profound effect on the behavior of the cells, particularly their migration, activation and survival. These potential effects might be moot if the cell were to rapidly die due to viral cytopathicity, but resting T cells survive for much greater lengths of time than activated T cells [1,22]. As previously mentioned, resting CD4 T cells are the dominant target of infection soon after transmission, the period when antiviral immunity is being established that will determine the outcome of infection [7]. Much of the latent reservoir is also established early in infection [99,100]. By manipulating the cells' activation state and the expression of receptors that support migration in and out of lymphoid tissues (and which also possess intracellular and extracellular signaling properties), HIV-1 could interfere with the establishment of antiviral immunity through suppression of Foxo1 activity.

The overall pattern of gene regulation in the productively infected naïve CD4 T cells was consistent with the observed suppression of Foxo1 activity by HIV-1. Although naïve T cells are a minority of infected T cells *in vivo*, they are important targets of infection [2,3,101,102]. We chose to examine gene regulation in this population because of its uniform expression of CD62L, whereas memory cells are heterogeneous in CD62L expression, with many T_{EM} expressing no CD62L. Future analysis of TCM will be useful in order to more fully understand Foxo1 dysregulation by HIV-1, and preliminary studies indicate a pattern of gene regulation by HIV-1 similar to naïve cells (unpublished data). One of the genes that Foxo1 maintains in resting T cells is KLF2, a second master regulator of T cell activation and migration [60,103,104], and we observed that KLF2 mRNA was strongly suppressed in infected cells. Prior studies have demonstrated that ectopic expression of KLF2 in proliferating and activated cells returns them to a quiescent state, and loss of KLF2 expression has been shown to result in increased T cell activation [57,105]. KLF2−/− mice lack naïve T cells in lymphoid organs, acquiring the homing characteristics of activated T cells [105]. In the present study the mRNA of several genes that are known to be transcriptionally activated by Foxo1 and/or KLF2 were lower in productively infected cells, including CD62L, IL-7rα, Fam65B and $S1P_1$, CD52, Myc and CCR5 [56,60,62,103,105,106]. mRNA for two genes that Foxo1 suppresses, CD69 and Cyclin D2, were increased in infected cells, again consistent with Foxo1 inactivation. Interestingly, the Foxo1-mediated suppression of Cyclin D2 transcription does not require Foxo1 DNA binding activity [107], evidence of Foxo1 gene regulation through interaction with protein binding partners [47]. Myc has been shown to suppress HIV-1 transcription [108] so its suppression in productively infected cells is quite interesting.

CD62L, KLF2, CD69, $S1P_1$, CCR5 and Fam65b are each involved in T cell migration. While CD62L is required for entry into lymph nodes, $S1P_1$ is required for egress in response to its ligand S1P present in blood [104,109]. KLF2 and Foxo1 both induce $S1P_1$ expression [45,60,62]. T cell responses to $S1P_1$ are impaired in HIV-1 infected individuals, perhaps contributing to lymphadenopathy [110]. $S1P_1$ and CD69 are mutual antagonists [110,111] and CD69 expression inhibits $S1P_1$-dependent egress from lymphoid organs until later in the activation cascade, when CD69 levels decline [112]. CD69 also regulates chemokine expression and T cell accumulation in the intestine [113]. Thus, by increasing CD69 and suppressing both CD62L and $S1P_1$, HIV-1 may disrupt both lymphoid tissue entry and exit functions of infected cells. Tat has been shown to induce CD69 expression through NF-κB activation [114]. However, we saw no NF-κB nuclear translocation, so Foxo1 suppression seems to be the operative in our system. The increase in CD69 which we observed was rather modest compared with the levels achieved following T cell receptor stimulation (Figure 1), and whether $S1P_1$ is being suppressed by CD69 binding to $S1P_1$ [115,116] awaits further study.

The mRNA of cell cycle regulator $p21^{CIP1}$ was also higher in productively infected cells. This finding is interesting in light of the findings that Foxo proteins are activators of $p21^{CIP1}$ transcription in neural cells [117] and that KLF2 upregulates p21 transcription in Jurkat T cells [118]. Based on these findings, we would expect lower p21 mRNA levels in HIV-1 infected cells. Our contrary finding may reflect cell-type specific differences or the possibility that transformed cells do not reproduce the regulatory pathways of primary cells. On the other hand, Myc was repressed in Foxo−/− mice [119], and Seoane et al. [117] also reported that Myc represses p21, so in this paradigm Myc repression in Foxo1-suppressed infected cells would result in increased p21 – the outcome we observed. To make the situation more complicated, overexpression of KLF2 represses Myc transcription in Jurkat cells [60,120], again, a finding hard to reconcile with our data; but, in a further apparent contradiction, a study KLF2−/− mice found no alteration in Myc in CD8 T cells [57] reviewed in [31]. Finally, HIV-1 Vpr can induce p21 transcription [121–123]. In macrophages, this p21 upregulation enhanced virus replication [123].

Studies are underway examining the contribution of Vpr to cellular gene regulation in resting T cells.

CCR7, Foxo1 and Foxo3a are also known transcriptional targets of Foxo1 or Foxo1 plus KLF2, and their mRNA levels remained unchanged during productive infection. Why expression of these genes was relatively unchanged remains to be investigated. Although CCR7 mRNA remained constant, CCR7 receptor staining was modestly reduced on productively infected cells, consistent with a recent report that Vpu modestly down-modulates CCR7 surface expression in activated T cells [67]. Here we report that HIV-1 modestly down-modulates CCR7 in resting T cells while not altering CCR7 mRNA levels.

The suppression of CCR5 mRNA in GFP+ bright cells was consistent with recent findings that KLF2 activated CCR5 expression and bound to the CCR5 promoter in resting T cells [61], but both of these reports are inconsistent with a study in KLF2 knockout mice [105]. CCR5 is the ligand for chemokines CCL3 and CCL4 (MIP1α and β) and its suppression would be expected to alter homing to inflammatory sites. Another migration-related gene suppressed in infected cells was Fam65b. Fam65b negatively regulates RhoA activity and chemokine-induced migration [124], and its transcription is activated in T cells by Foxo1 [64]. Together, the multitude of disruptions by Foxo1 suppression make proper homing to lymphoid tissues and effector sites appear unlikely, though functional tests will be required. A recent study found that quite low levels of KLF2 were sufficient to maintain CCR5 expression and infectability [61], and our data reveal exceptionally strong suppression of CCR5 mRNA in the GFP bright cells. HIV-1 Nef is known to down-modulate CCR5 [125,126], and the present work demonstrates a second mechanism (transcriptional repression) by which HIV-1 may reduce CCR5 in resting CD4 T cells. CCR5 receptor expression on resting CD4 T cells is difficult to quantify and further studies are underway. On the other hand, we did observe efficient down-modulation of CD4 surface expression in resting T cells (Figure 1) as well as Class I MHC down-modulation (unpublished data), but neither of their mRNA levels were affected by infection. GFP+ dim cells had about 1.5 times more CCR5 mRNA than the GFP− cells, which could be either preferential infection of cells that are slightly more activated or active upregulation in this subset. GFP+ dim cells display only early HIV-1 gene expression [22,127], so perhaps and early gene such as Tat or Nef increases CCR5 mRNA, while late HIV-1 gene expression is necessary for KLF2 suppression. It is interesting to note that in addition to binding to vascular endothelium, CD62L also seems important for regulating expression of the chemokine receptor CXCR4, the other HIV-1 co-receptor besides CCR5 [128]. Thus the potential for HIV-1 to disrupt cell trafficking via suppression of Foxo1 activity would appear to be wide ranging.

Finally, in light of the ability of HIV-1 to down-modulate CD62L, the use of CD62L to discriminate between central memory T cells and effector memory T cells during HIV-1 infection may be problematic. Our findings demonstrate that infected TCM (CD45RA-RO+CD62L+) that have down-modulated CD62L can, superficially at least, masquerade as infected T_{EM} (CD45RA-RO+CD62L−) in flow cytometry analysis. Additionally, TCM uniformly express CD62L, while TEM are sometimes represented as being uniformly CD62L-negative [129]. CCR7-negative T_{EM} are actually heterogeneous in their expression of CD62L (Figure S2 in File S1, [130]), so CCR7 expression or any of several other receptors [130] should be more useful markers for T_{CM} vs. T_{EM} discrimination.

Materials and Methods

Cells

Peripheral blood CD4+ T cells from healthy HIV-1-negative donors were isolated by negative selection using the Dynabeads Untouched Human CD4 T cell magnetic separation Kit (Life Technologies) per manufacturer direction as previously described [22]. Purified cells were routinely ≥99% small, CD4−, CD25−, CD38−,CD69−, and HLA-DR- quiescent T cells [22]. Blood was purchased from the New York Blood Center as de-identified samples. No protected health information was collected. The New York University Committee on Activities Involving Human Subjects (UCAIHS) determined that these samples do not constitute human research. Purified CD4+ T cells were cultured at 2×10^6 cells per ml in Gibco Advanced RPMI 1640 with 10% fetal bovine serum (HyClone) plus penicillin and streptomycin (Gibco) and 50 μM β-mercaptoethanol (Sigma). Where indicated, IL-7 (2 ng/ml, BioVision) or IL-4 (25 ng/ml) (R&D Systems) was added to the culture medium. Where indicated, cells were activated with Dynabeads Human T-Activator CD3/CD28 (Life Technologies), as per the manufacturer's instructions.

Viruses

Virus construction has been described previously [22,127,131]. NLENG1-IRES (Fig. 1, 2) is a replication competent HIV-1 NL4-3 backbone GFP reporter virus, identical to NLENY1-IRES and NLENC1-IRES [131] except that it contains the eGFP gene (Clontech) in place of eYFP or eCFP. Infections with this virus were restricted to a single round of infection by treatment with the protease inhibitor indinavir (2 μM). NLENG1-ESI (Figures 3, 4, 6) is an envelope mutant HIV-1 GFP reporter virus previously described [22,127]. NLENHSA-ESI (Figure 5) is an HIV-1 NL4-3 backbone HSA (mCD24) reporter virus constructed identically to NLENG1-ESI, except that it contains the gene for murine CD24 (Heat Stable Antigen – HSA) in place of GFP.

Infections

The titers of the virus stocks were determined using TaqMan qRT-PCR for HIV-1 RNA (target in integrase) and normalized to a nominal 400 virion equivalents per cell for infection. Infections were performed by spinoculation in the presence of 5 μg/ml DEAE dextran (Sigma) for 2 h at 1,200×g and 37°C [22,132]. Cells were then washed and plated. For FKHR TransAM experiments, IL-7 treated CD4 T cells were infected with NLENHSA-ESI. At 7 dpi., cells were ficolled in order to remove dead cells, then stained with a phycoerythrin (PE) labeled anti-mCD24 and bound to anti-PE magnetic microbeads (Miltenyi Biotec). Positive and negative cells were separated using the MACS system (Miltenyi Biotec). Purity was routinely >95%.

Cell treatments included PMA (2 nM, Fisher Scientific), LY294002 (5 μM, BioVision), PI-103 (5 μM, EMD Millipore), TAPI-1 (50 μM, Santa Cruz Biotechnology). Non-nucleoside reverse-transcriptase inhibitor Efavirenz (2 μg/ml) and Protease inhibitor Indinavir (2 μM) were obtained from the NIH AIDS Research and Reference Reagent Program. The Foxo1 inhibitor 5-amino-7-(cyclohexylamino)-1-ethyl-6-fluoro-4-oxo-1,4-dihydro-quinoline-3-carboxylic acid (AS1842856) [78], was purchased from EMD Millipore and used at a final concentration of 50 nM. DMSO controls were performed with a corresponding dilution of 1 in 20,000.

Tonsil cell infections. Tonsils were obtained as de-identified specimens from discarded pathologic specimens of children without known HIV-1 infection undergoing elective tonsillectomies at Children's Hospital Denver in accordance with the

Colorado Multiple Institutional Review Board (CMIRB), which reviewed this protocol on September 23, 2008 and determined that it does not constitute human subjects research. For this reason, informed consent is not required.

Tonsils were mechanically disaggregated in sterile phosphate buffered saline. The cell suspension was filtered through a 70 micron filter (Fisher Scientific, Denver, CO) and washed with PBS. Single cell suspensions were infected with NLENG1-IRES as described [133], then IL-4 (25 ng/ml) was added to the cultures and again on day 3 post infection. For flow cytometry, cells were stained with anti-CD3-PerCP, anti-CD8-PerCP-Cy5, anti-CD45RA-PE-Cy5, anti-CD62L-PE, (all from BD Pharmingen) and analyzed on a Becton Dickinson (BD) LSR II flow cytometer (UC Denver). Gating for GFP expression was on CD3+ $CD8^-$CD45RA+ cells.

Flow Cytometry

Flow cytometry was performed on a BD FACSort flow cytometer upgraded by Cytek Development, Fremont, CA, to contain 488-nm, 407-nm, and 637-nm lasers and 5 fluorescence detectors. Enhanced Green fluorescent protein (GFP) was detected in FL-1 using 510/21-nm and a 540-nm short-pass dichroic splitter. Compensation was applied during data collection on the basis of single-color controls. Data collection was with CellQuest Pro software for Mac OS X (BD Biosciences). Flow data were analyzed using FlowJo (v9 and v10) software for Mac OS X (Tree Star). T(x) population comoparison analysis was with FlowJo 9 [134]. Proliferation analysis was performed using eFluor670 (eBioscience). CD4 (PerCP-Cy5.5, SK3) and HLA-A2 (PerCP-Cy5.5, BB7.2) antibodies were purchased from BD Pharmingen. Memory and Naïve CD4 T cells were identified by positive CD45RA staining and/or negative CD45RO staining. CD45RA (Pacific Blue, HI100), CD45RO (Pacific Blue, UCHL1), CD62L (PerCP-Cy5.5 and APC, DREG-57), CD69 (PerCP-Cy5.5, FN50), and CCR7 (APC, TG8/CCR7) antibodies were purchased from BioLegend. Phosphatidylserine externalization was detected with Annexin-V Pacific Blue (Life Technologies) and cellular membrane permeability was assessed by 7-AAD (7-Aminoactinomycin D) (Life Technologies) incorporation. Cell sorting was performed using a BD FACSAria flow cytometer at the New York University Medical Center Flow Cytometry and Cell Sorting Center.

ImageStream

Foxo1 rabbit antibody (C59H4) was purchased from Cell Signaling and NF-κB (p65) rabbit antibody (C-20) was from Santa Cruz Biotechnology. CD45RO antibody was from BioLegend. Staining were performed following Cell Signaling protocol for intracellular staining, with modifications. Briefly, T cells were harvested at the indicated times and fixed with 2% paraformaldehyde (PFA) for 10 min at 37°C. Cells were then chilled on ice for 1 min and mixed while vortexing with 9 volumes of ice cold 100% methanol to a final concentration of 90% for permeabilization. Cells were incubated for 1 hour at −20°C and washed with incubation buffer (0.5% BSA in PBS). Cells were blocked in incubation buffer for 10 min. Staining were performed for either transcription factor plus mouse anti-CD45RO PerCP-Cy5.5 (CD45RO staining was performed after permeabilization to avoid fluorochrome degradation in methanol). Cells were incubated for 1 hour at room temperature, washed with 0.5% BSA PBS and stained with anti-rabbit DyLight 649 (BioLegend). Cells were incubated another hour at room temperature then washed. Prior to acquisition, cells were incubated at 10^6 cells per ml in DAPI staining solution (Life Technologies) for 15 min. Cells were then pelleted and resuspended in the same solution at 30×10^6 cells per ml for ImageStream acquisition. Acquisition was performed in the Flow Cytometry Resource Center at Rockefeller University (New York) using Amnis ImageStream-X and analysis was done with the Amnis IDEAS software and FlowJo (v10).

Single-color controls were acquired in order to construct a compensation matrix that was applied to all experimental samples. Similarity score between each transcription factor (Foxo1 or NF-κB) and DNA staining with DAPI was calculated using IDEAS software Similarity Feature. which is the log-transformed Pearson's correlation coefficient between the pixel values of two image pairs. The degree of nuclear localization of a protein is measured by the pixel intensity correlation between staining for that protein and DNA staining [135,136]. The higher the Similarity Score, the higher the level of nuclear localization.

Foxo1 TransAM

Foxo1 (FKHR) activity was quantified using the FKHR TransAM ELISA system from Active Motif. Briefly, T cells were treated and harvested as described in "Infections", then nuclear proteins were extracted using the Active Motif Nuclear Extraction Kit. Nuclear proteins were quantified with the NanoOrange Protein Quantitation Kit (Life Technologies). Samples were tested in triplicate wells of 3 µg total proteins per replicate. Foxo1 DNA binding activity to an oligonucleotide containing the Foxo1 target consensus sequence (5′-TTGTTTAC-3′) was measured following the Active Motif's instructions. Foxo1 binding specificity was verified by adding competitive specific or scrambled oligonucleotides provided in the kit. ELISA plate O.D. was read on a Molecular Devices SpectraMax M5 spectrophotometer with detection of absorbance at 450 nm and a reference wavelength of 655 nm.

Quantification of HIV-1 DNA

qPCR methods have been described previously [22]. Briefly, DNA from cells infected with benzonase-treated viruses was purified using a DNeasy Blood & Tissue Minikit or an AllPrep Minikit (Qiagen) with RNase A (Sigma) digestion. Quantitative real-time PCR for DNA analysis was performed using a QuantiTect Probe PCR kit (Qiagen). Primers and TaqMan probes were purchased from Integrated DNA Technologies (IDT). Amplification and detection were performed on a Chromo4 real-time PCR machine (Bio-Rad), and the data were analyzed using the manufacturer's Opticon Monitor 3 software.

Quantification of total HIV DNA was performed using:

forward primer: ZXF F (5′-AAG-TAGTGTGTGCCCGTCTGT-3′),

reverse primer: ZXF R (5′-GCTTCAGCAAGCCGAGTC-3′),

and probe: ZXF (5′-56-FAM-TGTGACTCT-ZEN-GGTAAC-TAGAGATCCCTCAGACCC-3IABlk_FQ-3′,

where FAM is 6-carboxyfluorescein, ZEN is an internal quencher (IDT), and 3IABlk_FQ is the 3′ Iowa black FQ quencher. Quantification of 2-LTR circles [22] was performed using:

forward primer: 2L-f2 (5′-TGTTGTGTGACTCTGGTAAC-TAGAGATCCC-3′),

reverse primer: 2L-r2 (5′-GATATCT-GATCCCTGGCCCTGG-3′),

probe: 2L-z2 (5′-56-FAM-CCACACACAAGGC-TACTTCCCTGATTGGCAG-3IABlk_FQ-3′).

CD4 gene DNA amplification (see primers in the qRT-PCR section) was used for normalization of the total number of HIV-1 DNA copies per cell. Standardization for quantification of total HIV-1 DNA was performed with 10-fold serial dilutions of genomic DNA extracted from Jurkat cells containing 2 integrated HIV-1 NL4-3 proviruses.

DNA qPCR used the following thermal cycling program: step 1: 95°C for 15 min; step 2: 94°C for 15 sec; step 3: 60°C for 30 sec; step 4: fluorescence data collection; and step 5: return to step 2×40.

qRT-PCR

RNA was isolated from virus-containing culture medium or infected cells using an RNeasy Minikit (Qiagen) with on-column DNase digestion (40 min). Quantitative real-time RT-PCR for RNA was performed using a QuantiTect Probe RT-PCR kit (Qiagen). All qRT-PCR used the following thermal cycling program: step 1: 50°C for 30 min; step 2: 94°C for 15 min; step 3: 94°C for 15 sec; step 4: 60°C for 30 sec; step 5: fluorescence data collection; and step 6: return to step 3×40.

Quantification of HIV-1 in supernatants (virus stock and experimental output). We used primers and TaqMan probes specific for a shared region of integrase RNA sequence. Quantification of HIV-1 RNA was performed against serial 10-fold dilutions of a synthetic RNA molecule containing the integrase target (67). Forward primer : FL-U Sense (5′-CAATTT-CACCAGTACTACAGTT-3′),

reverse primer: FL Sense (5′-GAATGC-CAAATTCCTGCTTGA-3′) (79),

probe: FL-U (5′-56-FAM-AAGGCCGCC-ZEN-TGTTGGTGGGCG-3IABlk_FQ-3′).

Control assays for DNA carryover were routinely performed and were either completely negative or contained ≤1/40,000 RNA molecules.

Quantification of fully spliced HIV RNA in infected cells. We used primers and TaqMan probes (Integrated DNA Technologies) detecting fully spliced RNA specific for NL4-3 HIV. Quantification of FS HIV RNA was performed against serial 10-fold dilutions of a synthetic RNA molecule containing the fully spliced (FS) target.

Forward primer: DNL287 (5′-GGAGACAGCGACGAA-GAGC-3′),

reverse primer: DNL288 (5′-CTCTCCACCTTCTTCTTC-TATTCC-3′),

probe: LA45-LA41: (5′-56-FAM-CATCAGAACAGTCA-GACTCATCAAGCTTCTCTATCAAAG-3IABlk_FQ-3′).

Quantification of cellular mRNA. With the exception of CD4 primers, which were from IDT, primers and TaqMan probes for mRNA quantification were from Life Technologies (Table S1 in File S1).

CD4 RNA the primers and probes:

Forward primer: CD4F2 Sense (5′- GCCAACTCTGACACC-CAC-3′),

reverse primer: CD4R2 Sense (5′- GACTCCTACATTG-CACTGAG-3′),

probe: CD4P2 (5′-56-FAM-CAGAGCCTG-ZEN-AC-CCTGACCTTGGAGA-3IABlk_FQ-3′).

Relative expression of cellular mRNAs in infected T cell subsets (Fig. 3C and D) was analyzed using the Comparative Ct method [137] and normalized to the average Ct of 2 endogenous housekeeping genes RPL13A and IPO8 [138]. Results were expressed in fold inductions in comparison to the reference sample of sorted GFP negative T cells.

Fold induction = $2^{-\Delta\Delta Ct}$.

$\Delta\Delta$Ct = ΔCt of sample–ΔCt of reference.

ΔCt = Ct of gene of interest–average Ct of house keeping genes.

Supporting Information

File S1 File S1 includes the following: Figure S1. CD62L expression is maintained in the presence of common gamma chain cytokines. Resting CD4+ T cells were cultured with no cytokine (Ø) or the indicated cytokine for 2 days then analyzed for CD45RA and CD62L expression by flow cytometry. Neg. control was with an isotype-matched non-specific antibody. IL-2 (50 u/ml), IL-4 (25 ng/ml), IL-7 (2 ng/ml), IL-15 (10 ng/ml). Data are representative of >3 independent experiments. **Figure S2. CD62L is down-modulated in HIV-1 expressing cells in both central memory and effector memory CD4+ T cells, and CCR7 is modestly down-modulated.** IL-7-treated resting CD4+ T cells were infected with a single round GFP virus and then analyzed as in Figure 1, with additional staining with CCR7 to distinguish central memory (T_{CM}) and effector memory (T_{EM}) cells. Data are representative of >3 independent experiments. **A.** CD62L is down-modulated on naïve (CD45RA+), central memory (TCM, CD45RA-CCR7+) and effector memory (T_{EM}, CD45RA-CCR7−) resting CD4+ T cells. A subset of TEM naturally lacks CD62L expression. **B.** CCR7 is slightly down-modulated on naïve and memory CD4+ T cells expressing HIV-1. Data are representative of >5 experiments which consistently show 20%–30% loss of CCR7 mean fluorescence intensity (MFI) in the HIV-1 expressing (GFP+) cells. Grey: isotype-matched IgG control antibody staining. Other histograms are color coded to match the legend font color. **C.** HIV-1 expression is highest in effector memory T cells as measured by GFP MFI. **Figure S3. Foxo1 inhibitor AS1842856 applied to productively infected GFP+ cells.** IL-7 treated resting CD4+ T cells were infected with a single round env-pseudotyped HIV-1 GFP reporter virus and sorted for GFP+ cells. On day 17 after infection, AS1842856 was applied and GFP expression was analyzed 3 days later. Cell viability was 14–20%. **Table S1.** TaqMan primer and probe sets for quantification of cellular RNA in Figure 3. **Table S2.** Values for RNA expression graphed in Figure 3. HIV-1 FS is fully spliced Rev-independent early viral RNA. HIV-1 FL is full length Rev-dependent late viral RNA.

Acknowledgments

The authors thank Svetlana Mazel, Stanka Semova, Darin Fogg and Richard Demarco for assistance with ImageStream data collection and analysis, Angela Kamer for statistical advice, and Vincent Sahi for advice regarding experimental methods.

Author Contributions

Conceived and designed the experiments: DNL BT. Performed the experiments: BT DNL CNC SM YL MP JF CSL. Analyzed the data: DNL BT. Contributed reagents/materials/analysis tools: DNL MM EC. Contributed to the writing of the manuscript: DNL BT.

References

1. Zhang ZQ, Wietgrefe SW, Li Q, Shore MD, Duan L, et al. (2004) Roles of substrate availability and infection of resting and activated CD4+ T cells in transmission and acute simian immunodeficiency virus infection. Proc Natl Acad Sci U S A 101: 5640–5645.
2. Ostrowski MA, Chun TW, Justement SJ, Motola I, Spinelli MA, et al. (1999) Both memory and CD45RA+/CD62L+ naive CD4(+) T cells are infected in human immunodeficiency virus type 1-infected individuals. J Virol 73: 6430–6435.
3. Zhang Z, Schuler T, Zupancic M, Wietgrefe S, Staskus KA, et al. (1999) Sexual transmission and propagation of SIV and HIV in resting and activated CD4+ T cells. Science 286: 1353–1357.

4. Schacker T, Little S, Connick E, Gebhard K, Zhang ZQ, et al. (2001) Productive infection of T cells in lymphoid tissues during primary and early human immunodeficiency virus infection. J Infect Dis 183: 555–562.
5. Li Q, Duan L, Estes JD, Ma ZM, Rourke T, et al. (2005) Peak SIV replication in resting memory CD4+ T cells depletes gut lamina propria CD4+ T cells. Nature 434: 1148–1152.
6. Mattapallil JJ, Douek DC, Hill B, Nishimura Y, Martin M, et al. (2005) Massive infection and loss of memory CD4+ T cells in multiple tissues during acute SIV infection. Nature 434: 1093–1097.
7. Hatziioannou T, Del Prete GQ, Keele BF, Estes JD, McNatt MW, et al. (2014) HIV-1-induced AIDS in monkeys. Science 344: 1401–1405.
8. Zack JA, Arrigo SJ, Weitsman SR, Go AS, Haislip A, et al. (1990) HIV-1 entry into quiescent primary lymphocytes: molecular analysis reveals a labile, latent viral structure. Cell 61: 213–222.
9. Pan X, Baldauf HM, Keppler OT, Fackler OT (2013) Restrictions to HIV-1 replication in resting CD4+ T lymphocytes. Cell Res 23: 876–885.
10. Zack JA, Kim SG, Vatakis DN (2013) HIV restriction in quiescent CD4(+) T cells. Retrovirology 10: 37.
11. Vella A, Teague TK, Ihle J, Kappler J, Marrack P (1997) Interleukin 4 (IL-4) or IL-7 prevents the death of resting T cells: stat6 is probably not required for the effect of IL-4. J Exp Med 186: 325–330.
12. Gomez J, Martinez AC, Gonzalez A, Garcia A, Rebollo A (1998) The Bcl-2 gene is differentially regulated by IL-2 and IL-4: role of the transcription factor NF-AT. Oncogene 17: 1235–1243.
13. Aronica MA, Goenka S, Boothby M (2000) IL-4-dependent induction of BCL-2 and BCL-X(L)IN activated T lymphocytes through a STAT6- and pi 3-kinase-independent pathway. Cytokine 12: 578–587.
14. Vella AT, Dow S, Potter TA, Kappler J, Marrack P (1998) Cytokine-induced survival of activated T cells in vitro and in vivo. Proc Natl Acad Sci U S A 95: 3810–3815.
15. Boise LH, Minn AJ, June CH, Lindsten T, Thompson CB (1995) Growth factors can enhance lymphocyte survival without committing the cell to undergo cell division. Proc Natl Acad Sci U S A 92: 5491–5495.
16. Estes JD (2013) Pathobiology of HIV/SIV-associated changes in secondary lymphoid tissues. Immunol Rev 254: 65–77.
17. Rathmell JC, Farkash EA, Gao W, Thompson CB (2001) IL-7 enhances the survival and maintains the size of naive T cells. J Immunol 167: 6869–6876.
18. Kinter A, Moorthy A, Jackson R, Fauci AS (2003) Productive HIV infection of resting CD4+ T cells: role of lymphoid tissue microenvironment and effect of immunomodulating agents. AIDS Res Hum Retroviruses 19: 847–856.
19. Unutmaz D, KewalRamani VN, Marmon S, Littman DR (1999) Cytokine signals are sufficient for HIV-1 infection of resting human T lymphocytes. J Exp Med 189: 1735–1746.
20. Ducrey-Rundquist O, Guyader M, Trono D (2002) Modalities of interleukin-7-induced human immunodeficiency virus permissiveness in quiescent T lymphocytes. J Virol 76: 9103–9111.
21. Steffens CM, Managlia EZ, Landay A, Al-Harthi L (2002) Interleukin-7-treated naive T cells can be productively infected by T-cell-adapted and primary isolates of human immunodeficiency virus 1. Blood 99: 3310–3318.
22. Trinité B, Ohlson EC, Voznesensky I, Rana SP, Chan CN, et al. (2013) An HIV-1 replication pathway utilizing reverse transcription products that fail to integrate. J Virol 87: 12701–12720.
23. Surh CD, Sprent J (2008) Homeostasis of naive and memory T cells. Immunity 29: 848–862.
24. Bradley LM, Haynes L, Swain SL (2005) IL-7: maintaining T-cell memory and achieving homeostasis. Trends Immunol 26: 172–176.
25. Yoder A, Yu D, Dong L, Iyer SR, Xu X, et al. (2008) HIV envelope-CXCR4 signaling activates cofilin to overcome cortical actin restriction in resting CD4 T cells. Cell 134: 782–792.
26. Wolf D, Witte V, Laffert B, Blume K, Stromer E, et al. (2001) HIV-1 Nef associated PAK and PI3-kinases stimulate Akt-independent Bad-phosphorylation to induce anti-apoptotic signals. Nat Med 7: 1217–1224.
27. Zhou F, Xue M, Qin D, Zhu X, Wang C, et al. (2013) HIV-1 Tat promotes Kaposi's sarcoma-associated herpesvirus (KSHV) vIL-6-induced angiogenesis and tumorigenesis by regulating PI3K/PTEN/AKT/GSK-3beta signaling pathway. PLoS One 8: e53145.
28. Swann SA, Williams M, Story CM, Bobbitt KR, Fleis R, et al. (2001) HIV-1 Nef blocks transport of MHC class I molecules to the cell surface via a PI 3-kinase-dependent pathway. Virology 282: 267–277.
29. Wu Y, Marsh JW (2001) Selective transcription and modulation of resting T cell activity by preintegrated HIV DNA. Science 293: 1503–1506.
30. Vatakis DN, Nixon CC, Zack JA (2010) Quiescent T cells and HIV: an unresolved relationship. Immunol Res 48: 110–121.
31. Yusuf I, Fruman DA (2003) Regulation of quiescence in lymphocytes. Trends Immunol 24: 380–386.
32. Tzachanis D, Lafuente EM, Li L, Boussiotis VA (2004) Intrinsic and extrinsic regulation of T lymphocyte quiescence. Leuk Lymphoma 45: 1959–1967.
33. Carrette F, Fabre S, Bismuth G (2009) FOXO1, T-cell trafficking and immune responses. Adv Exp Med Biol 665: 3–16.
34. Dejean AS, Hedrick SM, Kerdiles YM (2011) Highly specialized role of Forkhead box O transcription factors in the immune system. Antioxid Redox Signal 14: 663–674.
35. Hedrick SM, Hess Michelini R, Doedens AL, Goldrath AW, Stone EL (2012) FOXO transcription factors throughout T cell biology. Nat Rev Immunol 12: 649–661.
36. Medema RH, Kops GJ, Bos JL, Burgering BM (2000) AFX-like Forkhead transcription factors mediate cell-cycle regulation by Ras and PKB through p27kip1. Nature 404: 782–787.
37. Coffer PJ, Burgering BM (2004) Forkhead-box transcription factors and their role in the immune system. Nat Rev Immunol 4: 889–899.
38. Cui M, Huang Y, Zhao Y, Zheng J (2009) New insights for FOXO and cell-fate decision in HIV infection and HIV associated neurocognitive disorder. Adv Exp Med Biol 665: 143–159.
39. van Grevenynghe J, Cubas RA, DaFonseca S, Metcalf T, Tremblay CL, et al. (2012) Foxo3a: an integrator of immune dysfunction during HIV infection. Cytokine Growth Factor Rev 23: 215–221.
40. van Grevenynghe J, Procopio FA, He Z, Chomont N, Riou C, et al. (2008) Transcription factor FOXO3a controls the persistence of memory CD4(+) T cells during HIV infection. Nat Med 14: 266–274.
41. Leenders H, Whiffield S, Benoist C, Mathis D (2000) Role of the forkhead transcription family member, FKHR, in thymocyte differentiation. Eur J Immunol 30: 2980–2990.
42. Coffer PJ (2003) Transcriptional regulation of lymphocyte quiescence: as cunning as a FOX. Trends Immunol 24: 470–471; author reply 471.
43. van der Horst A, Burgering BM (2007) Stressing the role of FoxO proteins in lifespan and disease. Nat Rev Mol Cell Biol 8: 440–450.
44. Ouyang W, Liao W, Luo CT, Yin N, Huse M, et al. (2012) Novel Foxo1-dependent transcriptional programs control T(reg) cell function. Nature 491: 554–559.
45. Fabre S, Carrette F, Chen J, Lang V, Semichon M, et al. (2008) FOXO1 regulates L-Selectin and a network of human T cell homing molecules downstream of phosphatidylinositol 3-kinase. J Immunol 181: 2980–2989.
46. Tzivion G, Dobson M, Ramakrishnan G (2011) FoxO transcription factors; Regulation by AKT and 14-3-3 proteins. Biochim Biophys Acta 1813: 1938–1945.
47. van der Vos KE, Coffer PJ (2008) FOXO-binding partners: it takes two to tango. Oncogene 27: 2289–2299.
48. Kerdiles YM, Beisner DR, Tinoco R, Dejean AS, Castrillon DH, et al. (2009) Foxo1 links homing and survival of naive T cells by regulating L-selectin, CCR7 and interleukin 7 receptor. Nat Immunol 10: 176–184.
49. Ouyang W, Beckett O, Flavell RA, Li MO (2009) An essential role of the Forkhead-box transcription factor Foxo1 in control of T cell homeostasis and tolerance. Immunity 30: 358–371.
50. Hedrick SM (2009) The cunning little vixen: Foxo and the cycle of life and death. Nat Immunol 10: 1057–1063.
51. Sinclair LV, Finlay D, Feijoo C, Cornish GH, Gray A, et al. (2008) Phosphatidylinositol-3-OH kinase and nutrient-sensing mTOR pathways control T lymphocyte trafficking. Nat Immunol 9: 513–521.
52. Butcher EC, Picker LJ (1996) Lymphocyte homing and homeostasis. Science 272: 60–66.
53. Galkina E, Tanousis K, Preece G, Tolaini M, Kioussis D, et al. (2003) L-selectin shedding does not regulate constitutive T cell trafficking but controls the migration pathways of antigen-activated T lymphocytes. J Exp Med 198: 1323–1335.
54. Venturi GM, Tu L, Kadono T, Khan AI, Fujimoto Y, et al. (2003) Leukocyte migration is regulated by L-selectin endoproteolytic release. Immunity 19: 713–724.
55. Chao CC, Jensen R, Dailey MO (1997) Mechanisms of L-selectin regulation by activated T cells. J Immunol 159: 1686–1694.
56. Bai A, Hu H, Yeung M, Chen J (2007) Kruppel-like factor 2 controls T cell trafficking by activating L-selectin (CD62L) and sphingosine-1-phosphate receptor 1 transcription. J Immunol 178: 7632–7639.
57. Preston GC, Feijoo-Carnero C, Schurch N, Cowling VH, Cantrell DA (2013) The impact of KLF2 modulation on the transcriptional program and function of CD8 T cells. PLoS One 8: e77537.
58. Kuo CT, Veselits ML, Leiden JM (1997) LKLF: A transcriptional regulator of single-positive T cell quiescence and survival. Science 277: 1986–1990.
59. Schober SL, Kuo CT, Schluns KS, Lefrancois L, Leiden JM, et al. (1999) Expression of the transcription factor lung Kruppel-like factor is regulated by cytokines and correlates with survival of memory T cells in vitro and in vivo. J Immunol 163: 3662–3667.
60. Carlson CM, Endrizzi BT, Wu J, Ding X, Weinreich MA, et al. (2006) Kruppel-like factor 2 regulates thymocyte and T-cell migration. Nature 442: 299–302.
61. Richardson MW, Jadlowsky J, Didigu CA, Doms RW, Riley JL (2012) Kruppel-like factor 2 modulates CCR5 expression and susceptibility to HIV-1 infection. J Immunol 189: 3815–3821.
62. Haaland RE, Yu W, Rice AP (2005) Identification of LKLF-regulated genes in quiescent CD4+ T lymphocytes. Mol Immunol 42: 627–641.
63. Schmidt M, Fernandez de Mattos S, van der Horst A, Klompmaker R, Kops GJ, et al. (2002) Cell cycle inhibition by FoxO forkhead transcription factors involves downregulation of cyclin D. Mol Cell Biol 22: 7842–7852.
64. Rougerie P, Largeteau Q, Megrelis L, Carrette F, Lejeune T, et al. (2013) Fam65b is a new transcriptional target of FOXO1 that regulates RhoA signaling for T lymphocyte migration. J Immunol 190: 748–755.

65. Hung CH, Thomas L, Ruby CE, Atkins KM, Morris NP, et al. (2007) HIV-1 Nef assembles a Src family kinase-ZAP-70/Syk-PI3K cascade to downregulate cell-surface MHC-I. Cell Host Microbe 1: 121–133.
66. Marodon G, Landau NR, Posnett DN (1999) Altered expression of CD4, CD54, CD62L, and CCR5 in primary lymphocytes productively infected with the human immunodeficiency virus. AIDS Res Hum Retroviruses 15: 161–171.
67. Ramirez PW, Famiglietti M, Sowrirajan B, DePaula-Silva AB, Rodesch C, et al. (2014) Downmodulation of CCR7 by HIV-1 Vpu Results in Impaired Migration and Chemotactic Signaling within CD4(+) T Cells. Cell Rep 7: 2019–2030.
68. Levy DN, Fernandes LS, Williams WV, Weiner DB (1993) Induction of cell differentiation by human immunodeficiency virus 1 vpr. Cell 72: 541–550.
69. Moutsopoulos NM, Vazquez N, Greenwell-Wild T, Ecevit I, Horn J, et al. (2006) Regulation of the tonsil cytokine milieu favors HIV susceptibility. J Leukoc Biol 80: 1145–1155.
70. Wang Y, Zhang AC, Ni Z, Herrera A, Walcheck B (2010) ADAM17 activity and other mechanisms of soluble L-selectin production during death receptor-induced leukocyte apoptosis. J Immunol 184: 4447–4454.
71. Scheller J, Chalaris A, Garbers C, Rose-John S (2011) ADAM17: a molecular switch to control inflammation and tissue regeneration. Trends Immunol 32: 380–387.
72. Marschner S, Freiberg BA, Kupfer A, Hunig T, Finkel TH (1999) Ligation of the CD4 receptor induces activation-independent down-regulation of L-selectin. Proc Natl Acad Sci U S A 96: 9763–9768.
73. Wang J, Marschner S, Finkel TH (2004) CXCR4 engagement is required for HIV-1-induced L-selectin shedding. Blood 103: 1218–1221.
74. Wang L, Robb CW, Cloyd MW (1997) HIV induces homing of resting T lymphocytes to lymph nodes. Virology 228: 141–152.
75. Oswald-Richter K, Grill SM, Leelawong M, Unutmaz D (2004) HIV infection of primary human T cells is determined by tunable thresholds of T cell activation. Eur J Immunol 34: 1705–1714.
76. Francois F, Klotman ME (2003) Phosphatidylinositol 3-kinase regulates human immunodeficiency virus type 1 replication following viral entry in primary CD4+ T lymphocytes and macrophages. J Virol 77: 2539–2549.
77. Kutsch O, Benveniste EN, Shaw GM, Levy DN (2002) Direct and quantitative single-cell analysis of human immunodeficiency virus type 1 reactivation from latency. J Virol 76: 8776–8786.
78. Nagashima T, Shigematsu N, Maruki R, Urano Y, Tanaka H, et al. (2010) Discovery of novel forkhead box O1 inhibitors for treating type 2 diabetes: improvement of fasting glycemia in diabetic db/db mice. Mol Pharmacol 78: 961–970.
79. Shore AM, White PC, Hui RC, Essafi A, Lam EW, et al. (2006) Epstein-Barr virus represses the FoxO1 transcription factor through latent membrane protein 1 and latent membrane protein 2A. J Virol 80: 11191–11199.
80. Fu Z, Tindall DJ (2008) FOXOs, cancer and regulation of apoptosis. Oncogene 27: 2312–2319.
81. Huang H, Tindall DJ (2011) Regulation of FOXO protein stability via ubiquitination and proteasome degradation. Biochim Biophys Acta 1813: 1961–1964.
82. Calnan DR, Brunet A (2008) The FoxO code. Oncogene 27: 2276–2288.
83. Misse D, Gajardo J, Oblet C, Religa A, Riquet N, et al. (2005) Soluble HIV-1 gp120 enhances HIV-1 replication in non-dividing CD4+ T cells, mediated via cell signaling and Tat cofactor overexpression. AIDS 19: 897–905.
84. Borgatti P, Zauli G, Colamussi ML, Gibellini D, Previati M, et al. (1997) Extracellular HIV-1 Tat protein activates phosphatidylinositol 3- and Akt/PKB kinases in CD4+ T lymphoblastoid Jurkat cells. Eur J Immunol 27: 2805–2811.
85. Siekevitz M, Feinberg MB, Holbrook N, Wong-Staal F, Greene WC (1987) Activation of interleukin 2 and interleukin 2 receptor (Tac) promoter expression by the trans-activator (tat) gene product of human T-cell leukemia virus, type I. Proc Natl Acad Sci U S A 84: 5389–5393.
86. Rhee SS, Marsh JW (1994) HIV-1 Nef activity in murine T cells. CD4 modulation and positive enhancement. J Immunol 152: 5128–5134.
87. Ott M, Emiliani S, Van Lint C, Herbein G, Lovett J, et al. (1997) Immune hyperactivation of HIV-1-infected T cells mediated by Tat and the CD28 pathway. Science 275: 1481–1485.
88. Schrager JA, Marsh JW (1999) HIV-1 Nef increases T cell activation in a stimulus-dependent manner. Proc Natl Acad Sci U S A 96: 8167–8172.
89. Wang JK, Kiyokawa E, Verdin E, Trono D (2000) The Nef protein of HIV-1 associates with rafts and primes T cells for activation. Proc Natl Acad Sci U S A 97: 394–399.
90. Luo HR, Hattori H, Hossain MA, Hester L, Huang Y, et al. (2003) Akt as a mediator of cell death. Proc Natl Acad Sci U S A 100: 11712–11717.
91. Alexander W (2011) Inhibiting the akt pathway in cancer treatment: three leading candidates. P T 36: 225–227.
92. Denisova OV, Soderholm S, Virtanen S, Von Schantz C, Bychkov D, et al. (2014) Akt Inhibitor MK2206 Prevents Influenza pH1N1 Virus Infection In Vitro. Antimicrob Agents Chemother 58: 3689–3696.
93. Li Z, Yan S, Attayan N, Ramalingam S, Thiele CJ (2012) Combination of an allosteric Akt Inhibitor MK-2206 with etoposide or rapamycin enhances the antitumor growth effect in neuroblastoma. Clin Cancer Res 18: 3603–3615.
94. Zhang X, Tang N, Hadden TJ, Rishi AK (2011) Akt, FoxO and regulation of apoptosis. Biochim Biophys Acta 1813: 1978–1986.
95. Pal SK, Reckamp K, Yu H, Figlin RA (2010) Akt inhibitors in clinical development for the treatment of cancer. Expert Opin Investig Drugs 19: 1355–1366.
96. Kim D, Sun M, He L, Zhou QH, Chen J, et al. (2010) A small molecule inhibits Akt through direct binding to Akt and preventing Akt membrane translocation. J Biol Chem 285: 8383–8394.
97. Kim Y, Hollenbaugh JA, Kim DH, Kim B (2011) Novel PI3K/Akt inhibitors screened by the cytoprotective function of human immunodeficiency virus type 1 Tat. PLoS One 6: e21781.
98. Chugh P, Bradel-Tretheway B, Monteiro-Filho CM, Planelles V, Maggirwar SB, et al. (2008) Akt inhibitors as an HIV-1 infected macrophage-specific anti-viral therapy. Retrovirology 5: 11.
99. Zhang L, Chung C, Hu BS, He T, Guo Y, et al. (2000) Genetic characterization of rebounding HIV-1 after cessation of highly active antiretroviral therapy. J Clin Invest 106: 839–845.
100. Sedaghat AR, Siliciano JD, Brennan TP, Wilke CO, Siliciano RF (2007) Limits on replenishment of the resting CD4+ T cell reservoir for HIV in patients on HAART. PLoS Pathog 3: e122.
101. Eckstein DA, Penn ML, Korin YD, Scripture-Adams DD, Zack JA, et al. (2001) HIV-1 actively replicates in naive CD4(+) T cells residing within human lymphoid tissues. Immunity 15: 671–682.
102. Blaak H, van't Wout AB, Brouwer M, Hooibrink B, Hovenkamp E, et al. (2000) In vivo HIV-1 infection of CD45RA(+)CD4(+) T cells is established primarily by syncytium-inducing variants and correlates with the rate of CD4(+) T cell decline. Proc Natl Acad Sci U S A 97: 1269–1274.
103. Rollins BJ (2008) Innocents abroad: regulating where naive T cells go. Nat Immunol 9: 233–235.
104. Schwab SR, Cyster JG (2007) Finding a way out: lymphocyte egress from lymphoid organs. Nat Immunol 8: 1295–1301.
105. Sebzda E, Zou Z, Lee JS, Wang T, Kahn ML (2008) Transcription factor KLF2 regulates the migration of naive T cells by restricting chemokine receptor expression patterns. Nat Immunol 9: 292–300.
106. Berstein G, Abraham RT (2008) Moving out: mobilizing activated T cells from lymphoid tissues. Nat Immunol 9: 455–457.
107. Ramaswamy S, Nakamura N, Sansal I, Bergeron L, Sellers WR (2002) A novel mechanism of gene regulation and tumor suppression by the transcription factor FKHR. Cancer Cell 2: 81–91.
108. Jiang G, Espeseth A, Hazuda DJ, Margolis DM (2007) c-Myc and Sp1 contribute to proviral latency by recruiting histone deacetylase 1 to the human immunodeficiency virus type 1 promoter. J Virol 81: 10914–10923.
109. Garris CS, Blaho VA, Hla T, Han MH (2014) Sphingosine-1-phosphate receptor 1 signalling in T cells: trafficking and beyond. Immunology 142: 347–353.
110. Mudd JC, Murphy P, Manion M, Debernardo R, Hardacre J, et al. (2013) Impaired T-cell responses to sphingosine-1-phosphate in HIV-1 infected lymph nodes. Blood 121: 2914–2922.
111. Chu P, Pardo J, Zhao H, Li CC, Pali E, et al. (2003) Systematic identification of regulatory proteins critical for T-cell activation. J Biol 2: 21.
112. Shiow LR, Rosen DB, Brdickova N, Xu Y, An J, et al. (2006) CD69 acts downstream of interferon-alpha/beta to inhibit S1P1 and lymphocyte egress from lymphoid organs. Nature 440: 540–544.
113. Radulovic K, Rossini V, Manta C, Holzmann K, Kestler HA, et al. (2013) The early activation marker CD69 regulates the expression of chemokines and CD4 T cell accumulation in intestine. PLoS One 8: e65413.
114. Blazquez MV, Macho A, Ortiz C, Lucena C, Lopez-Cabrera M, et al. (1999) Extracellular HIV type 1 Tat protein induces CD69 expression through NF-kappaB activation: possible correlation with cell surface Tat-binding proteins. AIDS Res Hum Retroviruses 15: 1209–1218.
115. Bankovich AJ, Shiow LR, Cyster JG (2010) CD69 suppresses sphingosine 1-phosophate receptor-1 (S1P1) function through interaction with membrane helix 4. J Biol Chem 285: 22328–22337.
116. Fulcher D, Wong S (1999) Carboxyfluorescein succinimidyl ester-based proliferative assays for assessment of T cell function in the diagnostic laboratory. Immunol Cell Biol 77: 559–564.
117. Seoane J, Le HV, Shen L, Anderson SA, Massague J (2004) Integration of Smad and forkhead pathways in the control of neuroepithelial and glioblastoma cell proliferation. Cell 117: 211–223.
118. Wu J, Lingrel JB (2004) KLF2 inhibits Jurkat T leukemia cell growth via upregulation of cyclin-dependent kinase inhibitor p21WAF1/CIP1. Oncogene 23: 8088–8096.
119. Tejera MM, Kim EH, Sullivan JA, Plisch EH, Suresh M (2013) FoxO1 controls effector-to-memory transition and maintenance of functional CD8 T cell memory. J Immunol 191: 187–199.
120. Buckley AF, Kuo CT, Leiden JM (2001) Transcription factor LKLF is sufficient to program T cell quiescence via a c-Myc-dependent pathway. Nat Immunol 2: 698–704.
121. Chowdhury IH, Wang XF, Landau NR, Robb ML, Polonis VR, et al. (2003) HIV-1 Vpr activates cell cycle inhibitor p21/Waf1/Cip1: a potential mechanism of G2/M cell cycle arrest. Virology 305: 371–377.
122. Amini S, Saunders M, Kelley K, Khalili K, Sawaya BE (2004) Interplay between HIV-1 Vpr and Sp1 modulates p21(WAF1) gene expression in human astrocytes. J Biol Chem 279: 46046–46056.

123. Vazquez N, Greenwell-Wild T, Marinos NJ, Swaim WD, Nares S, et al. (2005) Human immunodeficiency virus type 1-induced macrophage gene expression includes the p21 gene, a target for viral regulation. J Virol 79: 4479–4491.
124. Rougerie P, Delon J (2012) Rho GTPases: masters of T lymphocyte migration and activation. Immunol Lett 142: 1–13.
125. Michel N, Allespach I, Venzke S, Fackler OT, Keppler OT (2005) The Nef protein of human immunodeficiency virus establishes superinfection immunity by a dual strategy to downregulate cell-surface CCR5 and CD4. Curr Biol 15: 714–723.
126. Landi A, Iannucci V, Nuffel AV, Meuwissen P, Verhasselt B (2011) One protein to rule them all: modulation of cell surface receptors and molecules by HIV Nef. Curr HIV Res 9: 496–504.
127. Gelderblom HC, Vatakis DN, Burke SA, Lawrie SD, Bristol GC, et al. (2008) Viral complementation allows HIV-1 replication without integration. Retrovirology 5: 60.
128. Duchesneau P, Gallagher E, Walcheck B, Waddell TK (2007) Up-regulation of leukocyte CXCR4 expression by sulfatide: an L-selectin-dependent pathway on CD4+ T cells. Eur J Immunol 37: 2949–2960.
129. Mueller SN, Gebhardt T, Carbone FR, Heath WR (2013) Memory T cell subsets, migration patterns, and tissue residence. Annu Rev Immunol 31: 137–161.
130. Sallusto F, Geginat J, Lanzavecchia A (2004) Central memory and effector memory T cell subsets: function, generation, and maintenance. Annu Rev Immunol 22: 745–763.
131. Levy DN, Aldrovandi GM, Kutsch O, Shaw GM (2004) Dynamics of HIV-1 recombination in its natural target cells. Proc Natl Acad Sci U S A 101: 4204–4209.
132. O'Doherty U, Swiggard WJ, Malim MH (2000) Human immunodeficiency virus type 1 spinoculation enhances infection through virus binding. J Virol 74: 10074–10080.
133. Meditz AL, Haas MK, Folkvord JM, Melander K, Young R, et al. (2011) HLA-DR+ CD38+ CD4+ T lymphocytes have elevated CCR5 expression and produce the majority of R5-tropic HIV-1 RNA in vivo. J Virol 85: 10189–10200.
134. Roederer M, Treister A, Moore W, Herzenberg LA (2001) Probability binning comparison: a metric for quantitating univariate distribution differences. Cytometry 45: 37–46.
135. George TC, Fanning SL, Fitzgerald-Bocarsly P, Medeiros RB, Highfill S, et al. (2006) Quantitative measurement of nuclear translocation events using similarity analysis of multispectral cellular images obtained in flow. J Immunol Methods 311: 117–129.
136. Maguire O, Collins C, O'Loughlin K, Miecznikowski J, Minderman H (2011) Quantifying nuclear p65 as a parameter for NF-kappaB activation: Correlation between ImageStream cytometry, microscopy, and Western blot. Cytometry A 79: 461–469.
137. Livak KJ, Schmittgen TD (2001) Analysis of relative gene expression data using real-time quantitative PCR and the 2(-Delta Delta C(T)) Method. Methods 25: 402–408.
138. Ledderose C, Heyn J, Limbeck E, Kreth S (2011) Selection of reliable reference genes for quantitative real-time PCR in human T cells and neutrophils. BMC Res Notes 4: 427.

HIV-1 Conserved Elements p24CE DNA Vaccine Induces Humoral Immune Responses with Broad Epitope Recognition in Macaques

Viraj Kulkarni[1], Antonio Valentin[2], Margherita Rosati[2], Morgane Rolland[3¤a¤b], James I. Mullins[3], George N. Pavlakis[2]*, Barbara K. Felber[1]*

1 Human Retrovirus Pathogenesis Section, Vaccine Branch, Center for Cancer Research, National Cancer Institute at Frederick, Frederick, Maryland, United States of America, 2 Human Retrovirus Section, Vaccine Branch, Center for Cancer Research, National Cancer Institute at Frederick, Frederick, Maryland, United States of America, 3 Departments of Microbiology, Medicine and Laboratory Medicine, University of Washington, Seattle, Washington, United States of America

Abstract

To target immune responses towards invariable regions of the virus, we engineered DNA-based immunogens encoding conserved elements (CE) of HIV-1 p24^{gag}. This conserved element vaccine is designed to avoid decoy epitopes by focusing responses to critical viral elements. We previously reported that vaccination of macaques with p24CE DNA induced robust cellular immune responses to CE that were not elicited upon wild type p55^{gag} DNA vaccination. p24CE DNA priming followed by p55^{gag} DNA boost provided a novel strategy to increase the magnitude and breadth of the cellular immune responses to HIV-1 Gag, including the induction of strong, multifunctional T-cell responses targeting epitopes within CE. Here, we examined the humoral responses induced upon p24CE DNA or p55^{gag} DNA vaccination in macaques and found that although both vaccines induced robust p24^{gag} binding antibody responses, the responses induced by p24CE DNA showed a unique broad range of linear epitope recognition. In contrast, antibodies elicited by p55^{gag} DNA vaccine failed to recognize p24CE protein and did not recognize linear epitopes spanning the CE. Interestingly, boosting of p24CE DNA primed animals with p55^{gag} DNA resulted in augmentation of antibodies able to recognize p24^{gag} as well as the p24CE proteins, thereby inducing broadest immunity. Our results indicate that an effectively directed vaccine strategy that includes priming with the conserved element vaccine followed by boost with the complete immunogen induces broad cellular and humoral immunity focused on the conserved regions of the virus. This novel and effective strategy to broaden responses could be applied against other antigens of highly diverse pathogens.

Editor: Geetha P. Bansal, Tulane University, United States of America

Funding: This work was supported in part by the Intramural Research Program of the National Cancer Institute, National Institutes of Health (NCI/NIH) (BKF, GNP) and by Public Health Services grant AI57005 (to JIM). The funders had no role in study design, data collection and analysis, decision to publish, or preparation of the manuscript.

Competing Interests: GNP and BKF are inventors on US Government-owned patents and patent applications related to DNA vaccines and gene expression optimization. GNP, JIM, BKF are inventors on an US Government and University of Washington co-owned patent application relating to material pertinent to this article. There are no further patents, products in development or marketed products to declare. This does not alter the authors' adherence to all the policies on sharing data and materials.

* Email: barbara.felber@nih.gov (BKF); george.pavlakis@nih.gov (GNP)

¤a Current address: United States Military HIV Research Program, Walter Reed Army Institute of Research, Silver Spring, Maryland, United States of America
¤b Current address: The Henry M. Jackson Foundation, Bethesda, Maryland, United States of America

Introduction

The development of an effective HIV vaccine is critical to control the AIDS pandemic. Protection against HIV is difficult to obtain in part because the virus readily mutates and generates viable alternatives to the epitopes targeted by the immune system of the host. To address the problem of viral variability many strategies have been tested [1–19]. We have focused in conserved elements from the HIV-1 proteome and have based our immunogen designs on (a) stringent conservation among all HIV sequences, (b) selection of epitopes associated with better virologic control in HIV-1 infected individuals, and (c) optimizing immunogen expression and proteolytic cleavage [11,12,16–25]. We focused on Gag as a prototype vaccine, because Gag-specific $CD8^+$ T cell responses were found to correlate with control of viremia in clade B and C infected individuals [26–29], to contribute to control HIV-1 after infection in the Step trial [30], and Gag-specific $CD4^+$ T cell responses were associated with virus control [31,32]. We selected 7 conserved elements (CE) within HIV-1 p24$^{gag.}$ which cover ~98% of the HIV-1 Group M viruses worldwide and represent 54% of the p24^{gag} protein. These p24CE sequences were collinearly arranged to express what we refer to as the p24CE immunogen [18]. Using *ex vivo* transfection of CE-encoding RNA into human dendritic cells, we were able to generate levels of CD4 and CD8 responses comparable to that of the full-length p55^{Gag} protein [25]. C57BL/6 mice immunized with p24CE plasmids developed immune responses of high magnitude and recognized more CE than those induced by the complete p55^{gag} DNA immunogen [18]. Vaccination of macaques with p24CE DNA vaccine showed that all of the 10 animals developed cellular responses against the CE, while only 50% of the macaques vaccinated with the full-length p55^{gag} DNA developed cellular responses targeting any of the CE [19]. Importantly, boosting CE-primed macaques with DNA expressing full-length p55^{gag} increased magnitude and poly-functionality of the CE responses, and breadth of Gag immunity, targeting epitopes within the highly conserved elements and also outside p24^{gag}, and demonstrating alteration of the hierarchy of epitope recognition in the presence of pre-existing CE-specific responses [19].

Although the p24CE vectors were primarily designed as a prototype T cell vaccine to induce optimal cell-mediated responses, the development of humoral immunity is critical to contain HIV transmission. Therefore, we explored whether the CE vaccine approach also elicits humoral immunity and defined the breath of the antibody responses observed. Although antibodies targeting the HIV Gag protein are not expected to prevent viral transmission, this study serves as proof-of-concept that can be translated to other viral antigens, such as Env. In the present work, we performed a detailed analysis of the antibodies induced by p24CE DNA vaccination in macaques [19], including peptide mapping of the different CE that are recognized by those antibody responses. We report that the p24CE DNA vaccine was able to induce robust humoral immune responses that recognized wild type HIV-1 p24^{gag}. Interestingly, we also found that the CE-induced responses were broad, sustained, and could be boosted by heterologous p55^{gag} DNA vaccination. Thus, our finding suggests that inclusion of conserved elements as a priming immunogen provides a novel and effective strategy to broaden responses against highly diverse pathogens like HIV by avoiding decoy epitopes, while focusing responses to critical viral elements for which fewer escape pathways exist. This study serves as proof-of-concept to assess immunogenicity of conserved elements in the macaque model, a concept that can be translated into other viral proteins, such as Env, where the combination of distinct antibody and cellular responses against invariable epitopes may provide an immunologic advantage for the containment of the virus.

Material and Methods

Ethics statement

The animals in this study were Indian rhesus macaques (Macaca mulatta) as described previously [19] and were housed at the Advanced BioScience Laboratories, Inc. (ABL) animal facility. All animals were cared for and procedures performed under a protocol approved by the ABL Animal Care and Use Committee (animal welfare assurance no. A3467-01; protocol no. AUP516) and USDA Certificate number 51-R-0059. Furthermore, the macaques in this study were managed according to the animal husbandry program of the ABL Animal Facility, which aims at providing consistent and excellent care to nonhuman primates at the vivarium. This program operates based on the laws, regulations, and guidelines promulgated by the United States Department of Agriculture (e.g., the Animal Welfare Act and its regulations, and the Animal Care Policy Manual), Institute for Laboratory Animal Research (e.g., Guide for the Care and Use of Laboratory Animals, 8th edition), Public Health Service, National Research Council, Centers for Disease Control, and the Association for Assessment and Accreditation of Laboratory Animal Care (AAALAC) International. The nutritional plan utilized by the ABL Animal Facility consisted of twice daily feeding of Labdiet 5045 High Protein Primate Diet and food intake was closely monitored by Animal Research Technicians. This diet was also supplemented with a variety of fruits, vegetables, and other edible objects as part of the environmental enrichment program established by the Veterinary staff and enrichment Technician. Pairing of animals as part of the environmental enrichment program was managed by the enrichment technician. All primary enclosures and animal rooms were cleaned daily with water and sanitized at least once every two weeks. All macaques (N = 10) used in this study were males, except for four females: M695, P572, P574, M437. Their average weight was 8.5 kg (range: 3.8–11.2 kg) and their average age was 7 years (range: 4–12 years). Vaccinations were performed under anesthesia (Ketamine administered at 10 mg/kg) and all efforts were made to minimize suffering. No adverse effects were found. None of the animals were euthanized as part of this study.

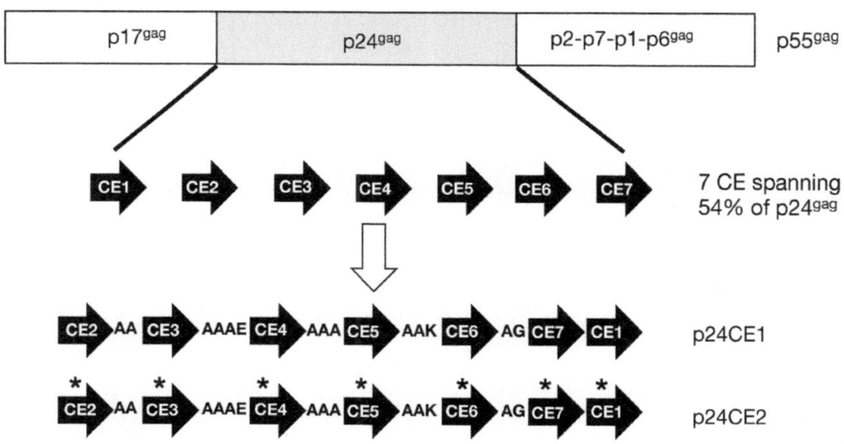

Figure 1. p24CE Expression plasmids. Cartoon depicting the HIV p55^{gag} protein and its proteolytic cleavage products p17^{gag}, p24^{gag} and the C-terminal p2, p7, p1 and p6 proteins. The 7 highly conserved elements (CE) identified within p24^{Gag} are indicated. The two p24CE constructs differ by 1 'toggle' AA per CE, indicated by asterisks. The 7 CE were connected via linkers and the p24CE proteins were expressed from the CMV promoter using the mammalian expression vector pCMV.kan [18].

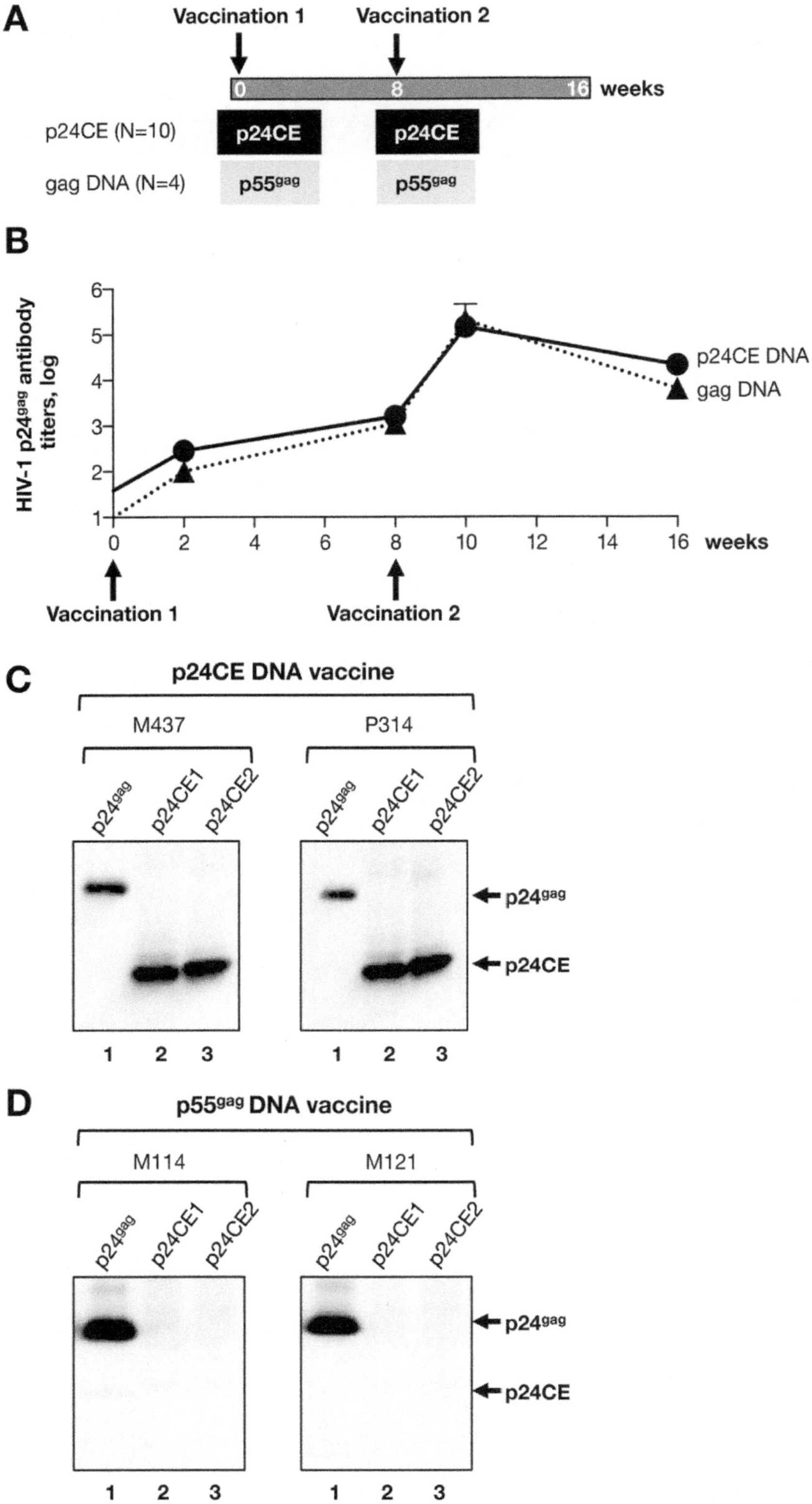

Figure 2. Induction of humoral immune responses upon p24CE DNA vaccination in macaques. (A) Cartoon depicts the vaccination schedule. Each macaque received 2 vaccinations with a mixture of p24CE1 and p24CE2 DNAs or $p55^{gag}$ DNA at week 0 and 8. Plasma samples were analyzed for bAb to Gag at the time of each vaccination and at the additional indicated time points. **(B)** Plasma bAb to HIV-1 $p24^{Gag}$ measured by ELISA. Mean and standard error of the reciprocal Gag antibody endpoint titers (in log_{10}) of 10 macaques vaccinated with p24CE DNA mixture and 4 macaques which received the $p55^{gag}$ DNA are shown. (**C, D**) Western immunoblot analysis was used to identify binding antibodies to HIV-1 $p24^{Gag}$ and the p24CE proteins present in plasma collected after the last vaccination. The membranes contain the soluble processed clade B $p24^{gag}$ protein (lane 1), p24CE1 (lane 2) and p24CE2 (lane 3) protein and were probed with plasma collected after the last vaccination. The data from 2 representative macaques from each vaccine group are shown: **(C)** p24CE DNA vaccinated animals M437 (plasma dilution 1:2000) and P314 (plasma dilution 1:1000) and **(D)** $p55^{gag}$ DNA vaccinated animals M114 and M121 (plasma dilution 1:2000 for both). The positions of $p24^{gag}$ and p24CE proteins are indicated.

Table 1. Peptide list and coverage of CE.

ID	Peptide[a]	CE	ID	Peptide[a]	CE
1	PIVQNLQGQMVHQAI		31	WMTSNPPIPVGEIYK	
2	NLQGQMVHQA**ISPRT**		32	NPPIPVGEIY**KRWII**	CE5
3	GQMVHQA**ISPRTLNA**	CE1	33	PVGEIY**KRWIILGLN**	CE5
4	HQA**ISPRTLNAWVKV**	CE1	34	Y**KRWIILGLNKIVR**	CE5
5	**SPRTLNAWVKV**IEEK	CE1	35	**WIILGLNKIVRMYSP**	CE5
6	**LNAWVKV**IEEKAFSP	CE1	36	**GLNKIVRMYSPVSI**L	CE5
7	**VKV**IEEKAFSPE**VIP**	CE2	37	**IVRMYSPVSI**LDIRQ	CE5
8	EEKAFSPE**VIPMFSA**	CE2	38	**YSPVSI**LDIRQGPK	CE5
9	FSPE**VIPMFSALSEG**	CE2	39	**VSI**LDIRQGPKEPFR	
10	**VIPMFSALSEGATPQ**	CE2	40	DIRQGPKEPFRD**YV**	
11	**FSALSEGATPQDLN**T	CE2	41	RQGPKEPFRD**YVDRF**	CE6
12	**SEGATPQDLN**TMLNT	CE2	42	KEPFRD**YVDRFFKTL**	CE6
13	**TPQDLN**TMLNT**VGGH**	CE2	43	RD**YVDRFFKTLRAEQ**	CE6
14	LNTMLNT**VGGHQAAM**	CE3	44	**DRFFKTLRAEQA**TQ	CE6
15	LNT**VGGHQAAMQMLK**	CE3	45	**FKTLRAEQA**TQDVKN	CE6
16	**GGHQAAMQMLKDTIN**	CE3	46	**RAEQA**TQDVKNWMT	CE6
17	**AAMQMLKDTINEEAA**	CE3	47	**EQA**TQDVKNWMTDTL	
18	**MLKDTINEEAAEWDR**	CE3	48	TQDVKNWMTDTLLVQ	
19	**TINEEAAEWDR**LHPV	CE3	49	KNWMTDTLLVQNANP	
20	**EAAEWDR**LHPVHAGP	CE3	50	TDTLLVQNANPDCKT	
21	**WDR**LHPVHAGPIPPG		51	LVQNANPDCKTILKA	
22	HPVHAGPIPPGQMR		52	ANPDCKTILKALGPG	
23	HAGPIPPGQMRE**PRG**		53	CKTILKALGPGATL	
24	IPPGQMRE**PRGSDIA**	CE4	54	ILKALGPGAT**LEEMM**	CE7
25	GQMRE**PRGSDIAGTT**	CE4	55	LGPGAT**LEEMMTACQ**	CE7
26	EP**RGSDIAGTTSTLQ**	CE4	56	AT**LEEMMTACQGVGG**	CE7
27	**SDIAGTTSTLQEQIA**	CE4	57	**EMMTACQGVGGPGHK**	CE7
28	**GTTSTLQEQIAW**MTS	CE4	58	**ACQGVGGPGHK**ARVL	CE7
29	**TLQEQIAW**MTSNPPI	CE4			
30	**EQIAW**MTSNPPIPVG	CE4			

[a]Amino acids indicated in bold cover the respective CE.

Vaccination regimens

The macaques were vaccinated as part of a previous study [19] with plasmids expressing p24CE1 and p24CE2 or COT-M p55^{gag} DNA, and all the vaccines contained IL-12 DNA, described in detail elsewhere [18,19]. The DNA vaccines were delivered via intramuscular injection followed by *in vivo* electroporation [19]. The animals received two vaccinations with p24CE DNA (N = 10) or p55^{gag} DNA (N = 4) (vaccination 1, vaccination 2) followed by a converse boost with p55^{gag} DNA or p24CE DNA (vaccination 3), respectively.

Antibody assays

Blood samples were collected at the day of each vaccination and 2 weeks later. Serial dilutions of plasma samples were tested by standard ELISA (Advanced Bioscience Lab, Rockville, MD) for binding antibodies to HIV-1 clade B p24^{gag} and the absorbance (OD) at 450 nm was determined. Binding titers were reported as the reciprocal of the highest dilution scoring positive (having a value greater than average values obtained with naive macaque plasma +3 standard deviations). Pepscan analysis was performed using 58 peptides covering HIV-1 consensus group M p24^{gag} (15-mers overlapping by 11 AA; #11057 AIDS Research and Reference Reagent Program, Germantown, MD) by standard ELISA. The plasma samples were tested at a dilution of 1:50 and absorbance (OD) was measured at 450 nm.

For Western blot analysis, 10^6 HEK293 cells were transfected with 1 μg of the p24CE DNAs or 5 μg of the HIV-1 molecular clone pNL4-3. Aliquots of the extracellular fractions containing p24^{gag} (pNL4-3; 1/250) or cell-associated fractions containing p24CE1 and p24CE2, respectively (1/50 of extract) were separated on 12% NuPAGE gels and blotted onto nitrocellulose membranes (Invitrogen, Carlsbad, CA). The membranes were incubated with plasma from vaccinated macaques, followed by anti-monkey–HRP labeled antibody (dilution 1:10,000), and the bands visualized using the enhanced chemiluminescence (ECL) Prime Western blotting detection reagent (GE HealthCare, Piscataway, NJ).

Table 2. Responses of individual CE to cellular an humoral immune responses.

Vaccine	Macaques (N = 10)		Cellular[a] and humoral immune responses to individual CE						
			CE1	CE2	CE3	CE4	CE5	CE6	CE7
Conserved Element p24CE DNA	L862	CMI[a]		+	+		+		
		pepscan	+		+				+
	M166	CMI[a]		+			+	+	
		pepscan	+	+	+		+		
	M695	CMI[a]			+		+	+	
		pepscan	+		+	+			
	R279	CMI[a]				+	+	+	
		pepscan	+	+	+				
	P314	CMI[a]			+	+	+		
		pepscan	+		+				
	M437	CMI[a]					+		
		pepscan	+		+				
	R315	CMI[a]					+		+
		pepscan	+		+				
	P302	CMI[a]			+		+	+	
		pepscan	+	+	+				+
	P307	CMI[a]			+		+	+	
		pepscan	+		+				
	P308	CMI[a]			+		+		
		pepscan	+		+				
Positive responses among 10 macaques		CMI[a]	0	2	6	2	10	5	1
		pepscan	10	3	10	1	1	0	2

[a]Cellular immune response data are from [19].

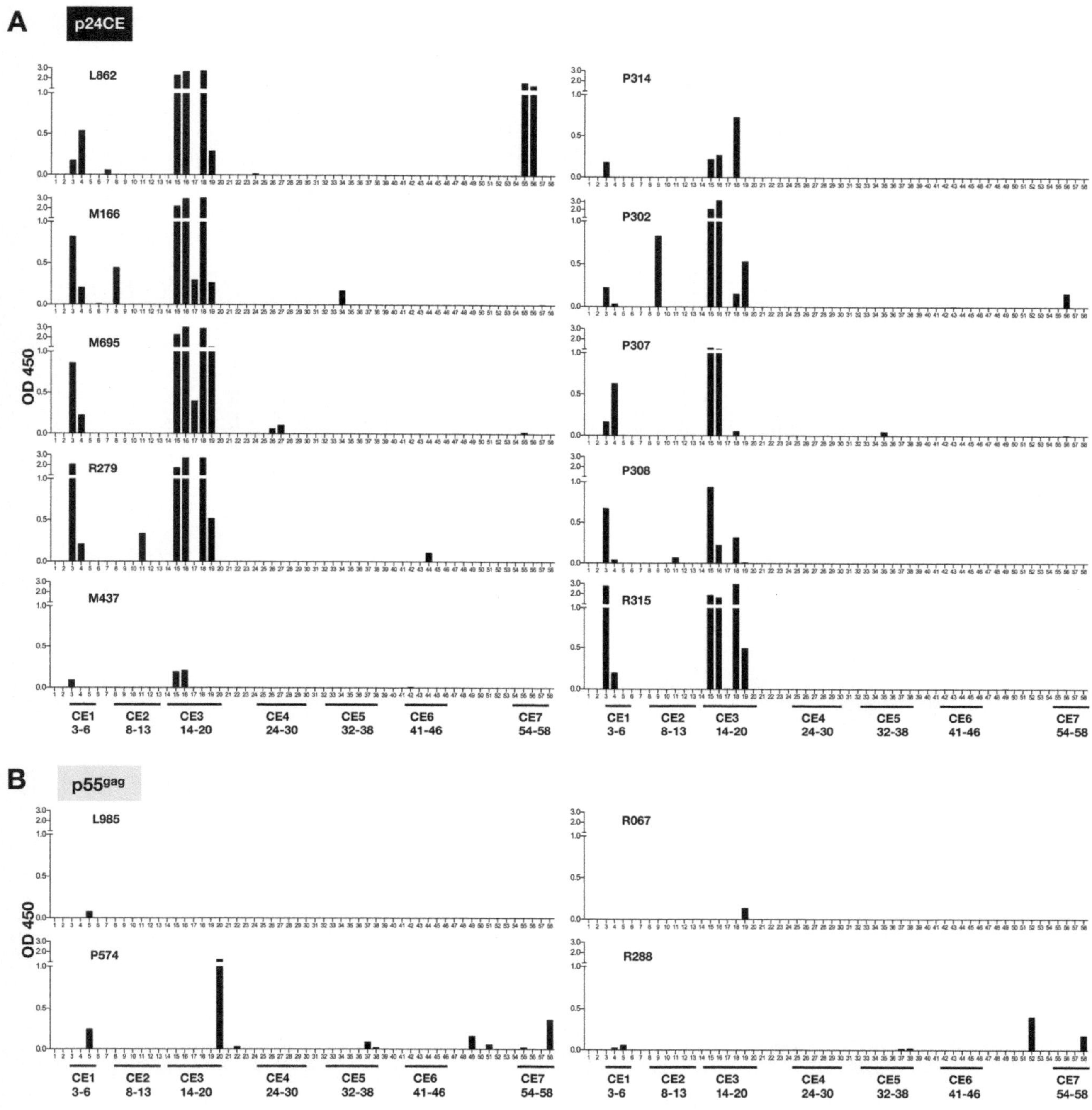

Figure 3. Pepscan analysis of humoral responses induced upon p24CE and p55^{gag} DNA vaccination in macaques. All macaques vaccinated with **(A)** p24CE DNA (N = 10) and **(B)** p55^{gag} DNA (N = 4) were subjected to Pepscan analysis against 58 peptides (15-mers overlapping by 11 AA) spanning p24^{gag}. Peptides corresponding to CE1 to CE7 are indicated and the peptides are listed below as detailed in **Table 1**. OD_{450} is reported after subtracting the mean OD_{450} of the values obtained from negative samples plus 3 SD.

Results

Development of humoral immune responses in macaques vaccinated with p24CE and p55^{gag} plasmid DNA

To focus the immune responses on nearly invariant regions of the HIV-1 proteome, we developed DNA immunogens encoding 7 highly conserved elements (CE) identified within HIV-1 p24^{gag} [18,19,23]. Two plasmids were constructed with each of the 7 CE elements, which differed by 1 'toggle' amino acid per CE to include a lesser conserved AA, and were arranged by taking into consideration the hydrophobicity of individual CE and spaced with linkers designed to maximize cleavage between the adjacent CE (**Figure 1**) as described previously [18,19,23]. Each 140-AA CE cassette, p24CE1 and p24CE2, was expressed from expression-optimized DNA vectors.

Rhesus macaques received two vaccinations with DNAs expressing either both p24CE1 and p24CE2 (N = 10) or p55^{gag} (N = 4), each delivered by intramuscular injection followed by *in vivo* electroporation as outlined in **Figure 2A** and previously

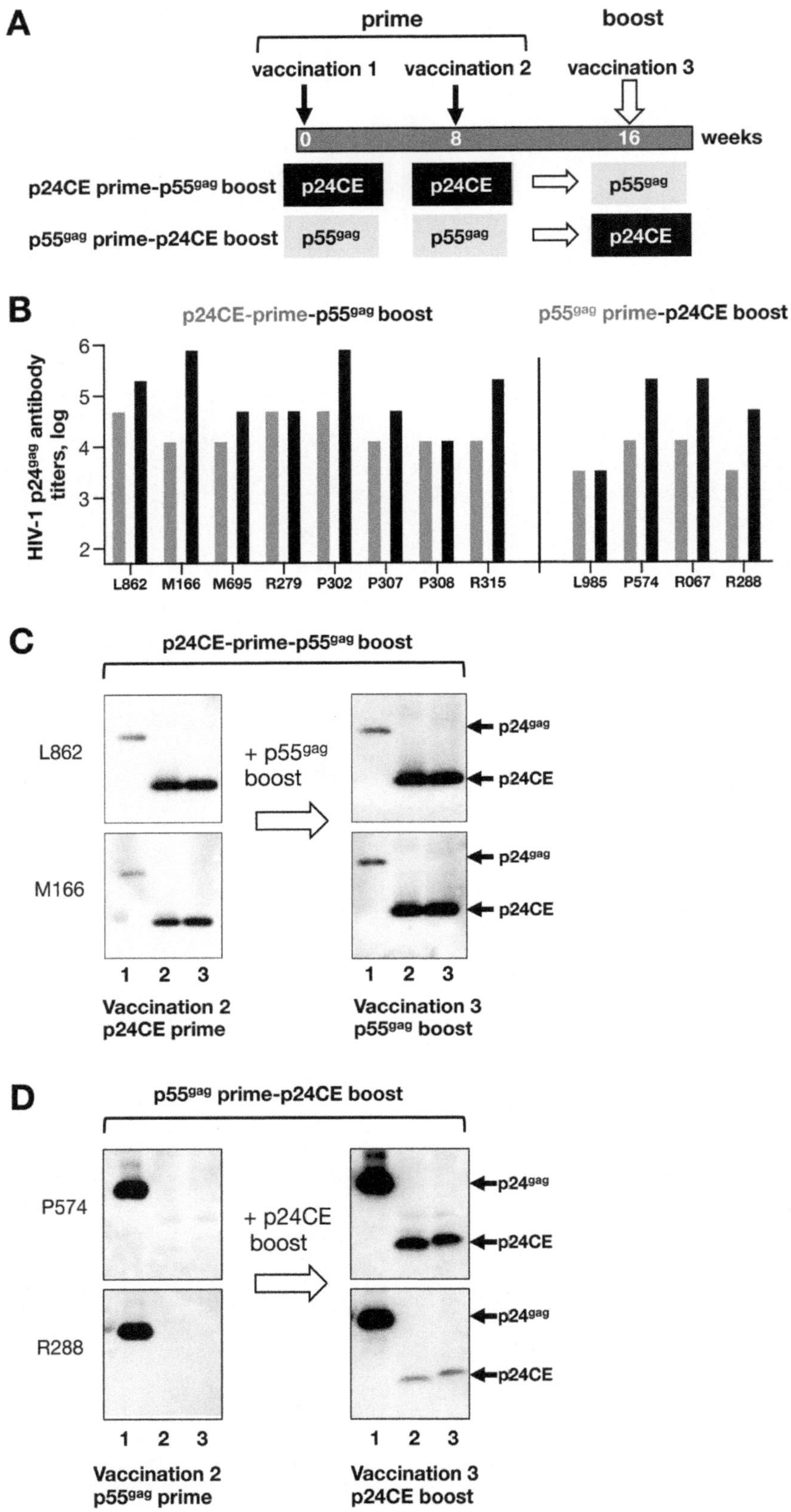

Figure 4. HIV-1 p55^{gag} DNA vaccination did not prime *de novo* CE humoral responses but increased pre-existing CE-specific responses. (A) Cartoon depicts the vaccination schedule. After receiving p24CE or p55^{gag} DNA as priming vaccination (see **Figure 2**) the animals received a heterologous boost vaccination (vaccination 3) with p55^{gag} DNA or p24CE DNA, respectively. **(B)** Comparison of plasma bAb to HIV-1 p24^{gag} ELISA titers at vaccination 3 and 2 weeks later. The reciprocal Gag antibody endpoint titers (in $\log_{10}$) from individual macaques vaccinated with the p24CE DNA mixture following by a p55^{Gag} DNA boost (N = 10; left panel) and macaques vaccinated with p55^{Gag} DNA followed by a p24CE DNA boost (N = 4; right panel) are shown. Data from day of 3rd vaccination are from Fig. 2B. **(C, D)** Western immunoblot analysis was used to test

macaque plasma for binding antibodies before (after vaccination 2) and after the boost (after vaccination 3). The membranes contain the soluble processed p24^{gag} (lane 1), p24CE1 (lane 2) or p24CE2 (lane 3) proteins and were probed with plasma collected 2 weeks after vaccinations 2 and 3. Data from 2 representative macaques are shown from each vaccine group. The membranes were probed with plasma from **(C)** macaques (L862, M166), which received the p24CE prime-p55^{gag} DNA boost (plasma dilution 1:2000) and from **(D)** macaques (P574, R288), which received the p55^{gag} prime-p24CE DNA boost regimen (plasma dilution 1:500).

reported [18,19]. Plasma samples were collected on the day of vaccination and 2 and 8 weeks later. We have previously reported that vaccination with p24CE DNA induced strong cellular immunity targeting new epitopes [18,19]. Here, we examined the development of Gag-specific humoral responses induced by the same immunization regimen. Animals vaccinated with p24CE DNA developed antibody responses against p24^{gag} and the kinetics of these responses were similar to those induced by p55^{gag} DNA vaccination (**Figure 2B**). p24^{gag} antibody responses were detectable upon a single DNA vaccination, and were efficiently boosted by the 2nd DNA immunization resulting in peak antibody titers (~5.3 log reciprocal end-point dilution) detected 2 weeks later. Similar levels of Gag-specific antibody responses were detected 8 weeks later in both groups of animals, indicating comparable persistence of humoral responses. These results demonstrate that p24CE DNA, an immunogen designed to elicit optimal T-cell responses, is able to induce humoral immune responses to p24^{gag} of similar magnitude as those induced by the p55^{gag} DNA vaccine.

The ability to recognize the p24CE proteins and processed p24^{gag} by the antibodies induced by either of the vaccination regimens was analyzed by Western immunoblots (**Figure 2C–D**). Plasma from macaques vaccinated with p24CE DNA contained antibodies that strongly reacted with processed p24^{gag} and both forms of the p24CE proteins (p24CE1 and p24CE2) (**Figure 2C**). As expected from the conservation within p24CE of the AA sequences from the HIV-1 M group, these antibodies strongly reacted with Gag from different subtypes, including subtypes A, B, C, and group M consensus (not shown). In contrast, plasma samples from macaques immunized with p55^{gag} DNA, although able to recognize the viral p24^{gag}, failed to bind to either of the two CE proteins (**Figure 2D**). Similar patterns of antibody recognition were found upon vaccination of mice [18]. Thus, antibodies induced by p24CE DNA vaccination recognized both the full-length p24^{Gag} and the p24CE proteins, but immunization with p55^{gag} DNA vaccination failed to produce antibodies specific for the CE proteins of p24^{gag}.

Humoral responses targeted four of the seven CE

To identify the linear epitopes recognized by the antibodies induced by the vaccination regimens, we performed a peptide scanning analysis (Pepscan) of plasma samples at the time of peak antibody responses (2 weeks after the 2nd vaccination) using a panel of peptides (15-mers overlapping by 11 AA) that cover the entire p24^{gag} protein (see **Table 1** for peptide sequences and association with CE). Data obtained with samples from macaques vaccinated with the p24CE DNA showed that each of the 10 animals developed antibodies that recognized CE1 and CE3 (**Table 2**). In addition, the number and locations of the peptides recognized suggest two distinct immunogenic epitopes within CE3. Three macaques (M166, R279 and P302) also developed responses to CE2, while two animals had responses to CE7 (L862, strong responses; P302, low responses) (**Figure 3A**). As expected, none of the macaques immunized with the p24CE recognized any peptide located outside the p24CE. In contrast, we found that the antibodies induced by p55^{gag} DNA vaccination failed to efficiently recognize linear epitopes within the p24^{gag} region (**Figure 3B**). Only one of the 4 animals (P574) had antibodies that recognized linear epitopes in CE1, CE3 and CE7, but we noted that different peptides were recognized compared to those in p24CE DNA vaccinated animals. Two macaques (P574 and R288) were able to recognize some peptides located in the 'variable' region between CE6 and CE7. These results demonstrate that vaccination with p24CE DNA triggered broad antibody responses that recognized several continuous epitopes within p24^{Gag}, whereas vaccination with p55^{gag} DNA failed to elicit antibodies against the linear segments in the conserved regions or in HIV-1 p24^{gag} in general.

Heterologous boost vaccination increased pre-existing antibody responses in p24CE and p55^{gag} DNA primed macaques

We next asked whether boosting with the heterologous DNA plasmid could increase pre-existing humoral responses. Animals from both groups received an additional DNA vaccination as outlined in **Figure 4A** and the responses were monitored by ELISA. Sustained antibody responses were observed at the day of the heterologous boost vaccination in both groups (**Figure 4B**, vaccination 3) as a result of the prior priming vaccination. Plasma samples collected 2 weeks later showed that these responses were further boosted by heterologous DNA vaccination in both vaccine groups. Boosting of p24CE DNA primed responses by p55^{gag} DNA resulted in an average 0.8 log increase in ELISA titers, and boosting of p55^{gag} DNA primed responses by p24CE DNA increase the Gag ELIA titers by 0.9 log.

The responses were further analyzed by Western immunoblot (**Figure 4C, D**). Prior to boost, macaques primed with p24CE recognized the naturally processed p24^{gag} as well as the p24CE1 and p24CE2 proteins (**Figure 4C**). Following the heterologous p55^{gag} DNA boost, stronger reactivity was found against both p24^{gag} and p24CE proteins and the data from two representative animals (L862 and M166) are shown (**Figure 4C**). Interestingly, although p55^{gag} priming was unable to induce detectable antibody responses to the CE proteins by Western blot analysis, it was able to boost preexisting CE-specific humoral responses.

Macaques primed with p55^{gag} DNA (2 weeks after the 2nd vaccination) developed humoral responses that strongly reacted with p24^{gag} but failed to recognize p24CE proteins (**Figure 4D**), as expected (see above **Figure 2D**). However, a single boost of these animals with p24CE DNA not only increased the reactivity to p24^{gag}, but it also elicited antibodies recognizing p24CE proteins as shown by Western immunoblot analysis from two representative animals (P574 and R288) (**Figure 4D**).

We also compared the antibody responses by Pepscan analysis of plasma samples collected after the prime (from **Figure 3**) and after the boost (**Figures 5 and 6**). In macaques primed with p24CE and boosted with p55^{gag} DNA (**Figure 5**), we observed no significant changes in the reactivity to linear epitopes except for M695, M437, P314 and R315, which showed increased recognition of 1 or 2 CE (M695:CE4; M437: CE1 and CE2; P314: CE1 and CE3) or new responses (R315: CE5 and CE7). Although p55^{gag} DNA vaccination did not induce antibodies against many linear peptides (see **Figure 3B**), it is noteworthy that it was able to alter responses in 4 of 10 animals, suggesting that it increased

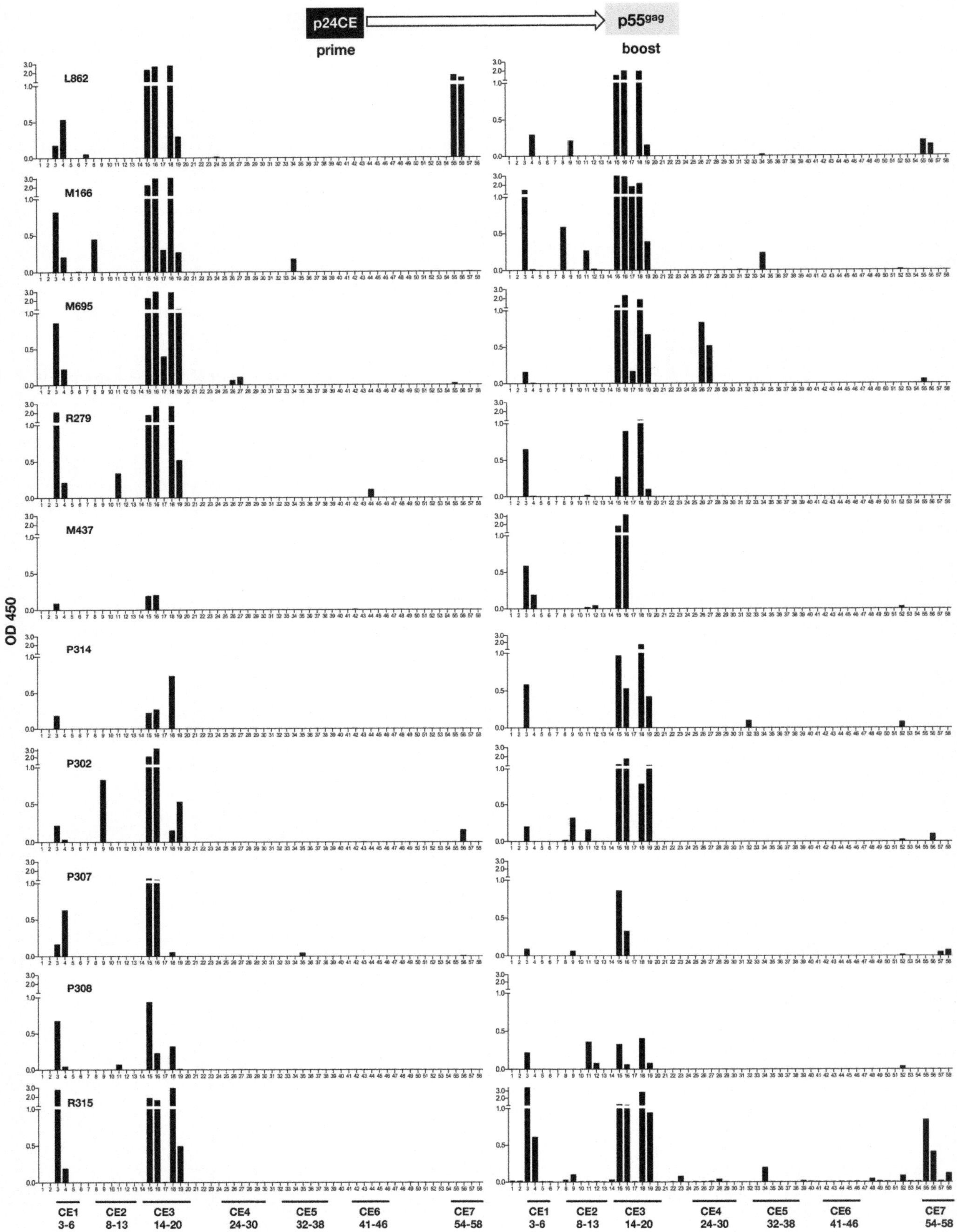

p24CE
prime
p55gag
boost
L862
M166
M695
R279
M437
P314
P302
P307
P308
R315
OD 450
CE1 3-6
CE2 8-13
CE3 14-20
CE4 24-30
CE5 32-38
CE6 41-46
CE7 54-58

Figure 5. Pepscan analysis of humoral responses induced upon heterologous prime-boost regimens of macaques primed with p24CE priming boosted p55^{gag} DNA boost vaccination. Plasma collected after the prime and after the boost vaccinations were subjected to Pepscan analysis against the 58 overlapping peptides described in **Figure 3**. Peptides corresponding to CE1 to CE7 are indicated and the peptides are listed below as detailed in **Table 1**. Samples were analyzed after the priming (data from Figure 3A, left panels) and boost vaccination (right panels).

pre-existing low peptide recognition rather than inducing *de novo* responses.

In contrast, p55^{gag} primed macaques boosted with p24CE DNA (**Figure 6**) showed *de novo* production of antibodies recognizing multiple CE in 3 of 4 macaques, with the linear peptide recognition pattern found from p24CE primed animals (see **Figure 3A**). These macaques (P574, R067 and R288) developed antibody responses mainly targeting CE1 and CE3, the two CE most commonly recognized upon the p24CE vaccination. Macaque L985 was the only animal that did not develop antibodies against CE after a single p24CE DNA boost.

Discussion

A successful vaccine against HIV-1 should induce both cellular and humoral immunity. We previously demonstrated that the p24CE vaccine induced strong cellular responses in both mice and macaques [18,19]. These responses were mediated by both CD4$^+$ and CD8$^+$ T cells with cytotoxic potential and targeted several of the CE encoded by the vaccine. In this report, we tested whether an immunogen designed to induce efficient cellular immune responses against conserved regions of HIV-1 p24^{gag} was also able to induce antibody responses in vaccinated rhesus macaques. We found that vaccination of macaques with p24CE also induced anti-Gag humoral responses with binding antibody titers and kinetics similar to those induced by p55^{gag} DNA vaccination. Interestingly, we found that the antibodies elicited by the p24CE DNA vaccine are able to recognize the processed p24^{gag}, whereas antibodies induced by p55^{gag} DNA vaccination failed to recognize the p24CE protein.

In addition, humoral responses induced by vaccination with the p24CE vectors targeted multiple linear epitopes within the CE, while antibodies induced by the p55^{gag} vaccine failed to recognize any of the conserved elements and in general only poorly induced antibodies able to recognize linear epitopes. Similar to the induction of cellular immunity [19], the p55^{gag} DNA vaccine was able to boost pre-existing CE-specific humoral responses in p24CE DNA primed animals. Table 2 shows a summary of the mapping of both cellular and humoral immune responses observed in the vaccinated animals. It is noteworthy that all the CEs selected for inclusion in the vaccine were immunogenic (humoral, cellular or both) in macaques, although the epitopes were selected based on association with better virologic control in HIV-1 infected individuals [23,24]. CE5 (YVDRFYKTLRAEQA) induced cell-mediated responses in all the vaccinated animals, but was poor in

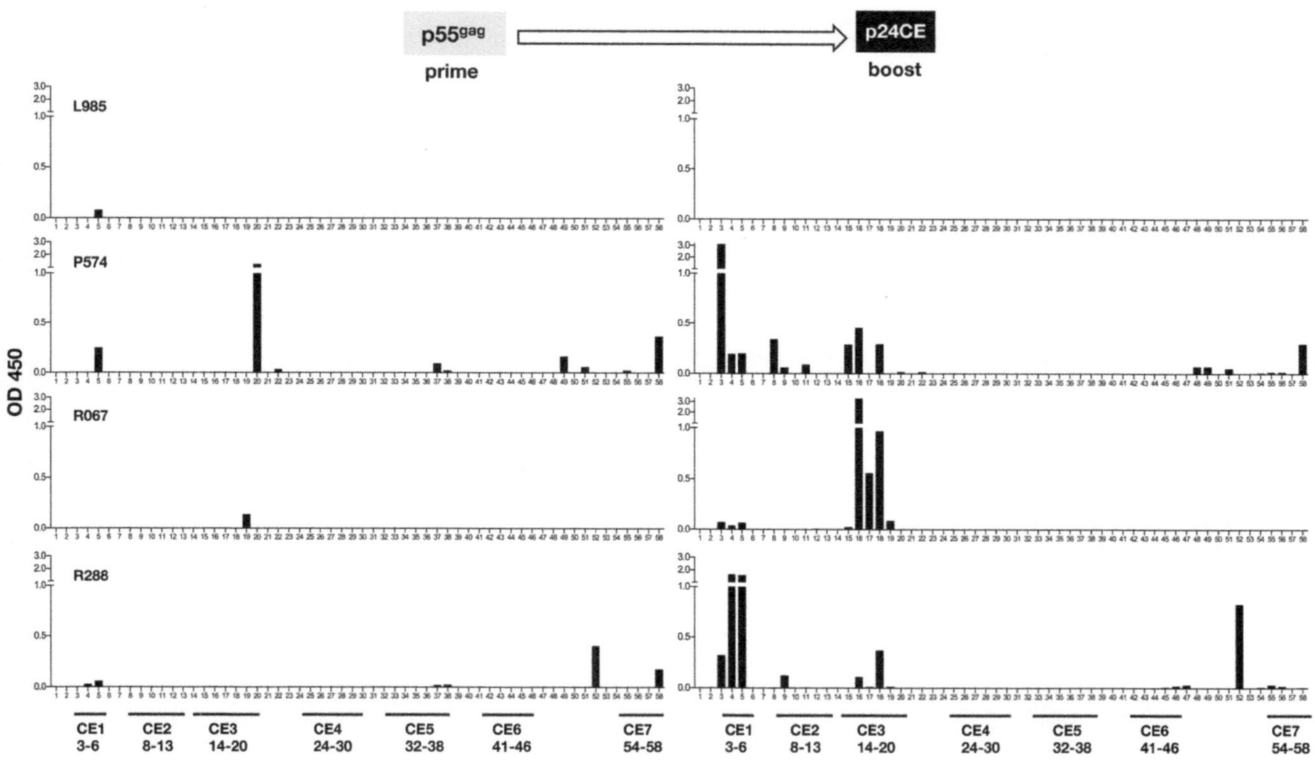

Figure 6. Pepscan analysis of humoral responses induced upon heterologous prime-boost regimens of macaques primed with p55^{gag} DNA and boosted with p24CE DNA. Plasma collected after the prime (left panels) and after the boost vaccinations (right panels) were subjected to Pepscan analysis as described in **Figures 3 and 5**.

inducing humoral responses. In contrast, CE1 (VIPMFSALSE-GATPQDLN) elicited humoral responses in all the animals but failed to induce cellular responses in any of the vaccinated macaques. Interestingly, all macaques developed antibody responses against CE3 (PRGSDIAGTTSTLQEQIGW), while several vaccinees (6 of the 10 macaques) also induced strong cellular immunity against this region, suggesting that CE3 is a good immunogen for both arms of the immune system in macaques. Hence, CE3, CE5 and CE6 (LEEMM-TACQGVGGPGHK) express the epitopes most efficiently recognized by the cellular immunity, while CE1 and CE3 are most efficient in inducing humoral responses.

In summary, these results demonstrate that an immunogen designed to induce cellular immune responses, and shown to do it efficiently in macaques [19], can also induce broad and distinct humoral immunity (this report). Although a correlation between humoral responses to Gag and improved virus control has been reported [33–35], future development of this vaccine concept will, logically, also include Env. It is further possible that analogous immunogens may benefit from both cellular immunity and the development of antibodies that otherwise may not be induced by the native molecule. Antibodies targeting linear epitopes could be useful in mediating protection either by binding to incoming viruses at mucosal surfaces or by mediating ADCC of infected cells. The combination of cellular and humoral responses targeting invariable regions of the virus may be beneficial to achieve protection against HIV-1 infection. Inclusion of conserved elements as a priming immunogen provides an effective vaccine to increase the breadth of the immune response. The concept of focusing responses to critical viral elements for which fewer escape pathways exist and of avoiding decoy epitopes could also be applied against other antigens of highly diverse pathogens.

Acknowledgments

We thank C. Bergamaschi for discussions, J. Bear and B. Chowdhury for technical support, I. Kalisz, D. Weiss, J. Treece and staff at Advanced Bioscience Laboratory for excellent support, and T. Jones for editorial assistance.

Author Contributions

Conceived and designed the experiments: GNP BKF JIM AV M. Rolland VK. Performed the experiments: VK AV M. Rosati. Analyzed the data: VK AV M. Rosati GNP BKF. Wrote the paper: AV BKF JIM GNP.

References

1. Nickle DC, Rolland M, Jensen MA, Pond SL, Deng W, et al. (2007) Coping with viral diversity in HIV vaccine design. PLoS Comput Biol 3: e75.
2. Nickle DC, Jojic N, Heckerman D, Jojic V, Kirovski D, et al. (2008) Comparison of immunogen designs that optimize peptide coverage: reply to Fischer et al. PLoS Comput Biol 4: e25.
3. Barouch DH, O'Brien KL, Simmons NL, King SL, Abbink P, et al. (2010) Mosaic HIV-1 vaccines expand the breadth and depth of cellular immune responses in rhesus monkeys. Nat Med 16: 319–323.
4. Santra S, Liao HX, Zhang R, Muldoon M, Watson S, et al. (2010) Mosaic vaccines elicit CD8+ T lymphocyte responses that confer enhanced immune coverage of diverse HIV strains in monkeys. Nat Med 16: 324–328.
5. Fischer W, Perkins S, Theiler J, Bhattacharya T, Yusim K, et al. (2007) Polyvalent vaccines for optimal coverage of potential T-cell epitopes in global HIV-1 variants. Nat Med 13: 100–106.
6. Fischer W, Liao HX, Haynes BF, Letvin NL, Korber B (2008) Coping with viral diversity in HIV vaccine design: a response to Nickle et al. PLoS Comput Biol 4: e15; author reply e25.
7. Doria-Rose NA, Learn GH, Rodrigo AG, Nickle DC, Li F, et al. (2005) Human immunodeficiency virus type 1 subtype B ancestral envelope protein is functional and elicits neutralizing antibodies in rabbits similar to those elicited by a circulating subtype B envelope. J Virol 79: 11214–11224.
8. Mullins JI, Nickle DC, Heath L, Rodrigo AG, Learn GH (2004) Immunogen sequence: the fourth tier of AIDS vaccine design. Expert Rev Vaccines 3: S151–159.
9. Nickle DC, Jensen MA, Gottlieb GS, Shriner D, Learn GH, et al. (2003) Consensus and ancestral state HIV vaccines. Science 299: 1515–1518; author reply 1515–1518.
10. Dahirel V, Shekhar K, Pereyra F, Miura T, Artyomov M, et al. (2011) Coordinate linkage of HIV evolution reveals regions of immunological vulnerability. Proc Natl Acad Sci U S A 108: 11530–11535.
11. Letourneau S, Im EJ, Mashishi T, Brereton C, Bridgeman A, et al. (2007) Design and pre-clinical evaluation of a universal HIV-1 vaccine. PLoS One 2: e984.
12. Rosario M, Bridgeman A, Quakkelaar ED, Quigley MF, Hill BJ, et al. (2010) Long peptides induce polyfunctional T cells against conserved regions of HIV-1 with superior breadth to single-gene vaccines in macaques. Eur J Immunol 40: 1973–1984.
13. De Groot AS, Rivera DS, McMurry JA, Buus S, Martin W (2008) Identification of immunogenic HLA-B7 "Achilles' heel" epitopes within highly conserved regions of HIV. Vaccine 26: 3059–3071.
14. Wilson CC, McKinney D, Anders M, MaWhinney S, Forster J, et al. (2003) Development of a DNA vaccine designed to induce cytotoxic T lymphocyte responses to multiple conserved epitopes in HIV-1. J Immunol 171: 5611–5623.
15. Kaufman DR, Li F, Cruz AN, Self SG, Barouch DH (2012) Focus and breadth of cellular immune responses elicited by a heterologous insert prime-boost vaccine regimen in rhesus monkeys. Vaccine 30: 506–509.
16. Almeida RR, Rosa DS, Ribeiro SP, Santana VC, Kallas EG, et al. (2012) Broad and cross-clade CD4+ T-cell responses elicited by a DNA vaccine encoding highly conserved and promiscuous HIV-1 M-group consensus peptides. PloS One 7: e45267.
17. Stephenson KE, SanMiguel A, Simmons NL, Smith K, Lewis MG, et al. (2012) Full-length HIV-1 immunogens induce greater magnitude and comparable breadth of T lymphocyte responses to conserved HIV-1 regions compared with conserved-region-only HIV-1 immunogens in rhesus monkeys. J Virol 86: 11434–11440.
18. Kulkarni V, Rosati M, Valentin A, Ganneru B, Singh AK, et al. (2013) HIV-1 p24gag derived conserved element DNA vaccine increases the breadth of immune response in mice. PLos One 8: e60245.
19. Kulkarni V, Valentin A, Rosati M, Alicea C, Singh AK, et al. (2014) Altered Immunodominance Hierarchy and Increased T-cell Breadth upon HIV-1 Conserved Element DNA Vaccination in Macaques. PLoS One 9: e86254.
20. Rosario M, Borthwick N, Stewart-Jones GB, Mbewe-Mvula A, Bridgeman A, et al. (2012) Prime-boost regimens with adjuvanted synthetic long peptides elicit T cells and antibodies to conserved regions of HIV-1 in macaques. AIDS 26: 275–284.
21. Ribeiro SP, Rosa DS, Fonseca SG, Mairena EC, Postol E, et al. (2010) A vaccine encoding conserved promiscuous HIV CD4 epitopes induces broad T cell responses in mice transgenic to multiple common HLA class II molecules. PLoS One 5: e11072.
22. Rosa DS, Ribeiro SP, Almeida RR, Mairena EC, Postol E, et al. (2011) A DNA vaccine encoding multiple HIV CD4 epitopes elicits vigorous polyfunctional, long-lived CD4+ and CD8+ T cell responses. PloS One 6: e16921.
23. Rolland M, Nickle DC, Mullins JI (2007) HIV-1 group M conserved elements vaccine. PLoS Pathog 3: e157.
24. Mothe B, Llano A, Ibarrondo J, Zamarreno J, Schiaulini M, et al. (2012) CTL responses of high functional avidity and broad variant cross-reactivity are associated with HIV control. PLoS One 7: e29717.
25. Niu L, Termini JM, Kanagavelu SK, Gupta S, Rolland MM, et al. (2011) Preclinical evaluation of HIV-1 therapeutic ex vivo dendritic cell vaccines expressing consensus Gag antigens and conserved Gag epitopes. Vaccine 29: 2110–2119.
26. Kiepiela P, Ngumbela K, Thobakgale C, Ramduth D, Honeyborne I, et al. (2007) CD8+ T-cell responses to different HIV proteins have discordant associations with viral load. Nat Med 13: 46–53.
27. Masemola A, Mashishi T, Khoury G, Mohube P, Mokgotho P, et al. (2004) Hierarchical targeting of subtype C human immunodeficiency virus type 1 proteins by CD8+ T cells: correlation with viral load. J Virol 78: 3233–3243.
28. Mothe B, Ibarrondo J, Llano A, Brander C (2009) Virological, immune and host genetics markers in the control of HIV infection. Dis Markers 27: 105–120.
29. Zuniga R, Lucchetti A, Galvan P, Sanchez S, Sanchez C, et al. (2006) Relative dominance of Gag p24-specific cytotoxic T lymphocytes is associated with human immunodeficiency virus control. J Virol 80: 3122–3125.
30. Janes H, Friedrich DP, Krambrink A, Smith RJ, Kallas EG, et al. (2013) Vaccine-induced gag-specific T cells are associated with reduced viremia after HIV-1 infection. J Infect Dis 208: 1231–1239.
31. Ranasinghe S, Cutler S, Davis I, Lu R, Soghoian DZ, et al. (2013) Association of HLA-DRB1-restricted CD4(+) T cell responses with HIV immune control. Nat Med 19: 930–933.
32. Ranasinghe S, Flanders M, Cutler S, Soghoian DZ, Ghebremichael M, et al. (2011) HIV-specific CD4 T cell responses to different viral proteins have discordant associations with viral load and clinical outcome. J Virol 86: 277–283.
33. French MA, Center RJ, Wilson KM, Fleyfel I, Fernandez S, et al. (2013) Isotype-switched immunoglobulin G antibodies to HIV Gag proteins may

provide alternative or additional immune responses to 'protective' human leukocyte antigen-B alleles in HIV controllers. AIDS 27: 519–528.

34. French MA, Tanaskovic S, Law MG, Lim A, Fernandez S, et al. (2010) Vaccine-induced IgG2 anti-HIV p24 is associated with control of HIV in patients with a 'high-affinity' FcgammaRIIa genotype. AIDS 24: 1983–1990.

35. Banerjee K, Klasse PJ, Sanders RW, Pereyra F, Michael E, et al. (2010) IgG subclass profiles in infected HIV type 1 controllers and chronic progressors and in uninfected recipients of Env vaccines. AIDS Res Hum Retroviruses 26: 445–458.

10

Attrition through Multiple Stages of Pre-Treatment and ART HIV Care in South Africa

Matthew P. Fox[1,2,3]*, Kate Shearer[2], Mhairi Maskew[2], Gesine Meyer-Rath[1,2], Kate Clouse[2,4], Ian Sanne[2,5]

1 Center for Global Health & Development, Boston University, Boston, Massachusetts, United States of America, **2** Health Economics and Epidemiology Research Office, Department of Internal Medicine, School of Clinical Medicine, Faculty of Health Sciences, University of the Witwatersrand, Johannesburg, South Africa, **3** Department of Epidemiology, Boston University School of Public Health, Boston, Massachusetts, United States of America, **4** Vanderbilt Institute for Global Health, Vanderbilt University, Nashville, Tennessee, United States of America, **5** Clinical HIV Research Unit, Department of Internal Medicine, School of Clinical Medicine, Faculty of Health Sciences, University of the Witwatersrand, Johannesburg, South Africa

Abstract

Introduction: While momentum for increasing treatment thresholds is growing, if patients cannot be retained in HIV care from the time of testing positive through long-term adherence to antiretroviral therapy (ART), such strategies may fall short of expected gains. While estimates of retention on ART exist, few cohorts have data on retention from testing positive through long-term ART care.

Methods: We explored attrition (loss or death) at the Themba Lethu HIV clinic, Johannesburg, South Africa in 3 distinct cohorts enrolled at HIV testing, pre-ART initiation, and ART initiation.

Results: Between March 2010 and August 2012 we enrolled 380 patients testing HIV+, 206 initiating pre-ART care, and 185 initiating ART. Of the 380 patients enrolled at testing HIV-positive, 38.7% (95%CI: 33.9–43.7%) returned for eligibility staging within ≤3 months of testing. Of the 206 enrolled at pre-ART care, 84.5% (95%CI: 79.0–88.9%) were ART eligible at their first CD4 count. Of those, 87.9% (95%CI: 82.4–92.2%) initiated ART within 6 months. Among patients not ART eligible at their first CD4 count, 50.0% (95%CI: 33.1–66.9%) repeated their CD4 count within one year of the first ineligible CD4. Among the 185 patients in the ART cohort, 22 transferred out and were excluded from further analysis. Of the remaining 163, 81.0% (95%CI: 74.4–86.5%) were retained in care through two years on treatment.

Conclusions: Our findings from a well-resourced clinic demonstrate continual loss from all stages of HIV care and strategies to reduce attrition from all stages of care are urgently needed.

Editor: Susan M. Graham, University of Washington, United States of America

Funding: The project described was also supported by Award Number K01AI083097 from the National Institute of Allergy And Infectious Diseases. This study is also made possible by the generous support of the American people through Cooperative Agreement AID 674-A-12-00029 from the United States Agency for International Development (USAID). The contents are the responsibility of the authors and do not necessarily reflect the views of the National Institute of Allergy and Infectious Diseases, the National Institutes of Health, USAID or the United States Government. The funders had no role in study design, data collection and analysis, decision to publish, or preparation of the manuscript.

Competing Interests: Co-author Matthew Fox is a PLOS ONE Editorial Board member. This does not alter the authors' adherence to PLOS ONE Editorial policies and criteria.

* Email: mfox@bu.edu

Introduction

Since modeling demonstrated that strategies of massive HIV testing and treating patients immediately after being found HIV-positive could substantially impact HIV incidence [1–10], enthusiasm for increasing treatment thresholds has grown. More recently, demonstration of a 96% reduction in transmission risk from an infected partner with a CD4 count between 350–500 cells to an uninfected partner with immediate HIV treatment vs. waiting until a CD4≤250 (HPTN-052) has increased the motivation to increase treatment thresholds [11]. Because the risk of HIV transmission is substantially reduced with decreasing viral load [11–14], the hope is that increasing treatment thresholds could have an important impact on reducing HIV incidence. The World Health Organization now recommends that national programs provide first-line treatment to anyone with a CD4 cell count of less than 500 cells [15], revised from earlier thresholds of 350 and 200.

While it is hoped that increasing treatment thresholds will have a benefit for patients taking treatment in addition to a reduction in transmission, if patients cannot be retained in HIV care continuously from the time of testing positive through long term adherence to antiretroviral therapy (ART), such strategies may fail to achieve the expected benefits to the individual, let alone any population benefits. In addition as increasing thresholds means more people will be eligible for treatment, it may also divert resources that are critically needed for linking patients who test HIV positive to care and treatment sites and for retaining patients in both pre-ART and ART care. Retention in both pre-ART [16] and ART care [17,18] have been shown to be sub-optimal.

Given the costs that are required for increasing treatment thresholds, it is important that we have a thorough understanding of retention in care under current guidelines so that we can monitor any differences associated with changing thresholds. While numerous estimates of retention on ART exist, few have data on retention from testing positive through pre-ART and on ART care within a single HIV care setting. We set out to estimate retention in three stages of HIV care within a single HIV care facility in Johannesburg, South Africa and to look for predictors of loss at each stage.

Methods

Study Site and Study Procedures

The study was conducted at the Themba Lethu HIV clinic in Johannesburg [19,20]. Themba Lethu is a comprehensive public-sector HIV care and management site that also receives PEPFAR support through a South African NGO called Right to Care. Themba Lethu is located at the Helen Joseph Hospital and provides both HIV testing as well as pre-ART and ART care, as per the South African national HIV treatment guidelines. The site currently has >8,500 patients in pre-ART care, >11,000 patients on ART and conducts roughly 840 HIV tests per month. At the study's start, guidelines called for treatment initiation at a CD4 count ≤200 or a WHO Stage IV condition [21]. In 2011 guidelines were updated to allow initiation with a CD4 count ≤ 350 [22].

At Themba Lethu, data on patients testing HIV positive at HIV counseling and testing (HCT) are kept in paper registers. Patients who test at the site are a mix of patients seeking self-initiated HCT as well as provider-initiated HCT from elsewhere in the hospital. Patients who test positive are sent from the HCT clinic to the HIV clinic for a blood draw for CD4 staging and asked to return in one week for the results. Those not eligible for ART begin in "wellness care" and have a paper file opened. Wellness patients are asked to return every six months for repeat CD4 testing, or more frequently when closer to the treatment threshold. Patients who are treatment eligible are asked to return for adherence and treatment readiness counseling over 2–3 weeks and then initiate treatment. Once a patient initiates ART, they are asked to return to the clinic every 1–3 months for the first twelve months for either drug pickups or medical visits.

Data on patients initiating ART care is kept in an electronic patient database. All pre-ART paper records are entered into the database at ART initiation. An effort is underway to enter all pre-ART records for all patients, but it is not complete. Accordingly, this study relied on both electronic and paper records to determine if patients returned for care.

To assess retention in all stages of HIV care we enrolled three distinct cohorts of patients at three different stages: a cohort of patients enrolled at the time of testing HIV-positive at HIV counseling and testing (referred to as the HCT cohort), a cohort of patients newly enrolled in pre-ART care after completing CD4 staging, regardless of ART eligibility, (referred to as the pre-ART cohort), and a cohort of patients newly initiating HIV treatment (referred to as the ART cohort). Patients who completed one stage of care were not followed after completing that stage of care. These cohorts roughly followed the published framework on pre-ART care [16] and additionally added a cohort post-ART initiation. Enrollment began on March 23, 2010 and was completed on August 19, 2012. We enrolled patients at care visits that were newly enrolled in pre-ART care (first CD4 count within 3 months of enrollment) and newly initiated on ART (on ART for no more than 1 month at the time of the interview). We attempted to recruit all patients eligible for care on the days where study staff were at the clinic, but as only one data collector was used who moved between part of the clinic (testing and treatment), enrollment was not done every day for each cohort. Due to sensitivity around receiving a positive HIV diagnosis, we enrolled HCT patients before they tested but limited our analysis to those who tested positive.

Patient follow-up

Patients from all three cohorts went through an informed consent process and completed a questionnaire to look for predictors of attrition beyond what would be captured in the treatment database. Patients also provided identifying information to allow us to track their clinic records including a South African national ID number when possible. Upon completion of the questionnaire, participants followed the standard clinic schedule of procedures. In order to not influence patient retention, no active follow-up of patients was conducted by the research team. When resources allow, clinic staff attempt to phone patients who do not return for care.

Upon database closure, we attempted to match all enrolled eligible patients to the HIV care database using national ID (when provided, 82.7% of patients), name and date of birth. We then searched in paper records and registers for patients who could not be found in the dataset. Because all ART patients should have a clinic record, one ART patient with no records was excluded from analysis. For the HCT and pre-ART cohorts, not having a clinic record would identify the patient as lost to follow-up. We excluded patients who withdrew from the study (n = 2), and in the pre-ART cohort, who did not have a CD4 count (n = 34), who transferred out (n = 21) or whose first CD4 count was recorded outside +/−3 months from either the date of first visit or the interview date (n = 37).

Analytic Methods

For the HCT cohort, loss to follow-up (LTF) was defined as not completing assessment for ART eligibility within 3 months of testing HIV positive. In the pre-ART cohort, LTF was defined as not initiating ART within 6 months of becoming eligible or, for those not eligible for ART, not repeating ART eligibility screening within 12 months of the previous ineligible staging. We note that the time frames used to allow patients to complete each stage of care are not necessarily ideal for patient care, but were chosen to balance the desires for fast, continual care but also to allow for the realities of patients' lives [23]. Finally, for ART patients we use the clinic's LTF definition of ≥3 months late for the next scheduled appointment. In the HCT cohort, the interview CD4 count was defined as the CD4 count closest to the interview date (84.3% were within +/−1 month).

We also present a secondary analysis using the time frames expected according to the clinic's guidelines of completion of ART eligibility assessment within 1 week of testing positive, ART initiation within 1 month of the first eligible CD4 count, and repeat ART eligibility screening within 6 months of the previous ineligible staging. Follow-up time accrued from beginning of the stage until the earliest of loss to follow-up, death, transfer, completing 24 months of follow-up or dataset closure (September 30, 2013). To determine the vital status of patients lost, we searched their national ID number in the national vital registration database.

For each cohort (stage of HIV care) we present descriptive statistics using medians and interquartile ranges (IQRs) for continuous variables and proportions for categorical variables. Our primary analysis was to measure the proportion of patients who did not complete each stage of HIV care (either through death or loss). In order to examine predictors of not completing each stage, we used modified Poisson regression with robust error estimation to estimate the risk of not completing the stage with corresponding 95% confidence intervals. Age and sex were included in all of the models as was CD4 count in the pre-ART and ART model. Other possible confounders associated with not completing the stage ($p<0.2$) in univariate analyses were also adjusted for in the multivariate analyses.

Ethical Clearance

Approval for analysis was granted by the Human Research Ethics Committee of the University of the Witwatersrand and by the Institutional Review Board of Boston University. Anonymized data can be requested from the corresponding author.

Results

Enrollment of patients into all three cohorts was conducted from March 2010 through August 2012. We enrolled 380 patients testing HIV-positive at HCT, 206 patients initiating pre-ART care, and 185 patients initiating HIV treatment. We had 45 refusals in the HCT cohort, 37 refusals in the wellness cohort and 26 refusals in the ART initiation cohort.

HIV Testing to Completing CD4 Staging

The first stage in the HIV care cascade requires patients to test for HIV. Those who test positive must have a blood draw for a CD4 count to determine ART eligibility and then return for the results. We enrolled 380 patients who tested HIV-positive. Of these, 56.1% were female, and the median age (IQR) was 35.8 (27.8–42.7) years (Table 1). A majority were unmarried (79.0%) and had some or completed high school (79.1%). Unemployment was common (37.7%) and over half (62.3%) required >30 minutes travel time to the clinic.

Of the 380 patients enrolled at HIV-testing, we found no evidence of a blood draw for 142 patients and these were all considered failures. Of the remaining 238, 147 completed the stage for a total of 38.7% (95% CI: 33.9–43.7%) returning to complete eligibility staging within 3 months of testing, our definition of timely stage completion (Figure 1a). A total of 47.4% (an additional 33) ever returned after testing. Of those 200 (52.6%) who either never had a blood draw or never returned to the clinic, 9.0% (N = 18) were known to have died. We note, however, that because patients who test HIV positive could go elsewhere for CD4 staging and enrollment in care, this may overstate total attrition.

Among the 180 who returned to the clinic and had a CD4 count value recorded, a high percentage (68.9%, N = 124) were ART eligible. Treatment initiation was high amongst this group at 87.1% (95% CI: 80.3–92.2%). Of the 16 that did not initiate, 1 died before treatment initiation. While numbers were small, of the 56 patients who were not ART eligible, 51.8% (N = 29) became ART eligible during follow-up and started treatment.

Exploring predictors of failing to complete CD4 staging within 3 months, we found that less education was predictive of attrition (those completing some high school were 20% less likely to not complete the stage as those with primary school or less) (Table 2) as was employment status (unemployed were 29% more likely to not complete the stage as those employed). While there were few non-South Africans in our sample (N = 20), South Africans were more likely to not complete staging within 3 months as non-South Africans (aRR: 1.80; 95% CI: 0.87–3.72).

Initiation of Pre-ART Care Through Treatment Initiation

The next stage in pre-ART HIV care requires patients who completed CD4 staging and were ART eligible to start treatment and those not ART eligible to complete routinely scheduled CD4 eligibility staging visits. We enrolled 206 patients who had recently completed CD4 staging. Of those, 69.9% were female and the median age (IQR) was 37.4 (31.7–43.5) years (Table 1). As with the testing cohort, few subjects were married (18.5%) and about 40% completed high school. Unemployment was 35.9% in this cohort and over two-thirds (72.3%) required >30 minutes travel time to the clinic.

Of the 206 patients, 84.5% (95% CI: 79.0–88.9%) were ART eligible at their first CD4 count. Of those 174, 87.9% (95% CI: 82.4–92.2%) (N = 153/174) successfully completed the stage by initiating ART within 6 months while a further 6 (3.5%) initiated ART more than 6 months after learning of their eligibility. Of the 15 who never initiated, 4 (26.7%) are confirmed to have died. Among the 32 not ART eligible at their first CD4 count, 50.0% (95% CI: 33.1–66.9%) successfully remained in the stage by repeating their CD4 count within one year. Taken together 82.0% (N = 169/206) were adherent to the care protocol after initial CD4 staging completion.

For pre-ART patients, we found that a higher first CD4 count was predictive of failure to complete the stage (>200 vs. <50, aRR: 2.43; 95%CI: 0.79–7.49). We also found some evidence that males were more likely to fail to complete the stage than females (aRR: 1.42; 95% CI: 0.73–2.74), the only stage for which we identified even a modest gender association. Living in a smaller household was associated with completing the stage (aRR for ≤3 people vs. ≥4 people: 0.56; 95% CI: 0.30–1.04).

Antiretroviral Therapy Initiation through 2 Years on ART

We enrolled 185 patients at treatment initiation. As enrollment occurred when the initiation CD4 threshold was <200, the median (IQR) CD4 count was 158 (95–198).

Of the 185, 22 patients transferred to another facility and are excluded from further analysis. After two years, among the remaining 163, 81.0% (95% CI: 74.4–86.5%)(N = 132) were retained through two years on treatment, while 23 were lost to follow-up and 8 died.

Patients without employment were somewhat more likely to not complete two years on treatment compared to those who reported employment in the formal and informal sectors or self-employment (aRR: 1.40; 95% CI: 0.67–2.94). We found very little else that was predictive of attrition from this stage, including age, sex, CD4 count and education, likely due to sample size.

Results using alternative definitions

While the results presented above for the HCT and pre-ART cohorts pertain to definitions of loss described by Fox et al. [23], we repeated this analysis utilizing clinic guidelines for these two groups, which differ slightly. For patients testing positive in the HCT cohort, we defined LTF as failure to complete ART eligibility assessment within 1 week of testing positive while for the pre-ART cohort, we defined LTF as not initiating ART within 1 month of becoming eligible or, for those not eligible for ART, not repeating ART eligibility screening within 6 months of the previous ineligible staging.

Using these modified definitions, estimates of LTF increased considerably. Of the 380 patients enrolled in the HCT cohort, only 17 (4.5%; 95% CI: 2.7–6.9%) completed eligibility staging

Table 1. Demographic and Clinical Characteristics of Three Cohorts of Patients Enrolled in Different Stages of HIV care in Johannesburg, South Africa.

	HCT Cohort			Pre-ART Cohort			ART Cohort		
Variable	**Total**	**Completed Stage**	**Did Not Complete Stage**	**Total**	**Completed Stage**	**Did Not Complete Stage**	**Total**	**Completed Stage**	**Did Not Complete Stage**
Total N	380 (100%)	147 (100%)	233 (100%)	206 (100%)	169 (100%)	37 (100%)	163 (100%)	132 (100%)	31 (100%)
Sex									
Missing	34	1	33	0	0	0	0	0	0
Male	152 (43.9%)	62 (42.5%)	90 (45.0%)	62 (30.1%)	51 (30.2%)	11 (29.7%)	33 (20.3%)	25 (18.9%)	8 (25.8%)
Female	194 (56.1%)	84 (57.5%)	110 (55.0%)	144 (69.9%)	118 (69.8%)	26 (70.3%)	130 (79.7%)	107 (81.1%)	23 (74.2%)
Age[†]									
Median (IQR) N	35.8 (27.8–42.7)	37.5 (32.1–43.8)	35.0 (26.1–42.1)	37.4 (31.7–43.5)	38.1 (31.7–43.8)	35.5 (31.8–39.6)	37.1 (31.5–43.9)	37.8 (31.8–43.4)	35.9 (28.5–46.0)
18–29.9	115 (30.3%)	31 (21.1%)	84 (36.1%)	40 (19.4%)	32 (18.9%)	8 (21.6%)	34 (20.9%)	26 (19.7%)	8 (25.8%)
30–34.9	57 (15.0%)	25 (17.0%)	32 (13.7%)	42 (20.4%)	33 (19.5%)	9 (24.3%)	29 (17.8%)	23 (17.4%)	6 (19.4%)
35–39.9	70 (18.4%)	31 (21.1%)	39 (16.7%)	42 (20.4%)	31 (18.3%)	11 (29.7%)	38 (23.3%)	31 (23.5%)	7 (22.6%)
40–44.9	67 (17.6%)	27 (18.4%)	40 (17.2%)	38 (18.5%)	35 (20.7%)	3 (8.1%)	25 (15.3%)	24 (18.2%)	1 (3.2%)
≥45	71 (18.7%)	33 (22.5%)	38 (16.3%)	44 (21.4%)	38 (22.5%)	6 (16.2%)	37 (22.7%)	28 (21.2%)	9 (29.0%)
Country of birth									
Missing	21	1	20	1	1	0	0	0	0
South Africa	339 (94.4%)	132 (90.4%)	207 (97.2%)	170 (82.9%)	137 (81.6%)	33 (89.2%)	140 (85.9%)	114 (86.4%)	26 (83.9%)
Other	20 (5.6%)	14 (9.6%)	6 (2.8%)	35 (17.1%)	31 (18.5%)	4 (10.8%)	23 (14.1%)	18 (13.6%)	5 (16.1%)
Marital status									
Missing	80	30	50	0	0	0	0	0	0
Unmarried[‡]	237 (79.0%)	102 (87.2%)	135 (73.8%)	168 (81.6%)	138 (81.7%)	30 (81.1%)	131 (80.4%)	104 (78.8%)	27 (87.1%)
Engaged or married	63 (21.0%)	15 (12.8%)	48 (26.2%)	38 (18.5%)	31 (18.3%)	7 (18.9%)	32 (19.6%)	28 (21.2%)	4 (12.9%)
Education level									
Missing	35	2	33	0	0	0	0	0	0
Primary school or less	72 (20.9%)	31 (21.4%)	41 (20.5%)	49 (23.8%)	40 (23.7%)	9 (24.3%)	34 (20.9%)	26 (19.7%)	8 (25.8%)
Some high school	130 (37.7%)	63 (43.5%)	67 (33.5%)	76 (36.9%)	61 (36.1%)	15 (40.5%)	80 (49.1%)	67 (50.8%)	13 (41.9%)
Completed high school or more	143 (41.5%)	51 (35.2%)	92 (46.0%)	81 (39.3%)	68 (40.2%)	13 (35.1%)	49 (30.1%)	39 (29.6%)	10 (32.3%)
Employment status[¥]									
Missing	35	2	33	0	0	0	0	0	0
Employed	215 (62.3%)	103 (71.0%)	112 (56.0%)	132 (64.1%)	114 (67.5%)	18 (48.7%)	100 (61.4%)	85 (64.4%)	15 (48.4%)
Unemployed	130 (37.7%)	42 (29.0%)	88 (44.0%)	74 (35.9%)	55 (32.5%)	19 (51.4%)	63 (38.6%)	47 (35.6%)	16 (51.6%)
Type of transport									
Missing	80	30	50	0	0	0	0	0	0
Used a taxi	213 (71.0%)	97 (82.9%)	116 (63.4%)	186 (90.3%)	151 (89.4%)	35 (94.6%)	137 (84.0%)	111 (84.1%)	26 (83.9%)
Did not use a taxi	87 (29.0%)	20 (17.1%)	67 (36.6%)	20 (9.7%)	18 (10.6%)	2 (5.4%)	26 (16.0%)	21 (15.9%)	5 (16.1%)

Table 1. Cont.

	HCT Cohort			Pre-ART Cohort			ART Cohort		
Variable	**Total**	**Completed Stage**	**Did Not Complete Stage**	**Total**	**Completed Stage**	**Did Not Complete Stage**	**Total**	**Completed Stage**	**Did Not Complete Stage**
Travel time to clinic									
Missing	80	30	50	0	0	0	2	1	1
≤30 minutes	113 (37.7%)	38 (32.5%)	75 (41.0%)	57 (27.7%)	48 (28.4%)	9 (24.3%)	34 (21.1%)	28 (21.4%)	6 (20.0%)
31–60 minutes	137 (45.7%)	61 (52.1%)	76 (41.5%)	86 (41.8%)	70 (41.4%)	16 (43.2%)	70 (43.5%)	58 (44.3%)	12 (40.0%)
>60 minutes	50 (16.7%)	18 (15.4%)	32 (17.5%)	63 (30.6%)	51 (30.2%)	12 (32.4%)	57 (35.4%)	45 (34.4%)	12 (40.0%)
Household size									
Missing	81	30	51	0	0	0	0	0	0
≤3 people	191 (63.9%)	71 (60.7%)	120 (65.9%)	127 (61.6%)	111 (65.7%)	16 (43.2%)	96 (58.9%)	74 (56.1%)	22 (71.0%)
≥4 people	108 (36.1%)	46 (39.3%)	62 (34.1%)	79 (38.4%)	58 (34.3%)	21 (56.8%)	67 (41.1%)	58 (43.9%)	9 (29.0%)
CD4 count (cells/mm^3)[Ɏ]									
Median (IQR) N	205 (99.5–344.5)	159 (75–245)	340 (160–505)	165 (85.5–256.5)	159 (85–247)	244.5 (151–446)	158 (95–198)	161.5 (106–199)	133 (91–178)
Missing	144	0	144	0	0	0	14	10	4
≤50	37 (15.7%)	27 (18.4%)	10 (11.2%)	29 (14.1%)	26 (15.4%)	3 (8.1%)	16 (10.7%)	14 (11.5%)	2 (7.4%)
51–100	22 (9.3%)	17 (11.6%)	5 (5.6%)	22 (10.7%)	20 (11.8%)	2 (5.4%)	25 (16.8%)	16 (13.1%)	9 (33.3%)
101–200	55 (23.3%)	46 (31.3%)	9 (10.1%)	67 (32.5%)	56 (33.1%)	11 (29.7%)	73 (49.0%)	63 (51.6%)	10 (37.0%)
>200	122 (51.7%)	57 (38.8%)	65 (73.0%)	88 (42.7%)	67 (39.6%)	21 (56.8%)	35 (23.5%)	29 (23.8%)	6 (22.2%)
WHO Stage at ART Initiation									
Stage I/II	–	–	–	–	–	–	98 (60.1%)	81 (61.4%)	17 (54.8%)
Stage III/IV	–	–	–	–	–	–	65 (39.9%)	51 (38.6%)	14 (45.2%)
BMI at ART Initiation									
Median (IQR)	–	–	–	–	–	–	22.8 (20.2–25.9)	22.6 (20.3–25.9)	22.9 (20.2–26.4)
Missing	–	–	–	–	–	–	10	8	2
<18.5	–	–	–	–	–	–	14 (9.2%)	11 (8.9%)	3 (10.3%)
18.5–24.9	–	–	–	–	–	–	94 (61.4%)	77 (62.1%)	17 (58.6%)
25–29.9	–	–	–	–	–	–	27 (17.7%)	23 (18.6%)	4 (13.8%)
≥30	–	–	–	–	–	–	18 (11.8%)	13 (10.5%)	5 (17.2%)
Anemia at ART Initiation									
Missing	–	–	–	–	–	–	10	10	0
None or mild							73 (47.7%)	58 (47.5%)	15 (48.4%)
Moderate or severe	–	–	–	–	–	–	80 (52.3%)	64 (52.5%)	16 (51.6%)

[†]Age at the time of the interview for the HCT cohort and the pre-ART cohort and at initiation for the ART cohort.
[‡]Unmarried includes patients who reported being single, divorced/separated, and widowed.
[¥]Employed includes patients who reported formal employment, informal employment, and self-employment. Unemployed includes those who reported no employment, studying, being retired, performing community service, and other.
[Ɏ]CD4 at the time of the interview for the HCT cohort, first CD4 count conducted for the pre-ART cohort and at baseline for the ART cohort.

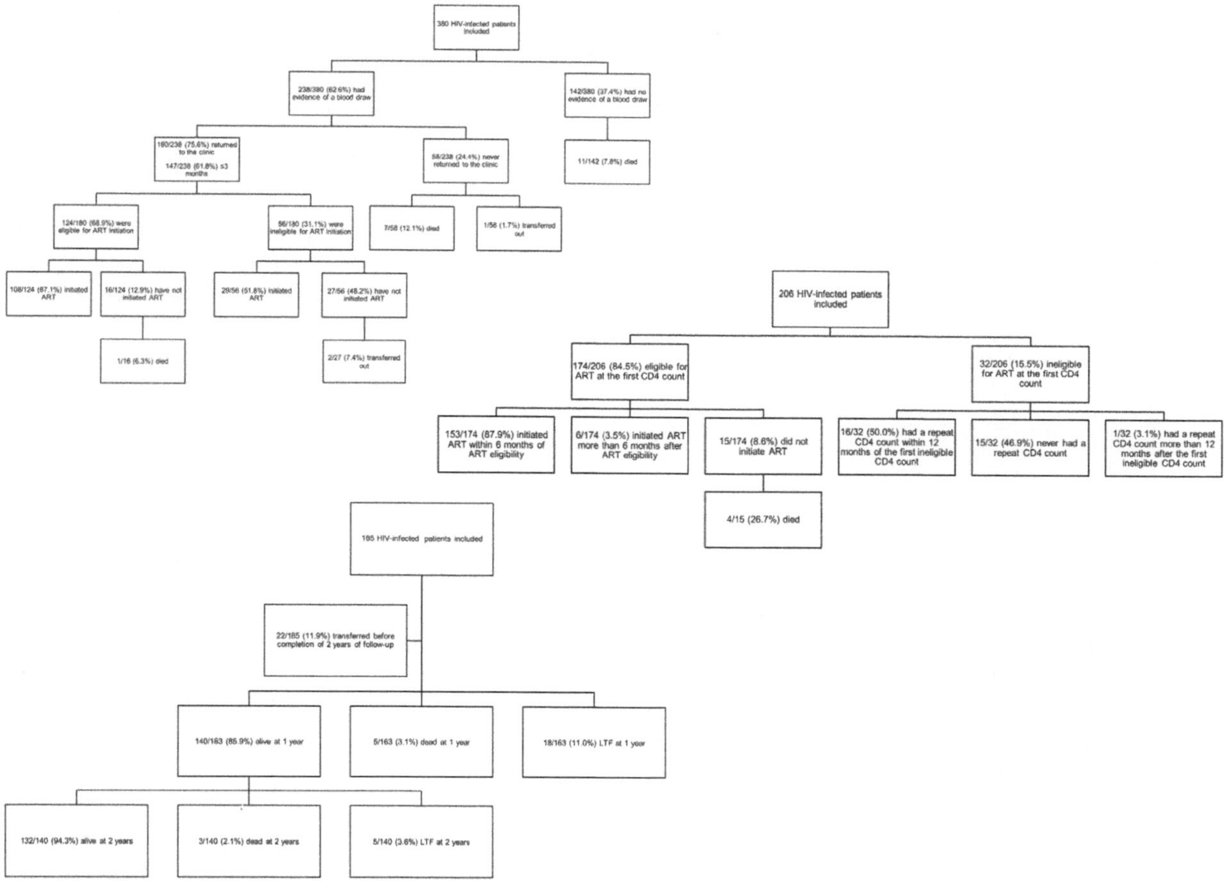

Figure 1. Flow Chart of Retention in Care of Three Cohorts of Patients Enrolled in Different Stages of HIV care in Johannesburg, South Africa.

within 1 week of testing positive. Likewise, in the pre-ART cohort, just 25.9% (95% CI: 19.8–32.8%) of ART eligible patients initiated ART within 1 month of their eligible CD4 count and only 34.4% (95% CI: 19.6–51.9%) returned within 6 months to repeat eligibility screening.

Discussion

Getting patients onto treatment earlier and maintaining them on ART lifelong has been an important goal of ART programs in an attempt to achieve benefits to the individual and their partners [24–27]. Our findings suggest that within our clinic population, 39% of patients who test positive complete CD4 staging within three months, 88% of patients who complete CD4 staging and are ART eligible initiate treatment within 6 months of eligibility and 81% of those starting treatment remain on treatment for two years. If we informally combine these three pieces of information by multiplying the probabilities, these estimates would suggest that approximately 28% of patients who test positive initiate treatment and remain on ART for at least the first two years. This does not account for attrition from those who are not treatment eligible at the time of entering pre-ART care, where monitoring is difficult and attrition is high. Thus, the overall picture of retention in this cohort is low in the pre-ART period, but better in the on-treatment era.

To put our estimates in context, we compared our results with the assumptions used in models of the potential benefits of test and treat strategies, approaches where massive testing is combined with treating all positives regardless of their CD4 count in order to reduce HIV incidence. In all these models, assumptions about retention on ART have varied. In the first analysis of universal test and treat, attrition was based on the Malawi national program, which saw an 8% immediate dropout rate and a 1–5% yearly dropout rate excluding deaths [1]. Another model estimated on ART attrition at 20% over the first year on treatment [4], in line with a previous review of on-ART retention [18]. A cost-effectiveness analysis of universal test and treat for discordant couples assumed a loss rate of 3.4/100 patient years, presumably during both pre-ART and ART periods [3]. While our attrition estimates include both death and loss to follow-up, these assumptions appear reasonably consistent with our findings and recent systematic reviews [18].

In terms of pre-ART linkage, one model used a linkage rate of 100% in order to test the maximum impact of universal test and treat and immediate ART initiation [2], while a second specified two-thirds of those testing positive completing linkage, a fair bit higher than our estimates [4]. A third model used a base-case scenario of 52% linkage, similar to that found in South Africa [28]. A fourth model assumed 41% loss between HIV testing and CD4 staging, and 54% loss between each 6-monthly pre-ART visit in their baseline scenario [29]. They found that increasing the proportion of patients receiving CD4 results was more cost-effective, while at expanded eligibility, improving ART retention was the most cost-effective option. Only universal test and treat with 80% testing and treatment initiation and zero ART dropout

Table 2. Predictors of Attrition from Different Stages of HIV care in Johannesburg, South Africa.

	HCT Cohort			Pre-ART Cohort			ART Cohort		
Variable	**Did not complete stage/N (%)**	**Unadjusted RR (95% CI)**	**Adjusted RR (95% CI)**	**Did not complete stage/N (%)**	**Unadjusted RR (95% CI)**	**Adjusted RR (95% CI)**	**Did not complete stage/N (%)**	**Unadjusted RR (95% CI)**	**Adjusted RR (95% CI)**
Sex									
Male	90/152 (59.2%)	1.04 (0.87, 1.25)	1.10 (0.91, 1.33)	11/62 (17.7%)	0.98 (0.52, 1.86)	1.42 (0.73, 2.74)	8/33 (24.2%)	1.37 (0.68, 2.78)	1.30 (0.58, 2.88)
Female	110/194 (56.7%)	**Reference**	**Reference**	26/144 (18.1%)	**Reference**	**Reference**	23/130 (17.7%)	**Reference**	**Reference**
Age									
18–29.9	84/115 (73.0%)	1.36 (1.07, 1.74)	1.36 (1.00, 1.83)	8/40 (20.0%)	1.47 (0.56, 3.86)	1.43 (0.55, 3.74)	8/34 (23.5%)	0.97 (0.42, 2.22)	1.22 (0.47, 3.16)
30–34.9	32/57 (56.1%)	1.05 (0.77, 1.44)	1.17 (0.83, 1.66)	9/42 (21.4%)	1.57 (0.61, 4.03)	1.55 (0.60, 3.98)	6/29 (20.7%)	0.85 (0.34, 2.12)	0.94 (0.33, 2.64)
35–39.9	39/70 (55.7%)	1.04 (0.77, 1.41)	1.16 (0.82, 1.64)	11/42 (26.2%)	1.92 (0.78, 4.73)	1.98 (0.85, 4.65)	7/38 (18.4%)	0.76 (0.31, 1.82)	0.83 (0.31, 2.25)
40–44.9	40/67 (59.7%)	1.12 (0.83, 1.49)	1.23 (0.87, 1.75)	3/38 (7.9%)	0.58 (0.16, 2.16)	0.76 (0.19, 2.96)	1/25 (4.0%)	0.16 (0.02, 1.22)	0.23 (0.03, 1.71)
≥45	38/71 (53.5%)	**Reference**	**Reference**	6/44 (13.6%)	**Reference**	**Reference**	9/37 (24.3%)	**Reference**	**Reference**
Country of birth									
South Africa	207/339 (61.1%)	2.04 (1.04, 4.00)	1.80 (0.87, 3.72)	33/170 (1941%)	1.70 (0.64, 4.49)	–	26/140 (18.6%)	0.85 (0.37, 2.00)	–
Other	6/20 (30.0%)	**Reference**	**Reference**	4/35 (11.4%)	**Reference**	–	5/23 (21.7%)	**Reference**	–
Marital status									
Unmarried	135/237 (57.0%)	**Reference**	**Reference**	30/168 (17.9%)	**Reference**	**Reference**	27/131 (20.6%)	**Reference**	–
Engaged or married	48/63 (76.2%)	1.34 (1.12, 1.60)	1.40 (1.11, 1.75)	7/38 (18.4%)	1.03 (0.49, 2.17)	–	4/32 (12.5%)	0.61 (0.23, 1.61)	–
Education level									
Primary school or less	41/72 (56.9%)	**Reference**	**Reference**	9/49 (18.4%)	**Reference**	–	8/34 (23.5%)	**Reference**	–
Some high school	67/130 (51.5%)	0.91 (0.70, 1.18)	0.80 (0.60, 1.06)	15/76 (19.7%)	1.07 (0.51, 2.26)	–	13/80 (16.3%)	0.69 (0.32, 1.51)	–
Completed matric or more	92/143 (64.3%)	1.13 (0.89, 1.43)	0.91 (0.69, 1.21)	13/81 (16.1%)	0.87 (0.40, 1.89)	–	10/49 (20.4%)	0.87 (0.38, 1.97)	–
Employment status									
Employed	112/215 (67.7%)	**Reference**	**Reference**	18/132 (13.6%)	**Reference**	**Reference**	15/100 (15.0%)	**Reference**	**Reference**
Unemployed	88/130 (52.1%)	1.30 (1.09, 1.55)	1.29 (1.06, 1.58)	19/74 (25.7%)	1.88 (1.06, 3.36)	1.56 (0.87, 2.80)	16/63 (25.4%)	1.69 (0.90, 3.18)	1.40 (0.67, 2.94)
Type of transport									
Used a taxi	116/213 (54.5%)	**Reference**	**Reference**	35/186 (18.8%)	**Reference**	–	26/137 (19.0%)	**Reference**	–
Did not use a taxi	67/87 (77.0%)	1.41 (1.20, 1.67)	1.37 (1.11, 1.70)	2/20 (10.0%)	0.53 (0.14, 2.05)	–	5/26 (19.2%)	1.01 (0.43, 2.40)	–
Travel time to clinic									
≤30 minutes	75/113 (66.4%)	1.04 (0.81, 1.33)	0.88 (0.67, 1.15)	9/57 (15.8%)	0.83 (0.38, 1.82)	–	6/33 (17.7%)	0.84 (0.35, 2.03)	–
31–60 minutes	76/137 (55.5%)	0.87 (0.67, 1.12)	0.88 (0.68, 1.13)	16/86 (18.6%)	0.98 (0.50, 1.92)	–	12/70 (17.1%)	0.81 (0.40, 1.67)	–
>60 minutes	32/50 (64.0%)	**Reference**	**Reference**	12/63 (19.1%)	**Reference**	–	12/57 (21.1%)	**Reference**	–
Household size									
≤3 people	120/191 (62.8%)	1.09 (0.90, 1.33)	–	16/127 (12.6%)	0.47 (0.26, 0.85)	0.56 (0.30, 1.04)	22/96 (22.9%)	1.71 (0.84, 3.47)	1.52 (0.69, 3.36)
≥4 people	62/108 (57.4%)	**Reference**	–	21/79 (26.6%)	**Reference**	**Reference**	9/67 (13.4%)	**Reference**	**Reference**
CD4 count (cells/mm^3)									

Table 2. Cont.

	HCT Cohort			Pre-ART Cohort			ART Cohort		
Variable	**Did not complete stage/N (%)**	**Unadjusted RR (95% CI)**	**Adjusted RR (95% CI)**	**Did not complete stage/N (%)**	**Unadjusted RR (95% CI)**	**Adjusted RR (95% CI)**	**Did not complete stage/N (%)**	**Unadjusted RR (95% CI)**	**Adjusted RR (95% CI)**
≤50	–	–	–	3/29 (10.3%)	**Reference**	**Reference**	2/16 (12.5%)	**Reference**	**Reference**
51–100	–	–	–	2/22 (9.1%)	0.88 (0.16, 4.82)	1.05 (0.19, 5.86)	9/25 (36.0%)	2.88 (0.71, 11.65)	2.01 (0.52, 7.79)
101–200	–	–	–	11/67 (16.4%)	1.59 (0.48, 5.27)	1.86 (0.58, 5.96)	10/73 (13.7%)	1.10 (0.27, 4.53)	1.00 (0.26, 3.85)
>200	–	–	–	21/88 (23.9%)	2.31 (0.74, 7.17)	2.43 (0.79, 7.49)	6/35 (17.1%)	1.37 (0.31, 6.07)	1.12 (0.25, 4.98)
WHO Stage at ART Initiation									
Stage I/II	–	–	–	–	–	–	17/98 (17.4%)	**Reference**	–
Stage III/IV	–	–	–	–	–	–	14/65 (21.5%)	1.24 (0.66, 2.34)	–
BMI at ART Initiation									
<18.5	–	–	–	–	–	–	3/14 (21.4%)	1.18 (0.40, 3.53)	–
18.5–24.9	–	–	–	–	–	–	17/94 (18.1%)	**Reference**	–
25–29.9	–	–	–	–	–	–	4/27 (14.8%)	0.82 (0.30, 2.23)	–
≥30	–	–	–	–	–	–	5/18 (27.8%)	1.54 (0.65, 3.63)	–
Anemia at ART Initiation									
None or mild	–	–	–	–	–	–	15/73 (20.6%)	**Reference**	–
Moderate or severe	–	–	–	–	–	–	16/80 (20.0%)	0.97 (0.52, 1.83)	–

would result in cost savings, and only after 20 years [29]. A compilation of a series of models [2] tested the impact of varying assumptions about linkage to care and showed that the rate of linkage impacts overall expected benefits and cost. In analyzing the impact that interventions to improve uptake and retention could have compared to simply extending eligibility, they found improvements to the care cascade were more beneficial than increasing eligibility alone.

Our study is one of the few where multiple stages of retention are traced within a single treatment site. A similar analysis was conducted by Kranzer [30], who found roughly 60% linkage from testing to staging and two-thirds of those ART eligible were initiated. A second, conducted by Clouse that looked at both pre- and post-ART retention found roughly 70% of patients testing positive linked to CD4 staging and 74% of those ART eligible initiated [16]'[31]. Our findings on pre-ART attrition also are similar to what was found in two systematic reviews which found 59%–72% of patients testing positive linking to care and 62%–68% of ART eligible patients initiated treatment. Our findings are similar to these overall but with higher rates of initiation among those ART eligible and somewhat lower rates of linkage to pre-ART care of those testing HIV positive. These findings demonstrate that particularly in the pre-ART period, attrition is poor. Our finding of retention on ART at two years is somewhat higher, but in the range of findings from two systematic reviews of retention, which suggest two year retention at about 70% [17,18,32].

Taken together these findings suggest that test-and-treat programs must focus on retention, particularly in the pre-ART period in order to reduce morbidity, mortality and transmission. While we found good retention in the post-ART period, this study does not tell us whether in a test-and-treat strategy, pre-ART attrition will shift to the post-ART period or whether such strategies will reduce cascade-wide attrition. Future efforts to implement these strategies must pay close attention to this issue and measure progress over time.

Our study has several limitations that could impact the interpretation of our results. First, because we did not follow a large number of patients from testing through long-term treatment it is not clear whether it is appropriate to combine the three observed estimates of retention to summarize total retention. If patients who complete one stage differ from those we enrolled at the next stage, we may over or under estimate total attrition. Further, if patients leave one stage of care but return again at a later time point, we likely overestimate attrition, and as such our estimates should be considered estimates of timely stage completion. Second, as most subjects who entered pre-ART care were not eligible for ART, we cannot estimate retention in this stage of care. This would likely underestimate total attrition across pre-ART care. Third, our study was conducted at a treatment site with testing onsite. It is not clear whether the linkage rates we observed would be as high if the site was a standalone testing site where patients then had to link to a new site for care. Fourth, because our study relied on clinic record linkage to determine stage completion, patients who returned for care but did not have their records located would appear as patients who did not return when in fact they did. This would also likely overestimate attrition. Fifth, we excluded 34 pre-ART patients due to lack of a CD4 count as we could not assess whether or not they completed the stage under our definitions because we did not know if they were ART eligible. If these patients differed from the patients who did have a CD4 count, our results could be biased. Finally, South Africa does not use a national identification number for care. While we did collect this information, because not all clinics routinely use or collect this identifier, and because there are so many options for care in South Africa, we could not tell if patients who left care presented for care at another site. Not being able to account for these "silent transfers" means that our estimates of attrition may be overestimates. On the other hand, if patients who transferred sites are more likely to be lost from care than those who remain at a single site, overall estimates of attrition may be underestimates.

In conclusion, we found that linkage from testing to pre-ART care was 39%, retention in pre-ART care was 88% and two-year on ART retention was 81%. Much of the pre-ART attrition was among patients with high CD4 counts. These findings suggest substantial attrition in the pre-ART period, higher than that used in many models of test-and-treat. Future revision of these models should include sensitivity analyses to gauge the impact of such assumptions on overall predicted benefits.

Acknowledgments

We express our gratitude to the directors and staff of the Themba Lethu Clinic (TLC) and to Right to Care, the NGO supporting the study site through a partnership with USAID. We also thank the Gauteng and National Department of Health for providing for the care of the patients at the TLC as part of the Comprehensive Care Management and Treatment plan. Most of all we thank the patients attending the clinic for their continued trust in the treatment provided at the clinic.

Author Contributions

Conceived and designed the experiments: MPF MM IS KS. Performed the experiments: MPF KS. Analyzed the data: MPF KS KC GMR. Contributed to the writing of the manuscript: MPF GMR KC IS KS MM.

References

1. Granich RM, Gilks CF, Dye C, De Cock KM, Williams BG (2009) Universal voluntary HIV testing with immediate antiretroviral therapy as a strategy for elimination of HIV transmission: a mathematical model. Lancet 373: 48–57.
2. Eaton JW, Johnson LF, Salomon JA, Bärnighausen T, Bendavid E, et al. (2012) HIV treatment as prevention: systematic comparison of mathematical models of the potential impact of antiretroviral therapy on HIV incidence in South Africa. PLoS Med 9: e1001245.
3. Walensky RP, Ross EL, Kumarasamy N, Wood R, Noubary F, et al. (2013) Cost-effectiveness of HIV treatment as prevention in serodiscordant couples. N Engl J Med 369: 1715–1725.
4. Bendavid E, Brandeau ML, Wood R, Owens DK (2010) Comparative effectiveness of HIV testing and treatment in highly endemic regions. Arch Intern Med 170: 1347–1354.
5. Bärnighausen T, Bloom DE, Humair S (2012) Economics of antiretroviral treatment vs. circumcision for HIV prevention. Proc Natl Acad Sci U S A 109: 21271–21276.
6. El-Sadr WM, Affrunti M, Gamble T, Zerbe A (2010) Antiretroviral therapy: a promising HIV prevention strategy? J Acquir Immune Defic Syndr 55 Suppl 2: S116–21.
7. Cohen MS, Mastro TD, Cates W (2009) Universal voluntary HIV testing and immediate antiretroviral therapy. Lancet 373: 1077; author reply 1080–1.
8. Montaner JSG, Hogg R, Wood E, Kerr T, Tyndall M, et al. (2006) The case for expanding access to highly active antiretroviral therapy to curb the growth of the HIV epidemic. Lancet 368: 531–536.
9. Hontelez JAC, Lurie MN, Bärnighausen T, Bakker R, Baltussen R, et al. (2013) Elimination of HIV in South Africa through expanded access to antiretroviral therapy: a model comparison study. PLoS Med 10: e1001534.
10. Hontelez JAC, de Vlas SJ, Tanser F, Bakker R, Bärnighausen T, et al. (2011) The impact of the new WHO antiretroviral treatment guidelines on HIV epidemic dynamics and cost in South Africa. PLoS One 6: e21919.
11. Cohen MS, Chen YQ, McCauley M, Gamble T, Hosseinipour MC, et al. (2011) Prevention of HIV-1 infection with early antiretroviral therapy. N Engl J Med 365: 493–505.
12. Montaner JSG, Lima VD, Barrios R, Yip B, Wood E, et al. (2010) Association of highly active antiretroviral therapy coverage, population viral load, and yearly new HIV diagnoses in British Columbia, Canada: a population-based study. Lancet 376: 532–539.

13. Das M, Chu PL, Santos G-M, Scheer S, Vittinghoff E, et al. (2010) Decreases in community viral load are accompanied by reductions in new HIV infections in San Francisco. PLoS One 5: e11068.
14. Donnell D, Baeten JM, Kiarie J, Thomas KK, Stevens W, et al. (2010) Heterosexual HIV-1 transmission after initiation of antiretroviral therapy: a prospective cohort analysis. Lancet 375: 2092–2098.
15. World Health Organization (2013) Antiretroviral therapy for HIV infection in adults and adolescents: Recommendations for a public health approach 2013 revisions. Geneva.
16. Rosen S, Fox MP (2011) Retention in HIV care between testing and treatment in sub-Saharan Africa: a systematic review. PLoS Med 8: e1001056.
17. Rosen S, Fox MP, Gill CJ (2007) Patient retention in antiretroviral therapy programs in sub-Saharan Africa: a systematic review. PLoS Med 4: e298.
18. Fox MP, Rosen S (2010) Patient retention in antiretroviral therapy programs up to three years on treatment in sub-Saharan Africa, 2007–2009: systematic review. Trop Med Int Heal 15 Suppl 1: 1–15.
19. Fox M, Maskew M, MacPhail A (2013) Cohort Profile: The Themba Lethu Clinical Cohort, Johannesburg, South Africa. Int J Epidemiol 42: 430–439.
20. Fox M, Shearer K, Maskew M, Macleod W, Majuba P, et al. (2012) Treatment outcomes after 7 years of public-sector HIV treatment. AIDS 26: 1823–1828.
21. National Department of Health SA (2004) National antiretroviral treatment guidelines, first edition. Pretoria, South Africa.
22. National Department of Health South Africa (2010) Clinical Guidelines for the Managment of HIV & AIDS in Adults and Adolescents. South Africa.
23. Fox MP, Larson B, Rosen S (2012) Defining retention and attrition in pre-antiretroviral HIV care: proposals based on experience in Africa. Trop Med Int Health 17: 1235–1244.
24. Severe P, Juste MAJ, Ambroise A, Eliacin L, Marchand C, et al. (2010) Early versus standard antiretroviral therapy for HIV-infected adults in Haiti. N Engl J Med 363: 257–265.
25. Fox MP, Sanne IM, Conradie F, Zeinecker J, Orrell C, et al. (2010) Initiating patients on antiretroviral therapy at CD4 cell counts above 200 cells/microl is associated with improved treatment outcomes in South Africa. AIDS 24: 2041–2050.
26. Cain LE, Logan R, Robins JM, Sterne JAC, Sabin C, et al. (2011) When to initiate combined antiretroviral therapy to reduce mortality and AIDS-defining illness in HIV-infected persons in developed countries: an observational study. Ann Intern Med 154: 509–515.
27. Kitahata MM, Gange SJ, Abraham AG, Merriman B, Saag MS, et al. (2009) Effect of early versus deferred antiretroviral therapy for HIV on survival. N Engl J Med 360: 1815–1826.
28. Govindasamy D, van Schaik N, Kranzer K, Wood R, Mathews C, et al. (2011) Linkage to HIV Care from a Mobile Testing Unit in South Africa by Different CD4 Count Strata. J Acquir Immune Defic Syndr 58: 344–352.
29. Klein DJ, Bershteyn A, Eckhoff PA (2014) Dropout and re-enrollment: implications for epidemiological projections of treatment programs. AIDS 28 Suppl 1: S47–59.
30. Kranzer K, Zeinecker J, Ginsberg P, Orrell C, Kalawe NN, et al. (2010) Linkage to HIV care and antiretroviral therapy in Cape Town, South Africa. PLoS One 5: e13801.
31. Kranzer K, Govindasamy D, Ford N, Johnston V, Lawn SD (2012) Quantifying and addressing losses along the continuum of care for people living with HIV infection in sub-Saharan Africa: a systematic review. J Int AIDS Soc 15: 17383.
32. Mugglin C, Estill J, Wandeler G, Bender N, Egger M, et al. (2012) Loss to programme between HIV diagnosis and initiation of antiretroviral therapy in sub-Saharan Africa: systematic review and meta-analysis. Trop Med Int Health 17: 1509–1520.

11

Phosphodiesterase 8a Supports HIV-1 Replication in Macrophages at the Level of Reverse Transcription

Thijs Booiman, Viviana Cobos Jiménez, Karel A. van Dort, Angélique B. van 't Wout[¤], Neeltje A. Kootstra*

Department of Experimental Immunology, Sanquin Research, Landsteiner Laboratory and Center for Infection and Immunity (CINIMA) at the Academic Medical Center of the University of Amsterdam, Amsterdam, The Netherlands

Abstract

Background: HIV-1 infected macrophages play a key role in HIV-1 infection. Even during anti-retroviral treatment, macrophages keep producing virus due to suboptimal tissue penetration and reduced efficacy of antiretrovirals. It is therefore of major importance to understand which host factors are involved in HIV-1 replication in macrophages. Previously, we have shown that genetic polymorphisms in phosphodiesterase 8a (PDE8A) are strongly associated with HIV-1 replication in these cells. Here we analyzed the mechanism and regulation of PDE8A in HIV-1 replication in macrophages.

Results: PDE8A mRNA expression strongly increases upon differentiation of monocytes into macrophages, which corresponds to the increased susceptibility of mature macrophages to HIV-1. In parallel, expression of microRNA miR-145-5p, predicted to target PDE8A mRNA, strongly decreased. The interaction of miR-145-5p with the 3′ UTR of PDE8A mRNA could be experimentally validated, suggesting that indeed miR-145-5p can regulate PDE8A expression levels. Knockdown of PDE8A in macrophages resulted in a decrease in total HIV-1 replication and proviral DNA levels. These observations confirm that PDE8A regulates HIV-1 replication in macrophages and that this effect is mediated through early steps in the viral replication cycle.

Conclusions: PDE8A is highly expressed in macrophages, and its expression is regulated by miR-145-5p. Our findings strongly suggest that PDE8A supports HIV-1 replication in macrophages and that this effect is mediated at the level of reverse transcription.

Editor: Massimo Caputi, Florida Atlantic University, United States of America

Funding: This work was supported by the Academic Medical Center of the University of Amsterdam and the Landsteiner Foundation of Blood Research (registration number 0526). The funders had no role in study design, data collection and analysis, decision to publish, or preparation of the manuscript.

Competing Interests: The authors have declared that no competing interests exist.

* Email: n.a.kootstra@amc.uva.nl

¤ Current address: Crucell Holland B. V., Leiden, The Netherlands

Introduction

Macrophages play a key role in HIV-1 infection. They are among the first cells that encounter HIV-1 upon transmission and once infected they facilitate spread of the virus to CD4+ T-cells [1–7]. Infected macrophages are relatively resistant to HIV-1 induced apoptosis and can efficiently evade host immunity [8,9]. Due to the ability of these cells to migrate into the tissue, the virus is disseminated throughout the body [10–14]. The introduction of combined antiretroviral therapy (cART) has reversed the fatal outcome of HIV-1 infection. Nonetheless, infected macrophages remain a source of residual virus production during treatment due to the low efficacy of cART, combined with the suboptimal tissue penetration of the drugs [10–15]. In addition to their contribution to the viral reservoir, HIV-1 infected macrophages play a crucial role in several AIDS related pathologies such as HIV-1 associated dementia, AIDS-related non-Hodgkin lymphoma and cardiovascular diseases [16–19]. It is therefore of major importance to specifically target HIV-1 replication in macrophages. *In vitro*, freshly isolated monocytes are almost refractory to HIV-1 infection and become permissive during differentiation into macrophages [20–23]. The differential susceptibility of monocytes and macrophages to HIV-1 is at least in part regulated by host factors [24–29]. Previously, we identified several host-genetic factors that were strongly associated with *in vitro* HIV-1 replication in macrophages [30,31]. We observed that four SNPs in the phosphodiesterase 8A (*PDE8A*) gene were highly associated with HIV-1 replication [31]. This suggests that PDE8A plays an important role in HIV-1 replication in macrophages. Indeed, a recent RNAi screen identified PDE8A as a HIV-1 dependency factor [32]. PDE8A is a phosphodiesterase that hydrolyzes cyclic adenosine monophosphate (cAMP) to AMP [33]. Several studies indeed have shown a role for cAMP in HIV-1 infection and it was demonstrated that cAMP can affect several steps of the viral replication cycle ranging from entry to proviral transcription [34].

Here we analyzed the regulation of *PDE8A* expression during monocyte differentiation and cytokine polarization. Furthermore, we investigated the effect of PDE8A knockdown on HIV-1 replication.

Results

PDE8A expression during differentiation and polarization of macrophages

Previously, we showed that genetic polymorphisms in the *PDE8A* gene are strongly associated with HIV-1 replication in macrophages [30,31]. *In vitro*, monocytes become highly susceptible to HIV-1 after differentiation into macrophages [20–23]. To determine whether PDE8A plays a role in the differential susceptibility of macrophages during differentiation, *PDE8A* mRNA expression was analyzed in freshly isolated monocytes and macrophages derived from 31 healthy blood donors. We observed on average a 70-fold increase in *PDE8A* expression upon differentiation of monocytes into macrophages, which suggests that PDE8A may be one of the factors that support the increased HIV-1 susceptibility of macrophages during differentiation (Figure 1A).

HIV-1 replication is strongly inhibited in macrophages stimulated with IFN-α, IFN-β, IFN-γ, IL-4, and IL-10 [22,24,35–41]. We analyzed whether differential expression of PDE8A during cytokine activation of macrophages may contribute to the decreased susceptibility of these cells to HIV-1 infection. Again, *PDE8A* mRNA expression increased during differentiation of monocytes into 5-day old macrophages (Figure 1B). Differentiation of monocytes in the presence of IFN-α, IFN-β, IFN-γ, or IL-10 did not change *PDE8A* expression, whereas the addition of IL-4 increased *PDE8A* expression (Figure 1B). This indicates that the restriction of HIV-1 replication observed in cytokine stimulated macrophages is not mediated by differential regulation of PDE8A expression.

PDE8A expression is regulated by miR-145-5p during differentiation of macrophages

miRNAs are known to play a key role in post-transcriptional regulation of gene expression and recently it was observed that miRNAs are differentially expressed during maturation of monocytes and polarization of macrophages by cytokines [42,43]. Therefore, we studied whether PDE8A expression is regulated by miRNAs during macrophage differentiation. miRNAs that target *PDE8A* mRNA were selected from miRNA-mRNA interactions that have been predicted and reported in the Ingenuity Knowledge Base, TarBase and miRecords and TargetScan [44–46]. Potential miRNAs regulating PDE8A expression were identified by pairing gene and miRNA expression data from monocytes and macrophages cultured for 5 days [43,47]. Of the 190 miRNAs that potentially could target *PDE8A*, we found that miR-145-5p, miR-577 and miR-1280 were significantly downregulated in 5-day cultured macrophages as compared to monocytes, while *PDE8A* expression was upregulated (Table 1). To confirm these results, we determined *PDE8A* and miRNA expression during differentiation of monocytes into macrophages in 8 additional donors. *PDE8A* expression increased significantly during the first day of differentiation and this effect was maintained during differentiation (Figure 2A). In contrast, expression of miR-145-5p decreased significantly during the first day of differentiation and miR-145-5p remained low during subsequent differentiation (Figure 2B). Expression of miR-577 could not be confirmed by qPCR, whereas down-regulation of expression of miR-1280 was not observed (data not shown). miR-145-5p is predicted to target the 3′UTR of the *PDE8A* mRNA transcript (Figure 2C). To confirm whether miR-145-5p can regulate PDE8A expression, we constructed a miR-145-5p overexpression vector and a luciferase reporter vector in which the 3′UTR of the *PDE8A* mRNA transcript was cloned into the 3′UTR of the luciferase gene. First, HEK293T cells were transfected with different concentrations of the miR-145-5p vector and miR-145-5p expression levels were analyzed 2 days after transfection by qPCR. We observed a dose dependent increase of miR-145-5p expression as compared to the empty vector control (Figure 2D). Next, we performed co-transfections of the miR-145-5p overexpression vector and the luciferase reporter vector containing the predicted miR-145-5p target sequence. We observed that miR-145-5p is able to down regulate luciferase activity in a dose dependent manner (Figure 2E). This suggests that miR-145-5p is indeed able to target the 3′UTR of *PDE8A* mRNA thereby regulating protein expression levels.

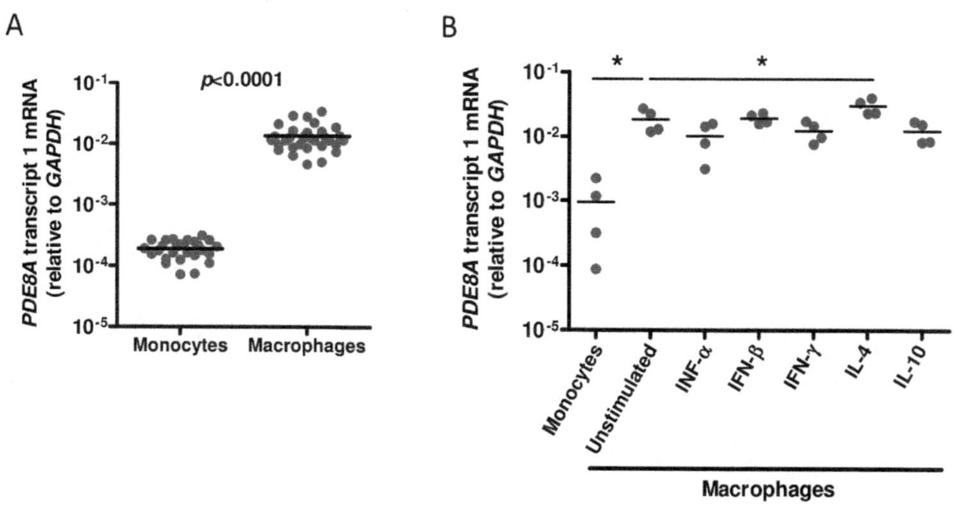

Figure 1. PDE8A expression during macrophage differentiation and polarisation. (A) *PDE8A* mRNA expression in freshly isolated monocytes and macrophages cultured for 7 days from 32 donors. (B) *PDE8A* mRNA expression in freshly isolated monocytes and macrophages from 4 donors cultured in the absence or presence of IFN-α (250 U/ml), IFN-β (250 U/ml), IFN-γ (2501U/ml), IL-4 (10 ng/ml), or IL-10 (100 U/ml) for 7 days. Statistical differences were analyzed using a paired T test: *p<0.05, **p<0.01, ***p<0.001.

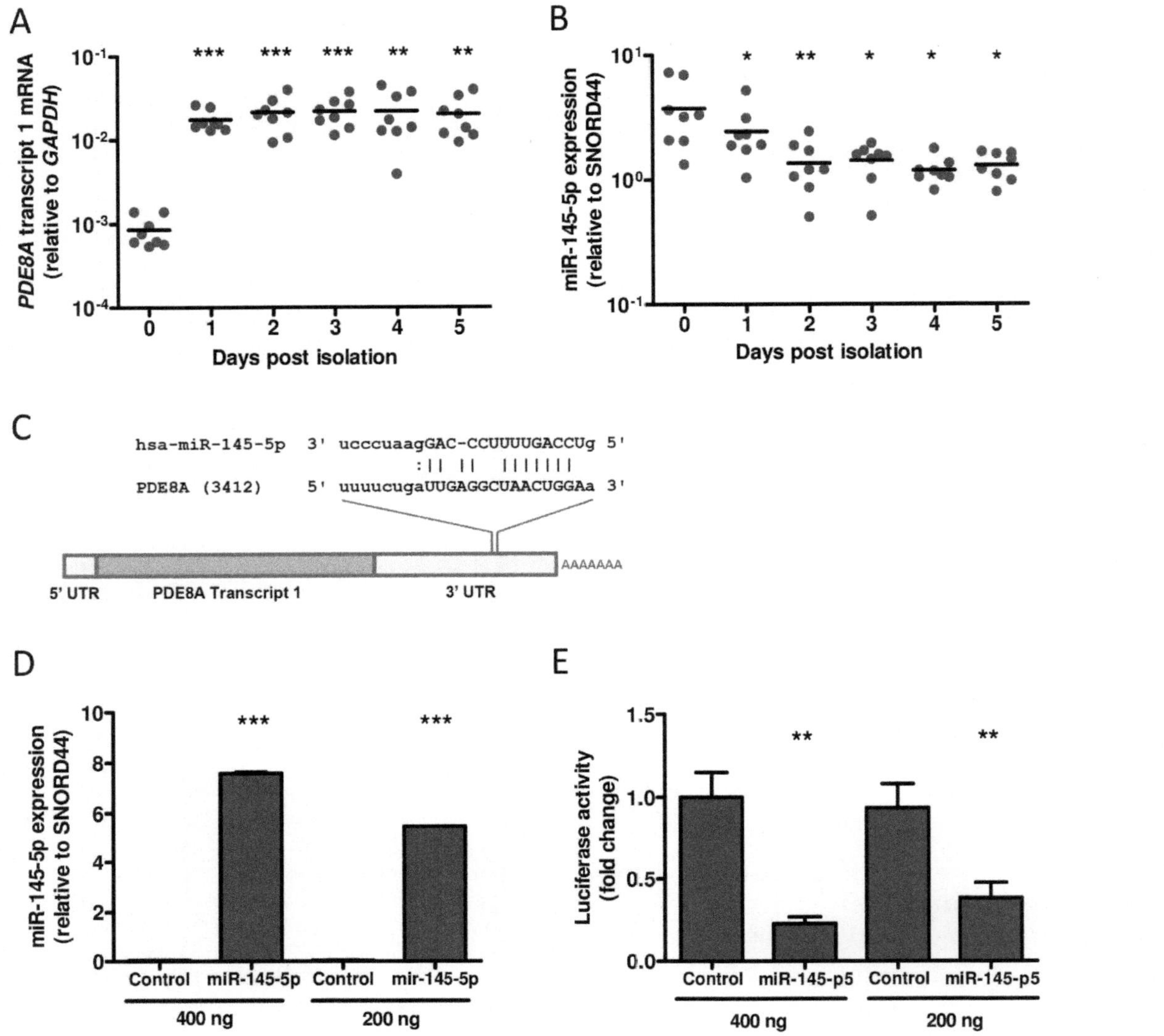

Figure 2. Regulation of PDE8A expression by miR-145-5p during differentiation of monocytes into macrophages. Confirmation of *PDE8A* mRNA (A) and miR-145-5p (B) expression during differentiation of monocytes into macrophages obtained from 8 donors. *PDE8A* mRNA or miR-145-5p expression during differentiation was compared with the expression at day 0 by using a paired T test: *$p<0.05$, **$p<0.01$, ***$p<0.001$. (C) Schematic overview of the *PDE8A* mRNA transcript 1 including the miR-145-5p binding site between base pair 3412 and 3435. (D) Expression levels of miR-145-5p determined by qPCR in HEK293T cells 2 days after transfection with an empty vector control or a vector containing a miR-145-5p expression cassette (n = 2, mean and SD). (E) Direct interaction between miR-145-5p and its target sequence in the *PDE8A* mRNA transcript was tested by co-transfection of p-hEF1a-miR-145-5p or an empty vector control and p-hEF1a-Luc-3'UTR PDE8A. Luciferase activity was measured 2 days post-transfection (n = 3, mean and SD). Statistical differences were analyzed using an un-paired T test: *$p<0.05$, **$p<0.01$, ***$p<0.001$.

Table 1. Potential miRNAs targeting PDE8A.

miRNA ID	Fold Change miRNA Day 5 vs Day 0 #	Source	Confidence	Gene Symbol	Fold Change mRNA Day 5 vs Day 0 #
hsa-miR-145-5p	0.102	TargetScan Human	High (predicted)	PDE8A	2.794
hsa-miR-1280	0.098	TargetScan Human	High (predicted)	PDE8A	2.794
hsa-miR-577	0.128	TargetScan Human	High (predicted)	PDE8A	2.794

#Fold change in expression in which day 5 is compared to day 0; >1 is an increase and <1 is a decrease in expression.

PDE8A affects HIV-1 replication at the level of reverse transcription

To determine which step of the replication cycle is affected by PDE8A we overexpressed a myc-tagged PDE8A in HEK293T cells and infected these cells with a VSV-G/NL4-3.Luc reporter virus. Overexpression of PDE8A resulted in a dose-dependent increase in luciferase activity (Figure 3A and 3B). This finding confirms our previous results and indicates that PDE8A supports HIV-1 replication. Next, we analyzed the effect of PDE8A overexpression on early steps of the viral replication cycle by analysis of proviral DNA levels during 48-hours post infection. HEK293T cells overexpressing PDE8A showed a dose dependent increase in *Pol* proviral DNA at 48-hours post infection (Figure 3C). The effect of PDE8A on *Pol* proviral DNA levels was already mediated within the first 24-hours post infection, whereas levels of strong stop proviral DNA as determined by *R/U5* qPCR were not affected (Figure 3D). Furthermore, PDE8A overexpression resulted in increased levels of integrated HIV-1 provirus as determined by Alu-PCR (Figure 3E). This indicates that PDE8A supports HIV-1 replication at the level of reverse transcription.

PDE8A supports HIV-1 replication in monocyte-derived macrophages

To determine the role of PDE8A in HIV-1 replication in macrophages, we analyzed the effect of PDE8A knockdown by shRNAs on the HIV-1 replication cycle in these cells. We selected two lentiviral vectors that were able to knockdown PDE8A expression (Figure S1A). Macrophages were transduced with the lentiviral vectors expressing either the shRNAs targeting PDE8A or a control shRNA which reduced *PDE8A* mRNA in most donors (Figure S1B). Subsequent infection with a VSV-G/NL-4-3.Luc reporter virus, resulted in a significant decrease in luciferase activity in the PDE8A knockdown cells (Figure 4A), demonstrating that HIV-1 replication in macrophages is supported by PDE8A. Next, the effect of PDE8A on proviral DNA synthesis was analyzed in macrophages. Knockdown of PDE8A expression resulted in a decrease in *Pol* proviral DNA levels at 48-hours post-infection (Figure 4B and 4C). This further confirms that PDE8A supports HIV-1 replication in macrophages and that this effect is mediated at the level of reverse transcription.

Discussion

The HIV-1 genome encodes only 15 proteins and therefore HIV-1 is heavily dependent on host proteins for its replication. Host cell proteins that are required for efficient replication of HIV-1 in macrophages are attractive targets for new therapeutic approaches and therefore it is crucial to better understand the interaction between HIV-1 and these host factors. In our previous work, we have identified polymorphisms in PDE8A that are strongly associated with PDE8A expression and *in vitro* HIV-1 replication in macrophages [30,31]. Here, we showed that *PDE8A* expression is highly upregulated during differentiation of monocytes into macrophages and that miR-145-5p may be involved in the regulation of PDE8A expression during differentiation. We demonstrated that PDE8A supports HIV-1 replication in macrophages and that this effect is mediated at the level of reverse transcription. These data suggest that PDE8A plays an important role in HIV-1 susceptibility of macrophages during differentiation [20–23].

PDE8A is a phosphodiesterase that regulates cAMP levels by hydrolyzing cAMP to AMP [33]. In the context of HIV-1 infection cAMP has been described as having opposing effects on the different steps of the viral replication cycle, which seems to be partially cell type dependent (reviewed by [34]). Here we show that increasing PDE8A expression levels are associated with higher concentrations of HIV-1 proviral DNA and subsequent higher levels of integrated HIV-1 provirus. This suggests that PDE8A supports HIV-1 replication at the level of reverse transcription. The increased proviral DNA synthesis in macrophages may be the result of low cAMP levels mediated by high PDE8A expression levels. Indeed, Thivierge *et al.* and Hayes *et al.* have shown that high cAMP levels decrease viral replication in macrophages [48,49]. Thivierge *et al.* attributed this effect to decreased expression of co-receptor CCR5 in cells with high cAMP levels [48], however they did not determine the effect of cAMP on the different steps in viral replication and only analyzed virus production in the culture supernatant. Here we used a VSV-G pseudotyped reporter virus to circumvent CD4 and CCR5 mediated entry and demonstrated that PDE8A affects HIV-1 replication independent of CCR5 expression levels. Hayes *et al.* demonstrated that high cAMP levels decreased HIV-1 mRNA expression and viral replication in macrophages, but this may have been the result of decreased proviral DNA synthesis as the effect of high cAMP levels on proviral DNA synthesis was not determined in this study [49].

PDE8 isoforms exhibit an extremely high affinity for cAMP and it is therefore suggested that PDE8 enzymes have an important role in protecting any associated protein from fluctuations in basal cAMP concentrations [50]. Besides the direct effect of PDE8A on total cellular cAMP levels, it is also possible that PDE8A affects the replication cycle via a binding partner like RAF-1. It has been demonstrated that RAF-1 plays a role in HIV-1 infection in dendritic cells, and that it is required for the induction of proviral transcription [51]. PDE8A associates with RAF-1 and prevents its inactivation by phosphorylation by protein kinase A (PKA) [52]. However, we observed that knockdown of RAF-1 did not affect the ability of PDE8A to support HIV-1 replication (data not shown). This indicates that the effect of PDE8A on HIV-1 replication described here is not mediated through RAF-1.

Conclusions

Here we demonstrated that PDE8A supports HIV-1 replication in macrophages at the level of reverse transcription. PDE8A is highly expressed in macrophages and can be regulated by miR-145-5p during differentiation. Macrophages are considered to be a source of residual viral replication even under cART. Since PDE enzymes are considered promising targets for pharmacological intervention [53–56], blocking of PDE8A may specifically interfere with HIV-1 replication in primary macrophages.

Methods

Ethics statement

This study has been conducted in accordance with the ethical principles set out in the declaration of Helsinki, and was approved by the Medical Ethics Committee of the Academic Medical Center and the Ethics Advisory Body of the Sanquin Blood Supply Foundation in Amsterdam, The Netherlands. Written informed consent was obtained from all participants.

Cell culture

Peripheral blood mononuclear cells (PBMC) were obtained from buffy coats from healthy blood donors. PBMC were isolated by Ficoll-Isopaque density gradient centrifugation and subsequently monocytes were isolated by magnetic-activated bead

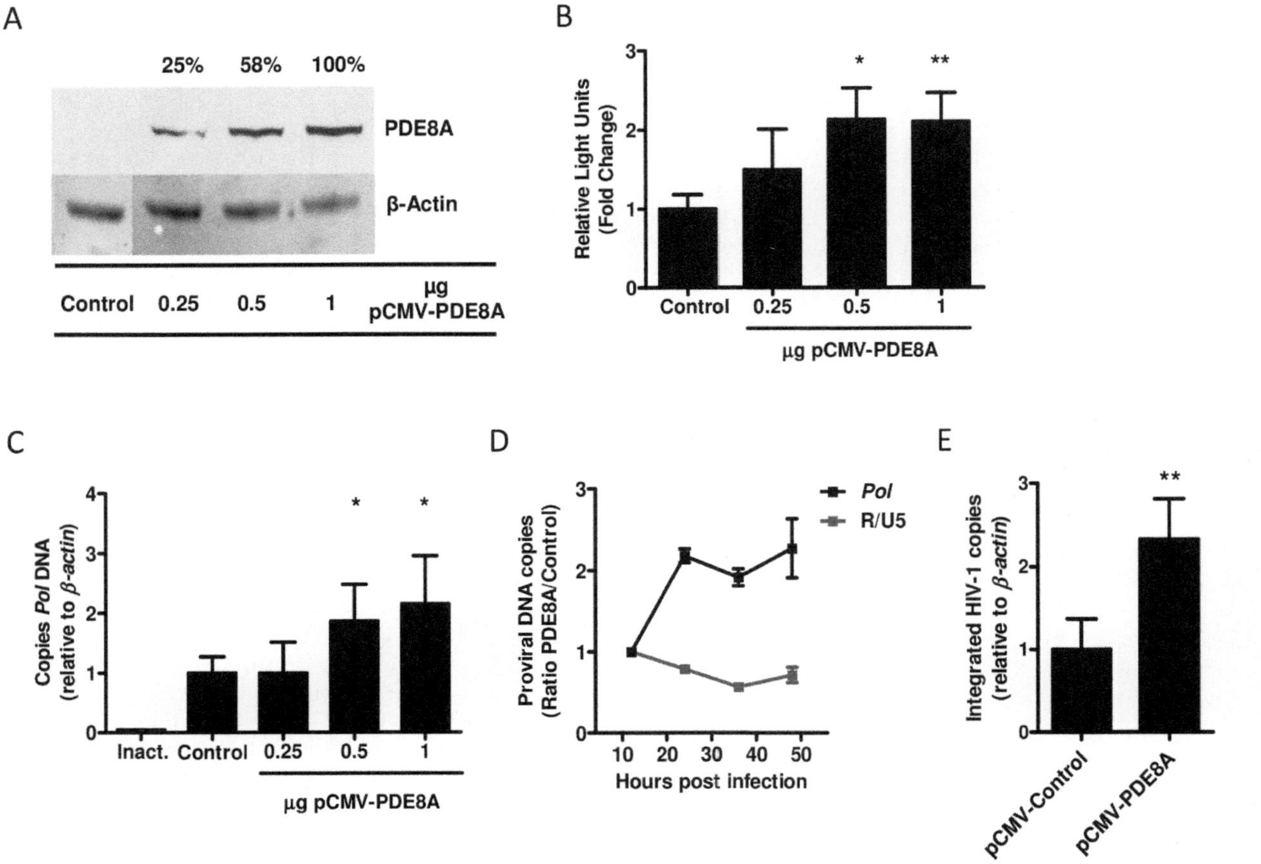

Figure 3. PDE8A supports HIV-1 replication at the level of reverse transcription. (A) HEK293T cells were transfected with different concentrations of pCMV6-PDE8A or an empty vector control. PDE8A expression was analyzed forty-eight hours after transfection by western blot. (B) HEK293T cells were transfected with different concentrations of pCMV6-PDE8A or an empty vector control and infected with VSV-G/NL4-3.Luc 48 hours after transfection. Luciferase activity was measured 2 days after infection (n = 3, mean and SD). (C) HEK293T cells were transfected with different concentrations of pCMV6-PDE8A or an empty vector control and infected with VSV-G/NL4-3-Ba-L 48 hours after transfection. Proviral DNA levels were analyzed forty-eight hours after infection by qPCR. Proviral DNA levels are expressed relative to the control after correction for β-actin levels in the same sample (n = 3, mean and SD). (D) HEK293T cells were transfected with 1 μg of pCMV6-PDE8A or 1 μg of empty vector control and infected with VSV-G/NL4-3-Ba-L 48 hours after transfection. *R/U5* and *Pol* proviral DNA levels were analyzed by qPCR during 48 hours post-infection. *R/U5* and *Pol* levels are expressed as the ratio of the expression in cells transfected with pCMV-PDE8A divided by the expression in cells that were transfected with the empty vector control and corrected for β-actin levels (n = 2, mean and SD). (E) HEK293T cells were transfected with 1 μg of pCMV6-PDE8A or 1 μg of the empty vector control and infected with VSV-G/NL4-3-Ba-L 48 hours after transfection. Integrated HIV-1 copies were determined 48 hours post infection by Alu-PCR and expressed relative to the control after correction for β-actin levels in the same sample (n = 2, mean and SD). Statistical differences were analyzed using an un-paired T test: *p<0.05, **p<0.01, ***p<0.001.

technology using CD14+ magnetic microbeads (Miltenyi Biotec, Bergisch Gladbach, Germany). Monocytes were differentiated in Iscove's modified Dulbecco medium (IMDM) supplemented with 10% (v/v) heat-inactivated human pool serum (HPS), penicillin (100 U/ml), streptomycin (100 μg/ml) and cyproxin (5 μg/ml) in the presents or absence of IFN-α (250 U/ml), IFN-β (250 U/ml), IFN-γ (250 U/ml), IL-4 (10 ng/ml), or IL-10 (100 U/ml) and maintained in a humidified 10% CO_2 incubator at 37°C. HEK293T cells were cultured in Dulbecco's Modified Eagle Medium without Hepes (DMEM) (Lonza, Basel, Switzerland) supplemented with 10% (v/v) inactivated fetal calf serum (FCS), penicillin (100 U/ml) and streptomycin (100 μg/ml), and maintained in a humidified 10% CO_2 incubator at 37°C [57].

Plasmids

For PDE8A overexpression and testing knockdown efficiency of the shRNAs targeting PDE8A, a vector expressing a MYC-tagged PDE8A under the control of the CMV promotor (Origene, Rockville, MD, USA) was used. The vector containing the miR-145-5p overexpression cassette was created by cloning the stem-loop sequence of human miR-145-5p (miRBase accession number MI0000461) including approximately 100 base pairs up- and down-stream of the stem-loop in a HIV-1 based lentiviral expression vector pLV-hEF1a in which expression is driven by the human Elongation Factor 1 alpha promotor (p-LV-hEF1a-miR-145-5p) [58,59]. The luciferase reporter vector containing the 3′UTR of the PDE8A mRNA transcript, which is targeted by miR-145-5p was constructed as follows: The miR-145-5p target sequence from 3′UTR of the PDE8A mRNA transcript, including flanking regions of 40 base pairs, was cloned into the 3′UTR sequence of a luciferase reporter gene in a pLV-pHEF1a-Luciferase vector in which expression is driven by the human Elongation Factor 1 alpha promotor (p-hEF1a-Luc-3′UTR PDE8A) [58,59]. Primers used for cloning are listed in Table S1.

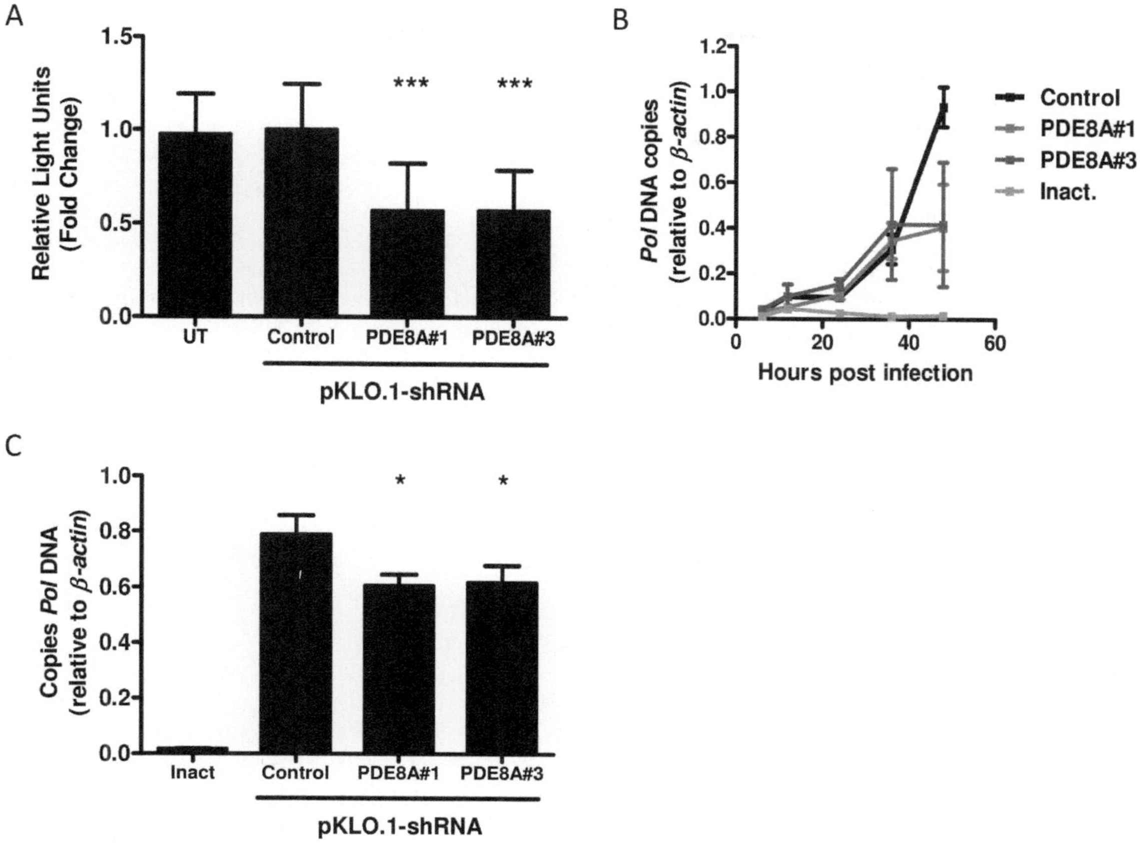

Figure 4. The effect of PDE8A knockdown on HIV-1 replication in macrophages. (A) To analyze the effect of PDE8A knockdown on HIV-1 replication in macrophages, monocytes from 4 donors were cultured for 5 days and transduced with lentiviral vectors expressing shRNA control or two shRNA's targeting PDE8A. Forty-eight hours after the lentiviral transduction, macrophages were infected with VSV-G/NL4-3.Luc and luciferase activity was measured at day 2 after infection. The results are given as the mean fold luciferase expression from 4 donors, relative to the medium control. UT: Untransduced control. Statistical differences were analyzed by mixed linear model, repeated covariance: diagonal (IBM SPSS Statistics 20). (B) To determine the effect of PDE8A knockdown on *Pol* proviral DNA levels, monocytes in which PDE8A was downregulated by lentiviral transduction were infected with VSV-G/NL4-3-Ba-L. *Pol* proviral DNA levels were analyzed by qPCR during 48 hours post-infection and expressed relative to β-actin. Results are given as mean and sd from 2 donors. (C) Monocytes in which PDE8A was downregulated by lentiviral transduction were infected with VSV-G/NL4-3-Ba-L. Two days post-infection, proviral DNA levels were analyzed by qPCR for *Pol*. Proviral DNA levels are expressed relative to the control after correction to β-actin for input. Results shown are representative for 3 donors. Inact.: Inactivated virus. Statistical differences were analyzed using a paired T test: *$p<0.05$, **$p<0.01$, ***$p<0.001$.

Virus production

YU2 and VSV-G pseudotyped NL4-3.Luc.R-E- luciferase reporter virus were produced by transfection of respectively pYU2 or pNL4-3.Luc.R-E- with pCMV-VSV-G in HEK293T cells. Lentiviral vectors were produced by co-transfection of pLV-CMV-GFP [58,59] or pLKO.1 constructs expressing shRNA candidates from the MISSION TRC-Hs 1.0 library (PDE8A TRCN48874, PDE8A TRCN48876 and control SHC001; Sigma-Aldrich St. Louis, MO, USA) [60] and pCMV-VSV-G, pMDLgp and pRSV-Rev in HEK293T cells [61]. Transfections were performed with the calcium phosphate method. In short, plasmid DNA was diluted in 0.042M HEPES containing 0.15M $CaCl_2$, subsequently mixed with an equal volume of 2× HEPES buffered saline pH 7.2, incubated at room temperature for 15 min and added to the culture medium. After 24 h incubation in a humidified 3% CO_2 incubator at 37°C, the culture medium was replaced and cultures were continued at 10% CO_2 at 37°C. Virus was harvested at 48 and 72 h after transfection and passed through a 0.22 μm filter. HIV-1 virus titers were quantified by determining the TCID50 on TZMBL, HEK293T or U87 cells [62]. Lentiviral vector supernatant was concentrated by centrifugation at 50,000xg for 2 hours directly after harvesting. Equal amounts of lentiviral vector as determined by p24 ELISA were used to inoculate target cells.

Infection of 293T cells

Cells were transfected as described previously with pCMV6-PDE8A [31]. Twenty-four hours post transfection cells were detached using trypsin (Invitrogen, Carlsbad, CA) and seeded in 24-wells plates to determine proviral DNA levels and in 96-wells plates to determine total HIV-1 replication. To determine proviral DNA levels, cells were inoculated at a multiplicity of infection (MOI) of 0.01 with VSV-G pseudotyped NL4-3-B-aL which was treated with DNAse (200 ng/ml) (RQ1; Promega Corp., Madison WI, USA) for 45 min at 37°C in medium containing 6 mM $MgCl_2$. As a control, a heat-inactivated (30 min; 56 C) inoculum was used. During 48-hours hours post infection, total DNA was isolated using the L6 method [63]. Proviral DNA was measured by qPCR using primers and probes detecting *R/U5* or *Pol* products (Table S1). To determine the effect of PDE8A on total HIV-1 replication, cells were inoculated at an MOI of 0.01 with VSV-G pseudotyped NL4-3.Luc.R-E- luciferase reporter virus. Forty-eight hours post infection, luciferase activity was determined as a measure for HIV-1 replication, by adding 25 μl substrate (0.83 mM ATP, 0.83 mM D-luciferin (Duchefa, Haarlem, The Netherlands), 18.7 mM $MgCl_2$, 0.78 μM $Na_2H_2P_2O_7$, 38.9 mM Tris pH 7.8, 0.39% (v/v) glycerol, 0.03% (v/v) Triton X-100, and 2.6 μM dithiothreitol) directly to the culture medium. Luminescence was measured for 1 s per well using a luminometer (Berthold, Bad Wildbad, Germany).

Lentiviral vector transduction and HIV-1 infection of primary cells

Monocytes were cultured for 5 days and transduced with lentiviral vectors expressing shRNA control or two shRNA's targeting PDE8A. Medium was replaced with IMDM without serum or antibiotics and two hours later, macrophages were inoculated with lentiviral vectors at a MOI of 10. Sixteen hours post transduction, medium was replaced with IMDM supplemented with 10% (v/v) heat-inactivated human pool serum (HPS), penicillin (100 U/ml), streptomycin (100 μg/ml) and cyproxin (5 μg/ml). Forty-eight hours post transduction, macrophages were infected with VSV-G pseudotyped luciferase reporter virus at a MOI of 0.2 to analyze total replication. In addition, macrophages were inoculated at a MOI of 0.012 with DNAse-treated YU2 to analyze the effect on proviral DNA levels. Forty-eight hours post transfection luciferase activity was measured as described above.

Nucleic acid isolation and quantitative PCR

Total RNA was extracted using the High Pure RNA Isolation kit (Roche, Basel, Switzerland) or TriPure Isolation Reagent (Roche). Reverse transcription of mRNA was performed using the Roche Transcriptor First Strand cDNA Synthesis kit (Roche) using a maximum of 1 μg total RNA and oligo(dT) primers. Reverse transcription of miRNAs was performed using the qScript microRNA cDNA synthesis kit (Quanta BioScineces Inc., Gaithersburg, MD). Resulting cDNA was used for quantitative PCR (qPCR) analysis using SYBR Green I Master or Probes Master (Roche) and target specific primers (Table S1). For quantification of miR-145-5p and SNORD44 control, specifically designed primers (Table S1) were used in combination with the PerfeCTa Universal PCR Primer, including the Human positive control (SNORD44) primers (Quanta BioSciences Inc.). Integrated HIV-1 DNA was measured by two-step Alu-PCR as described previously [51]. In short, during the first step Alu-LTR sequences were amplified with an HIV-1-specific primer (LTR R region) and a primer that anneals to the abundant genomic Alu repeats. The HIV-1-specific primer was extended with a marker region at the 5′ end, which was used for specificity in the second-round PCR. The second step consisted out of a nested quantitative real-time PCR in which PCR products from the first step were amplified with primers annealing to the aforementioned marker region and a HIV-1 specific primer (LTR U5 region) (Table S1). To account for the signal contributed by unintegrated HIV-1 DNA, the first-round PCR was also done with the HIV-1-specific primer alone as a control. HIV-1 integration was normalized relative to β-actin DNA. qPCRs were performed on a Lightcycler 480 II (Roche) and gene expression values were obtained using Roche's LightCycler relative quantification software (release 1.5.0).

Western blot analysis

The effect of PDE8A overexpression and subsequent knockdown by shRNAs on protein levels was analyzed by western blot. Two days post transfection, HEK293T cells were lysed in RIPA-buffer (150 mM NaCl, 1% Triton X-100, 0.5% sodium deoxycholate, 0.1% SDS, 50 mM Tris, pH 8.0) containing Complete EDTA free protease inhibitor (Roche). After adding NuPAGE LDS 4× sample buffer (Invitrogen) and 0.1 M DTT, samples were heated at 95°C for 10 min. The Odyssey Protein Weight Marker was used as a size reference (LI-COR, Lincoln, NE, USA). Proteins were separated by SDS-PAGE (NuPAGE 10% Bis-Tris precast gel and MES SDS running buffer (Invitrogen) and transferred to a nitrocellulose membrane (Protran, Schleicher & Schuell, Dassel, Germany) using NuPAGE transfer buffer. After blocking for 2 hours with PBS containing 5% Protifar (Nutricia, Schiphol, The Netherlands) and 0.5% bovine serum albumin, the blot was incubated with OP10L anti-c-Myc antibody to detect MYC-tagged PDE8A (1:5000; Calbiochem, San Diego, CA, USA), and SC-1616 anti-β-actin antibody (1:200; Santa Cruz Biotechnology, Santa Cruz, CA, USA) to detect β-actin. IRDye 800CW conjugated Goat anti-Mouse IgG (1:15000; 926-32210, LI-COR, Lincoln, NE, USA) and IRDye 680LT conjugated Donkey anti-Goat IgG (1:15000; 926–32224, LI-COR) were used as secondary antibodies to visualize expression using the Odyssey infrared image system (LI-COR). Image J software was used to quantify protein expression.

miRNA target selection

Selected microRNAs that were predicted to target PDE8A mRNA were identified with the microRNA Target Filter tool from IPA (Ingenuity Systems Inc., Redwood City, CA, USA). Expression of miRNAs in monocytes and macrophages was characterized by next-generation sequencing with the SOLiD system and qPCR, EMBL-EBI ArrayExpress public database (http://www.ebi.ac.uk/arrayexpress/) accession number: EMTAB-1969 [43]. miRNA expression from 1 donor was paired with the mean expression of PDE8A from 2 donors obtained from gene expression data in similar samples (GSE35495), SubSeries GSE49240 (samples GSM1195728–39), part of the SuperSeries GSE35495 [47]; miRNAs were selected if expression levels were lower in macrophages, compared to monocytes.

Statistical analysis

For statistical analysis the paired and unpaired T-test or the mixed linear model, repeated covariance: diagonal were used (IBM SPSS Statistics 20).

Supporting Information

Figure S1 (A) Western Blot analysis of HEK293T cells in which the efficiency of the lentiviral vectors containing shRNAs against an MYC-tagged PDE8A or a control shRNA was determined. (B) Efficiency of *PDE8A* mRNA downregulation was analyzed by transduction of macrophages with lentiviral vectors expressing shRNAs against *PDE8A* or a control shRNA. *PDE8A* mRNA expression was determined 2 days post-transduction by qPCR. Statistical differences were analyzed using a paired T test.

Acknowledgments

We are grateful to all blood donors from Sanquin Blood Bank for their participation in this study. Finally, we would like to thank Theo Geijtenbeek for critical reading of the manuscript.

Author Contributions

Conceived and designed the experiments: TB NAK. Performed the experiments: TB VCJ KVD. Analyzed the data: TB VCJ ABW NAK. Wrote the paper: TB VCJ NAK.

References

1. Carr JM, Hocking H, Li P, Burrell CJ (1999) Rapid and efficient cell-to-cell transmission of human immunodeficiency virus infection from monocyte-derived macrophages to peripheral blood lymphocytes. Virology 265: 319–329.
2. Gendelman HE, Orenstein JM, Martin MA, Ferrua C, Mitra R, et al. (1988) Efficient isolation and propagation of human immunodeficiency virus on recombinant colony-stimulating factor 1-treated monocytes. J Exp Med 167: 1428–1441.
3. Groot F, Welsch S, Sattentau QJ (2008) Efficient HIV-1 transmission from macrophages to T cells across transient virological synapses. Blood 111: 4660–4663.
4. Gupta P, Collins KB, Ratner D, Watkins S, Naus GJ, et al. (2002) Memory CD4(+) T cells are the earliest detectable human immunodeficiency virus type 1 (HIV-1)-infected cells in the female genital mucosal tissue during HIV-1 transmission in an organ culture system. J Virol 76: 9868–9876.
5. Ho DD, Rota TR, Schooley RT, Kaplan JC, Allan JD, et al. (1985) Isolation of HTLV-III from cerebrospinal fluid and neural tissues of patients with neurologic syndromes related to the acquired immunodeficiency syndrome. N Engl J Med 313: 1493–1497.
6. Mann DL, Gartner S, Le SF, Buchow H, Popovic M (1990) HIV-1 transmission and function of virus-infected monocytes/macrophages. J Immunol 144: 2152–2158.
7. Nicholson JKA, Cross GD, Callaway CS, McDougal JS (1986) In vitro infection of human monocytes with human T lymphotropic virus type III/lymphadenopathy-associated virus (HTLV-III/LAV). J Immunol 137: 323–329.
8. Olivetta E, Federico M (2006) HIV-1 Nef protects human-monocyte-derived macrophages from HIV-1-induced apoptosis. Exp Cell Res 312: 890–900.
9. Swingler S, Mann AM, Zhou J, Swingler C, Stevenson M (2007) Apoptotic killing of HIV-1-infected macrophages is subverted by the viral envelope glycoprotein. PLoS Pathog 3: 1281–1290.
10. Zhang H, Dornadula G, Beumont M, Livornese L Jr, Van UB, et al. (1998) Human immunodeficiency virus type 1 in the semen of men receiving highly active antiretroviral therapy. N Engl J Med 339: 1803–1809.
11. Poles MA, Boscardin WJ, Elliott J, Taing P, Fuerst MM, et al. (2006) Lack of decay of HIV-1 in gut-associated lymphoid tissue reservoirs in maximally suppressed individuals. J Acquir Immune Defic Syndr 43: 65–68.
12. Lambotte O, Chaix ML, Gasnault J, Goujard C, Lebras P, et al. (2005) Persistence of replication-competent HIV in the central nervous system despite long-term effective highly active antiretroviral therapy. AIDS 19: 217–218.
13. Guadalupe M, Sankaran S, George MD, Reay E, Verhoeven D, et al. (2006) Viral suppression and immune restoration in the gastrointestinal mucosa of human immunodeficiency virus type 1-infected patients initiating therapy during primary or chronic infection. J Virol 80: 8236–8247.
14. Chun TW, Nickle DC, Justement JS, Meyers JH, Roby G, et al. (2008) Persistence of HIV in gut-associated lymphoid tissue despite long-term antiretroviral therapy. J Infect Dis 197: 714–720.
15. Mayer KH, Boswell S, Goldstein R, Lo W, Xu C, et al. (1999) Persistence of human immunodeficiency virus in semen after adding indinavir to combination antiretroviral therapy. Clin Infect Dis 28: 1252–1259.
16. Crowe SM, Westhorpe CL, Mukhamedova N, Jaworowski A, Sviridov D, et al. (2010) The macrophage: the intersection between HIV infection and atherosclerosis. J Leukoc Biol 87: 589–598.
17. Gonzalez-Scarano F, Martin-Garcia J (2005) The neuropathogenesis of AIDS. Nat Rev Immunol 5: 69–81.
18. Hsue PY, Hunt PW, Schnell A, Kalapus SC, Hoh R, et al. (2009) Role of viral replication, antiretroviral therapy, and immunodeficiency in HIV-associated atherosclerosis. AIDS 23: 1059–1067.
19. Huysentruyt LC, McGrath MS (2010) The role of macrophages in the development and progression of AIDS-related non-Hodgkin lymphoma. J Leukoc Biol 87: 627–632.
20. Rich EA, Chen IS, Zack JA, Leonard ML, O'Brien WA (1992) Increased susceptibility of differentiated mononuclear phagocytes to productive infection with human immunodeficiency virus-1 (HIV-1). J Clin Invest 89: 176–183. doi: 10.1172/JCI115559.
21. Naif HM, Shan L, Alali M, Sloane A, Wu L, et al. (1998) CCR5 expression correlates with susceptibility of maturing monocytes to human immunodeficiency virus type 1 infection. J Virol 72: 830–836.
22. Schuitemaker H, Kootstra NA, Koppelman MH, Bruisten SM, Huisman HG, et al. (1992) Proliferation-dependent HIV-1 infection of monocytes occurs during differentiation into macrophages. J Clin Invest 89: 1154–1160.
23. Sonza S, Maerz A, Deacon N, Meanger J, Mills J, et al. (1996) Human immunodeficiency virus type 1 replication is blocked prior to reverse transcription and integration in freshly isolated peripheral blood monocytes. J Virol 70: 3863–3869.
24. Cobos Jiménez V, Booiman T, de Taeye SW, van Dort KA, Rits MA, et al. (2012) Differential expression of HIV-1 interfering factors in monocyte-derived macrophages stimulated with polarizing cytokines or interferons. Sci Rep 2: 763. doi: 10.1038/srep00763.
25. Hrecka K, Hao C, Gierszewska M, Swanson SK, Kesik-Brodacka M, et al. (2011) Vpx relieves inhibition of HIV-1 infection of macrophages mediated by the SAMHD1 protein. Nature 474: 658–661. doi: 10.1038/nature10195.
26. Lahouassa H, Daddacha W, Hofmann H, Ayinde D, Logue EC, et al. (2012) SAMHD1 restricts the replication of human immunodeficiency virus type 1 by depleting the intracellular pool of deoxynucleoside triphosphates. Nat Immunol 13: 223–228. doi: 10.1038/ni.2236.
27. Goldstone DC, Ennis-Adeniran V, Hedden JJ, Groom HC, Rice GI, et al. (2011) HIV-1 restriction factor SAMHD1 is a deoxynucleoside triphosphate triphosphohydrolase. Nature. doi: 10.1038/nature10623.
28. White TE, Brandariz-Nunez A, Valle-Casuso JC, Amie S, Nguyen LA, et al. (2013) The retroviral restriction ability of SAMHD1, but not its deoxynucleotide triphosphohydrolase activity, is regulated by phosphorylation. Cell Host Microbe 13: 441–451. doi: 10.1016/j.chom.2013.03.005.
29. Allouch A, David A, Amie SM, Lahouassa H, Chartier L, et al. (2013) p21-mediated RNR2 repression restricts HIV-1 replication in macrophages by inhibiting dNTP biosynthesis pathway. Proc Natl Acad Sci U S A 110: E3997–E4006. doi: 10.1073/pnas.1306719110.
30. Bol SM, Moerland PD, Limou S, van RY, Coulonges C, et al. (2011) Genome-Wide Association Study Identifies Single Nucleotide Polymorphism in DYRK1A Associated with Replication of HIV-1 in Monocyte-Derived Macrophages. PLoS One 6: e17190. 10.1371/journal.pone.0017190 [doi].
31. Bol SM, Booiman T, Bunnik EM, Moerland PD, van DK, et al. (2011) Polymorphism in HIV-1 dependency factor PDE8A affects mRNA level and HIV-1 replication in primary macrophages. Virology 420: 32–42. S0042-6822(11)00376-X [pii];10.1016/j.virol.2011.08.013 [doi].
32. Zhou H, Xu M, Huang Q, Gates AT, Zhang XD, et al. (2008) Genome-scale RNAi screen for host factors required for HIV replication. Cell Host Microbe 4: 495–504. S1931-3128(08)00330-2 [pii];10.1016/j.chom.2008.10.004 [doi].
33. Fisher DA, Smith JF, Pillar JS, St Denis SH, Cheng JB (1998) Isolation and characterization of PDE8A, a novel human cAMP-specific phosphodiesterase. Biochem Biophys Res Commun 246: 570–577. S0006-291X(98)98684-3 [pii];10.1006/bbrc.1998.8684 [doi].
34. Moreno-Fernandez ME, Rueda CM, Velilla PA, Rugeles MT, Chougnet CA (2012) cAMP during HIV infection: friend or foe? AIDS Res Hum Retroviruses 28: 49–53. 10.1089/AID.2011.0265 [doi].
35. Naif H, Ho-Shon M, Chang J, Cunningham AL (1994) Molecular mechanisms of IL-4 effect on HIV expression in promonocytic cell lines and primary human monocytes. J Leukoc Biol 56: 335–339.
36. Montaner LJ, Griffin P, Gordon S (1994) Interleukin 10 inhibits initial reverse transcription of human immunodeficiency virus type 1 and mediates a virostatic latent state in primary blood-derived human macrophages in vitro. J Gen Virol 75: 3393–3400.
37. Montaner LJ, Bailer RT, Gordon S (1997) IL-13 acts on macrophages to block the completion of reverse transcription, inhibit virus production, and reduce virus infectivity. J Leukoc Biol 62: 126–132.
38. Montaner LJ, da Silva RP, Sun J, Sutterwala S, Hollinshead M, et al. (1999) Type 1 and type 2 cytokine regulation of macrophage endocytosis: differential activation by IL-4/IL-13 as opposed to IFN-gamma or IL-10. J Immunol 162: 4606–4613.
39. Kootstra NA, van 't Wout A, Huisman HG, Miedema F, Schuitemaker H (1994) Interference of interleukin-10 with human immunodeficiency virus type 1 replication in primary monocyte-derived macrophages. J Virol 68: 6967–6975.
40. Cassol E, Cassetta L, Rizzi C, Alfano M, Poli G (2009) M1 and M2a polarization of human monocyte-derived macrophages inhibits HIV-1 replication by distinct mechanisms. J Immunol 182: 6237–6246. 182/10/6237 [pii];10.4049/jimmunol.0803447 [doi].
41. Cassol E, Cassetta L, Alfano M, Poli G (2010) Macrophage polarization and HIV-1 infection. J Leukoc Biol 87: 599–608. jlb.1009673 [pii];10.1189/jlb.1009673 [doi].
42. Graff JW, Dickson AM, Clay G, McCaffrey AP, Wilson ME (2012) Identifying functional microRNAs in macrophages with polarized phenotypes. J Biol Chem 287: 21816–21825. M111.327031 [pii];10.1074/jbc.M111.327031 [doi].
43. Cobos Jiménez V, Bradley EJ, Willemsen AM, van Kampen AH, Baas F, et al. (2014) Next-generation sequencing of microRNAs uncovers expression signatures in polarized macrophages. Physiol Genomics 46: 91–103. physiolgenomics.00140.2013 [pii];10.1152/physiolgenomics.00140.2013 [doi].
44. Vergoulis T, Vlachos IS, Alexiou P, Georgakilas G, Maragkakis M, et al. (2012) TarBase 6.0: capturing the exponential growth of miRNA targets with experimental support. Nucleic Acids Res 40: D222–D229. gkr1161 [pii];10.1093/nar/gkr1161 [doi].

45. Xiao F, Zuo Z, Cai G, Kang S, Gao X, et al. (2009) miRecords: an integrated resource for microRNA-target interactions. Nucleic Acids Res 37: D105–D110. gkn851 [pii];10.1093/nar/gkn851 [doi].
46. Garcia DM, Baek D, Shin C, Bell GW, Grimson A, et al. (2011) Weak seed-pairing stability and high target-site abundance decrease the proficiency of lsy-6 and other microRNAs. Nat Struct Mol Biol 18: 1139–1146. nsmb.2115 [pii];10.1038/nsmb.2115 [doi].
47. Martinez FO, Helming L, Milde R, Varin A, Melgert BN, et al. (2013) Genetic programs expressed in resting and IL-4 alternatively activated mouse and human macrophages: similarities and differences. Blood 121: e57–e69. blood-2012-06-436212 [pii];10.1182/blood-2012-06-436212 [doi].
48. Thivierge M, Le Gouill C, Tremblay MJ, Stankova J, Rola-Pleszczynski M (1998) Prostaglandin E2 induces resistance to human immunodeficiency virus-1 infection in monocyte-derived macrophages: downregulation of CCR5 expression by cyclic adenosine monophosphate. Blood 92: 40–45.
49. Hayes MM, Lane BR, King SR, Markovitz DM, Coffey MJ (2002) Prostaglandin E(2) inhibits replication of HIV-1 in macrophages through activation of protein kinase A. Cell Immunol 215: 61–71. S0008874902000175 [pii].
50. Soderling SH, Bayuga SJ, Beavo JA (1998) Cloning and characterization of a cAMP-specific cyclic nucleotide phosphodiesterase. Proc Natl Acad Sci U S A 95: 8991–8996.
51. Gringhuis SI, van der Vlist V, van den Berg LM, den DJ, Litjens M, et al. (2010) HIV-1 exploits innate signaling by TLR8 and DC-SIGN for productive infection of dendritic cells. Nat Immunol 11: 419–426. ni.1858 [pii];10.1038/ni.1858 [doi].
52. Brown KM, Day JP, Huston E, Zimmermann B, Hampel K, et al. (2013) Phosphodiesterase-8A binds to and regulates Raf-1 kinase. Proc Natl Acad Sci U S A 110: E1533–E1542. 1303004110 [pii];10.1073/pnas.1303004110 [doi].
53. Francis SH, Houslay MD, Conti M (2011) Phosphodiesterase inhibitors: factors that influence potency, selectivity, and action. Handb Exp Pharmacol 47–84. 10.1007/978-3-642-17969-3_2 [doi].
54. Schwartz BG, Kloner RA (2010) Drug interactions with phosphodiesterase-5 inhibitors used for the treatment of erectile dysfunction or pulmonary hypertension. Circulation 122: 88–95. 122/1/88 [pii];10.1161/CIRCULATIONAHA.110.944603 [doi].
55. Giembycz MA, Field SK (2010) Roflumilast: first phosphodiesterase 4 inhibitor approved for treatment of COPD. Drug Des Devel Ther 4: 147–158.
56. Zhang HT (2009) Cyclic AMP-specific phosphodiesterase-4 as a target for the development of antidepressant drugs. Curr Pharm Des 15: 1688–1698.
57. Pear WS, Nolan GP, Scott ML, Baltimore D (1993) Production of high-titer helper-free retroviruses by transient transfection. Proc Natl Acad Sci U S A 90: 8392–8396.
58. Follenzi A, Ailles LE, Bakovic S, Geuna M, Naldini L (2000) Gene transfer by lentiviral vectors is limited by nuclear translocation and rescued by HIV-1 pol sequences. Nat Genet 25: 217–222. 10.1038/76095 [doi].
59. Kootstra NA, Munk C, Tonnu N, Landau NR, Verma IM (2003) Abrogation of postentry restriction of HIV-1-based lentiviral vector transduction in simian cells. Proc Natl Acad Sci U S A 100: 1298–1303. 10.1073/pnas.0337541100 [doi];0337541100 [pii].
60. Root DE, Hacohen N, Hahn WC, Lander ES, Sabatini DM (2006) Genome-scale loss-of-function screening with a lentiviral RNAi library. Nat Methods 3: 715–719. nmeth924 [pii];10.1038/nmeth924 [doi].
61. Dull T, Zufferey R, Kelly M, Mandel RJ, Nguyen M, et al. (1998) A third-generation lentivirus vector with a conditional packaging system. J Virol 72: 8463–8471.
62. van 't Wout AB, Schuitemaker H, Kootstra NA (2008) Isolation and propagation of HIV-1 on peripheral blood mononuclear cells. Nat Protoc 3: 363–370.
63. Kootstra NA, Schuitemaker H (1999) Phenotype of HIV-1 lacking a functional nuclear localization signal in matrix protein of gag and Vpr is comparable to wild-type HIV-1 in primary macrophages. Virology 253: 170–180.

12

Expression of the IL-7 Receptor Alpha-Chain Is Down Regulated on the Surface of CD4 T-Cells by the HIV-1 Tat Protein

Denny McLaughlin[1], **Elliott Faller**[1,4], **Scott Sugden**[1], **Paul MacPherson**[1,2,3,4]*

1 Department of Biochemistry, Microbiology and Immunology, Faculty of Medicine, University of Ottawa, Ottawa, Ontario, Canada, **2** Department of Medicine, Faculty of Medicine, University of Ottawa, Ottawa, Ontario, Canada, **3** Division of Infectious Diseases, Ottawa Hospital General Campus, Ottawa, Ontario, Canada, **4** Ottawa Hospital Research Institute, Ottawa, Ontario, Canada

Abstract

HIV infection elicits defects in CD4 T-cell homeostasis in both a quantitative and qualitative manner. Interleukin-7 (IL-7) is essential to T-cell homeostasis and several groups have shown reduced levels of the IL-7 receptor alpha-chain (CD127) on both CD4 and CD8 T-cells in viremic HIV+ patients. We have shown previously that soluble HIV Tat protein specifically down regulates cell surface expression of CD127 on human CD8 T-cells in a paracrine fashion. The effects of Tat on CD127 expression in CD4 T-cells has yet to be described. To explore this effect, CD4 T-cells were isolated from healthy individuals and expression levels of CD127 were examined on cells incubated in media alone or treated with Tat protein. We show here that, similar to CD8 T-cells, the HIV-1 Tat protein specifically down regulates CD127 on primary human CD4 T-cells and directs the receptor to the proteasome for degradation. Down regulation of CD127 in response to Tat was seen on both memory and naive CD4 T-cell subsets and was blocked using either heparin or anti-Tat antibodies. Tat did not induce apoptosis in cultured primary CD4 T-cells over 72 hours as determined by Annexin V and PI staining. Pre-incubation of CD4 T-cells with HIV-1 Tat protein did however reduce the ability of IL-7 to up regulate Bcl-2 expression. Similar to exogenous Tat, endogenously expressed HIV Tat protein also suppressed CD127 expression on primary CD4 T-cells. In view of the important role IL-7 plays in lymphocyte proliferation, homeostasis and survival, down regulation of CD127 by Tat likely plays a central role in immune dysregulation and CD4 T-cell decline. Understanding this effect could lead to new approaches to mitigate the CD4 T-cell loss evident in HIV infection.

Editor: Simona Stager, INRS - Institut Armand Frappier, Canada

Funding: Funding for this study was provided by CIHR, grant number 200709HOP-180274-VVP-ADYP-39720 (http://www.cihr-irsc.gc.ca/). The funders had no role in study design, data collection and analysis, decision to publish, or preparation of the manuscript.

Competing Interests: The authors have declared that no competing interests exist.

* Email: pmacpherson@toh.on.ca

These authors contributed equally to this work.

Introduction

CD4 T-cell depletion is a hallmark of HIV disease progression. The exact mechanisms by which HIV causes CD4 T-cell loss, however, have yet to be fully elucidated. While direct cytopathic effects of HIV and activation of HIV-specific natural killer cells and cytotoxic T-cells are two important means by which HIV-infected CD4 T-cells may be eliminated, these mechanisms likely explain only a portion of the loss given less than 0.2% of the peripheral CD4 T-cell population is productively infected [1,2,3]. Chronic immune activation with T-cell exhaustion [4], impaired T-cell production [5], and increased CD4 T-cell susceptibility to apoptosis have also been suggested to account for the dramatic decline in CD4 T-cells in infected individuals [6]. Of note, quiescent CD4 T-cells are particularly susceptible to death by caspase-1 mediated pyroptosis induced by accumulation of incomplete HIV reverse transcripts resulting from abortive infection [7,8].

Interleukin (IL)-7 is pivotal to T-cell survival and homeostasis and plays an important role in maintaining constant numbers of naïve and memory CD4 and CD8 T-lymphocytes in the peripheral circulation [9]. IL-7 promotes T-cell proliferation by stimulating entry into the cell cycle[10,11,12,13] and enhances T-cell survival by up regulating the anti-apoptotic factors Bcl-2 and Bcl-xL [14] while inhibiting the pro-apoptotic factors Bad and Bax [15]. IL-7 signals through the IL-7 receptor, a heterodimeric complex comprised of a unique α-chain (CD127) and the common γ-chain (CD132) that is shared with the receptors for IL-2, -4, -9, -15, and -21. CD127 is highly expressed on naïve and memory CD4 and CD8 T-cells [16,17]. In the absence of IL-7 signaling there is a substantial depletion of T-cells from the peripheral circulation [18].

We and others have shown decreased expression of the IL-7R α-chain (CD127) on CD4 and CD8 T-cells in HIV-infected individuals [19,20,21,22,23,24,25,26]. Loss of this receptor sub-unit has been shown to correlate with CD4 T-cell decline [24] and disease progression in HIV-infected patients [22,24,26,27]. Notably, reduced CD127 expression on the surface of CD4 T-cells in viremic HIV+ patients results in decreased responsiveness to the anti-apoptotic effects of IL-7 [28] likely contributing to CD4 T-cell apoptosis and depletion. Together, these data suggest suppression of CD127 expression on CD4 T-cells during HIV infection results in homeostatic imbalance and contributes to the loss of circulating CD4 T-cells.

We have previously shown down regulation of CD127 on the surface of CD8 T-cells is mediated at least in part by soluble HIV Tat protein [27]. Tat, a small 14 kdal HIV regulatory polypeptide, acts in a paracrine fashion to alter the function of neighboring cells [29,30]. This small protein is secreted by HIV-infected cells and can be found in the media during in vitro infection [31,32] as well as in the serum of HIV-infected patients [33]. Secreted Tat is rapidly internalized by a variety of cell types [32,34,35] by binding via its arginine-rich basic domain to heparan sulfate proteoglycans on the cell surface [35,36,37] and is then internalized by endocytosis [35,38,39,40]. When added to purified CD8 T-cells isolated from healthy HIV-negative donors, soluble Tat protein induces a significant reduction in CD127 surface expression compared to cells maintained in medium alone [27]. We have recently demonstrated soluble Tat protein enters CD8 T-cells by endocytosis and exits late endosomes through a process dependent on the usual acidification of these vesicles [41]. Once inside the cytoplasm, Tat translocates to the inner leaflet of the plasma membrane where it binds directly to the cytoplasmic tail of CD127 [41]. This interaction with Tat induces receptor aggregation or capping and removal from the cell surface through a process dependent on microtubules [41]. Finally, Tat directs CD127 to the proteasome for degradation. Through this mechanism, Tat decreases the half-life of CD127 in CD8 T-cells by more than three-fold [41]. Importantly, not only does Tat down regulate CD127 on CD8 T-cells, but this down regulation prevents accumulation of intracellular perforin in response to IL-7 [27]. The significant role the HIV Tat protein plays in removing CD127 from the surface of CD8 T-cells lead us and others to ask if it had the same effect on CD4 T-cells. By decreasing CD127 expression on the surface of CD4 T-cells, Tat could disrupt IL-7 signaling leading to reduced Bcl-2 expression and increased CD4 T-cell apoptosis and depletion. As hypothesized, we found that similar to CD8-T cells, CD127 is down regulated from the surface of CD4 T-cells by the HIV-1 Tat protein and degraded by the proteasome. This down regulation was dose dependant and resulted in a significant reduction in IL-7 induced Bcl-2 production. In addition to extracellular Tat having this effect, we also demonstrate that Tat produced endogenously also down regulates CD127 expression on CD4 T-cells.

Materials and Methods

Ethics statement

This work was reviewed and approved by the Ottawa Hospital Research Ethics Board and informed written consent was obtained from all participants. No children were used in this study. Written consent was obtained from all participants after reading a 5 page document describing phlebotomy, study outline, and research goals.

Isolation and culture of Primary CD8+ and CD4+ T-Cells

Peripheral blood mononuclear cells (PBMC) were isolated by Ficoll-Paque density centrifugation from blood of healthy adult volunteers with no known risk factors for HIV infection. CD8+ T-cells were positively selected as previously described using the MACS Microbead CD8+ Cell AutoMACS Isolation System (Miltenyi Biotec, Bergisch Gladbach, Germany) according to the manufacturer's directions [27]. Purified CD8 T-cells were resuspended at 10^6 cells/ml in RPMI 1640 (Hyclone, Logan, Utah) medium supplemented with 20% fetal calf serum (FCS; Cansera, Rexdale, Ont. Canada) plus 100 units/ml penicillin, 100 µg/ml streptomycin and 0.2 M L-glutamine (RPMI-20). The negative cell fraction was also suspended in RPMI-20 and incubated in a polystyrene tissue culture flask (BD Falcon) at 37°C for 75 minutes to allow CD4+ monocytes to adhere to the surface. The medium containing nonadhered lymphocytes was then decanted into a new tube and CD4 T-cells were isolated in the same manner as for the CD8 T-cells using anti-CD4 antibody conjugated ferromagnetic beads (Miltenyi Biotec). Purified CD4 T-cells were resuspended in RPMI-20 at 10^6 cells/ml. In order to confirm purity the cells were analyzed for CD4 and CD14 expression and were consistently >97% pure CD4 T-cells.

The isolated T-cells were maintained in medium alone or suspended in medium containing purified HIV-1 Tat protein (Advanced Bioscience Laboratories, Inc. Kensington, MD) or recombinant human IL-7 (Invitrogen Biosource. Carlsbad, CA) as specified. All cultures were incubated at 37°C in 5% CO_2.

To block Tat's effect, purified Tat protein was pre-incubated with heparin (Organon; 10 µl/ml to give final concentration of 100 USP units/ml) or rabbit anti-Tat polyclonal antibodies (Diatheva; ANT000) at a final concentration 140 µg/ml. Inhibitors were purchased from Sigma Aldrich, St Louis, MA. Cells were pre-incubated with and without proteasome inhibitors (5 µM MG132, 10 µM Lactacystin), lysosome inhibitors (10 µM Leupeptin, 10 µg/ml Pepstatin) and 100 µM cyclohexamide for 1 hour prior to incubation with and without 10 µg/ml Tat protein.

Flow cytometry

Cells were incubated with the indicated flourochrome-labeled antibodies for 20 minutes in the dark at room temperature and analyzed immediately using a Coulter Epics ALTRA flow cytometer (Fullerton, CA). Live cells were gated on the basis of side and forward scatter and at least 10,000 events were recorded for each sample. The following antibodies were obtained from Immunotech Beckman Coulter (Marseille, France): anti-CD127-phycoerythrin (PE) (R34.34), anti-CD3-fluorescein isothiocyanate (FITC) (UCHT1), anti-CD4-FITC (13B.2), anti-CD8-phycoerythrin-Cy5 (PC5) (B9.11), anti-CD14-FITC (RM052), anti-CD25-PC5 (B1.49.9), anti-CD28-PC5 (CD28.2), anti-CD45RA-FITC (ALB11), anti-CD45RO-FITC (UCHL1), anti-CD56-PC5 (N901NHK-1), and anti-CD62L-FITC (DREG56). Anti-CD132-PE (555900) was obtained from BD Biosciences (Mississauga, Ontario, Canada). All antibodies were used at saturating concentrations and the corresponding isotype controls were included.

Cell viability assays

Purified CD4 T-cells were incubated in medium alone or with Tat protein (10 µg/ml) in a humidified incubator at 37°C with 5% CO_2. Camptothecin (10 µM, Sigma-Aldrich) was used as a positive control for apoptosis. At 24 and 72 hours, cells were stained with Annexin V-FITC and propidium iodide (PI) using the Apoptosis Detection Kit I (BD Biosciences) according to the manufacturer's directions.

Intracellular staining for BCL-2

Purified CD4 T-cells were pre-incubated at a concentration of 1×10^6 cells/ml either in RPMI-20 alone or with Tat protein (10 µg/ml) for 48 hours. Recombinant human IL-7 (10 ng/ml) was then added and the cells were incubated at 37°C for an additional 72 hours. Following treatment, the cells were fixed in 2% paraformaldehyde in phosphate buffered saline (PBS) (PFA) at room temperature for 10 minutes. The samples were then washed

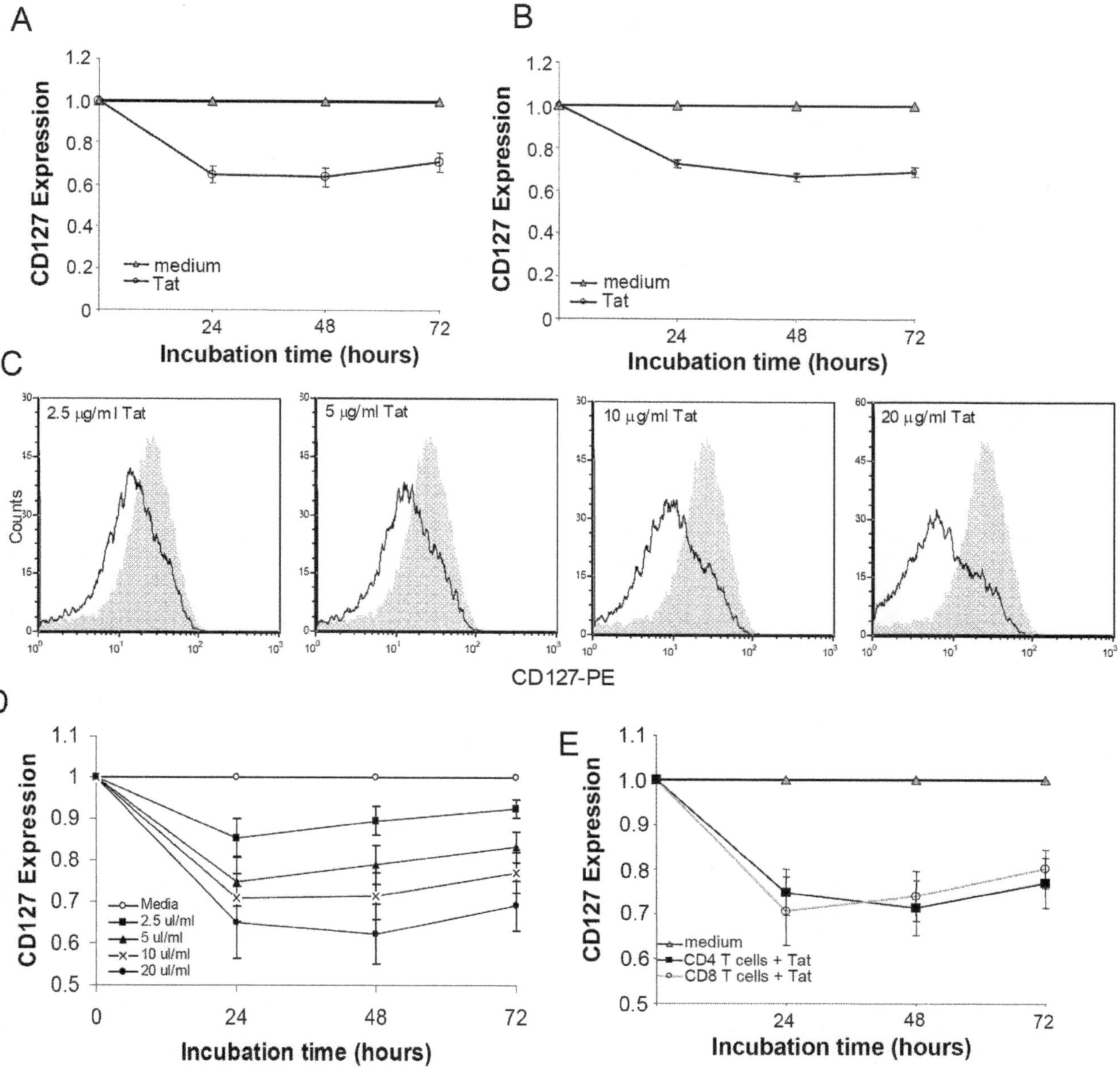

Figure 1. HIV-1 Tat protein down regulates CD127 surface expression on CD4 T-cells. Purified CD4 T-cells from healthy HIV-negative volunteers were incubated with Tat protein or in medium alone, stained for CD127 and analyzed by flow cytometry. (A) Percent change in CD127+ CD4 T-cells cultured with Tat (10 µg/ml) compared with media controls (n = 17; $p<0.01$). (B) Change in mean channel fluorescence relative to media controls for the same cultures ($p<0.01$). (C) Representative flow cytometry histograms from one individual showing progressive down regulation of CD127 surface expression at 48 hours with increasing amounts of Tat protein (black line) compared to medium (grey fill). (D) Composite data (n = 6; $p<0.02$) showing time and dose response to Tat in percent change in CD127+ CD4 T cells compared to media controls. (E) Purified CD4 and CD8 T-cells from the same healthy HIV-negative volunteers (n = 5) were incubated for up to 72 hours with HIV-1 Tat protein (10 µg/ml) or in medium alone. Percent changes in surface CD127 expression compared to medium controls are shown ($p<0.01$ for Tat-treated samples; $p>0.5$ between T-cell subsets). Graphs show mean values ± standard error of the mean (SEM).

twice with PBS containing 1% bovine serum albumin (BSA) and permeabilized by resuspending in cold methanol for 10 minutes at 4°C. The cells were again washed twice as above and resuspended in 100 µl PBS with 1% BSA. The cells were then stained with FITC-conjugated mouse anti-human Bcl-2 monoclonal antibodies (Bcl-2/100; BD Biosciences) or FITC labeled mouse IgG, κ isotype control (MOPC-21; BD-Biosciences) for 45 minutes at room temperature in the dark. The cells were then washed as above, resuspended in PFA and immediately analyzed by flow cytometry.

Primary CD4 T Cell Nucleofection

Primary CD4 T-cells were isolated as described above and cultured overnight in RPMI-20. The next day cells were stimulated with anti-CD3/anti-CD28 antibody conjugated ferro-magnetic beads using the T-cell activation/expansion kit from Miltenyi Biotec (Bergisch Gladbach, Germany). After 24 hours, beads were removed by magnetic separation and CD4 T-cells were nucleofected using the human T-cell nucleofector kit (Lonza, Basel, Switzerland). Briefly, 5×10^6 CD4 T-cells per condition

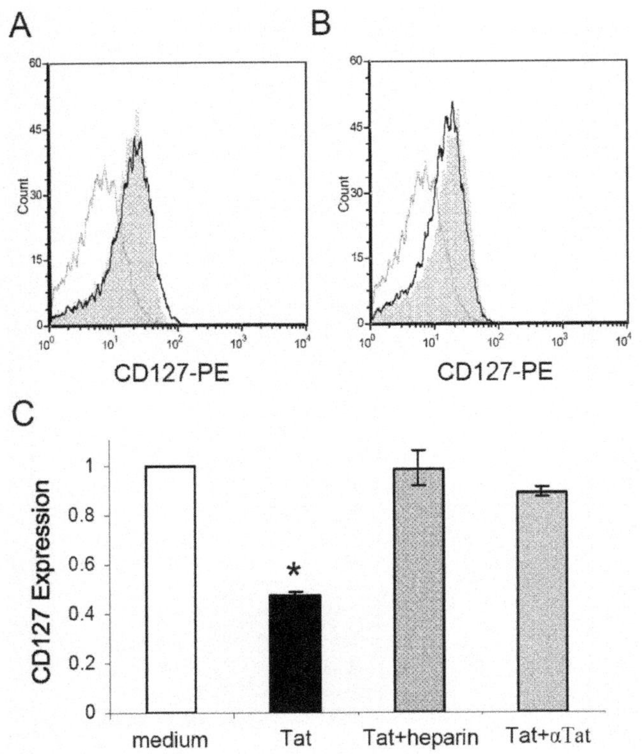

Figure 2. Tat-induced CD127 down regulation is blocked by heparin and anti-Tat antibodies. Purified Tat protein (2 µg) was pre-incubated with 20 USP heparin or 20 µg anti-Tat polyclonal antibodies (equimolar ratio with Tat) for 30 minutes before being added to CD4 T-cells (n = 4). Representative flow cytometry histograms show CD127 surface expression on CD4 T-cells after 24 hours incubation with (A) 10 µg/ml Tat (grey line), Tat plus heparin (black line) or in medium alone (grey fill); and (B) 10 µg/ml Tat (grey line), Tat plus anti-Tat antibodies (black line) or in medium alone (grey fill). (C) Composite data (n = 5) showing CD127 expression relative to medium controls for Tat, Tat plus heparin, and Tat plus anti-Tat antibodies after 24 hours incubation. * denotes p value <0.05 compared to media. The relative changes are mean values ± SEM.

were resuspended in 100 µL of human T-cell nucleofection solution containing 1.5 µg of Tat-expressing pcDNA3.1$^{(-)}$ or empty vector control, and co transfected with 0.25 µg of pGFPmax plasmid using the nucleofector II device (Lonza, Basel, Switzerland) protocol U-014. Following nucleofection, cells were allowed to recover at a concentration of 2.5×10^6 cells/ml for 4 hours in serum-free RPMI-1640 before being transferred into RPMI-20 at a concentration of 1×10^6 cells/ml. Surface CD127 expression was monitored at 24 hour intervals by flow cytometry. GFP florescence was used as an internal control for transfection efficiency.

Statistical analysis

All statistical analyses were performed using Microsoft Excel software. Statistical significance was measured by Students two tailed *t*-test for paired samples. Given the sample sizes of the groups, parallel nonparametric analyses were also carried out using the Wilcoxon matched pair test with 95% confidence intervals (one tailed). Statistical significance as defined by a p value greater or less than 0.05 remained the same for all comparisons irrespective of parametric or nonparametric analysis. All flow cytometry data were analysed using the FCS Express 3.0 software (De NovoSoftware, Thornhill, ON, Canada).

Results

Soluble HIV Tat protein down regulates surface CD127 expression on CD4 T-cells

Given the effect of soluble HIV-1 Tat protein on CD127 expression on CD8 T-cells, we wanted to determine if this HIV regulatory protein had the same effect on CD4 T-cells. To investigate this, CD4 T-cells were isolated from healthy volunteers and incubated in RPMI-20 with or without purified Tat protein (10 µg/ml) and analyzed by flow cytometry at 24 hour intervals. While CD127 surface expression varied little on cells cultured in medium alone over at least 72 hours, cells incubated in medium containing soluble Tat protein demonstrated a significant reduction in surface CD127 expression both in terms of percent positive cells and in mean channel fluorescence (Figures 1A and 1B). In the presence of exogenous Tat protein, there was a 35%±4% reduction in CD127+ CD4 T-cells relative to controls at 24 hours. This decrease leveled off at 48 hours and showed some signs of recovery by 72 hours although CD127+ cells still remained 30%±4.4% lower relative to controls.

The effect of Tat on CD127 surface expression was both time and dose dependent. Increasing amounts of Tat from 2.5 to 20 µg/ml showed a progressively greater reduction in CD127 surface expression as measured by both mean channel fluorescence (Figure 1C) and percent positive cells (Figure 1D). At 24 hours, 2.5 µg/ml Tat induced a 14.7%±4.8% decrease in CD127 expression whereas 20 µg/ml induced a 35%±8.5% reduction. Interestingly, peak suppression of CD127 occurred within 24 hours in the presence of 2.5, 5 and 10 µg/ml of Tat while peak suppression occurred at 48 hours in the presence of 20 µg/ml Tat. This may suggest Tat consumption plays a role in the recovery of CD127 at later time points.

We next asked whether soluble Tat protein reduced surface CD127 expression to the same extent comparing CD8 and CD4 T-cells. To answer this, CD8 and CD4 T-cells were purified from the same individuals (n = 5) and incubated in RPMI-20 alone or in the presence of HIV-1 Tat protein (10 µg/ml) for up to 72 hours. As seen in figure 1E, Tat down regulated CD127 expression equally on both T-cell populations. CD127 surface expression on CD4 T-cells decreased and remained within one standard deviation of that on CD8 T-cells throughout the entire incubation period (p>0.52).

We showed previously Tat dependant down regulation of CD127 on T-cells was not caused by bacterial contaminants such as LPS in the protein preparation [27]. To further test this we added *E. coli* Endotoxin (100 µg/ml CSE) to cultured CD4 T-cells and found this had no impact on CD127 surface expression (data not shown).

HIV-1 Tat-Induced down regulation of CD127 surface expression can be blocked with heparin or anti-Tat antibodies

To ensure the down regulation of surface CD127 expression on CD4 T-cells was specifically due to Tat, we pre-incubated Tat protein with either heparin or polyclonal anti-Tat antibodies to see if this would block the effect. Heparin has been shown to bind directly to Tat protein and prevent its uptake by cells from the culture medium [36,42]. Purified Tat protein was pre-incubated for 30 minutes with an equimolar concentration of anti-Tat polyclonal antibodies (140 µg/ml) or with 100 USP/ml heparin. The Tat preparations were then added to purified CD4 T-cells and the samples were incubated for 24 hours (figure 2). Whereas cells incubated with heparin or with anti-Tat antibodies alone demonstrated no change in CD127 surface expression, 10 µg/ml

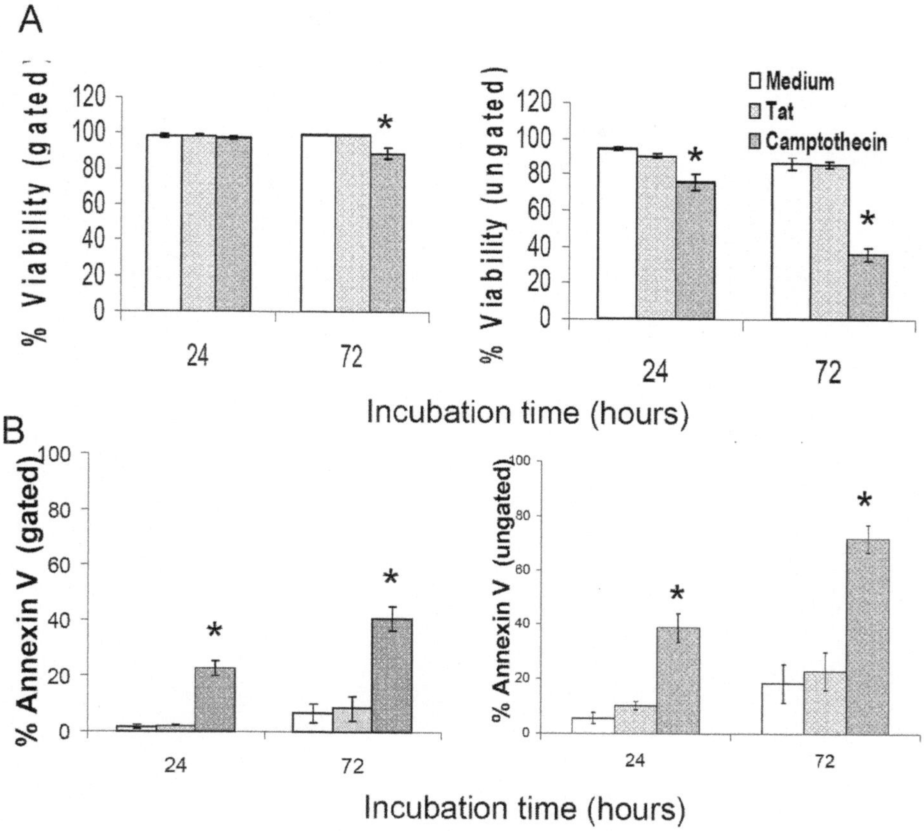

Figure 3. Tat protein does not affect the viability of purified CD4 T-cells. Purified CD4 T-cells from healthy HIV-negative volunteers (n = 4) were incubated in medium alone or with Tat protein (10 μg/ml) for up to 72 hours and then stained with propidium iodide or annexin V-FITC and analyzed by flow cytometry. Analyses were performed on the total ungated population as well as on only live cells based on forward and side scatter. (A) Propidium iodide exclusion showed no significant difference in viability between cells cultured in Tat or medium alone. (B) Apoptosis as indicated by positive annexin V staining averaged <10% in the gated population at 72 hours and was no different comparing cells cultured in medium alone or with Tat protein. Camptothecin (10 μM) induces apoptosis and was used as a positive control. * denotes p value <0.05 compared to media. Graphs show mean values ± SEM.

Tat protein induced a 52%±7% decrease in CD127. In contrast, Tat protein pre-bound with heparin had no effect on CD127 expression (1.4%±2.1% decrease relative to media control; p = 0.61). Similarly, polyclonal anti-Tat antibodies pre-bound to Tat also inhibited Tat's ability to down regulate CD127 (11%±5.4% reduction relative to media control; p = 0.54). These data then confirm the down regulation of CD127 on the surface of CD4 T-cells is due specifically to the HIV Tat protein. The fact that anti-Tat antibodies inhibit the effect further demonstrates CD127 suppression is not due to bacterial contaminants in the Tat protein preparation.

HIV-1 Tat-Induced down regulation of CD127 surface expression is not caused by cell death or apoptosis

There have been conflicting reports regarding the effect of HIV-1 Tat on both promoting and inhibiting apoptosis in T-cells [43,44,45]. To ensure that the reduction in CD127 surface expression evident on Tat treated cells was not the result of apoptosis or cell death, purified CD4 T-cells were cultured in the presence of Tat protein (10 μg/ml) and stained with propidium iodide and annexin V at 24 and 72 hours. Cell viability as indicated by propidium iodide exclusion in the total ungated cell population was maintained at >85%±3.5% over 72 hours for cells incubated in RPMI-20 alone or in the presence of Tat protein. Within the live gate based on forward and side scatter viability was >99%±0.1% at 72 hours and again was not different comparing cells incubated in medium alone or in the presence of Tat protein (Figure 3A). Apoptosis as indicated by positive annexin V staining remained <10%±4.3% over 72 hours in the gated population regardless of the presence of Tat protein in the medium. In the ungated total population the difference in annexin V staining comparing Tat-treated cells to media control was only 4.5%, less than the standard error of 7.1% (Figure 3B). Thus, Tat-induced down regulation of CD127 surface expression is not the result of cell death or apoptosis.

CD127 surface expression is down regulated by HIV-1 Tat protein on both naïve and memory CD4 T-cell subsets

The memory subset of CD4 T-cells has been shown to be particularly sensitive to CD127 down regulation in HIV-infected individuals [23,46,47]. This raised the question as to whether the HIV-1 Tat protein would have a more profound effect on this subset compared to naïve cells. Purified CD4 T-cells were incubated in RPMI-20 alone or with Tat protein (10 μg/ml) and CD127 expression was analyzed by flow cytometry gating on the different CD4 T-cell subsets. Naïve cells were defined as $CD45RA^{+}CD62L^{+}$ and memory cells were defined as $CD45RO^{+}$. As seen in figure 4, soluble HIV Tat protein down regulated CD127 surface expression equally on naïve and memory CD4 T-cells compared to controls. Both demonstrated a 32%±2.8%

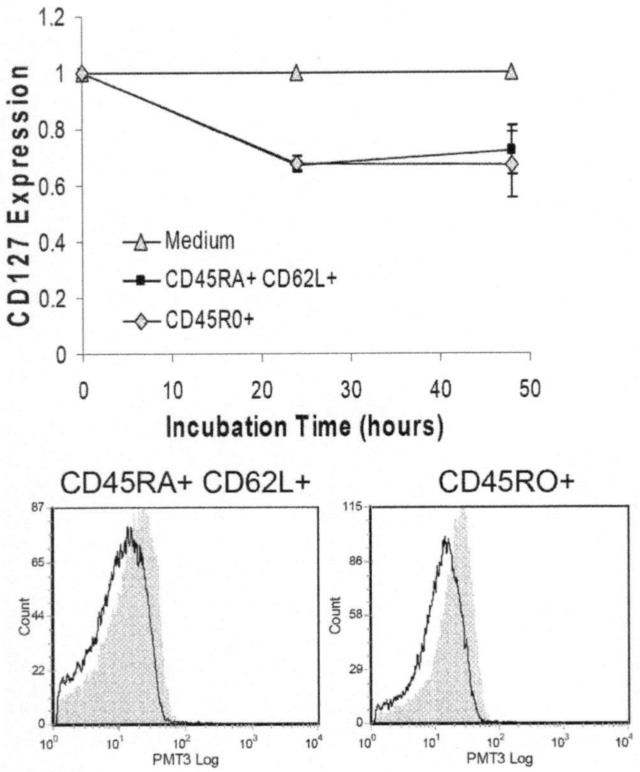

Figure 4. Tat down regulates CD127 surface expression equally on naïve and memory CD4 T-cell subsets. Purified CD4 T-cells from healthy HIV-negative volunteers (n = 4) were incubated in medium alone or with Tat protein (10 μg/ml) for up to 48 hours. CD127 surface expression was then measured by flow cytometry on naïve CD4 T-cells defined as CD45RA+ and CD62L+, and on memory cells defined as CD45RO+. There was little difference between the subsets ($p>0.33$). The changes relative to medium controls ($p<0.02$) are shown (mean values ± SEM). Representative histograms show CD127 expression on indicated populations at 24 hours comparing media (grey fill) to CD4 T-cells treated with Tat protein (black line).

decrease in CD127 at 24 hours, equivalent to what was seen in the total CD4 T-cell population.

HIV Tat specifically down regulates CD127 and does not affect other cell surface proteins

Internalization of soluble HIV-1 Tat protein by uninfected neighbouring CD4 T-cells occurs via clathrin-mediated endocytosis [40]. In view of this it is possible that transduction of Tat across the cell membrane could induce a non-specific and generalized down regulation of cell surface proteins. To explore this possibility, CD4 T-cells were incubated in RPMI-20 alone or with Tat protein (10 μg/ml) and then analyzed by flow cytometry for expression of a series of cell surface markers. Cells were stained for CD127, CD45RA (a marker of naïve T-cells), CD62L (a secondary lymphoid tissue homing receptor expressed on T-cells), and CD3 (an essential component of the T-cell receptor complex). Cells were also examined for the expression of CD132, the common γ-chain that associates with CD127 to form the IL-7 receptor heterodimer. Whereas Tat induced the down regulation of CD127 surface expression by 38.2%±14.2% at 48 hours relative to controls, it had no effect on the expression of the other cell surface proteins examined (Figure 5A). CD3 showed the maximum variance, only a 3.2%±2.3% difference relative to controls (Figure 5A). Similarly, Tat had no effect on the expression of CD132 (Figure 5B). After 48 hours in the presence of Tat, CD132 increased by only 3.1%±1.5% compared to controls. Thus it appears Tat specifically down regulates CD127 and does not affect at least a number of other cell surface proteins.

CD127 down regulation by HIV-1 Tat protein is not due to CD4 T-cell activation

T-cell activation has been shown to down regulate CD127 surface expression on CD8 and CD4 T-cells [24,48,49]. Indeed, levels of $CD127^{-}$ T-cells were shown to be directly correlated with CD8 T-cell activation [24] and in a study of 42 HIV-infected individuals receiving antiretroviral therapy, Benito et al. demonstrated CD127 down regulation was associated with activation of CD4 T-cells [49]. This raised the question as to whether Tat down regulates CD127 on the cell surface by activating CD4 T-cells. To address this question, purified CD4 T-cells were incubated in RPMI-20 alone or with Tat protein (10 μg/ml) and then examined by flow cytometry for expression of CD127 as well as the established activation markers CD25 and CD56. CD28 is constitutively expressed on naïve T-cells where it provides costimulatory signals and is down regulated upon T-cell stimulation. As seen in figure 6 and consistent with the previous data, Tat induced a significant down regulation of CD127 on the surface of CD4 T-cells. In contrast, CD28, CD25 and CD56 remained unchanged relative to controls in the presence of Tat protein. Thus Tat does not appear to induce a generalized activation of CD4 T-cells leading to the down regulation of CD127.

Tat-induced down regulation of CD127 surface expression is reversible

CD127 is down regulated on CD4 T-cells in HIV infected patients and partially recovers following viral suppression with antiretroviral therapy [26]. A cohort study of patients with primary, chronic and long-term non-progressive HIV-1 infection showed that CD127 down regulation on CD4 T-cells was rapidly reversible and returned to normal levels less than 24 hours after incubation ex vivo in fresh medium [26]. To investigate whether CD127 down regulation by Tat was reversible, purified CD4 T-cells were incubated in RPMI-20 alone or with Tat protein (10 μg/ml). At 24 and 48 hours, the cells were washed and resuspended in fresh RPMI-20 without Tat. As shown in figure 7, once Tat was removed from the medium CD127 recovered on the cell surface within 24 hours. This clearly indicates Tat's effect on CD127 is reversible and that Tat is continually required to maintain suppression of CD127.

Tat has a direct effect on CD127 expression and does not require de novo protein synthesis

We next questioned whether soluble HIV Tat protein had a direct effect on CD127 surface expression or whether induction of a second factor was required to down regulate the receptor. To investigate this, purified CD4 T-cells were incubated in RPMI-20 alone, with Tat protein (10 μg/ml), with cyclohexamide (CHX) or with Tat protein plus CHX (figure 8). Cells treated with CHX alone represent the normal decay rate of CD127 from the cell surface in the absence of new protein synthesis. As seen in figure 8, cells incubated with CHX alone showed a 16.5%±7.3% decrease in CD127 surface expression over 24 hours. Tat protein alone induced a 39.6%±5.6% decrease in CD127. When CHX was included with Tat, there was a 46.5%±1.9% drop in CD127 surface expression indicating de novo protein synthesis is not required for Tat to have its effect.

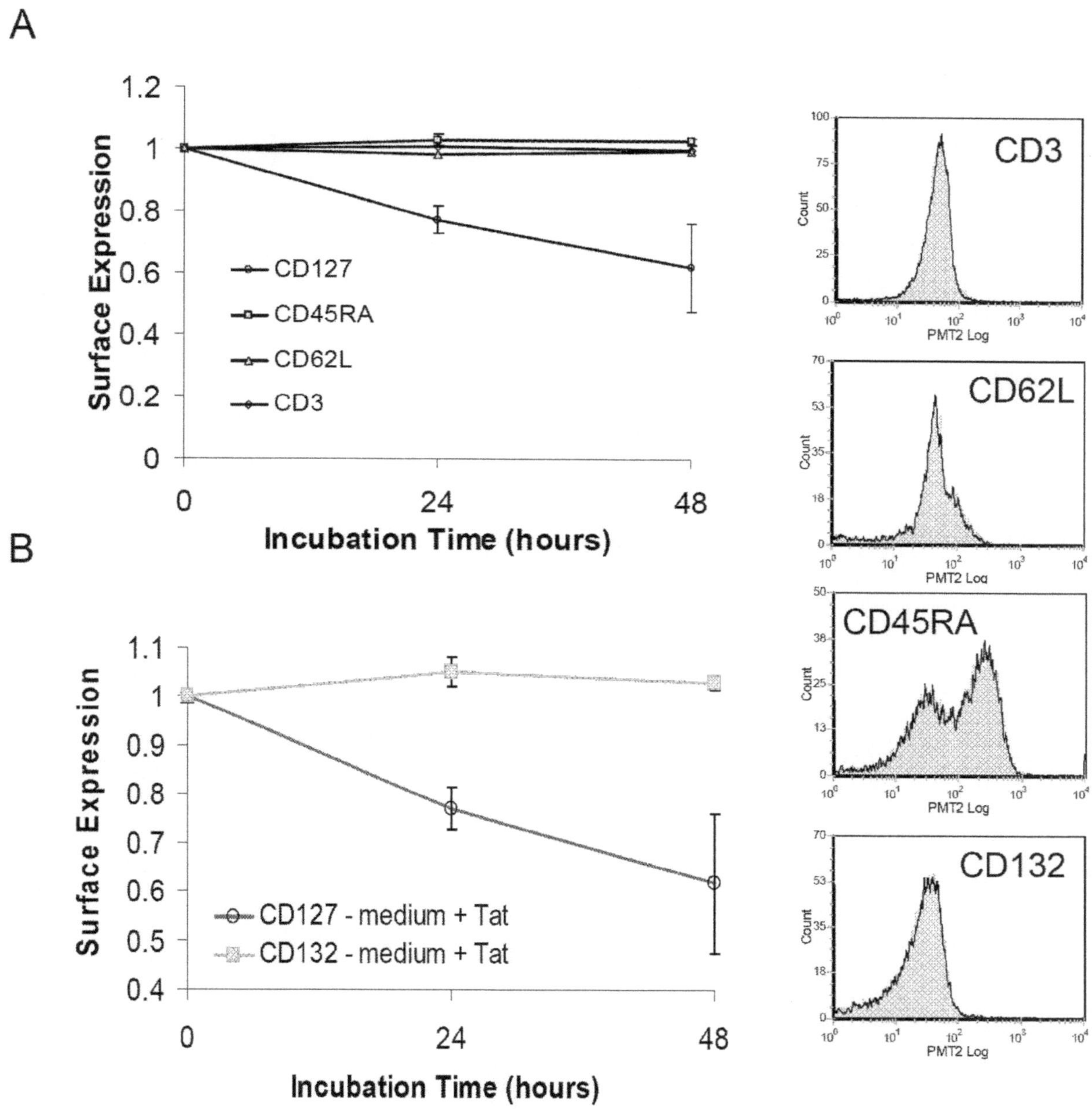

Figure 5. Tat does not affect other CD4 T-cell surface proteins. Purified CD4 T-cells from healthy HIV-negative volunteers (n = 4) were incubated in medium alone or with Tat protein (10 µg/ml) for up to 48 hours and then analyzed by flow cytometry. (A) Changes in positive staining for the indicated surface proteins relative to medium controls ($p > 0.09$ for all proteins other than CD127 where $p < 0.04$). (B) Change in CD132+ CD4 T-cells relative to medium controls ($p > 0.12$ at 48 hours). Graph represents mean values ± SEM. Representative flow histograms show CD4 T-cells from one individual incubated in media (grey fill) or media plus Tat (black line) at 48 hours.

New protein synthesis is required for CD127 recovery following down regulation by Tat

As shown above, CD127 recovers on the cell surface once soluble Tat protein is removed from the medium. To determine if this recovery of CD127 requires new protein synthesis, CD4 T-cells were first incubated with soluble Tat for 24 hours and then washed and re-incubated in medium alone or medium containing cycloheximide. As shown in figure 9A, cells maintained in medium containing Tat protein maintained suppression of CD127 for up to 72 hours while those washed and transferred to fresh medium alone after 24 hours recovered surface CD127 expression. However, when Tat protein was removed from the medium and the cells were then incubated in cycloheximide, CD127 failed to recover. Thus Tat induces an absolute loss of CD127 from the cell and new protein synthesis is required to replace CD127 on the cell surface. Previously we have shown HIV-1 Tat protein removes CD127 from the surface of CD8 T cells and directs it to the proteasome for degradation [41]. To determine if this is also the case in primary CD4 T cells, the cells were pre-incubated with proteasome (MG132, lactacystin) or lysosome inhibitors (leupeptin, pepstatin) for 1 hour and then incubated with HIV-1 Tat protein for 24 hours. As seen in figure 9B, Tat-induced down regulation of CD127 (33+/−3%, p value <0.01 compared to medium) was inhibited by both lactacystin and MG132, showing only a 16+/−3% (p value = 0.02 compared to Tat treated cells) and 8+/−5% (p value compared to Tat treated cells <0.01)

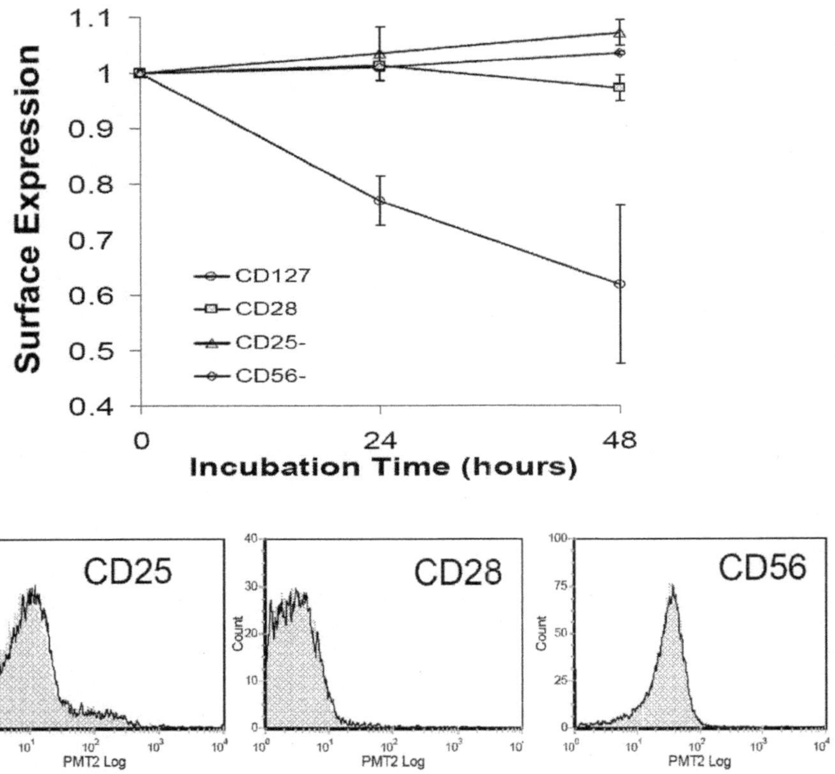

Figure 6. Tat-induced CD127 down regulation is not due to CD4 T-cell activation. Purified CD4 T-cells from healthy HIV-negative volunteers (n = 4) were incubated in medium alone or with Tat protein (10 µg/ml) for up to 48 hours and then analyzed by flow cytometry. The changes in surface protein expression relative to medium controls are shown (p>0.19 for all proteins other than CD127 where p<0.04 at 48 hours). Graph represents mean values ± SEM. Representative flow histograms show CD4 T-cells from one individual incubated in media (grey fill) or media plus Tat (black line) at 48 hours.

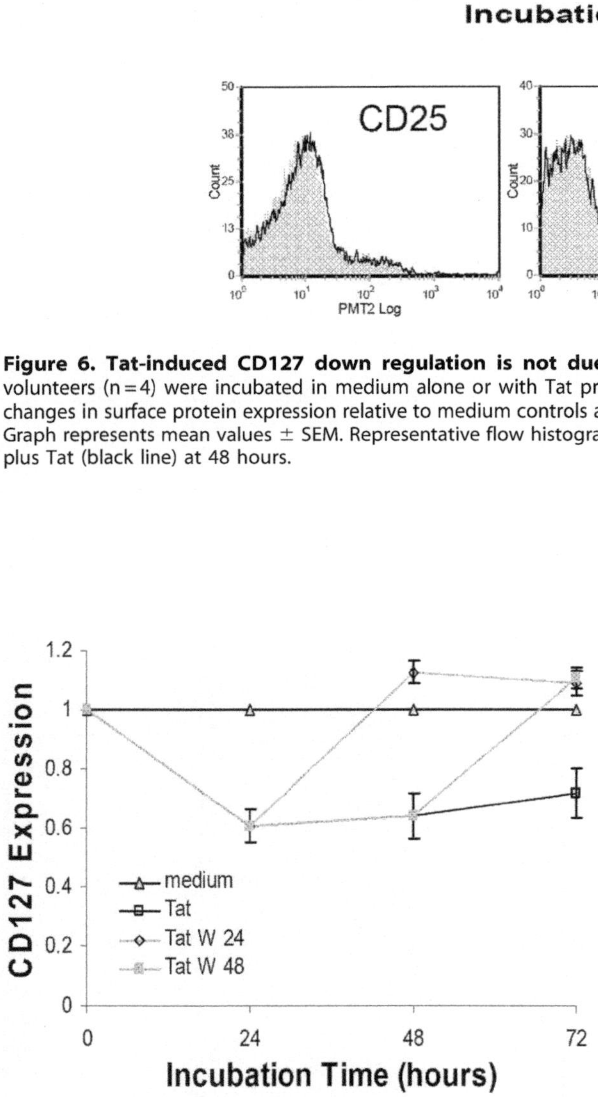

Figure 7. CD127 surface expression recovers on CD4 T-cells after Tat is removed from the culture medium. Purified CD4 T-cells from healthy HIV-negative volunteers (n = 4) were incubated in medium alone or with Tat protein (10 µg/ml). At 24 (Tat W 24) and 48 (Tat W 48) hours the cells were washed twice in PBS and resuspended in fresh medium in the absence of Tat protein. Cells were analyzed for CD127 surface expression by flow cytometry at the times indicated. The changes relative to medium controls are shown (mean values ± SEM).

reduction in CD127 respectively. In contrast, cells pretreated with the lysosome inhibitors pepstatin (31+/−3 %, p value = 0.35, compared to Tat treated cells) or leupeptin (34+/−6%, p value = 0.41) still down regulated CD127 in response to extracelluar Tat similar to cells treated with Tat alone.

Endogenously expressed HIV Tat protein down regulates CD127 expression

HIV-1 Tat is secreted from infected CD4 cells and is readily internalized by uninfected bystander cells. Since less than 0.2% of peripheral CD4 T cells are productively infected with HIV [1,2,3], exogenous Tat protein may exert a wider influence on the CD4 T cell population. To address whether endogenously expressed Tat protein also down regulates CD127 surface expression, we expressed Tat in primary human CD4 T cells by transient transfection (Figure 10A). This was achieved by first stimulating the cells with anti-CD3/anti-CD28 beads for 24 hours followed by transfection with the pcDNA3.1$^{(-)}$ empty vector or pcDNA3.1$^{(-)}$ expressing Tat. CD127 expression was then measured by flow cytometry at 24 hours. As seen in figure 10B, CD4 T cells transfected with the Tat expressing plasmid had lower CD127 expression (18+/−3, p value = 0.01) compared to CD4 T cells transfected with the empty vector.

HIV-1 Tat protein inhibits IL-7-induced up regulation of Bcl-2

IL-7 signaling plays an essential role in CD4 T-cell proliferation and homeostasis and has been specifically shown to up regulate

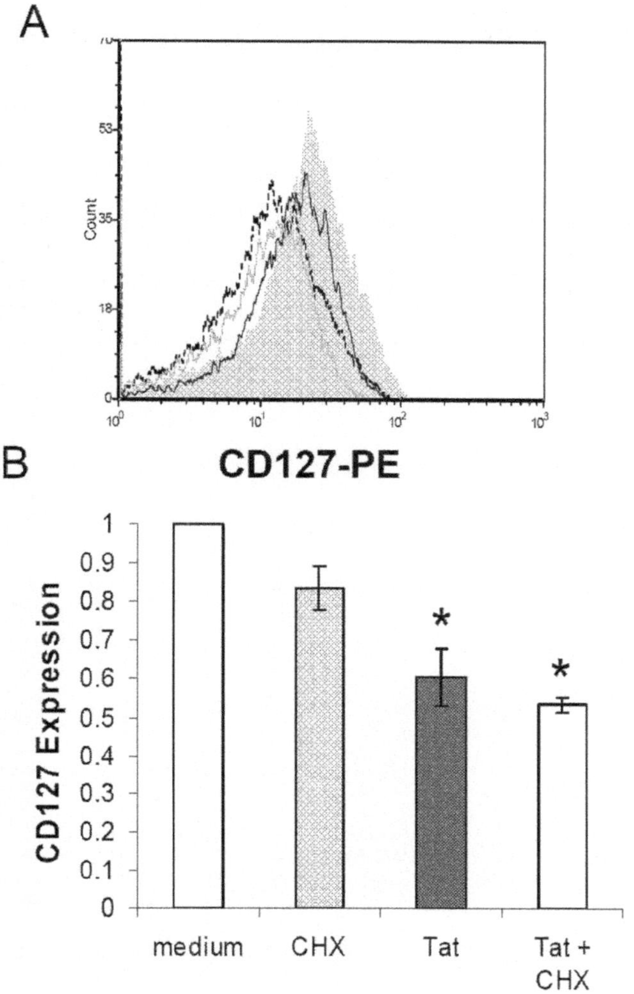

Figure 8. de novo protein synthesis is not required for Tat-induced down regulation of CD127. Purified CD4 T-cells from healthy HIV-negative volunteers were incubated in medium alone, with cyclohexamide (100 μM; CHX), Tat protein (10 μg/ml) or Tat plus CHX for 24 hours and then analyzed by flow cytometry. (A) Representative histogram showing CD127 surface expression on CD4 T-cells cultured in the presence of CHX alone (black line), Tat alone (dashed line) and CHX plus Tat (grey line) compared to medium control (grey fill). (B) Composite data from n = 4 demonstrating inhibition of protein synthesis with CHX does not prevent Tat-induced CD127 down regulation at the cell surface. CHX alone had no significant effect on CD127 expression (p = 0.07). There was no significant variance in surface CD127 expression between Tat and Tat + CHX treatments (p = 0.38) whereas both treatments showed significant down regulation of CD127 relative to medium (* denotes p<0.009). The percent changes relative to medium controls are shown (mean values ± SEM).

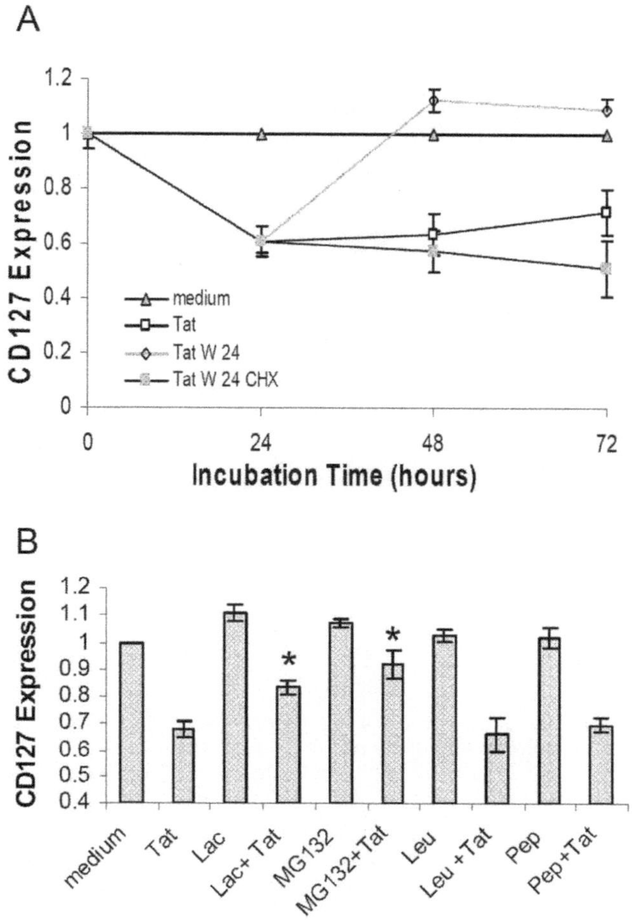

Figure 9. de novo protein synthesis is required for recovery of CD127 surface expression on CD4 T-cells following Tat-induced down regulation. Purified CD4 T-cells from healthy HIV-negative volunteers (n = 4) were incubated in medium alone or with Tat protein (10 μg/ml). (A) After 24 hours, cells incubated with Tat were washed twice and resuspended in fresh medium alone (Tat W 24) or in medium plus 100 μM CHX (Tat W 24 CHX). Cells were analyzed for CD127 surface expression by flow cytometry at the times indicated. (B) Cells were pre-incubated with and without proteasome inhibitors (5 μM MG132, 10 μM Lactacystin) and lysosome inhibitors (10 μM Leupeptin, 10 μg/ml Pepstatin) for 1 hour followed by incubation with 10 μg/ml Tat protein. After 24 hours, CD127 surface expression was measured by flow cytometry. The changes relative to medium controls are shown (mean values ± SEM). * denotes p value less than 0.05 compared to Tat treated control.

expression of the anti-apoptotic molecule B cell leukemia/lymphoma 2 (Bcl-2) [50,51]. Because Tat protein down regulates the IL-7 receptor alpha-chain on the surface of CD4 T-cells, we wanted to determine whether this effect was functionally significant. To investigate this, purified CD4 T cells were pre-incubated in RPMI-20 alone or with Tat protein (10 μg/ml) for 48 hours and then stimulated with IL-7 (10 ng/ml). While IL-7 as expected induced the expression of Bcl-2, pre-incubation with Tat protein significantly blunted IL-7's effect. The cells pre-incubated with Tat protein before administration of IL-7 showed diminished up regulation of Bcl-2 as demonstrated by mean channel fluorescence of Bcl-2 positive stained cells. The maximum effect is a 25% decrease in the MCF from cells treated with IL-7 alone compared to cells pretreated with Tat protein followed by IL-7 that was statistically significant (pvalue = 0.04) (Figure 11).

Discussion

HIV-1 influences T-cell function and homeostasis throughout the course of infection leading to quantitative effects within the CD4 T-cell population and qualitative effects in both CD4 and CD8 T cells. Homeostatic maintenance within the CD4 T cell population is largely dependent upon IL-7 signaling. IL-7 prolongs T cell survival through induction of the anti-apoptotic factors Bcl-2 and Bcl-xL as well as inhibition of the pro-apoptotic factors Bad and Bax [15]. IL-7, in combination with IL-15, has also been

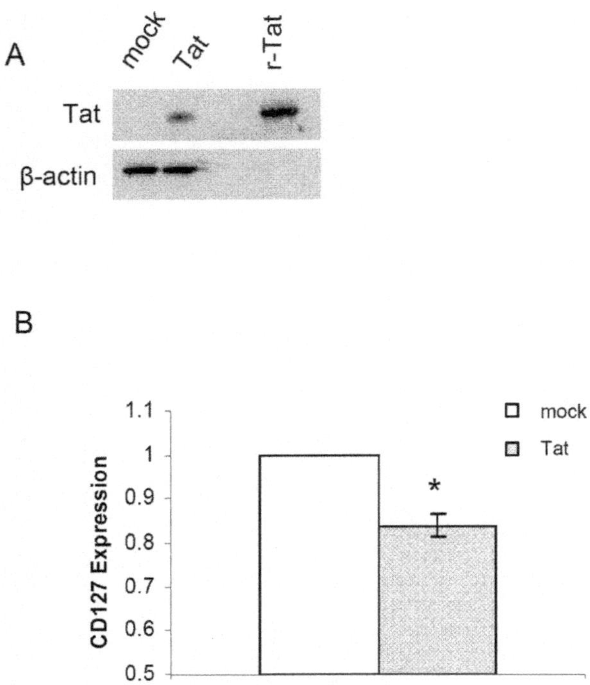

Figure 10. Endogenous production of Tat protein within CD4 T-cells prevents recovery of CD127 on the cell surface. Isolated CD4 T cells were stimulated with anti-CD3/anti-CD28 beads for 24 hours and then nucleofected with either pcDNA3.1$^{(-)}$ empty vector (mock) or pcDNA3.1$^{(-)}$ expressing Tat. (A) Tat protein expression was confirmed by western blot analysis. Cell lysates were prepared 24 hours following transfection, separated by SDS-PAGE and then analyzed by Western for Tat expression using α-Tat antibodies (clone 1102-Immunodiagnostics). Beta-actin was used as a loading control and purified recombinant Tat (r-Tat) was included to confirm the size and identity of endogenously expressed Tat protein. (B) Surface CD127 expression on CD4 T cells was measured after 24 hours by flow cytometry. Percent change in CD127 expression relative to empty pcDNA3.1$^{(-)}$ control is shown (n = 4; mean values ± SEM). * denotes p value less than 0.05 compared to mock control.

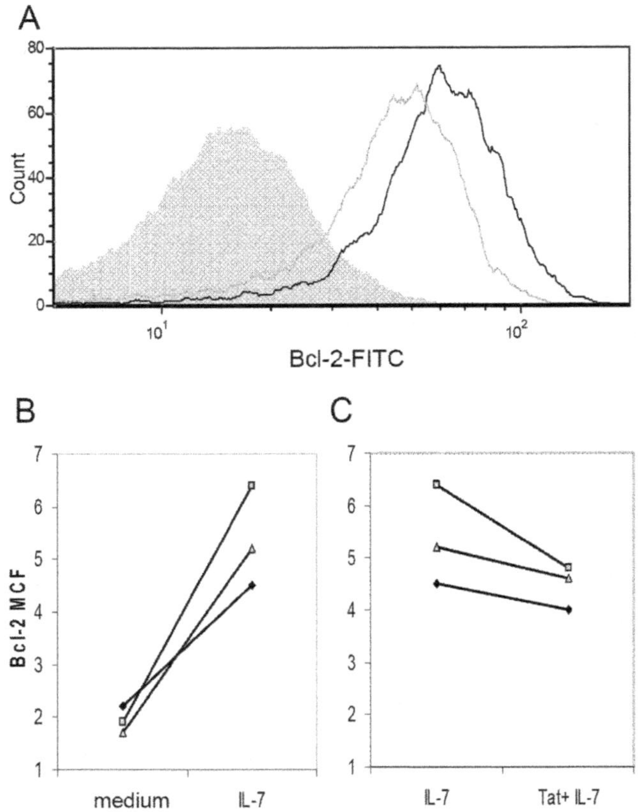

Figure 11. Soluble HIV-1 Tat protein inhibits IL-7 induced Bcl-2 expression in CD4 T-cells. Purified CD4 T-cells from healthy HIV-negative volunteers were pre-incubated in medium alone or in medium containing Tat protein (10 μg/ml) for 48 hours. Cells were then stimulated with IL-7 (10 ng/ml) for an additional 72 hours and then fixed, stained for Bcl-2 expression and analyzed by flow cytometry. (A) Representative flow cytometry histogram showing Bcl-2 expression in untreated CD4 T-cells (grey fill), following IL-7 stimulation (black line), and following IL-7 stimulation of Tat pre-treated cells (grey line). (B, C) Bcl-2 expression as measured by mean channel fluorescence (MCF) in (B) CD4 T cells treated with IL-7 compared to medium controls, and (C) cells pre-incubated in medium or with Tat prior to IL-7 stimulation (n = 5).

shown to initiate proliferation in human memory CD4 T cells and its absence results in substantial depletion and lack of regeneration in this lymphocyte population [18]. IL-7 is also important in T-cell development [52] and initiation of cellular responses [53,54].

IL-7 signaling is dependent upon heterodimerization of the IL-7 receptor complex consisting of the subunits CD132 and CD127 [55]. Down regulation of CD127 surface expression on CD4 and CD8 T-cells is associated with HIV infection [22,24,26,27]. Viremia results in increased plasma IL-7 levels [56,57] which are inversely correlated with CD4 T-cell counts during HIV infection [9]. The decreased expression of CD127 on CD4 and CD8 T-cells in HIV+ patients results in poor responses to IL-7 including decreased induction of anti-apoptotic factors [28] and CD25 expression [58]. Reduced CD127 expression and subsequent impaired IL-7 signaling would be expected to have significant effects on T-cell homeostasis and function.

Tat is secreted by infected CD4+ cells and can affect the function of uninfected neighboring bystander cells [32]. We have shown previously that soluble Tat protein specifically down regulates CD127 expression on the surface of CD8 T-cells. Tat is initially internalized by CD8 T cells via endocytosis, exits the endosome through a process dependent upon the usual acidification of these vesicles, and then localizes to the inner leaflet of the cell membrane where it associates with the cytoplasmic tail of CD127 inducing receptor clustering, internalization and subsequent proteosomal degradation [41]. This loss of CD127 expression leads to inhibition of CD8 T-cell proliferation and perforin synthesis which normally follow IL-7 stimulation.

We show here that the HIV Tat protein also down regulates CD127 on the surface of CD4 T cells. This in addition to its effect on CD8 T cells expands the range of influence for this soluble accessory viral protein. Tat's effect on CD127 surface expression is similar comparing CD4 and CD8 T-cells, is dose- and time-dependent, is reversible, and is not the result of nonspecific T cell activation, necrosis or apoptosis. Furthermore, Tat selectively down regulates CD127 leaving the common Υ-chain (CD132) and a number of other surface markers unaffected. We also demonstrated the specificity of Tat's effect on CD127 with both heparin and anti-Tat antibodies. These experiments further indicate the effect is not due to bacterial contaminates in the Tat protein preparation. Finally we also showed Tat dependant down regulation of CD127 has a functional impact on CD4 T cells, and compromises IL-7 dependant up regulation of Bcl-2. The very similar effect of Tat on CD127 expression in both CD4 and CD8 T cells suggests a likely common mechanism. Whether this mechanism operates in other lymphocyte populations expressing the IL-7 receptor is a matter of speculation. However, the fact that Tat has been shown to have the opposite effect and up regulates CD127 on monocyte-derived macrophages [60] suggests this viral protein may exert it effect through cell-specific signaling pathways.

CD4 T cells are infected by HIV and we show here endogenously produced Tat protein also down regulates CD127 expression. However, since only 0.2% of CD4 T cells in the peripheral circulation are infected, release of Tat from infected cells and the ability of soluble Tat to down regulate CD127 on bystander cells extends the influence of this HIV accessory protein on the CD4 T cell population. Down regulation of CD127 and the resultant decrease in IL-7 signaling in turn leads to reduced expression of the anti-apoptotic protein Bcl-2. Through this mechanism Tat is able to disrupt CD4 T cell homeostasis. Indeed, recent studies have shown that naïve CD4 T-cells that are not productively infected are destroyed by innate immune cells through type 1 interferon activation of caspase-1 [7,8]. By this process, abortive infection causes accumulation of incomplete HIV DNA transcripts, leading to interferon type 1 activation of caspase-1 resulting in cell death by pyroptosis, a highly inflammatory form of apoptosis [7,8]. It is possible that lower expression of CD127 induced at least in part by HIV-1 Tat protein contributes to this destructive process by making cells more susceptible to cell death through down regulation of Bcl-2.

While free Tat protein has been measured in the blood plasma of HIV-infected individuals at concentrations ranging 4–550 nM [33,59], we have used considerably higher concentrations (10 μg/mL or 670 μM) in our in vitro experiments. Considerable caution, however, should be exercised when comparing in vivo fluids to in vitro assays. First, the Tat protein used in our experiments is recombinant protein produced in *E coli* and as such is not post-translationally modified. Tat is acetylated in eukaryotic cells at Lys28 and Lys50 and these modifications have been shown to enhance Tat activity in transcription assays [60,61]. Further, protein produced in *E coli* and purified over columns is unlikely to retain 100% biological activity. Clearly, in vivo concentrations of post-translationally modified Tat secreted from neighboring HIV-infected CD4 cells and in vitro concentrations of recombinant Tat protein purified in the laboratory from *E. coli* may not be comparable. In addition to these considerations, the micro-environment in vivo is distinct from that in vitro. Indeed, the concentration of Tat in primary and secondary lymphoid tissue is unknown but given lymphoid tissues contain the highest concentration of actively infected CD4 cells [62,63,64,65], it is likely the concentration of extracellular Tat in the lymphoid microenvironment is considerably higher than that of peripheral blood. In addition, Tat is not only trapped by cell surface glycans in the extracellular matrix [66] but is also rapidly taken up by neighboring cells in blood and lymphoid tissue. Thus the amount of free Tat measured in blood plasma may be only a fraction of the Tat protein available to cells in vivo. Finally, cell-cell interactions in vivo that allow efficient transfer of Tat protein from HIV-infected to uninfected cells are not likely to be efficiently recapitulated in vitro.

Therapeutic advantages have been explored in regards to HIV-1 Tat. In fact, a phase I clinical trial using a Tat variant as a vaccine showed safe induction of a balanced T_h1/T_h2 immune response and anti-Tat antibody production [67]. A Phase II trial has further shown that anti-Tat vaccination increased the viability and immune function of T cells [68]. This could have occurred in part by blocking the effect that Tat has on CD127 expression. Indeed, in the present study we have shown that exogenous Tat protein decreased the IL-7 induced induction of the anti-apoptotic protein Bcl-2 (Figure 11). Thus by blocking Tat, a therapeutic anti-Tat vaccination may have been able to restore at least to some extent T cell function and homeostasis. Our data support ongoing research in this area and the further development and investigation of anti-Tat vaccines.

Author Contributions

Conceived and designed the experiments: EF DM PM. Performed the experiments: DM EF SS. Analyzed the data: DM EF SS. Contributed reagents/materials/analysis tools: PM. Wrote the paper: DM EF PM.

References

1. Embretson J, Zupancic M, Beneke J, Till M, Wolinsky S, et al. (1993) Analysis of human immunodeficiency virus-infected tissues by amplification and in situ hybridization reveals latent and permissive infections at single-cell resolution. Proc Natl Acad Sci U S A 90: 357–361.
2. Chun TW, Carruth L, Finzi D, Shen X, DiGiuseppe JA, et al. (1997) Quantification of latent tissue reservoirs and total body viral load in HIV-1 infection. Nature 387: 183–188.
3. Clark DR, de Boer RJ, Wolthers KC, Miedema F (1999) T cell dynamics in HIV-1 infection. Adv Immunol 73: 301–327.
4. Hazenberg MD, Hamann D, Schuitemaker H, Miedema F (2000) T cell depletion in HIV-1 infection: how CD4+ T cells go out of stock. Nat Immunol 1: 285–289.
5. McCune JM (2001) The dynamics of CD4+ T-cell depletion in HIV disease. Nature 410: 974–979.
6. Fevrier M, Dorgham K, Rebollo A (2011) CD4+ T cell depletion in human immunodeficiency virus (HIV) infection: role of apoptosis. Viruses 3: 586–612.
7. Doitsh G, Galloway NL, Geng X, Yang Z, Monroe KM, et al. (2014) Cell death by pyroptosis drives CD4 T-cell depletion in HIV-1 infection. Nature 505: 509–514.
8. Monroe KM, Yang Z, Johnson JR, Geng X, Doitsh G, et al. (2014) IFI16 DNA sensor is required for death of lymphoid CD4 T cells abortively infected with HIV. Science 343: 428–432.
9. Sasson SC, Zaunders JJ, Kelleher AD (2006) The IL-7/IL-7 receptor axis: understanding its central role in T-cell homeostasis and the challenges facing its utilization as a novel therapy. Curr Drug Targets 7: 1571–1582.
10. Welch PA, Namen AE, Goodwin RG, Armitage R, Cooper MD (1989) Human IL-7: a novel T cell growth factor. J Immunol 143: 3562–3567.
11. Armitage RJ, Namen AE, Sassenfeld HM, Grabstein KH (1990) Regulation of human T cell proliferation by IL-7. J Immunol 144: 938–941.
12. Westermann J, Aicher A, Qin Z, Cayeux Z, Daemen K, et al. (1998) Retroviral interleukin-7 gene transfer into human dendritic cells enhances T cell activation. Gene Ther 5: 264–271.
13. Soares MV, Borthwick NJ, Maini MK, Janossy G, Salmon M, et al. (1998) IL-7-dependent extrathymic expansion of CD45RA+ T cells enables preservation of a naive repertoire. J Immunol 161: 5909–5917.
14. Jiang Q, Li WQ, Hofmeister RR, Young HA, Hodge DR, et al. (2004) Distinct regions of the interleukin-7 receptor regulate different Bcl2 family members. Mol Cell Biol 24: 6501–6513.
15. Mazzucchelli R, Durum SK (2007) Interleukin-7 receptor expression: intelligent design. Nat Rev Immunol 7: 144–154.
16. Sudo T, Nishikawa S, Ohno N, Akiyama N, Tamakoshi M, et al. (1993) Expression and function of the interleukin 7 receptor in murine lymphocytes. Proc Natl Acad Sci U S A 90: 9125–9129.
17. Tan JT, Dudl E, LeRoy E, Murray R, Sprent J, et al. (2001) IL-7 is critical for homeostatic proliferation and survival of naive T cells. Proc Natl Acad Sci U S A 98: 8732–8737.
18. Kondrack RM, Harbertson J, Tan JT, McBreen ME, Surh CD, et al. (2003) Interleukin 7 regulates the survival and generation of memory CD4 cells. J Exp Med 198: 1797–1806.
19. Boutboul F, Puthier D, Appay V, Pelle O, Ait-Mohand H, et al. (2005) Modulation of interleukin-7 receptor expression characterizes differentiation of CD8 T cells specific for HIV, EBV and CMV. Aids 19: 1981–1986.
20. Colle JH, Moreau JL, Fontanet A, Lambotte O, Joussemet M, et al. (2006) CD127 expression and regulation are altered in the memory CD8 T cells of HIV-infected patients–reversal by highly active anti-retroviral therapy (HAART). Clin Exp Immunol 143: 398–403.
21. Koesters SA, Alimonti JB, Wachihi C, Matu L, Anzala O, et al. (2006) IL-7Ralpha expression on CD4(+) T lymphocytes decreases with HIV disease progression and inversely correlates with immune activation. Eur J Immunol 36: 336–344.

22. MacPherson PA, Fex C, Sanchez-Dardon J, Hawley-Foss N, Angel JB (2001) Interleukin-7 receptor expression on CD8(+) T cells is reduced in HIV infection and partially restored with effective antiretroviral therapy. J Acquir Immune Defic Syndr 28: 454–457.
23. Mercier F, Boulassel MR, Yassine-Diab B, Tremblay C, Bernard NF, et al. (2008) Persistent human immunodeficiency virus-1 antigenaemia affects the expression of interleukin-7Ralpha on central and effector memory CD4+ and CD8+ T cell subsets. Clin Exp Immunol 152: 72–80.
24. Paiardini M, Cervasi B, Albrecht H, Muthukumar A, Dunham R, et al. (2005) Loss of CD127 expression defines an expansion of effector CD8+ T cells in HIV-infected individuals. J Immunol 174: 2900–2909.
25. Rethi B, Fluur C, Atlas A, Krzyzowska M, Mowafi F, et al. (2005) Loss of IL-7Ralpha is associated with CD4 T-cell depletion, high interleukin-7 levels and CD28 down-regulation in HIV infected patients. Aids 19: 2077–2086.
26. Sasson SC, Zaunders JJ, Zanetti G, King EM, Merlin KM, et al. (2006) Increased plasma interleukin-7 level correlates with decreased CD127 and Increased CD132 extracellular expression on T cell subsets in patients with HIV-1 infection. J Infect Dis 193: 505–514.
27. Faller EM, McVey MJ, Kakal JA, MacPherson PA (2006) Interleukin-7 receptor expression on CD8 T-cells is downregulated by the HIV Tat protein. J Acquir Immune Defic Syndr 43: 257–269.
28. Vingerhoets J, Bisalinkumi E, Penne G, Colebunders R, Bosmans E, et al. (1998) Altered receptor expression and decreased sensitivity of T-cells to the stimulatory cytokines IL-2, IL-7 and IL-12 in HIV infection. Immunol Lett 61: 53–61.
29. Pugliese A, Vidotto V, Beltramo T, Petrini S, Torre D (2005) A review of HIV-1 Tat protein biological effects. Cell Biochem Funct 23: 223–227.
30. Huigen MC, Kamp W, Nottet HS (2004) Multiple effects of HIV-1 trans-activator protein on the pathogenesis of HIV-1 infection. Eur J Clin Invest 34: 57–66.
31. Frankel AD, Pabo CO (1988) Cellular uptake of the tat protein from human immunodeficiency virus. Cell 55: 1189–1193.
32. Ensoli B, Buonaguro L, Barillari G, Fiorelli V, Gendelman R, et al. (1993) Release, uptake, and effects of extracellular human immunodeficiency virus type 1 Tat protein on cell growth and viral transactivation. J Virol 67: 277–287.
33. Poggi A, Carosio R, Fenoglio D, Brenci S, Murdaca G, et al. (2004) Migration of V delta 1 and V delta 2 T cells in response to CXCR3 and CXCR4 ligands in healthy donors and HIV-1-infected patients: competition by HIV-1 Tat. Blood 103: 2205–2213.
34. Helland DE, Welles JL, Caputo A, Haseltine WA (1991) Transcellular transactivation by the human immunodeficiency virus type 1 tat protein. J Virol 65: 4547–4549.
35. Fittipaldi A, Giacca M (2005) Transcellular protein transduction using the Tat protein of HIV-1. Adv Drug Deliv Rev 57: 597–608.
36. Rusnati M, Coltrini D, Oreste P, Zoppetti G, Albini A, et al. (1997) Interaction of HIV-1 Tat protein with heparin. Role of the backbone structure, sulfation, and size. J Biol Chem 272: 11313–11320.
37. Tyagi M, Rusnati M, Presta M, Giacca M (2001) Internalization of HIV-1 tat requires cell surface heparan sulfate proteoglycans. J Biol Chem 276: 3254–3261.
38. Ferrari A, Pellegrini V, Arcangeli C, Fittipaldi A, Giacca M, et al. (2003) Caveolae-mediated internalization of extracellular HIV-1 tat fusion proteins visualized in real time. Mol Ther 8: 284–294.
39. Fittipaldi A, Ferrari A, Zoppe M, Arcangeli C, Pellegrini V, et al. (2003) Cell membrane lipid rafts mediate caveolar endocytosis of HIV-1 Tat fusion proteins. J Biol Chem 278: 34141–34149.
40. Vendeville A, Rayne F, Bonhoure A, Bettache N, Montcourrier P, et al. (2004) HIV-1 Tat enters T cells using coated pits before translocating from acidified endosomes and eliciting biological responses. Mol Biol Cell 15: 2347–2360.
41. Faller EM, Sugden SM, McVey MJ, Kakal JA, MacPherson PA (2010) Soluble HIV Tat protein removes the IL-7 receptor alpha-chain from the surface of resting CD8 T cells and targets it for degradation. J Immunol 185: 2854–2866.
42. Albini A, Benelli R, Presta M, Rusnati M, Ziche M, et al. (1996) HIV-tat protein is a heparin-binding angiogenic growth factor. Oncogene 12: 289–297.
43. Li CJ, Friedman DJ, Wang C, Metelev V, Pardee AB (1995) Induction of apoptosis in uninfected lymphocytes by HIV-1 Tat protein. Science 268: 429–431.
44. Dabrowska A, Kim N, Aldovini A (2008) Tat-induced FOXO3a is a key mediator of apoptosis in HIV-1-infected human CD4+ T lymphocytes. J Immunol 181: 8460–8477.
45. Gibellini D, Re MC, Ponti C, Maldini C, Celeghini C, et al. (2001) HIV-1 Tat protects CD4+ Jurkat T lymphoblastoid cells from apoptosis mediated by TNF-related apoptosis-inducing ligand. Cell Immunol 207: 89–99.
46. Koesters SA, Alimonti JB, Wachihi C, Matu L, Anzala O, et al. (2006) IL-7Ralpha expression on CD4+ T lymphocytes decreases with HIV disease progression and inversely correlates with immune activation. Eur J Immunol 36: 336–344.
47. Dunham RM, Cervasi B, Brenchley JM, Albrecht H, Weintrob A, et al. (2008) CD127 and CD25 expression defines CD4+ T cell subsets that are differentially depleted during HIV infection. J Immunol 180: 5582–5592.
48. Schluns KS, Lefrancois L (2003) Cytokine control of memory T-cell development and survival. Nat Rev Immunol 3: 269–279.
49. Benito JM, Lopez M, Lozano S, Gonzalez-Lahoz J, Soriano V (2008) Down-regulation of interleukin-7 receptor (CD127) in HIV infection is associated with T cell activation and is a main factor influencing restoration of CD4(+) cells after antiretroviral therapy. J Infect Dis 198: 1466–1473.
50. Golden-Mason L, Burton JR Jr, Castelblanco N, Klarquist J, Benlloch S, et al. (2006) Loss of IL-7 receptor alpha-chain (CD127) expression in acute HCV infection associated with viral persistence. Hepatology 44: 1098–1109.
51. von Freeden-Jeffry U, Solvason N, Howard M, Murray R (1997) The earliest T lineage-committed cells depend on IL-7 for Bcl-2 expression and normal cell cycle progression. Immunity 7: 147–154.
52. Namen AE, Lupton S, Hjerrild K, Wignall J, Mochizuki DY, et al. (1988) Stimulation of B-cell progenitors by cloned murine interleukin-7. Nature 333: 571–573.
53. Alderson MR, Sassenfeld HM, Widmer MB (1990) Interleukin 7 enhances cytolytic T lymphocyte generation and induces lymphokine-activated killer cells from human peripheral blood. J Exp Med 172: 577–587.
54. Jicha DL, Mule JJ, Rosenberg SA (1991) Interleukin 7 generates antitumor cytotoxic T lymphocytes against murine sarcomas with efficacy in cellular adoptive immunotherapy. J Exp Med 174: 1511–1515.
55. Goodwin RG, Friend D, Ziegler SF, Jerzy R, Falk BA, et al. (1990) Cloning of the human and murine interleukin-7 receptors: demonstration of a soluble form and homology to a new receptor superfamily. Cell 60: 941–951.
56. Albuquerque AS, Cortesao CS, Foxall RB, Soares RS, Victorino RM, et al. (2007) Rate of increase in circulating IL-7 and loss of IL-7Ralpha expression differ in HIV-1 and HIV-2 infections: two lymphopenic diseases with similar hyperimmune activation but distinct outcomes. J Immunol 178: 3252–3259.
57. Beq S, Rannou MT, Fontanet A, Delfraissy JF, Theze J, et al. (2004) HIV infection: pre-highly active antiretroviral therapy IL-7 plasma levels correlate with long-term CD4 cell count increase after treatment. AIDS 18: 563–565.
58. Colle JH, Moreau JL, Fontanet A, Lambotte O, Joussemet M, et al. (2006) Regulatory dysfunction of the interleukin-7 receptor in CD4 and CD8 lymphocytes from HIV-infected patients–effects of antiretroviral therapy. J Acquir Immune Defic Syndr 42: 277–285.
59. Westendorp MO, Frank R, Ochsenbauer C, Stricker K, Dhein J, et al. (1995) Sensitization of T cells to CD95-mediated apoptosis by HIV-1 Tat and gp120. Nature 375: 497–500.
60. Col E, Caron C, Seigneurin-Berny D, Gracia J, Favier A, et al. (2001) The histone acetyltransferase, hGCN5, interacts with and acetylates the HIV transactivator, Tat. J Biol Chem 276: 28179–28184.
61. Kiernan RE, Vanhulle C, Schiltz L, Adam E, Xiao H, et al. (1999) HIV-1 tat transcriptional activity is regulated by acetylation. EMBO J 18: 6106–6118.
62. Di Mascio M, Paik CH, Carrasquillo JA, Maeng JS, Jang BS, et al. (2009) Noninvasive in vivo imaging of CD4 cells in simian-human immunodeficiency virus (SHIV)-infected nonhuman primates. Blood 114: 328–337.
63. Goonetilleke N, Liu MK, Salazar-Gonzalez JF, Ferrari G, Giorgi E, et al. (2009) The first T cell response to transmitted/founder virus contributes to the control of acute viremia in HIV-1 infection. J Exp Med 206: 1253–1272.
64. Lerner P, Guadalupe M, Donovan R, Hung J, Flamm J, et al. The gut mucosal viral reservoir in HIV-infected patients is not the major source of rebound plasma viremia following interruption of highly active antiretroviral therapy. J Virol 85: 4772–4782.
65. Vanderford TH, Bleckwehl C, Engram JC, Dunham RM, Klatt NR, et al. Viral CTL escape mutants are generated in lymph nodes and subsequently become fixed in plasma and rectal mucosa during acute SIV infection of macaques. PLoS Pathog 7: e1002048.
66. Chang HC, Samaniego F, Nair BC, Buonaguro L, Ensoli B (1997) HIV-1 Tat protein exits from cells via a leaderless secretory pathway and binds to extracellular matrix-associated heparan sulfate proteoglycans through its basic region. Aids 11: 1421–1431.
67. Bellino S, Francavilla V, Longo O, Tripiciano A, Paniccia G, et al. (2009) Parallel conduction of the phase I preventive and therapeutic trials based on the Tat vaccine candidate. Rev Recent Clin Trials 4: 195–204.
68. Ensoli B, Bellino S, Tripiciano A, Longo O, Francavilla V, et al. (2010) Therapeutic immunization with HIV-1 Tat reduces immune activation and loss of regulatory T-cells and improves immune function in subjects on HAART. PLoS One 5: e13540.

13

Invariant Natural Killer T (iNKT) Cells in HAART-Treated, HIV-Positive Patients with Bone and Cardiovascular Impairment

Camilla Tincati[1], Matteo Basilissi[1], Elisabetta Sinigaglia[2], Esther Merlini[1], Giovanni Carpani[2], Antonella d'Arminio Monforte[1], Giulia Marchetti[1]*

1 Department of Health Sciences, Clinic of Infectious Diseases and Tropical Medicine, "San Paolo" Hospital, University of Milan, Milan, Italy, **2** Blood Transfusion Unit, "San Paolo" Hospital, Milan, Italy

Abstract

Background: Invariant Natural Killer T (iNKT) cells represent a determinant in the course of infections and diseases, however, their role in the pathogenesis of non-infectious co-morbidities in HIV-positive patients is unknown.

Methods: Flow cytometry was used to investigate iNKT cell frequency, phenotype and function in HIV-infected patients on HAART with bone and/or cardiovascular disorders and in HIV-positive controls free from co-morbidities.

Results: iNKT cells from subjects with bone and cardiovascular impairment expressed high levels of CD161 and predominantly secreted TNF. iNKT cells from individuals with bone disease alone did not show any distinctive phenotypical or functional characteristics. The functional capacity of iNKT cells in patients with cardiovascular disorder was impaired with no cytokine release upon stimulation.

Conclusion: iNKT cells may have a role in non-infectious co-morbidities in treated HIV disease, possibly through the exacerbation of inflammation. Further studies are needed to investigate iNKT cells in the pathogenesis of non-communicable disorders in HIV infection.

Editor: Derya Unutmaz, New York University, United States of America

Funding: Grants from Italian Ministry of Health (GR-2009-1592029) and the Fellowship Program 2012 (9Ab87b2822). The funders had no role in study design, data collection and analysis, decision to publish, or preparation of the manuscript.

Competing Interests: The authors have declared that no competing interests exist.

* Email: giulia.marchetti@unimi.it

Introduction

HIV-positive patients on virologically-suppressive treatment are at risk of non-infectious co-morbidities [1]. Indeed, HIV infection is characterized by a state of persistent inflammation/immune activation [2–4] known to predict clinical progression [5–8]; such abnormalities are a distinctive characteristic of a senescent immune system [9] which may accelerate the aging process in the HIV-infected population [10–12]. In keeping with these observations, HIV-positive patients with reduced Bone Mineral Density (BMD) have been shown to feature a hyperactivated peripheral T-cell phenotype [13]; similarly, HIV-infected subjects with increased carotid Intima Media Thickness (IMT) and/or positive history for cardiovascular disease show expansion of activated CD8+CD38+ cells [14–17]. Most interestingly, T-cell activation has been described an independent risk factor for osteopenia/osteoporosis [13] and subclinical carotid abnormalities [17,18].

While T-cell and monocyte activation has been extensively investigated in the setting of non-infectious co-morbidities in course of treated HIV disease and postulated as a possible marker of "immunosenescence" in this patient population, very few studies have investigated the role of other lymphoid cells in the pathogenesis of non-infectious co-morbidities in HIV-infected subjects.

Invariant natural killer T (iNKT) cells are a rare population of T cells that possess qualities of both the innate and adaptive arms of the immune response; iNKT cells recognize glycolipid antigens presented by the non-classical MHC molecule CD1d [19–21] and represent key components in the pathogenesis of many clinical conditions [22–30].

Frequency and function of iNKT cells are impaired in the course of HIV disease [31–35]. Indeed, iNKT cells express both CD4 and the CXCR4/CCR5 co-receptors, thus representing a target for the virus [36]. Accordingly, the CD4+ iNKT cell subset is preferentially depleted in HIV disease [31,33,34,37] with a parallel loss of IL-4 and IFN-γ production [38] and such defects are only partially restored by HAART [38–40]. Interestingly, the production of Th1 cytokines from iNKT cells, such as IFN-γ and TNF has been inversely correlated with cell surface expression of CD161 [32], thus suggesting that this molecule may represent a marker of iNKT exhaustion in course of HIV [32].

iNKT cells have also been implicated in atherogenesis [41–43]; indeed, in the mouse model, CD4+ iNKT cells are recruited to the atherosclerotic lesions within arterial walls [44,45] and contribute to the formation of fatty streaks [45–47]. Of note, CD1d is also expressed in human atherosclerotic lesions [48,49] and lower frequencies of iNKT were found in circulating blood of patients with symptomatic atherosclerosis [49,50]. More specifically, iNKT cells infiltrating human atherosclerotic tissue express CD4, CD161 and produce IFN-γ [51] and seem to be implicated in plaque stability through the interaction with vascular smooth muscle cells [51].

Furthermore, in the mouse model, α-GalCer-activated iNKT cells have been demonstrated to increase the frequency of osteoclast progenitor cells and favour their maturation into osteclasts [52]. The pro-osteocalstogenic effect of iNKT cells is positively regulated by TNF, while IFN-γ negatively affects this process [52]. While specific iNKT subsets have been linked to overt cardiovascular disease in humans [49,50], to our knowledge, clinical findings on iNKT and osteopenia/osteoporosis in humans have yet to be described.

In this report we investigated iNKT cell frequency, phenotype and function in HIV-positive patients on virologically-suppressive HAART with bone and/or cardiovascular impairment.

Our study is the first to show that iNKT cells from HIV-infected individuals with cardiovascular and bone co-morbidities express high levels of CD161 and predominantly secrete TNF, suggesting a role in the pathogenesis of immunosenescent disorders in treated HIV infection.

Materials and Methods

Study Patients

We consecutively recruited HIV-positive patients on virologically-suppressive HAART (HIV-RNA<40 cp/ml) with available Bone Mineral Density (BMD; Dual-energy X-ray Absorptiometry-DXA) and carotid Intima Media Thickness (IMT; ultrasonography) measures for the screening of non-communicable disorders. The research has been approved by the Ethical Committee of San Paolo Hospital, Milan. All study participants provided written informed consent. All study participants provided written informed consent.

Bone disease was defined by the presence of osteopenia or osteoporosis upon DXA scan: According to WHO criteria, osteopenia and osteoporosis were defined by T-scores at the lumbar spine and/or femoral neck that were <-1 SD and ≥-2.5 and <-2.5, respectively [53]. Cardiovascular disease was defined by either right and/or left carotid IMT>1 mm [54,55] or presence of a carotid plaque upon ultrasonographic evaluation.

On the basis of lumbar/femoral BMD and carotid IMT values, patients were divided into the following 4 groups: a) Double Positive (DP) patients with both bone and cardiovascular impairment (n = 10); subjects with Bone Disease (BD) (n = 10) or Cardiovascular Disease (CD) (n = 10) alone; Double Negative (DN) patients with neither bone nor cardiovascular disorders (n = 10).

Human Lymphocyte separation and stimulation assays

Human peripheral blood (8 mL) was collected into EDTA tubes and PBMCs were isolated using ficoll-paque (Biocoll separating solution, BIOSPA). Cells of all patients were cultured in R10 medium alone (composition per 100 mL R10:88 mL RPMI, 10 mL fetal bovine serum, 1 mL [100 UI/mL] L-glutamine, and 1 mL [100 UI/mL] penicillin/streptomycin; Euroclone, Italy) (unstimulated, US), or in medium supplemented with Phorbol 12-myristate 13-acetate (PMA, 50 ng/mL; Sigma-Aldrich, Milan, Italy)/ionomycin (500 ng/mL; Sigma-Aldrich, Milan, Italy). In a subgroup of 20 patients PBMCs were stimulated also with α-GalactosylCeramide (α-GalCer, 200 ng/mL; Enzo Life Sciences, NY, USA). Dose response curves were performed to determine the optimal concentration of both stimuli.

Flow Cytometry

Parameters for inclusion of Natural Killer T surface phenotype and functional data. As iNKT cell levels are very low in peripheral blood, particularly during HIV infection, 1 million of total events (and never less than 500,000) were acquired for each sample. Moreover, as previously performed [32] a minimum of 20 events collected within the iNKT gate was required for the data to be considered for functional data analysis.

Surface staining. For the measurement of iNKT cell frequency and CD161 expression, freshly-isolated PBMCs were incubated with CD1d-tetramer-α-GalCer-PE (α-GalCer) (Proimmune, Oxford, UK), anti-CD3-PE Cy7 (Beckman Coulter, Fullerton, California, USA), anti-CD161-FITC (Mylteni Biotec, Bologna, Italy) anti-Vα24-biotin (Beckman Coulter, Fullerton, California, USA), for 30 minutes at 4°C. Cells were then washed with buffer (PBS with 0.5% bovine serum albumin and 2 mmol/EDTA) and stained with streptavidin-Qdot 655 (Invitrogen, Carlsbad, California, USA) for 30 minutes at 4°C, in the dark. Cells were washed again and run on a FACS CANTO 2.6 cytometer (BD Bioscences, San Jose, California, USA).

Intracellular staining. For the measurement of intracellular cytokine production, a separate aliquot of PBMCs was incubated with R10 (unstimulated), PMA and ionomycin (n = 40) or α-GalCer (n = 20), as described above. After 1 h at 37°C in 5% CO_2, Brefeldin A (BRFA) (10 μg/mL; Sigma-Aldrich, Milan, Italy,) was added. After incubation for 14 h, the cells were washed and surface stained as described above, with the exception of anti-CD161. Cells were washed again and incubated with 1 mL of FACS Lysing Solutions (BD Bioscences, San Jose, California, USA) for 45 minutes at room temperature, in the dark and washed prior to intracellular staining with anti-TNF-α-FITC (BD Bioscences, San Jose, California, USA)/IFN-γ-FITC (Beckman Coulter, Fullerton, California, USA). After 30 minutes of incubation at 4°C in the dark, samples were washed, run on a FACS CANTO 2.6 cytometer and analyzed with FACS Diva 6.1.3 software.

Statistical analysis

Data were analyzed with GraphPad 5 PRISM software. Fisher's exact test, Chi-squared test, Mann-Whitney *U*-test, Kruskall-Wallis followed by Dunn's post hoc analysis and Wilcoxon tests were used for statistics. Differences were considered statistically significant at $p<0.05$.

Results

Patient characteristics

Forty HIV-positive patients with available BMD and carotid IMT measurements were consecutively recruited at the Clinic of Infectious and Tropical Diseases, San Paolo Hospital, University of Milan. Subjects were divided into the following 4 groups (Table 1): 10 Double Positive (DP) patients; 10 Bone Disease (BD); 10 Cardiovascular Disease (CD); 10 Double Negative (DN) patients (Table 1). 3 patients in the BD group were diagnosed with osteoporosis and 7 subjects in the CD group presented a carotid plaque upon ultrasonography.

Table 1. Patient characteristics.

Characteristic	DP (n = 10)	BD (n = 10)	CD (n = 10)	DN (n = 10)
Age, years (IQR)	50 (44–57)	44 (38–62)	45 (43–54)	42 (38–50)
Sex, F (%)	3 (30)	3(30)	3 (30)	5 (50)
Duration of HIV infection, mths (IQR)	82 (67–323)	96 (44–183)	198 (141–263)	189 (71–225)
HIV epidemiology, n (%)				
MSM	2 (20)	2 (20)	3 (30)	4 (40)
Heterosex	6 (60)	3 (30)	3 (30)	6 (60)
IVD use	2 (20)	3 (30)	4 (40)	0 (0)
HCV-Ab, n (%)	1 (10)	3 (30)	3 (30)	0 (0)
Nadir CD4, cells/mmc (IQR)	89 (60–222)	210 (109–362)	232 (80–280)	321 (54–397)
White blood cells (1000/mmc)	5.6 (4.7–7.9)	5.6 (5.1–6.5)[c]	6.0 (5.4–8.1)[e]	4.7 (4.5–5.6)
Neutrophils (%)	56 (48.0–64.0)	56 (50.0–59.0)	56 (49.0–68.0)	52 (45.0–64.0)
Lymphocytes (%)	32 (26.0–39.0)	34 (30.0–40.0)	37 (24.0–41.0)	34 (26.0–40.0)
Monocytes (%)	7.8 (7.2–9.1)	7.2 (6.3–8.0)	8.2 (7.7–8.8)	9 (6.8–11.4)
Eosinophils (%)	2.7 (1.6–4.1)	1.8 (1.3–2.6)	1.9 (1.4–2.6)	1.6 (1.0–3.6)
Basophils (%)	0.6 (0.4–0.6)	0.7 (0.5–0.7)	0.5 (0.4–0.6)	0.5 (0.3–0.6)
Lymphocytes (n)	1928 (1375–2049)	1862 (1332–2179)	1919 (1675–2551)	1733 (1317–2239)
Zenith HIV RNA, log10 cp/mL (IQR)	5.4 (4.6–5.9)	5.6 (4.9–5.9)	5.3 (5.2–5.7)	5.0 (4.5–5.4)
AIDS diagnosis n (%)	4 (40)	3 (30)	0 (0)	3 (30)
Current CD4 counts, cells/mmc (IQR)	515 (308–575)	583 (379–716)	570 (517–798)	532 (354–614)
Current CD4 counts, %	26 (23–30)	33 (26–39)	32 (24–39)	30 (22–40)
Current HIV RNA, log10 cp/mL (IQR)	1.59	1.59	1.59	1.59
HAART duration, mths (IQR)	72 (63–149)	88 (45–123)	164 (56–180)	76 (52–130)
HAART regimen				
PI (%)	2 (20)	3 (30)	3 (30)	6 (60)
NNRTI (%)	6 (60)	6 (60)	6 (60)	4 (40)
Other (%)	2 (20)	1 (10)	1 (10)	0 (0)
Tenofovir use (%)	7 (70)	8 (80)	8 (80)	9 (90)
DXA (IQR)				
T-score femoral neck	−1.55 (−2.00−−1.10)[a,f]	−1.80 (−2.15−−1.35)[c,d]	−0.25 (−0.90−1.35)	−0.55 (−0.95−0.80)
T-score lumbar spine	−1.75 (−2.15−−1.48)[a,f]	−2.10 (−2.73−−1.45)[c,d]	−0.25 (0.25–1.08)	0.00 (−0.25−0.43)
Carotid IMT, mm (IQR)				
Left	1.04 (0.93–1.11)[a,b]	0.82 (0.65−0.96)	1.05 (0.98–1.21)[e]	0.85 (0.80−0.93)
Right	1.05 (0.96–1.25)[a]	0.87 (0.65−0.97)[c]	1.11 (1.00–1.38)[e]	0.89 (0.83−0.91)

DP: Double Positive; BD: Bone Disease; CD: Cardiovascular Disease; DN: Double Negative. MSM: Males Who Have Sex With Males. IVD: Intravenous Drug. HCV: Hepatitis C Virus. HAART: Highly Active Antiretroviral Therapy; PI: Protease Inhibitor; NNRTI: Non-Nucleoside Retroscriptase Inhibitor. DXA: Dual-energy X-ray absorptiometry. IMT: Intima Media Thickness. Data presented as: median (interquartile range, IQR) for continuous variables; absolute number (percentage) for categorical variables. $p<0.05$: [a]DP vs DN; [b]DP vs BD; [c]BD vs DN; [d]BD vs CD; [e]CD vs DN; [f]CD vs DP.

Study subgroups were comparable in terms of demographic and HIV-related parameters (Table 1).

Differences in BMD and IMT values were registered among groups as per inclusion criteria (Table 1).

HIV-infected DP patients display high levels of CD161-expressing iNKT cells

We used a tetramer-based gating strategy (Fig. 1A) to measure iNKT cell frequencies in HIV-positive patients with bone and cardiovascular impairment (Double Positive, DP) and in HIV-infected subjects free from co-morbidities (Double Negative, DN).

The frequency of iNKT cells in peripheral blood was similar in the two patient groups (DP:.007% [IQR:.003–.021]; DN:.005% [IQR:.003–.015]; $p = .88$; Fig. 1C); interestingly, however, DP patients exhibited significantly higher CD161-expressing iNKT cells in comparison to DN patients (DP: 87.8% [IQR: 80.6–92] vs DN: 56.3% [IQR 37.4–76.1]; $p = .001$; Fig. 1D), suggesting an exhausted iNKT phenotype in HIV-infected subjects with bone and cardiovascular impairment.

HIV-positive DP patients display high TNF production from iNKT cells both constitutively and following stimulation

Given that iNKT cells are able to produce a wide range of Th1 and Th2 cytokines, we determined the functional status of circulating iNKT by measuring TNF and IFN-γ directly *ex vivo* and after stimulation with PMA/ionomycin (Figure 1E, F) and the iNKT-specific stimulus α-GalCer (Fig. 1G, H).

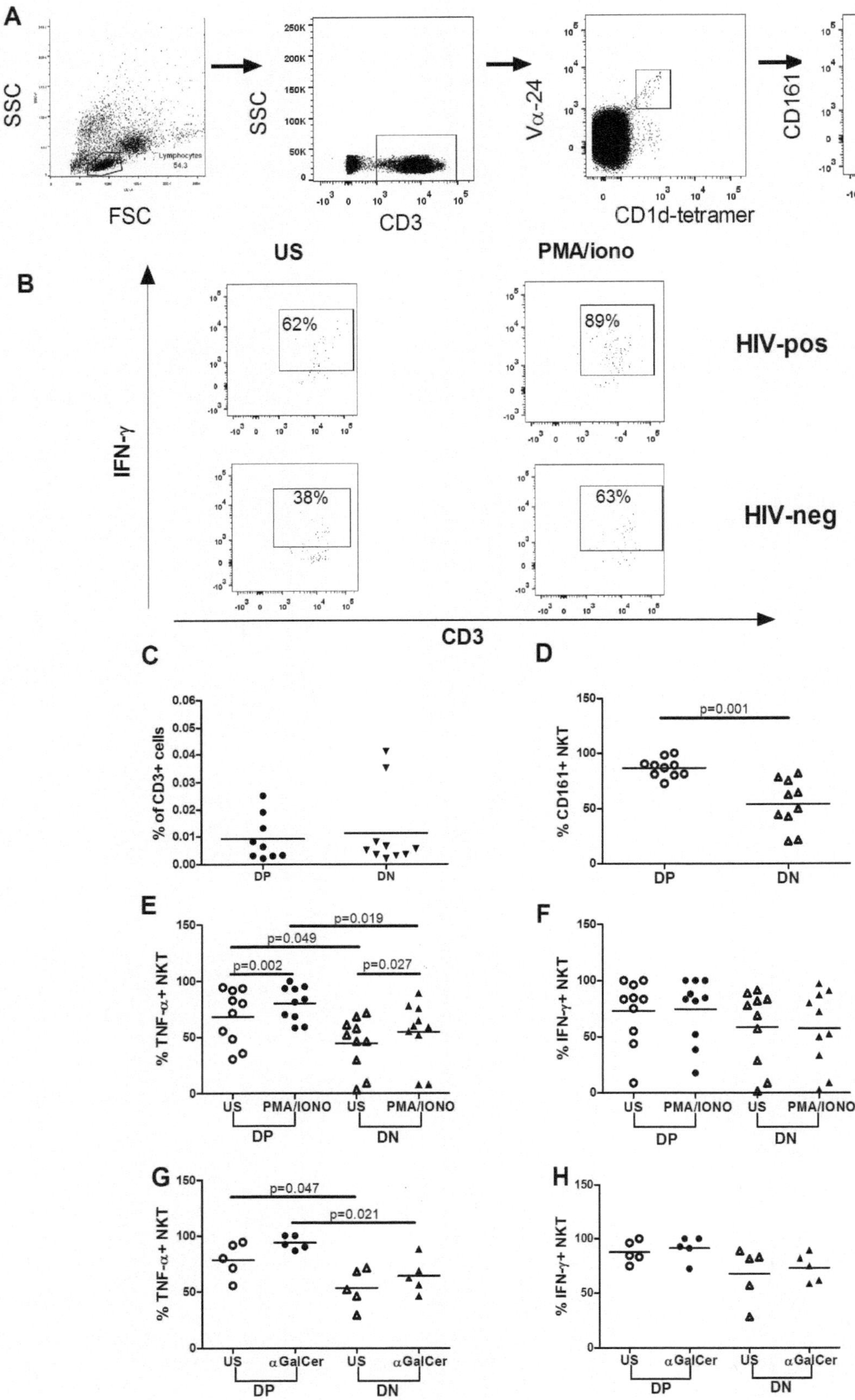

Figure 1. iNKT cell phenotype and function in HIV-positive "Double Positive" (DP) and "Double Negative" (DN) patients. Gating strategy of flow cytometry analysis for staining of iNKT cell frequencies, phenotype and intracellular cytokine production in a representative HIV-positive individual (A); an example of staining for intracellular cytokines is also shown of a representative HIV-negative subject (B). PBMCs were gated on lymphocytes, and iNKT cells were visualized as CD3+, Vα24+ and CD1d-tetramer+. An example of CD161 surface staining is shown in the far right

plot. iNKT frequency were comparable in DP and DN groups (C). iNKT cell phenotype was analyzed through the *ex vivo* expression of CD161 in DP (n = 10) and DN (n = 10) patients (D). DP subjects exhibited significantly higher levels of CD161 on iNKT cell surface compared to DN patients (p = .001). iNKT cell function was measured through the production of TNF and IFN-γ *ex vivo* (US) and following stimulation with PMA/ionomycin (n = 10 per group) (E, F) and α-GalCer (n = 5 per group) (G, H). Although DP and DN patients significantly increased TNF production upon PMA/ionomycin stimulation (p = .002 and p = .027 respectively), DP subjects showed higher TNF release both prior to (p = .049) and following PMA/ionomycin (E). Study groups exhibited similar frequencies of IFN-γ-producing iNKT cells both *ex vivo* and after stimulation with PMA/ionomycin (F). DP patients were characterized by significantly higher TNF release both prior to (p = .047) and following stimulation with α-GalCer (p = .021) (G). Similar results were obtained in terms of IFN-γ production, with a trend to higher cytokine production in DP subjects following iNKT-specific stimulation (p = .059) (H). FSC, Forward Scatter: SSC, Side Scatter. Each symbol represents an individual.

Both DP and DN patients displayed a significant increase in TNF production following PMA/ionomycin (p = .002 and p = .027 respectively; Fig. 1E). Interestingly however, DP patients showed higher, spontaneous release of TNF both prior to stimulation (75.8% [IQR: 46.3–92.1] vs 49.1% [IQR: 24.4–62.9]; p = .049; Fig. 1E) and following PMA/ionomycin stimulation (DP: 82.6% [IQR: 65.9–93.9]; DN 59.4% [IQR: 41–76.1]; p = .019; Fig. 1E).

The functional capacity of iNKT in terms of INF-γ production did not differ between groups. Indeed, neither DP nor DN patients displayed a significant response to PMA/ionomycin (DP us: 83.3% [IQR: 52.2–87.1]; DP stim: DP: 84% [IQR: 48.6–100]; p = .58; DN us: 73.3% [IQR: 24–84.7]; DN stim: 62.2% [IQR: 27.2–88]; p = .38; Fig. 1F); moreover, INF-γ release from iNKT cells was comparable between subjects both prior to (p = .24) and following PMA/ionomycin (p = .19; Fig. 1F).

Given the differences in TNF production upon PMA/ionomycin, we decided to evaluate iNKT functional capacity in response to iNKT-specific stimulation with αGalCer in 5 patients per group.

In keeping with the above mentioned findings, significantly higher spontaneous TNF release was noted in DP patients (DP: 80% [IQR: 63.5–93.1]; DN: 52% [IQR: 37.8–69.8]; p = .047; Fig. 1G), who tended to significant TNF production after α-GalCer (p = .063). Accordingly, TNF release from α-GalCer-activated iNKT cells was greater in DP subjects (DP: 92.3% [IQR: 88.3–100]; DN: 62.3% [IQR: 51.1–78.5]; p = .021; Fig. 1G).

While no differences were observed in terms of IFN-γ production upon PMA/ionomycin, a non-significant trend to higher cytokine release was noted following α-GalCer stimulation in DP compared to DN subjects (92.9% [IQR: 82–100]; 75% [IQR: 60.3–89.5] respectively; p = .059; Fig. 1G).

Taken together, these findings suggest that iNKT cells from HIV-infected patients with concurrent bone and cardiovascular disease selectively produce high levels of TNF, both constitutively and upon stimulation.

HIV-positive BD patients display normal iNKT cell frequencies and CD161 expression

Given that HIV-positive patients with bone and cardiovascular impairment present higher levels of CD161-expressing and TNF-producing iNKT cells, we aimed to investigate the phenotype and functional capacity of these cells in the two disorders separately.

We thus measured the frequency of total and CD161-expressing iNKT cells in patients with Bone Disease (BD) and compared them to patients free from co-morbidities (DN subjects).

Differently from what observed in patients with both bone and cardiovascular disease, the frequency of total (BD:.007% [IQR:.005–.019]; DN.005% [IQR:.003–.015], p = .34 Figure 2A), and CD161-expressing iNKT cells (BD: 62.3% [IQR: 50.7–90.7]; DN 56.3% [IQR 37.4–76.1]; p = .25; Fig. 2B) were comparable in the two groups.

HIV-positive BD patients display high levels of TNF and IFN-γ from iNKT cells following stimulation

The functional capacity of iNKT cells in patients with bone disease was measured through the production of TNF and IFN-γ prior to and following stimulation with PMA/ionomycin (Fig. 2C, D) and α-GalCer (Fig. 2E, F).

Both BD and DN patients displayed a significant increase in TNF-producing cells following stimulation with PMA/ionomycin (BD us: 72.8% [IQR: 48.7–77.6]; BD stim: 76.7% [IQR: 60.2–89], p = .002: see above for DN values; Fig. 2C). A non-significant trend to higher spontaneous TNF release was observed in BD patients (p = .075) with no differences between study individuals upon PMA/ionomycin (p = .11) (Fig. 2C).

In reference to IFN-γ production, BD patients alone responded significantly to PMA/ionomycin (BD us: 70.5% [IQR: 31.1–83.3], BD stim: 81.6% [IQR: 48.3–89.4]; p = .049; Fig. 2D), with no differences among groups prior to and following stimulation (Fig. 2D).

Upon iNKT-specific α-GalCer activation, BD patients displayed a non-significant trend to an increase in TNF production (BD us: 76.5% [IQR: 66.7–84]; BD stim: 87.5% [IQR: 78.2–99.1]; (p = .063), (Fig. 2E), with a tendency to higher cytokine release compared to DN subjects (p = .056; see above for DN values) (Fig. 2E). Of note, the finding of higher spontaneous TNF release in the BD patient group prior to α-GalCer stimulation which was not detected prior to PMA/ionomycin may reflect the smaller sample size in the former experimental condition (n = 5 vs n = 10, respectively) (Fig. 2E).

Similarly, BD patients were characterized by a non-significant trend to higher IFN-γ production (DB us: 83.3% [IQR: 75–88.7]; BD: stim: 87.5% [IQR: 84.1–97.1]; p = .063; Fig. 2F) with no differences in cytokine release upon specific iNKT-activation (p = .095; Fig. 2F).

Taken together, the present findings suggest that HIV-positive subjects with bone impairment, display a tendency to a more activated functional profile of iNKT cells compared to DN individuals.

HIV-positive CD patients display normal iNKT cell frequencies and CD161 expression

We next evaluated the frequency of total and CD161-expressing iNKT cells in HIV-infected patients with CD.

Similarly to what registered in patients with bone impairment alone, CD and DN subjects displayed similar iNKT frequencies (CD: 0.004% [IQR: 0.002–0.005]; see above for DN values p = .17: Figure 2G) and proportion of CD161-expressing cells (CD: 47.1% [IQR: 41–79.5]; see above for DN values p = 1.0) (Fig. 2H).

HIV-positive CD patients display a highly activated and functionally exhausted iNKT-cell phenotype

iNKT cell function was measured *ex vivo* and following PMA/ionomycin (Fig. 2I, J) and α-GalCer stimulation (Fig. 2K, L).

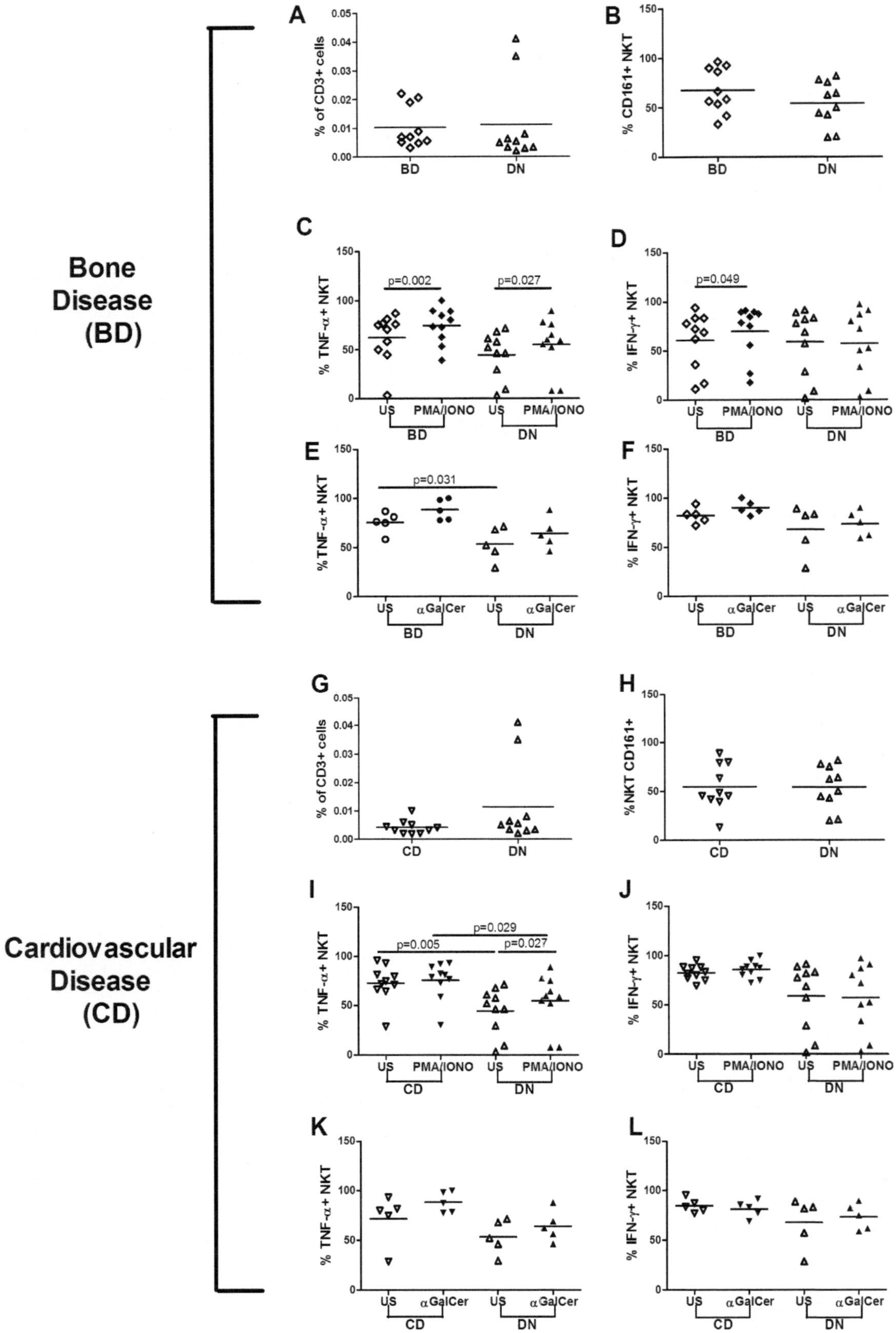

Figure 2. iNKT cell phenotype and function in HIV-positive "Bone Disease" (BD), "Cardiovascular Disease" (CD) and "Double Negative" (DN) patients. iNKT frequency was comparable among BD and DN groups (A). BD (n = 10) and DN (n = 10) showed similar CD161-expressing iNKT cell frequencies (B) and a significant increase in TNF production following PMA/ionomycin stimulation (p = .002 and p = .027 respectively). Despite a trend to higher spontaneous TNF release in BD patients (p = .075), comparable cytokine levels were recorded upon PMA/

ionomycin (C). BD patients alone responded to PMA/ionomycin with significant IFN-γ production following stimulation (p = .0488) (D). Significantly higher TNF production was detected in BD subjects (p = .031) prior to α-GalCer stimulation. Upon α-GalCer stimulation, BD patients displayed a trend to significant increases in TNF release (p = .063), leading to higher cytokine levels in this population (p = .056) (E). No significant differences were noted in terms of IFN-γ production following α-GalCer, although BD patients tended to significant cytokine production (p = .063) (F). CD and DN showed comparable iNKT cell frequencies (G). CD (n = 10) and DN (n = 10) showed similar CD161-expressing iNKT cell frequencies (H). CD subjects showed higher TNF release both prior to (p = .005) and following stimulation with PMA/ionomycin (p = .029). Of note, DN patients alone responded to stimulation by significantly increasing TNF release from iNKT cells aspecific stimulation (p = .027) (I). In keeping with these results, the CD group displayed a trend to higher IFN-γ release after PMA/ionomycin stimulation (p = .052) (J). No statistical differences were noted between groups in terms of iNKT function following specific activation with α-GalCer (K, L). Horizontal lines indicate median values. Each symbol represents an individual.

Compared to DN subjects, patients with CD presented significantly higher TNF levels both prior to (CD us: 73.7% [IQR: 66.2–84.7]; DN see above; p = .005; Fig. 2I) and following mitogen stimulation (CD post PMA/ionomycin: 80.2% [IQR: 69.6–90.2]; DN see above p = .029; Fig. 2I). Of note however, healthy patients alone were able to induce significant TNF release upon PMA/ionomycin, suggesting a highly activated and exhausted iNKT phenotype in HIV-patients with cardiovascular disease.

Similarly, CD patients presented a non-significant trend to higher post-stimulation IFN-γ production from iNKT cells (86.9% [IQR: 79.3–90.8]; p = .052; Fig. 2J; see above for DN values) despite similar spontaneous cytokine release between groups (CD: 82.85% [IQR: 76.7–88.3]; see above for DN values p = .15; Fig. 2J).

The study of the functional capacity of iNKT cells following specific stimulation with α-GalCer revealed comparable TNF and IFN-γ production between subjects in all experimental conditions (Fig. 2K, 2L).

Discussion

The objective of the present study was to assess whether HIV-positive individuals on virologically-suppressive HAART with bone and cardiovascular co-morbidities are characterized by specific iNKT cell phenotype and function.

The key finding of our analysis is the expansion of CD161-expressing and, TNF-secreting iNKT cells in subjects with coexisting bone and cardiovascular impairment; a less clear iNKT fingerprint was found in patients affected by single co-morbidities.

HIV-related T-lymphocyte activation has been postulated as a possible driving force of premature osteopenia/osteoporosis [13] and coronary heart disease [14–18]. HIV infection is also featured by impaired iNKT cell frequency [31,33,34,36,37] and function [32,35]. In HIV-negative cohorts, iNKT cells have been involved in the pathogenesis of cardiovascular disease; recently a correlation between the loss of an anti-inflammatory subset of gut-residing CD4+ iNKT cells and systemic immune activation has been described in HIV infection [37], providing evidence for the contribution of this particular cell subset in the pathogenesis of HIV disease and non-communicable co-morbidities.

This is the first report to describe a peculiar iNKT phenotype in HIV-positive patients with concomitant early bone and cardiovascular disease, consisting of heightened CD161 expression. In our cohort, DP patients appear to be older and present a lower CD4 T-cell nadir, albeit not statistically significant when compared to the other subject groups; these findings are in line with literature data showing a higher prevalence of non-infectious co-morbidities in the aging population and in patients with a history of advanced HIV infection [10], thus reinforcing our findings on a peculiar iNKT phenotype in this setting. Interestingly, when analyzing subjects with either bone or cardiovascular impairment, we did not observe differences in terms of iNKT surface expression of CD161 between diseased and healthy individuals. Given that CD161 up-regulation reflects a more mature iNKT cell phenotype [56,57], our finding suggests the preferential expansion of senescent circulating iNKT cells in HIV-infected patients with multiple co-morbidities and not in individuals with only one non-communicable disorder, although the smaller sample size may affect data analysis in the latter groups.

CD161 is also expressed on NK and CD8+ T cells [58]. Interestingly CD161+ NK cells have been reported to infiltrate the human atherosclerotic plaque [51]; to our knowledge, studies on CD161-expressing CD8+ T cells in bone and cardiovascular co-morbidities in course of physiological aging are currently lacking and it would be interesting to assess the role of this subset in these settings.

Heightened CD161 expression was also associated with increased iNKT TNF release in patients with bone and cardiovascular impairment. This is in contrast to previous reports describing an inverse correlation between CD161 and cytokine production from iNKT cells [32]; however participants in the present study were all on virologically-suppressive HAART and may have undergone iNKT restoration [38–40]. Indeed, our findings suggest that these cells are capable of producing high levels of TNF, which, in turn, may represent the major driver of iNKT-mediated inflammation and exacerbate bone/cardiovascular co-morbidities.

In order to evaluate the role of iNKT cells in the pathogenesis of bone and cardiovascular disease alone, we investigated their functional capacity in patients with either bone or cardiovascular impairment.

In keeping with the evidence of a pro-inflammatory milieu in the pathogenesis of non-infectious diseases in course of HIV [1,10,11], subjects with bone impairment showed a trend to higher spontaneous *ex vivo* TNF secretion and a significant IFN-γ increase release after stimulation, Given the limited number of patients enrolled and the weak statistical significance of such findings we cannot draw definitive conclusions on the role of iNKT cells in bone disease. iNKT cell expression of other members of the TNF superfamily such as RANKL, known to be involved in bone homeostasis, should be explored in such setting.

Finally, we concentrated on the role of iNKT cells in the pathogenesis of cardiovascular disease. Individuals with atherosclerosis displayed higher TNF secretion, both constitutively and after stimulation. However, upon stimulation, iNKT cells from patients with vascular damage were not able to further release TNF, possibly suggesting exhausted functional capacity.

In line with the role of IFN-γ–producing iNKT cells in the pathogenesis of atherosclerosis and plaque stability [45,51], we also found a trend to higher IFN-γ secreting iNKT in patients with endothelial damage; this finding did not reach statistical significance, possibly due to limited sample size.

In the attempt to control for differences in antigen presenting cells in the PBMC mixtures, white blood cell count and formula were analyzed in our study population. The finding of similar percentages of circulating monocytes in all study patients suggests that iNKT phenotype and function may not be affected by diverse monocyte frequencies, albeit not ruling out possible differences other antigen presenting cells.

Several limitations exist in this study. First, the lack of HIV-negative controls; second, individuals with co-morbidities represent a heterogeneous population ranging from patients with preclinical damage (i.e. osteopenia/increased IMT) to subjects with overt disease (i.e. osteoporosis/carotid plaque). In this respect however, our findings were confirmed even when comparing patients with advanced disease (osteoporosis, n = 3; carotid plaque, n = 7) to individuals free from both co-morbidities. Further, our finding of similar iNKT function following mitogen and CD1d-antigen (α-GalCer) stimulation is in contrast to previous literature reports showing enhanced iNKT response to the former stimulus [32], and possibly reflects the different sample size used in the 2 experimental conditions. Finally the present work cannot establish a cause-effect relationship between activated iNKT and co-morbidities in the absence of a temporal relationship; moreover we cannot exclude that T-cell immune activation is driving the changes within the iNKT subset, as recently suggested by Fernandez et al. [59]. Future studies should also assess whether CD4- and CD8-expressing iNKT cells play a different role in the pathogenesis of non-infectious co-morbidities.

Despite these limitations, we show an increase in CD161-expressing and TNF secreting iNKT cells in HIV-positive individuals with bone and cardiovascular impairment, setting the basis for future studies specifically designed to investigate the role of iNKT cells in the pathogenesis of non-communicable co-morbidities in course of HIV infection.

Acknowledgments

We thank the staff and patients who participated in this study. We are grateful to Francesca Rogers for reviewing the manuscript.

Author Contributions

Conceived and designed the experiments: CT GM. Performed the experiments: MB ES. Analyzed the data: MB EM CT. Contributed reagents/materials/analysis tools: EM GC ES. Contributed to the writing of the manuscript: CT MB GM ADM.

References

1. Deeks SG, Lewin SR, Havlir DV (2013) The end of AIDS: HIV infection as a chronic disease. Lancet 382: 1525–1533.
2. Baker J, Ayenew W, Quick H, Hullsiek KH, Tracy R, et al. (2010) High-density lipoprotein particles and markers of inflammation and thrombotic activity in patients with untreated HIV infection. J Infect Dis 201: 285–292.
3. Funderburg NT, Mayne E, Sieg SF, Asaad R, Jiang W, et al. (2010) Increased tissue factor expression on circulating monocytes in chronic HIV infection: relationship to in vivo coagulation and immune activation. Blood 115: 161–167.
4. Neuhaus J, Jacobs DR, Baker JV, Calmy A, Duprez D, et al. (2010) Markers of inflammation, coagulation, and renal function are elevated in adults with HIV infection. J Infect Dis 201: 1788–1795.
5. Giorgi JV, Liu Z, Hultin LE, Cumberland WG, Hennessey K, et al. (1993) Elevated levels of CD38+ CD8+ T cells in HIV infection add to the prognostic value of low CD4+ T cell levels: results of 6 years of follow-up. The Los Angeles Center, Multicenter AIDS Cohort Study. J Acquir Immune Defic Syndr 6: 904–912.
6. Liu Z, Cumberland WG, Hultin LE, Prince HE, Detels R, et al. (1997) Elevated CD38 antigen expression on CD8+ T cells is a stronger marker for the risk of chronic HIV disease progression to AIDS and death in the Multicenter AIDS Cohort Study than CD4+ cell count, soluble immune activation markers, or combinations of HLA-DR and CD38 expression. J Acquir Immune Defic Syndr Hum Retrovirol 16: 83–92.
7. Giorgi JV, Hultin LE, McKeating JA, Johnson TD, Owens B, et al. (1999) Shorter survival in advanced human immunodeficiency virus type 1 infection is more closely associated with T lymphocyte activation than with plasma virus burden or virus chemokine coreceptor usage. J Infect Dis 179: 859–870.
8. Hunt PW, Martin JN, Sinclair E, Bredt B, Hagos E, et al. (2003) T cell activation is associated with lower CD4+ T cell gains in human immunodeficiency virus-infected patients with sustained viral suppression during antiretroviral therapy. J Infect Dis 187: 1534–1543.
9. Franceschi C, Capri M, Monti D, Giunta S, Olivieri F, et al. (2007) Inflammaging and anti-inflammaging: a systemic perspective on aging and longevity emerged from studies in humans. Mech Ageing Dev 128: 92–105.
10. Deeks SG (2011) HIV infection, inflammation, immunosenescence, and aging. Annu Rev Med 62: 141–155.
11. Desai S, Landay A (2010) Early immune senescence in HIV disease. Curr HIV/AIDS Rep 7: 4–10.
12. Desquilbet L, Margolick JB, Fried LP, Phair JP, Jamieson BD, et al. (2009) Relationship between a frailty-related phenotype and progressive deterioration of the immune system in HIV-infected men. J Acquir Immune Defic Syndr 50: 299–306.
13. Gazzola L, Bellistri G, Tincati C, Ierardi V, Savoldi A, et al. (2013) Association between peripheral T-Lymphocyte activation and impaired bone mineral density in HIV-infected patients. J Transl Med 11: 1–10.
14. Tincati C, Bellistrì GM, Casana M, Merlini E, Comi L, et al. (2009) CD8+ hyperactivation and senescence correlate with early carotid intima-media thickness in HIV+ patients with no cardiovascular disease. J Acquir Immune Defic Syndr 51: 642–644.
15. Merlini E, Luzi K, Suardi E, Barassi A, Cerrone M, et al. (2012) T-cell phenotypes, apoptosis and inflammation in HIV+ patients on virologically effective cART with early atherosclerosis. PLoS One 7: e46073.
16. Kaplan RC, Sinclair E, Landay AL, Lurain N, Sharrett AR, et al. (2011) T cell activation and senescence predict subclinical carotid artery disease in HIV-infected women. J Infect Dis. 203: 452–463.
17. Kaplan RC, Sinclair E, Landay AL, Lurain N, Sharrett AR, et al. (2011) T cell activation predicts carotid artery stiffness among HIV-infected women. Atherosclerosis 217: 207–213.
18. Longenecker CT, Funderburg NT, Jiang Y, Debanne S, Storer N, et al. (2013) Markers of inflammation and CD8 T-cell activation, but not monocyte activation, are associated with subclinical carotid artery disease in HIV-infected individuals. HIV Med 14: 385–390.
19. Bendelac A (1995) CD1: presenting unusual antigens to unusual T lymphocytes. Science 269: 185–186.
20. Bendelac A, Rivera MN, Park SH, Roark JH (1997) Mouse CD1-specific NK1 T cells: development, specificity, and function. Annu Rev Immunol 15: 535–562.
21. Kawano T, Cui J, Koezuka Y, Toura I, Kaneko Y, et al. (1997) CD1d-restricted and TCR-mediated activation of valpha14 NKT cells by glycosylceramides. Science 278: 1626–1629.
22. de Lalla C, Galli G, Aldrighetti L, Romeo R, Mariani M, et al. (2004) Production of profibrotic cytokines by invariant NKT cells characterizes cirrhosis progression in chronic viral hepatitis. J Immunol 173: 1417–1425.
23. Joyee AG, Qiu H, Wang S, Fan Y, Bilenki L, et al. (2007) Distinct NKT cell subsets are induced by different Chlamydia species leading to differential adaptive immunity and host resistance to the infections. J Immunol 178: 1048–1058.
24. Terabe M, Matsui S, Noben-Trauth N, Chen H, Watson C, et al. (2000) NKT cell-mediated repression of tumor immunosurveillance by IL-13 and the IL-4R-STAT6 pathway. Nat Immunol 1: 515–520.
25. Snyder-Cappione JE, Nixon DF, Chi JC, Nguyen ML, Kirby CK, et al. (2013) Invariant natural killer T (iNKT) cell exhaustion in sarcoidosis. Eur J Immunol 43: 2194–2205.
26. Subleski JJ, Jiang Q, Weiss JM, Wiltrout RH (2011) The split personality of NKT cells in malignancy, autoimmune and allergic disorders. Immunotherapy 3: 1167–1184.
27. Juno JA, Keynan Y, Fowke KR (2012) Invariant NKT cells: regulation and function during viral infection. PLoS Pathog 8: e1002838.
28. Reilly EC, Thompson EA, Aspeslagh S, Wands JR, Elewaut D, et al. (2012) Activated iNKT cells promote memory CD8+ T cell differentiation during viral infection. PLoS One 7: e37991.
29. Smyth MJ, Thia KY, Street SE, Cretney E, Trapani JA, et al. (2000) Differential tumor surveillance by natural killer (NK) and NKT cells. J Exp Med 191: 661–668.
30. Snyder-Cappione JE, Nixon DF, Loo CP, Chapman JM, Meiklejohn DA, et al. (2007) Individuals with pulmonary tuberculosis have lower levels of circulating CD1d-restricted NKT cells. J Infect Dis 195: 1361–1364.
31. Sandberg JK, Fast NM, Palacios EH, Fennelly G, Dobroszycki J, et al. (2002) Selective loss of innate CD4(+) V alpha 24 natural killer T cells in human immunodeficiency virus infection. J Virol 76: 7528–7534.
32. Snyder-Cappione JE, Loo CP, Carvalho KI, Kuylenstierna C, Deeks SG, et al. (2009) Lower cytokine secretion ex vivo by natural killer T cells in HIV-infected individuals is associated with higher CD161 expression. AIDS 23: 1965–1970.
33. Motsinger A, Haas DW, Stanic AK, Van Kaer L, Joyce S, et al. (2002) CD1d-restricted human natural killer T cells are highly susceptible to human immunodeficiency virus 1 infection. J Exp Med 195: 869–879.
34. van der Vliet HJ, von Blomberg BM, Hazenberg MD, Nishi N, Otto SA, et al. (2002) Selective decrease in circulating V alpha 24+V beta 11+ NKT cells during HIV type 1 infection. J Immunol 168: 1490–1495.

35. Moll M, Kuylenstierna C, Gonzalez VD, Andersson SK, Bosnjak L, et al. (2009) Severe functional impairment and elevated PD-1 expression in CD1d-restricted NKT cells retained during chronic HIV-1 infection. Eur J Immunol 39: 902–911.
36. Fleuridor R, Wilson B, Hou R, Landay A, Kessler H, et al. (2003) CD1d-restricted natural killer T cells are potent targets for human immunodeficiency virus infection. Immunology 108: 3–9.
37. Ibarrondo FJ, Wilson SB, Hultin LE, Shih R, Hausner MA, et al. (2013) Preferential depletion of gut CD4-expressing iNKT cells contributes to systemic immune activation in HIV-1 infection. Mucosal Immunol 6: 591–600.
38. Vasan S, Poles MA, Horowitz A, Siladji EE, Markowitz M, et al. (2007) Function of NKT cells, potential anti-HIV effector cells, are improved by beginning HAART during acute HIV-1 infection. Int Immunol 19: 943–951.
39. van der Vliet HJ, van Vonderen MG, Molling JW, Bontkes HJ, Reijm M, et al. (2006) Cutting edge: Rapid recovery of NKT cells upon institution of highly active antiretroviral therapy for HIV-1 infection. J Immunol 177: 5775–5778.
40. Yang OO, Wilson SB, Hultin LE, Detels R, Hultin PM, et al. (2007) Delayed reconstitution of CD4+ iNKT cells after effective HIV type 1 therapy. AIDS Res Hum Retroviruses 23: 913–922.
41. Major AS, Wilson MT, McCaleb JL, Ru Su Y, Stanic AK, et al. (2004) Quantitative and qualitative differences in proatherogenic NKT cells in apolipoprotein E-deficient mice. Arterioscler Thromb Vasc Biol 24: 2351–2357.
42. Tupin E, Nicoletti A, Elhage R, Rudling M, Ljunggren HG, et al. (2004) CD1d-dependent activation of NKT cells aggravates atherosclerosis. J Exp Med 199: 417–422.
43. To K, Agrotis A, Besra G, Bobik A, Toh BH (2009) NKT cell subsets mediate differential proatherogenic effects in ApoE−/− mice. Arterioscler Thromb Vasc Biol 29: 671–677.
44. Ostos MA, Recalde D, Zakin MM, Scott-Algara D (2002) Implication of natural killer T cells in atherosclerosis development during a LPS-induced chronic inflammation. FEBS Lett 519: 23–29.
45. Nakai Y, Iwabuchi K, Fujii S, Ishimori N, Dashtsoodol N, et al. (2004) Natural killer T cells accelerate atherogenesis in mice. Blood 104: 2051–2059.
46. VanderLaan PA, Reardon CA, Sagiv Y, Blachowicz L, Lukens J, et al. (2007) Characterization of the natural killer T-cell response in an adoptive transfer model of atherosclerosis. Am J Pathol 170: 1100–1107.
47. Aslanian AM, Chapman HA, Charo IF (2005) Transient role for CD1d-restricted natural killer T cells in the formation of atherosclerotic lesions. Arterioscler Thromb Vasc Biol 25: 628–632.
48. Melián A, Geng YJ, Sukhova GK, Libby P, Porcelli SA (1999) CD1 expression in human atherosclerosis. A potential mechanism for T cell activation by foam cells. Am J Pathol 155: 775–786.
49. Kyriakakis E, Cavallari M, Andert J, Philippova M, Koella C, et al. (2010) Invariant natural killer T cells: linking inflammation and neovascularization in human atherosclerosis. Eur J Immunol 40: 3268–3279.
50. Andoh Y, Fujii S, Iwabuchi K, Yokota T, Inoue N, et al. (2006) Lower prevalence of circulating natural killer T cells in patients with angina: a potential novel marker for coronary artery disease. Coron Artery Dis 17: 523–528.
51. Chan WL, Pejnovic N, Hamilton H, Liew TV, Popadic D, et al. (2005) Atherosclerotic abdominal aortic aneurysm and the interaction between autologous human plaque-derived vascular smooth muscle cells, type 1 NKT, and helper T cells. Circ Res 96: 675–683.
52. Hu M, Bassett JH, Danks L, Howell PG, Xu K, et al. (2011) Activated invariant NKT cells regulate osteoclast development and function. J Immunol 186: 2910–2917.
53. Kanis JA (2002) Diagnosis of osteoporosis and assessment of fracture risk. Lancet 359: 1929–1936.
54. Salonen JT, Salonen R (1993) Ultrasound B-mode imaging in observational studies of atherosclerotic progression. Circulation 87: II56–65.
55. Chambless LE, Heiss G, Folsom AR, Rosamond W, Szklo M, et al. (1997) Association of coronary heart disease incidence with carotid arterial wall thickness and major risk factors: the Atherosclerosis Risk in Communities (ARIC) Study, 1987–1993. Am J Epidemiol 146: 483–494.
56. Berzins SP, Cochrane AD, Pellicci DG, Smyth MJ, Godfrey DI (2005) Limited correlation between human thymus and blood NKT cell content revealed by an ontogeny study of paired tissue samples. Eur J Immunol 35: 1399–1407.
57. Sandberg JK, Stoddart CA, Brilot F, Jordan KA, Nixon DF (2004) Development of innate CD4+ alpha-chain variable gene segment 24 (Valpha24) natural killer T cells in the early human fetal thymus is regulated by IL-7. Proc Natl Acad Sci U S A 101: 7058–7063.
58. Tarazona R, DelaRosa O, Alonso C, Ostos B, Espejo J, et al. (2000) Increased expression of NK cell markers on T lymphocytes in aging and chronic activation of the immune system reflects the accumulation of effector/senescent T cells. Mech Ageing Dev 121: 77–88.
59. Fernandez CS, Kelleher AD, Finlayson R, Godfrey DI, Kent SJ (2014) NKT cell depletion in humans during early HIV infection. Immunol Cell Biol 92: 578–590.

HIV Testing Implementation in Two Urban Cities: Practice, Policy, and Perceived Barriers

Camden J. Hallmark[1]*, Jennifer Skillicorn[2], Thomas P. Giordano[3,4], Jessica A. Davila[3,4], Marlene McNeese[1], Nestor Rocha[5], Avemaria Smith[5], Stacey Cooper[5], Amanda D. Castel[2]

1 Houston Department of Health and Human Services, Houston, Texas, United States of America, **2** Department of Epidemiology and Biostatistics, School of Public Health and Health Services, George Washington University, Washington, DC, United States of America, **3** Center for Innovations in Quality, Effectiveness and Safety, Michael E. DeBakey VA Medical Center, Houston, Texas, United States of America, **4** Department of Medicine, Baylor College of Medicine, Houston, Texas, United States of America, **5** HIV/AIDS, Hepatitis, STD, and TB Administration, District of Columbia Department of Health, Washington, DC, United States of America

Abstract

Background: Although funding has supported the scale up of routine, opt-out HIV testing in the US, variance in implementation mechanisms and barriers in high-burden jurisdictions remains unknown.

Methods: We conducted a survey of health care organizations in Washington, DC and Houston/Harris County to determine number of HIV tests completed in 2011, policy and practices associated with HIV testing, funding mechanisms, and reported barriers to testing in each jurisdiction and to compare results between jurisdictions.

Results: In 2012, 43 Houston and 35 DC HIV-testing organizations participated in the survey. Participants represented 85% of Department of Health-supported testers in DC and 90% of Department of Health-supported testers in Houston. The median number of tests per organization was 568 in DC and 1045 in Houston. Approximately 50% of organizations in both DC and Houston exclusively used opt-in consent and most conducted both pre- and post-test counseling with HIV testing (80% of organizations in DC, 70% in Houston). While the most frequent source of funding in DC was the Department of Health, Houston organizations primarily billed the patient or third-party payers. Barriers to testing most often reported were lack of funding, followed by patient discomfort/refusal with more barriers reported in DC.

Conclusions: Given unique policies, resources and programmatic contexts, DC and Houston have taken different approaches to support routine testing. Many organizations in both cities reported opt-in consent approaches and pre-test counseling, suggesting 2006 national HIV testing recommendations are not being followed consistently. Addressing the barriers to testing identified in each jurisdiction may improve expansion of testing.

Editor: Eliseo A. Eugenin, Rutgers University, United States of America

Funding: This study was supported by a supplement to the National Institutes of Health-funded Baylor College of Medicine-University of Texas Houston Center for AIDS Research (Grant Number P30AI036211, www.nih.gov, TPG, JAD), the District of Columbia Developmental Center for AIDS Research (Grant Number P30AI087714, www.nih.gov, JS, ADC), the Centers for Disease Control and Prevention (Grant Number 5U62PS000775-03, www.cdc.gov, CJH, MM), and the facilities and resources of the Department of Veterans Affairs (www.va.gov, TPG, JAD). The opinions expressed are those of the authors and not the National Institutes of Health, the Department of Veterans Affairs or the Centers for Disease Control and Prevention. The funders had no role in study design, data collection and analysis, decision to publish, or preparation of the manuscript.

Competing Interests: The authors have declared that no competing interests exist.

* Email: camden.hallmark@houstontx.gov

Introduction

HIV testing is an important step of the HIV care continuum and a critical component of prevention programs throughout the United States (US). Nationally, an estimated 18% of infected persons remain undiagnosed. [1] Awareness of HIV infection decreases risk-taking behaviors, [2] with earlier initiation of care resulting in decreased HIV-associated morbidity and mortality. [3,4] In 2006, the US Centers for Disease Control and Prevention (CDC) released revised recommendations for routine, opt-out HIV screening in healthcare settings. Specifically, the revised recommendations include screening patients for HIV using an opt-out approach, the elimination of a separate written consent for HIV testing, and optional pre-testing prevention counseling. [5]

CDC funding has since supported the scale up of routine, opt-out screening nationwide, [6] yet implementation varies widely by jurisdiction as each determines how to expand testing given diverse contexts. Initiatives to scale up testing have included social marketing campaigns in Miami, FL and Oakland, CA, door-to-door testing outreach in San Diego, CA and Philadelphia, PA, [7] and policy change to mandate the offer of HIV testing in primary care settings in New York State. [8] Some models, such as that of the Bronx Knows HIV Testing Initiative, have demonstrated success through combination approaches in partnership with the local community and clinical providers. [7,9]

This article reports on some of the similarities and differences in HIV testing observed in two jurisdictions highly impacted by HIV, Washington DC and Houston, TX. The jurisdictions are two of the twelve urban areas that represent 44% of the nation's AIDS cases. [10] DC has a generalized epidemic with 14,465 living HIV/AIDS cases and a prevalence of 2.7%, and Houston has 19,943 living HIV/AIDS cases and a concentrated epidemic with a prevalence of 0.6%. [11–13] Each jurisdiction's local epidemic and the associated policies, programmatic priorities, and resources that influence testing implementation are reported in Table 1.

Policy in both jurisdictions has been relatively permissive of the expansion of routine HIV testing. Statutes relevant to the 2006 recommendations in DC and Texas were either neutral or consistent with all routine, opt-out recommendations. [14] Specifically, in DC, there are no regulations requiring written consent or pre/post-test counseling. The Insurance Coverage for HIV Testing in Emergency Departments (ED) Amendment Act, which was passed in 2008, attempts to facilitate third party coverage of testing in DC EDs. Under Texas Health and Safety Code, informed consent for HIV testing may be verbal as long as test explanation and consent are documented in a patient's medical record. Additionally, an opt-out approach is required by statute for pregnant women, where HIV screening is required at the first visit and during the third trimester. No statute requires pre-test prevention counseling and post-test counseling is only required upon delivery of a positive test result. [15–17]

Since 2006, the DC Department of Health (DOH) has supported targeted testing and routine, opt-out HIV testing implementation as a standard of care in health care settings. [18,19] The DOH began this initiative by providing free rapid test kits and funding to testing programs at community-based organizations (CBOs), clinics, DC Department of Corrections, hospitals, and EDs. Between 2007 and 2008, DC expanded testing to additional hospitals, primary medical settings, managed care organizations, and CBOs. [20] The "Ask for the Test/Offer the Test" initiative launched in 2009 to educate providers on how to establish routine HIV testing protocols that emphasize the use of standard blood panels. The DOH also engaged the DC Department of Health Care Finance on promoting standard HIV testing as part of the DC Medicaid and Alliance programs. In

Table 1. HIV Prevalence, Testing Policies and Programs by City.

	Washington, DC	Houston, TX[a]
Local Data		
Population (persons ≥13 yrs; Census estimates for 2010)	528,109	3,249,542
Number of living HIV/AIDS Cases ≥13 yrs (reported as of 2010)	14,465	19,943
HIV/AIDS Prevalence Rate (as of 2010)	2.7	0.6
Type of epidemic	Generalized	Concentrated
Testing Guidance & Policies		
Initiation of support for routine testing (year)	2006	2008
HIV testing consent and counseling regulations or statutes	No	Chapter 81 of Texas Health and Safety Code[b]
Mandatory HIV testing	Mandatory testing of convicted sex offenders within the criminal justice system	Mandatory testing of all offenders upon entry and release within Texas Department of Criminal Justice Texas law allows for mandatory testing in county and municipal jails
		Texas law allows for mandatory testing in county and municipal jails
Established HIV testing reimbursement and billing laws or regulations (year)	Insurance Coverage for HIV Testing in Emergency Departments Amendment Act (2008)	No specific laws on reimbursement or billing
Programming & Resources		
Estimated number of annual publically-funded HIV tests conducted	129,464 (2011)	107,458 (2011)
Testing campaigns/Programmatic initiatives/ Research activities to scale-up HIV testing	Come Together DC Get Screened for HIV (2006)	HIP HOP for HIV Awareness (2007)
	Ask for the Test/Offer the Test (2009)	Expanded Testing Initiative (2008)
	Enhanced Comprehensive HIV Prevention Planning Initiative (2010)	Routine Screening for HIV- Memorial Hermann Health System and Project RUSH at Harris Health System (2008)
	HIV Prevention Trials Network 065 (intervention community) (2010)	Enhanced Comprehensive HIV Prevention Planning Initiative (2010)
		HIV Prevention Trials Network 065 (control community) (2010)

[a]Jurisdiction is Houston/Harris County. Population data are for Harris County.
[b]Since 1999, opt-out HIV testing has been required by Texas law during pregnancy at the first prenatal visit and at delivery. As of 2010, opt-out HIV testing is required during the third trimester. If no record of third trimester testing is found, opt-out testing at time of delivery is required. For all other persons (not incarcerated), general written consent for HIV testing is allowable. Informed consent may be verbal as long as test explanation and consent is documented in patient's medical record. Opt-in versus opt-out approach is not specified.

2010, DC DOH received funding from NIH as an intervention community for the HIV Prevention Trials Network (HPTN) Study 065 to support enhanced routine HIV testing and assess the feasibility of a test and treat strategy. [21] DC's DOH funded over 129,000 HIV tests in 2011, including the provision of over 122,000 rapid test kits.

In Houston, the CDC-funded Expanded Testing Initiative (ETI) started in 2008 when the Houston Department of Health and Human Services (HDHHS) began supporting routine, opt-out HIV testing in the EDs of two large hospitals and two community health centers. The Initiative grew to encompass four large EDs by 2009. With funding from the Texas Department of State Health Services (DSHS), routine testing was further expanded in 2010 to five additional EDs and twelve additional community health centers. Targeted testing was also funded by the HDHHS at CBOs for outreach to high risk populations and geographic areas. In 2011, the HDHHS funded over 107,000 tests in the Houston area.

Both DC and Houston health departments have provided support for the provision and funding of HIV testing in community and health care settings, including implementation of social marketing campaigns. HIV testing and promotion of HIV testing was further scaled up with the influx of HIV prevention activities funded by the CDC's Enhanced Comprehensive HIV Prevention Planning (ECHPP) Project in both DC and Houston. ECHPP was a 3-year demonstration project designed to improve program planning and implementation in support of the National HIV/AIDS Strategy. [22]

As part of ECHPP efforts, partnerships were formed between academic institutions and public health departments to improve program planning of HIV prevention activities in both DC and Houston. These partnerships ensured that local research capacity was improved and policy and programming stakeholders were invested in the study's outcomes, both of which are enabling factors for success in operational research. [23] While operational research has been utilized in low-income countries, [23,24] it has been suggested that US jurisdictions could greatly benefit from applying an operational research approach to identify barriers and inform policy and decision-making in HIV prevention programs. [25] Therefore, in response to ECHPP's goal of improving implementation, we used descriptive operational research to gain knowledge of HIV testing implementation and organizational-level testing barriers in Washington, DC and Houston, Texas. Although implementation and barriers have been assessed among EDs, health centers, or clinics, [26–28] assessment across different types of organizations and jurisdictions has been limited. This study examined implementation mechanisms, testing volume, and organizational barriers for two cities with a high HIV/AIDS burden and provides a comprehensive jurisdictional-level perspective on HIV testing.

Methods

Survey instrument

Surveys were designed to gather organizational-level data on sites conducting HIV testing in each jurisdiction in 2011. Selected survey questions were adapted from the National Association of Community Health Centers survey on HIV testing, [29] a method used previously in similar research. [30] In both DC and Houston, organizations were questioned regarding their policies, funding, implementation practices, testing volume, and barriers to testing for calendar year 2011. Testing volume in 2011 was assessed by each organization providing counts by test type. Review of administrative and/or clinical data was the primary methodology used for gathering this data (80.0% of organizations in DC and 81.4% of organizations in Houston), followed by estimates from organizational staff members (17.1% DC and 11.6% Houston). Barriers to HIV testing were assessed by asking respondents to indicate the extent to which they agreed with possible barriers using a 5-point scale ranging from no barrier (1) to major barrier (5). Possible barriers included attitudinal conflicts, staff capacity, and available resources and funding.

Sampling Frame

Sampling frames were designed to best fit the model of HIV prevention activities unique to each jurisdiction. In DC, the sampling strategy was developed through a partnership between DC DOH and researchers at the George Washington University as part of ECHPP. In 2011, DC DOH's HIV/AIDS, Hepatitis, STD, and TB Administration (HAHSTA)'s prevention model primarily supported HIV testing through distribution of HIV rapid test kits at no cost to approximately forty organizations. With stakeholder and DOH input, it was determined that these organizations conducted the vast majority of testing within the city. Therefore, organizations were identified for survey inclusion if their HIV testing services were HAHSTA-supported. These organizations included CBOs, clinics, and hospitals.

In Houston, the sampling frame and sampling tool were designed jointly by staff and researchers from HDHHS, Houston Area HIV Services Ryan White Planning Council's Office of Support, and Baylor-UTHouston Center for AIDS Research, also as part of ECHPP. The HDHHS funded two distinct HIV testing services at 10 organizations in 2011: 1) targeted HIV testing by CBOs that included prevention counseling, and 2) routine, opt-out HIV testing in EDs and county clinics. HIV testing in Houston was supported by a diverse mix of both public and private support, thus sampled organizations included both those that were and were not financially supported by the HDHHS. Utilizing a methodology described previously, [31] an exhaustive list of known HIV testing organizations was created from stakeholder input. The list included CBOs, substance abuse treatment centers, homeless shelters, hospitals, clinics and universities. This list was then prioritized to focus on obtaining information from HDHHS HIV prevention contractors, major public and private hospitals and clinics, and known HIV testing organizations.

Survey Administration

In DC, surveys were emailed to HIV testing coordinators at each organization. Confidential surveys were administered online using Research Electronic Data Capture (REDCap). If no response was received within one month of invitation, paper surveys were mailed in addition to follow up phone calls. Participants were compensated for survey completion.

In Houston, each organization was emailed a formal invitation letter, followed by phone calls if there was no response via email. Initial contact was with HIV program directors, nurse managers, and/or lab directors. Respondents were selected based on their authority to make HIV testing program decisions and/or their knowledge of HIV testing activities within the organization. When possible, surveys were completed by an in-person interview, otherwise a telephone interview was conducted. Participants were not compensated for survey completion.

Data Analysis

In DC, data collection and storage were via REDCap. Data analysis was conducted using SAS 9.2 (SAS Institute, Cary, NC). In Houston, all data were entered and managed in Excel. Data analysis was conducted using SAS 9.3 (SAS Institute, Cary, NC).

Summary data from both jurisdictions were compiled via Excel and analyzed collaboratively by researchers from both jurisdictions.

Consent

This study was approved by the Institutional Review Boards of The George Washington University, the District of Columbia Department of Health (Washington, DC) and the Baylor College of Medicine (Houston). In Houston, the Institutional Review Board approved verbal consent, with completion of the survey as documentation of consent. Consent was also documented in a secure database by the interviewer. Written consent would have been the only record linking the participant and survey; therefore, the potential harm resulting from a breach of confidentiality would have increased since no other personal identifiers were gathered. In DC, the Institutional Review Board approved the use of written consent. The survey instructions asked participants to mark "yes" or "no" to indicate their consent to the survey prior to answering any further questions. In both jurisdictions, the survey was voluntary and deemed no more than minimal risk to participants.

Results

Respondents & Organizational Characteristics

In DC, 41 organizations were contacted for study inclusion. Of these, 35 (85.4%) organizations participated in the survey, representing 103 facilities that conducted HIV testing. Many of the DC organizations were community-based organizations/community service organizations (40.0%) (Table 2).

In Houston, 84 organizations were contacted for study inclusion. Of these, 55 (65.5%) organizations participated in the survey. Forty-three participating organizations, representing 114 facilities in the Houston/Harris County area, conducted HIV testing. This analysis focused only on the 43 organizations conducting HIV testing of which over half (51.2%) were outpatient clinics or university health centers (Table 2).

Policy and Practices, Funding, and Testing Volume

The majority of organizations reported that a specific individual coordinated HIV testing efforts for the organization. DC organizations more frequently reported a coordinator than did Houston (82.9% and 62.8%, respectively) (Table 2). Similarly, 82.9% of surveyed organizations in DC reported having a written policy for HIV testing, while only 46.5% of surveyed organizations in Houston reported having a policy for their organization.

The two jurisdictions reported similar approaches to provider education about HIV testing. The top three sources of provider education for DC were continuing education (74.3%), DOH or clinic training (65.7%), and peer-to-peer best practices (57.1%). Houston organizations most frequently identified DOH or clinic training (58.1%), manuals/guidelines/literature (48.8%), and continuing education (46.5%).

A similar proportion of organizations exclusively used an opt-in consent approach in DC and Houston (51.4% and 48.8% respectively). However, a substantial number of organizations in Houston used a combination of opt-in and opt-out approaches (44.2%). Further analysis revealed that 11.6% (n = 5) of organizations in Houston using a combination approach only used opt-out consent during pregnancy. While only three (7.0%) organizations in Houston reported using only the opt-out approach, 48.6% of the surveyed organizations in DC exclusively used an opt-out approach.

Despite CDC recommendations that removed the need for pre-test counseling, most organizations in both jurisdictions reported conducting both pre- and post-test counseling with HIV testing (80.0% in DC and 69.8% in Houston). Very few organizations reported conducting only post-test counseling (11.4% in DC and 16.3% in Houston).

For all HIV testing conducted by surveyed organizations, the most frequent funding sources for DC were the DOH (74.3%), research monies (34.3%), and federal funding other than that from CDC and DOH (33.3%). In contrast, Houston organizations most frequently identified the payer as the patient or the patient's insurance (65.1%), Medicaid (53.5%), Medicare (32.6%), and other sources (32.6%) such as the organization's general revenue or funds received as donations. Funding specifically for routine, opt-out HIV testing also varied between the two cities. The most frequent funding source in DC was the DOH (68.6%), while Houston organizations primarily paid for HIV testing by billing the patient or patient's insurance (54.5%) or Medicaid (50.0%).

The median total number of HIV tests performed per organization in 2011 was higher in Houston than in DC (1045 and 568 respectively). While the total number of rapid tests performed in DC was higher than in Houston (78,765 in DC vs. 40,910 in Houston), the median number of rapid tests performed per organization was lower in DC than in Houston (593 vs. 1478). Similarly, although the median number of venipuncture tests per organization was higher in DC (1200 in DC vs. 585 in Houston), the total number of venipuncture tests was higher in Houston than in DC (169,635 in Houston vs. 4,558 in DC).

Barriers to HIV Testing

On a scale of 1 (no barrier) to 5 (major barrier), the highest reported barriers to HIV testing in both DC and Houston were patient discomfort/refusal (median score = 2) and lack of funding for testing (median score = 3). When categorizing all items dichotomously (no barrier vs. any barrier), DC organizations most frequently selected "HIV not a problem for client population" (68.6% of organizations), "lack of funding" (60.0%), and "patient discomfort or refusal for testing" (59.4%) as barriers (Figures 1–3). Houston organizations most frequently selected "lack of funding" (59.5% of organizations), "patient discomfort or refusal for testing" (51.2%), and "staff knowledge, skill, experience" (41.9%).

In comparison to Houston organizations, DC organizations more frequently reported every area as a barrier except for staff knowledge, skill, experience (41.9% Houston vs. 32.4% DC) and provider/staff resistance (20.9% vs. 20.6%) (Figures 1–3). However, 11 Houston organizations (25.6%) scored "other" barriers to testing at 3 or higher, including managing data and/or paperwork associated with testing and funding for testing (n = 4) and challenges in contacting patients for results delivery and/or care referrals (n = 3). The largest variances observed between the two jurisdictions were "HIV is not a problem for the client population" (20.9% Houston vs. 68.6% DC), "limited staff time to provide testing" (30.2% vs. 52.9%), and "limited staff size to provide testing" (37.2% vs. 58.8%).

We examined whether barriers to testing implementation differed by organization type (CBOs, hospitals, and clinics; data not shown). Lack of funding was reported frequently across all organizational types. Clinics were particularly challenged by cost or reimbursement for testing and patient refusal, while CBOs reported staff size as a barrier. Among hospitals, the highest ranked barrier to testing in both jurisdictions was the perception that HIV was not a problem in their client population. In DC, barriers to testing were most frequently reported among hospitals in comparison to other site types. The most frequent barriers among DC hospitals included the perception that HIV is not a problem in the client population (83.3% of organizations), staff

Table 2. HIV Testing Policy, Funding, and Implementation Practices.

	Washington, DC (N = 35)		Houston, TX (N = 43)	
	N	%	N	%
Type of organization				
Hospital	12	34.3%	11	25.6%
Community-based or community service organization[a]	14	40.0%	10	23.3%
Clinic or university health center	9	25.7%	22	51.2%
Individual at organization who coordinates HIV testing efforts				
Yes	29	82.9%	27	62.8%
No	6	17.1%	16	37.2%
Have a written policy for HIV testing				
Yes	29	82.9%	20	46.5%
No	6	17.1%	23	53.5%
How providers are educated about HIV testing[c]				
Continuing education	26	74.3%	20	46.5%
DOH or clinic training	23	65.7%	25	58.1%
Peer-to-peer best practices	20	57.1%	17	39.5%
Manuals, guidelines, or literature	16	45.7%	21	48.8%
Web seminars	12	34.3%	11	25.6%
Consulting site visits	6	17.1%	11	25.6%
In-person or video conferences	5	14.3%	10	23.3%
Other	1	2.9%	1	2.3%
None reported	2	5.7%	9	20.9%
Type of consent procedure for HIV testing[b]				
Opt in approach ONLY	18	51.4%	21	48.8%
Opt out approach ONLY	17	48.6%	3	7.0%
Combination of opt in and opt out	0	0.0%	19	44.2%
Type of HIV counseling offered with testing				
Pre-test counseling only	1	2.9%	1	2.3%
Post-test counseling only	4	11.4%	7	16.3%
Both pre and post-test counseling	28	80.0%	30	69.8%
Neither pre nor post-test counseling	1	2.9%	5	11.6%
Other	1	2.9%	0	0.0%
Funding used by organization for HIV testing[c]				
Local Health Department Funding (DC, Houston)	26	74.3%	10	23.3%
Texas DSHS	N/A	N/A	8	18.6%
CDC Funding	9	25.7%	3	7.0%
Other Federal Funding (Ryan White, Other HRSA, SAMHSA, VA)	11	31.4%	7	16.3%
Private Grant Funding	7	20.0%	8	18.6%
Research (HPTN 065/TLC Plus HIV testing or other research study)	12	34.3%	2	4.7%
Medicaid	10	28.6%	23	53.5%
Medicare	4	11.4%	14	32.6%
Patient/patient's insurance	10	28.6%	28	65.1%
Other [d]	1	2.9%	14	32.6%
None reported	12	34.3%	0	0.0%
Funding used by organization for routine, opt out testing (among those doing opt out testing)[c]	*n = 35*		*n = 22*	
Local Health Department Funding (DC, Houston)	24	68.6%	4	18.2%
Texas DSHS	N/A	N/A	5	22.7%
CDC Funding	5	14.3%	0	0.0%
Other Federal Funding (Ryan White, Other HRSA, SAMHSA, VA)	6	17.1%	1	4.5%
Private Grant Funding	5	14.3%	6	27.3%

Table 2. Cont.

	Washington, DC (N = 35)		Houston, TX (N = 43)	
	N	%	N	%
Research (HPTN 065/TLC Plus HIV testing or other research study)	5	14.3%	0	0.0%
Medicaid	9	25.7%	11	50.0%
Medicare	4	11.4%	3	13.6%
Patient/patient's insurance	7	20.0%	12	54.5%
Other [e]	1	2.9%	9	40.9%
None reported	6	17.1%	0	0.0%
HIV tests performed in 2011				
	Median (Range)	Total No. of Tests	Median (Range)	Total No. of Tests
Rapid tests (DC n = 30; Houston n = 21)	593 (5–10,673)	78,765	1,478 (4–9,945)	40,910
Venipuncture tests (DC n = 3; Houston n = 34)	1200 (36–3,322)	4,558	585 (1.5–46,590)[f]	169,635
Total tests (DC n = 22; Houston n = 41)	568 (20–10,673)	41,085	1,045 (1.5–47,209)[f]	210,565

[a]Community service organizations include homeless services, substance abuse recovery centers, life skills programs, housing assistance programs, faith-based organizations, and other community-oriented service organizations.
[b]Five organizations participating in the Houston survey only use opt-out consent during pregnancy as required by Texas law but do not use opt-out consent otherwise. Therefore, the bulk of consent used for these organizations would be opt-in. Results if these organizations are re-classified into the "opt-in approach only" category: 26 (60.5%) organizations use opt-in approach only, 3 (7.0%) organizations use opt-out approach only, and 14 (32.6%) organizations use a combination of opt-in and opt-out consent.
[c]Respondents could check more than one response.
[d]Other responses in DC include general revenue (n = 1). Other responses in Houston include donations (n = 12) and general revenue (n = 2).
[e]Other responses in DC include general revenue (n = 1). Other responses in Houston include donations (n = 8) and general revenue (n = 2). One Houston organization selected both donations and general revenue for a total of n = 9 organizations selecting "other".
[f]One Houston organization estimated 1–2 tests were completed. The average, 1.5 tests, was recorded as the response.

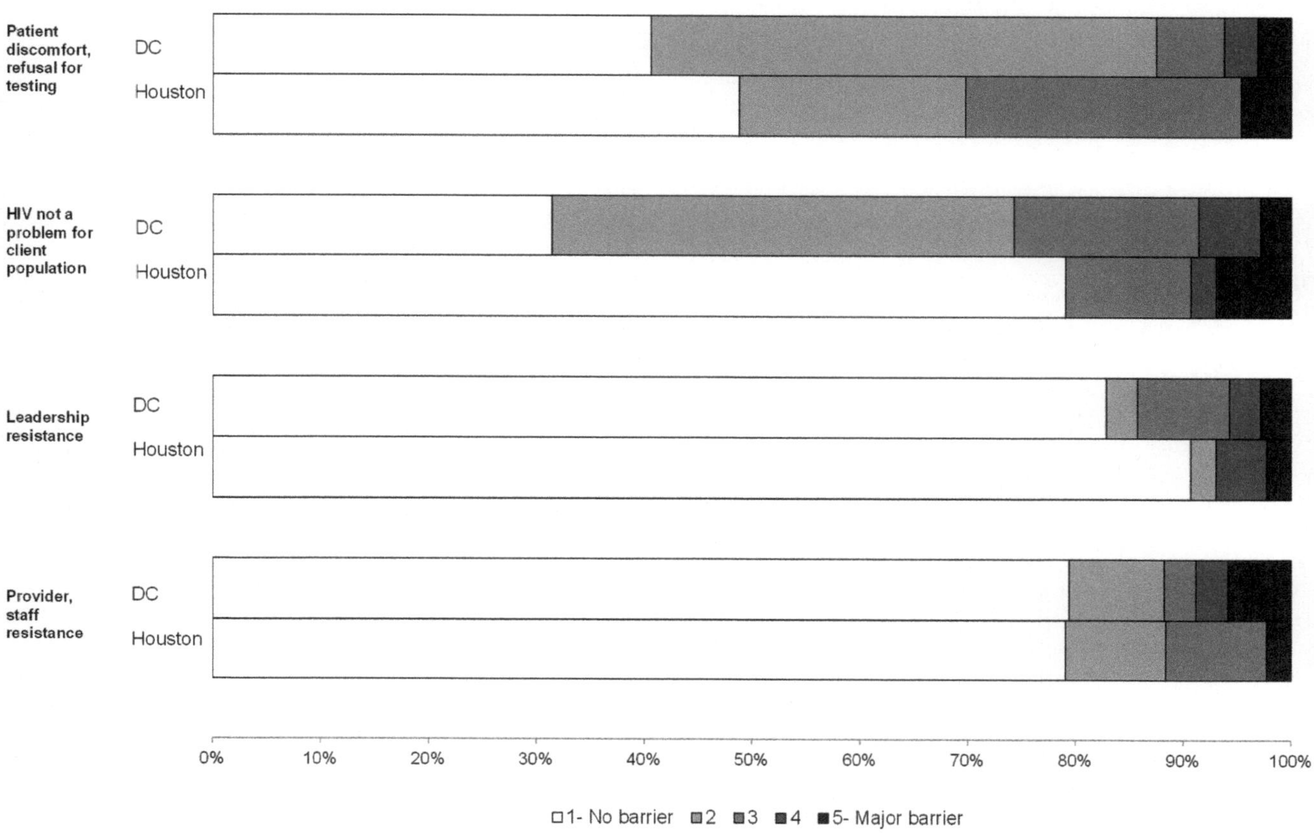

Figure 1. Attitudinal barriers to HIV testing by City.

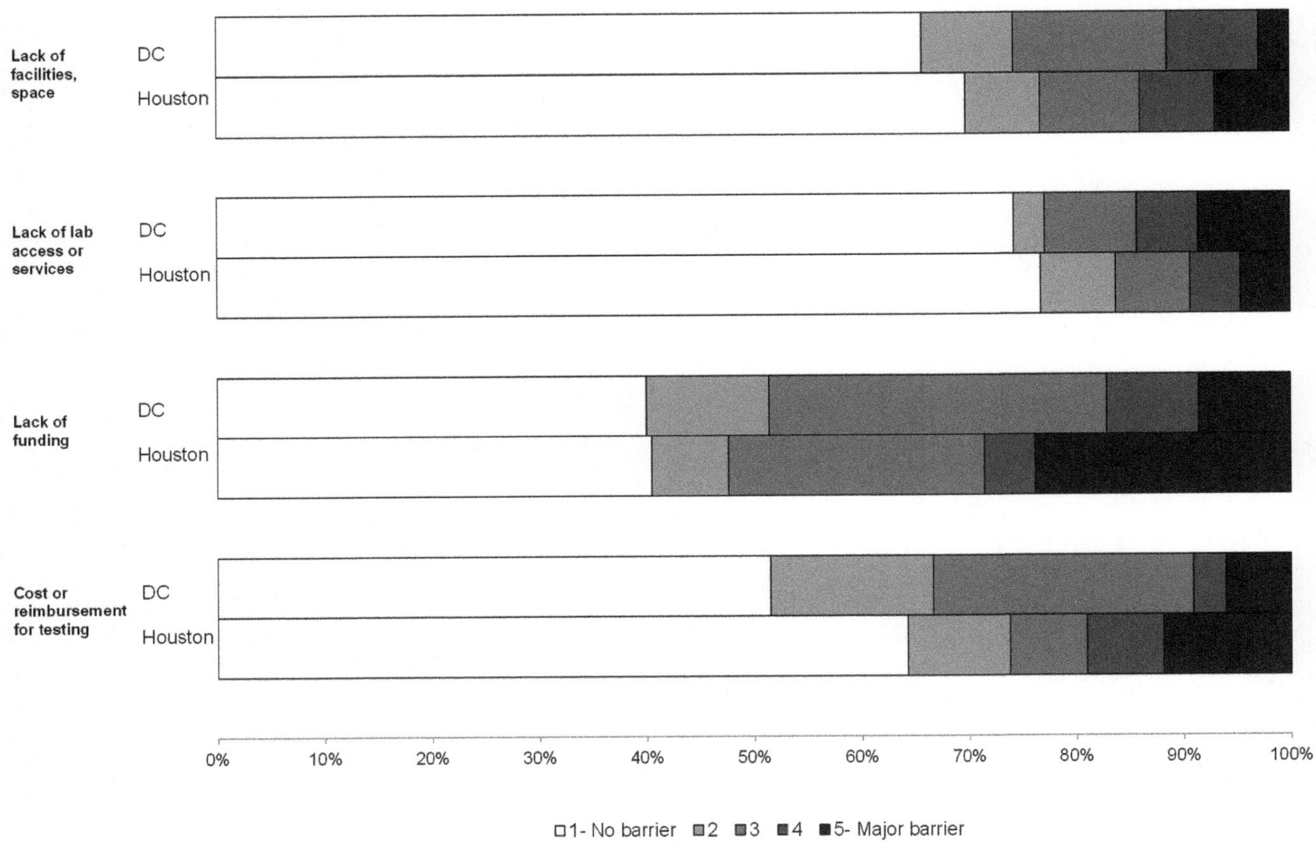

Figure 2. Resources and funding barriers to HIV testing by City.

time (75.0%), staff size (75.0%), and lack of funding (66.7%). In contrast, in Houston, hospitals reported the fewest barriers, while clinics reported the most. The most frequent barriers among Houston clinics included lack of funding (68.2%), refusal to get tested (63.6%), cost/reimbursement (50.0%), and staff knowledge/skill/experience (50.0%).

Discussion

Utilizing a framework of operational research for HIV prevention, [25] this study identified differences and similarities in the approaches two high prevalence cities have taken to implement routine HIV testing. While both jurisdictions reported a high level of provider education on HIV testing, many organizations in both cities reported opt-in consent approaches and pre-test counseling, suggesting the 2006 CDC recommendations are not being followed consistently. The cause of inconsistency merits further research since statutes do not pose a substantial barrier in either jurisdiction. [14] Previous implementation research has shown that this inconsistency may be due to 1) a lack of awareness or misunderstanding of the recommendations, [27,32,33] 2) disagreement with the recommendations, [34] and/or 3) organizational barriers that impede application of the recommendations. [27,28,30,35,36] Both cities may benefit from further research into why organizations continue to use both pre- and post-test counseling and do not use opt-out testing.

The two jurisdictions have taken different approaches to support and fund the expansion of routine testing. DC DOH's approach has involved considerable funding for the distribution of free rapid test kits to local implementation sites including clinics, hospitals and CBOs. This is in contrast to the HDHHHS' approach which has encouraged performing venipuncture tests as part of routine visits and funding large volumes of HIV testing in hospitals and clinics with rapid results of standard testing. [37] This divergence of approaches is reflected in the greater total number of rapid tests being utilized in DC and much greater total number of venipuncture tests being performed in Houston.

Funding sources for testing also varied between the two jurisdictions which could have implications for the long term sustainability and scalability of these testing programs. Houston testing organizations reported much more third party billing and reimbursement from Medicaid, Medicare, and private insurance as a primary means to support their testing programs, compared to DC sites which relied much more heavily on direct support from DC DOH. Because of this, Houston organizations may be better positioned to more quickly adapt and benefit from expanded coverage through the Affordable Care Act (ACA), especially now that routine testing is rated a recommended service for coverage by the US Public Health Services Task Force (USPHSTF). However, this strong reliance on third party reimbursement does leave these organizations more vulnerable to reimbursement challenges and inadequate reimbursement rates that may not cover the total cost of testing provision. The monitoring of HIV testing post-ACA and USPHSTF implementation will allow for further exploration of the impact of these policies on testing programs.

Overall, few barriers to testing implementation were reported by organizations in both jurisdictions however, among those reported, lack of funding and organizational capacity to conduct testing were key barriers. Capacity barriers, such as staff size and

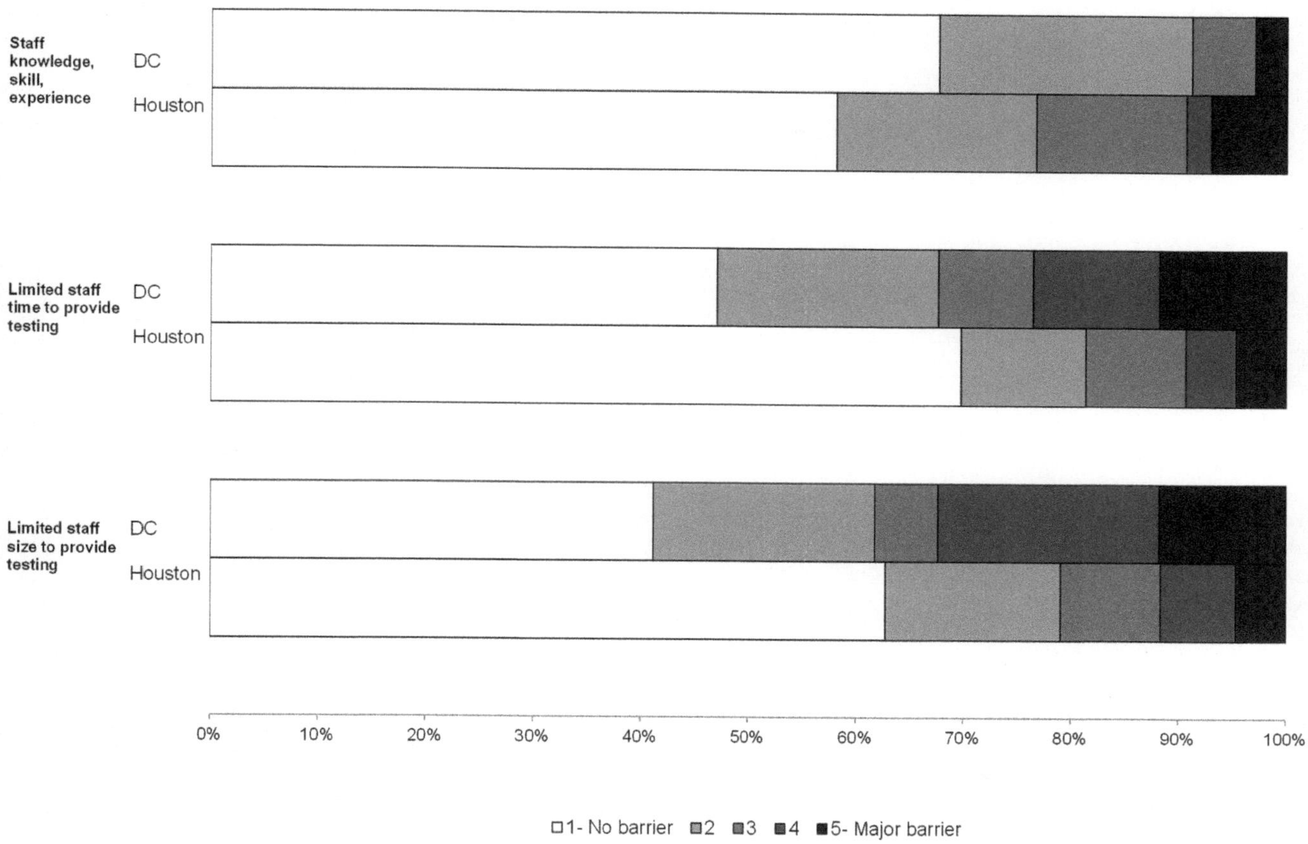

Figure 3. Staff capacity barriers to HIV testing by City.

time were moderate barriers for the surveyed organizations and may have been related to lack of funding to support these efforts at the organizational level, particularly among organizations in DC. Although multiple methods of routine HIV testing have been promoted in DC, there is more reliance on rapid testing, which can be more time and labor-intensive than venipuncture testing. Time-related barriers and competing priorities have been extensively reported in literature, [26–28,30,32,35,38,39] but research has found that providers cite consent and counseling requirements as time-intensive even when statutes have removed these barriers in a jurisdiction. [26] Interestingly, despite the generalized epidemic and high HIV prevalence in DC, a commonly reported barrier included the perception that HIV was not a problem among the patient population. This perception may depend on the age of the population being served as a previous survey conducted by DC DOH found that almost 40% of providers did not perceive HIV to be a problem among those 50 years of age and older [Michael Kharfen, personal communication]. Barriers elicited in this study suggest that DC may benefit from campaigns that emphasize the necessity of HIV testing, while Houston may benefit from increasing testing knowledge and skill among providers. Patient discomfort or refusal for testing was a barrier in both cities and has been reported by providers elsewhere [26,27,39] with clients often refusing due to low-perceived risk for HIV, recent testing elsewhere, [40,41] fear of loss, fatalism, confidentiality concerns, and structural barriers. [36] Future qualitative research in both DC and Houston, focusing first on the commonly reported barriers presented here, may best elicit additional barriers and facilitators of sustained HIV testing.

This study determined current implementation practices and perceived barriers to HIV testing, a crucial step to design interventions and guide policy to improve HIV testing in cities with a high burden of HIV, such as DC and Houston. In 2010, New York State enacted a statute requiring primary care settings to offer HIV testing to all patients between the ages of 13 to 64. Since this law was enacted, one study found that only 65% of emergency departments implemented HIV testing as required by the law. [8] While changes to policy guidance at the jurisdictional level may increase testing, [42] statute alone is not the solution. [8,35] Further increases in testing uptake may be realized with policy change and implementation at the organizational level, [43,44] especially in jurisdictions with low uptake such as some organizations in Houston. Organizational leadership to drive local policy formulation, revision, and implementation is critical. Other facilitators include organizational buy-in from both providers and administration, [27,28] written procedures for HIV testing, [30] provider trainings, [27] and dedicated staff and funding. [35]

There are a number of limitations to this study. The survey was a convenience sample that could be subject to non-response bias. The self-reported responses were limited to the organizational knowledge, perceptions and/or experiences of the person completing the survey, thus the responses may not accurately reflect the practices or opinions of all providers or staff members. The primary limitation of the parts of this study that compared DC and Houston was differences in survey administration between the two cities. Non-response was potentially influenced in Houston (65.5% vs. 85.4% in DC) by the lack of compensation for survey completion. The differing routes of survey administration (in-person in Houston and online in DC) may have also led to variances in social desirability or comprehension of the survey questions. In addition, social desirability may have biased the results, especially in reporting of testing barriers. Furthermore, our ability to statistically analyze barrier data was limited as many of the barriers received low rankings. Finally, generalizability of these findings may be limited, particularly in jurisdictions that have statutes in conflict with the 2006 CDC recommendations. Results presented herein may be useful to such jurisdictions after their statutes transition.

Despite both DC and Houston having high HIV prevalence, each jurisdiction has tailored their HIV testing strategies to meet particular funding options, resources, and statutes. The range of approaches was appropriate given the distinct context of the epidemic in each jurisdiction. Reported implementation practices, such as types of tests used and the funding mechanisms most often used to pay for HIV testing, highlight this variation. Regardless of different implementation approaches, our results suggest many organizations in at least two high burden jurisdictions have not aligned with all aspects of national testing recommendations. Research has shown that neither awareness of CDC guidelines nor jurisdictional policy change alone fully scales up testing to the levels recommended in the 2006 guidelines. [8,32,39] It is likely that a multi-faceted approach is needed that includes awareness campaigns, policy change, and reduction of jurisdictional and organizational-specific barriers. Few multi-faceted approaches have been rigorously evaluated to determine if they can widely span multiple jurisdictions with diverse epidemics, policy, and resources. Further implementation research and dissemination of implementation research findings is critical to the expansion of routine HIV testing and early diagnosis of HIV infection.

Acknowledgments

The authors would like to acknowledge Christina Shaw, Divina Oweis, Jennifer Hadayia, Dr. John Chen, Dr. Monisha Arya, and Lena Williams for their contributions to the Houston survey tool design and/or data collection, and Wenze Tang, Sarah Willis, Morgan Bennett, and Kristen Camuso for their assistance with the design and analysis of the DC data. Portions of this manuscript were presented at the First National Centers for AIDS Research/AIDS Prevention Centers Enhanced Comprehensive HIV Prevention Planning Meeting, November 19, 2012, Washington DC.

Author Contributions

Conceived and designed the experiments: CJH JS TPG JAD MM ADC. Performed the experiments: CJH JS. Analyzed the data: CJH JS TPG JAD ADC. Contributed reagents/materials/analysis tools: JS TPG MM. Wrote the paper: CJH JS TPG JAD MM NR AS SLC ADC.

References

1. The Centers for Disease Control and Prevention (2012) Monitoring Selected National HIV Prevention and Care Objectives by Using HIV Surveillance Data-United States and 6 U.S. Dependent Areas- 2010. Available: www.cdc.gov/hiv/topics/surveillance/resources/reports. Accessed 2013 Jul 18.
2. Marks G, Crepaz N, Senterfitt JW, Janssen RS (2005) Meta-analysis of high-risk sexual behavior in persons aware and unaware they are infected with HIV in the United States: implications for HIV prevention programs. J Acquir Immune Defic Syndr 39: 446–453.
3. Palella FJ Jr, Delaney KM, Moorman AC, Loveless MO, Fuhrer J, et al. (1998) Declining morbidity and mortality among patients with advanced human immunodeficiency virus infection. HIV Outpatient Study Investigators. N Engl J Med 338: 853–860. doi: 10.1056/NEJM199803263381301.
4. Chadborn TR, Delpech VC, Sabin CA, Sinka K, Evans BG (2006) The late diagnosis and consequent short-term mortality of HIV-infected heterosexuals (England and Wales, 2000–2004). AIDS Lond Engl 20: 2371–2379. doi: 10.1097/QAD.0b013e32801138f7.
5. Branson BM, Handsfield HH, Lampe MA, Janssen RS, Taylor AW, et al. (2006) Revised recommendations for HIV testing of adults, adolescents, and pregnant women in health-care settings. MMWR Recomm Rep Morb Mortal Wkly Rep Recomm Rep Cent Dis Control.
6. The Centers for Disease Control and Prevention (2011) Results of the Expanded HIV Testing Initiative–25 jurisdictions, United States, 2007–2010. MMWR Morb Mortal Wkly Rep 60: 805–810.
7. Nunn A, Yolken A, Cutler B, Trooskin S, Wilson P, et al. (2014) Geography Should Not Be Destiny: Focusing HIV/AIDS Implementation Research and Programs on Microepidemics in US Neighborhoods. Am J Public Health 104: 775–780. doi: 10.2105/AJPH.2013.301864.
8. Egan DJ, Cowan E, Fitzpatrick L, Savitsky L, Kushner J, et al. (2014) Legislated Human Immunodeficiency Virus Testing in New York State Emergency Departments: Reported Experience from Emergency Department Providers. AIDS Patient Care STDs 28: 91–97. doi: 10.1089/apc.2013.0124.
9. Myers JE, Braunstein SL, Shepard CW, Cutler BH, Mantsios AR, et al. (2012) Assessing the Impact of a Community-Wide HIV Testing Scale-Up Initiative in a Major Urban Epidemic: JAIDS J Acquir Immune Defic Syndr 61: 23–31. doi: 10.1097/QAI.0b013e3182632960.
10. U.S. Department of Health and Human Services. NHAS-HHS-12.pdf. 12 Cities Proj. Available: http://blog.aids.gov/wp-content/uploads/NHAS-HHS-12.pdf. Accessed 2013 Jan 8.
11. District of Columbia Department of Health HIV/AIDS, Hepatitis, STD and TB Administration (HAHSTA). HIV/AIDS, Hepatitis, STD, and TB Administration (HAHSTA) Annual Report 2011. Available: http://www.doh.dc.gov/hahsta.
12. United States Census Bureau. American FactFinder. U.S. Department of Commerce. Available: http://factfinder2.census.gov. Accessed 2013 Jan 7.
13. Houston Area Ryan White Planning Council and Houston Area HIV Prevention Community Planning Group (2013) HIV/AIDS in the Houston Area: The 2013 Houston Area Integrated Epidemiological Profile for HIV/AIDS Prevention and Care Services Planning. Available: http://www.rwpchouston.org/Publications/2013%20Epi%20Profile%20-%20APPROVED%20-%2005-09-13.pdf. Accessed 2013 Jul 18.
14. Mahajan AP, Stemple L, Shapiro MF, King JB, Cunningham WE (2009) Consistency of state statutes with the Centers for Disease Control and Prevention HIV testing recommendations for health care settings. Ann Intern Med 150: 263–269.
15. Prevention, Control, and Reports of Diseases. Tex Health Saf Code Chapter 81. Communicable Diseases. Available: http://www.statutes.legis.state.tx.us/Docs/HS/htm/HS.81.htm. Accessed 2013 Jan 7.
16. DC Regulations. Available: http://www.dcregs.dc.gov. Accessed 2013 Jan 7.
17. National HIV/AIDS Clinicians' Consultation Center. Available: http://www.nccc.ucsf.edu/consultation_library/state_hiv_testing_laws. Accessed 2013 Jan 7.
18. (n.d.) How-to Guide for DC Medical Providers, Routine HIV Screening Implementation Handbook. Government of the District of Columbia, HIV/AIDS, Hepatitis, STD, Tuberculosis Administration (HAHSTA).
19. Castel AD, Magnus M, Peterson J, Anand K, Wu C, et al. (2012) Implementing a novel citywide rapid HIV testing campaign in Washington, D.C.: findings and lessons learned. Public Health Rep 127: 422–431.
20. HIV Prevention Trials Network [HPTN] 065 (2010) TLC-Plus: A Study to Evaluate the Feasibility of an Enhanced Test, Link to Care, Plus Treat Approach for HIV Prevention in the United States. Division of AIDS (DAIDS), U.S. National Institute of Allergy and Infectious Diseases (NIAID), U.S. National Institutes of Health (NIH). Available: http://www.hptn.org/web%20documents/HPTN065/065Protocol_V2_15Jul10.pdf.
21. District of Columbia Department of Health HIV/AIDS, Hepatitis, STD and TB Administration (HAHSTA) (2011) Enhanced Comprehensive HIV/AIDS Prevention Planning (ECHPP) Workbooks. Available: http://www.cdc.gov/hiv/strategy/echpp/index.htm.
22. The Centers for Disease Control and Prevention. Enhanced Comprehensive HIV Prevention Planning (ECHPP) Project. Available: http://www.cdc.gov/hiv/pdf/prevention_demonstration_echpp.pdf. Accessed 2013 Jul 18.
23. Zachariah R, Harries AD, Ishikawa N, Rieder HL, Bissell K, et al. (2009) Operational research in low-income countries: what, why, and how? Lancet Infect Dis 9: 711–717. doi: 10.1016/S1473-3099(09)70229-4.
24. Zachariah R, Ford N, Maher D, Bissell K, Van den Bergh R, et al. (2012) Is operational research delivering the goods? The journey to success in low-income countries. Lancet Infect Dis 12: 415–421. doi: 10.1016/S1473-3099(11)70309-7.
25. Herbst JH, Glassman M, Carey JW, Painter TM, Gelaude DJ, et al. (2012) Operational research to improve HIV prevention in the United States. J Acquir Immune Defic Syndr. 59: 530–536. doi: 10.1097/QAI.0b013e3182479077.
26. Myers JJ, Koester KA, Dufour M-SK (2011) Barriers and facilitators to enhancing HIV testing in publicly funded primary care clinics: findings from San Francisco. AIDS Educ Prev Off Publ Int Soc AIDS Educ 23. doi: 10.1521/aeap.2011.23.3_supp.84.
27. Johnson CV, Mimiaga MJ, Reisner SL, VanDerwarker R, Mayer KH (2011) Barriers and facilitators to routine HIV testing: perceptions from Massachusetts Community Health Center personnel. AIDS Patient Care STDs 25: 647–655. doi: 10.1089/apc.2011.0180.
28. Mumma BE, Suffoletto BP (2011) Less encouraging lessons from the front lines: barriers to implementation of an emergency department-based HIV screening program. Ann Emerg Med 58: S44–48. doi: 10.1016/j.annemergmed.2011.03.022.

29. Charlebois ED, Myers JJ, Harcourt J, Morfit S, Gaffney S, et al. (2003) National survey of health center HIV testing, prevention, care and treatment practices. AIDS Policy Research Center & Center for AIDS Prevention Studies: AIDS Research Institute, University of California, San Francisco. Available: http://www.nachc.com/client/documents/clinical/Clinical_HIV_NACHC_2003_Final_Report.pdf.
30. Mimiaga MJ, Johnson CV, Reisner SL, Vanderwarker R, Mayer KH (2011) Barriers to routine HIV testing among Massachusetts community health center personnel. Public Health Rep 126: 643–652.
31. Giordano TP, Hallmark CJ, Davila JA, Arya M, Chen GJ, et al. (2013) Assessing HIV testing and linkage to care activities and providing academic support to public health authorities in Houston, TX. J Acquir Immune Defic Syndr 64 Suppl 1: S7–13. doi: 10.1097/QAI.0b013e3182a90183.
32. Mohajer MA, Lyons M, King E, Pratt J, Fichtenbaum CJ (2012) Internal Medicine and Emergency Medicine Physicians Lack Accurate Knowledge of Current CDC HIV Testing Recommendations and Infrequently Offer HIV Testing. J Int Assoc Physicians AIDS Care 11: 101–108. doi: 10.1177/1545109711430165.
33. Arya M, Bush AL, Kallen MA, Rodriguez-Barradas MC, Giordano TP (2013) Are VA primary care providers aware of HIV testing recommendations for Veterans? Findings at an urban VA primary care clinic. Mil Med 178: e483–488. doi: 10.7205/MILMED-D-12-00222.
34. Merchant RC, Waxman MJ, Maher JG, Clark MA, Celada MT, et al. (2012) Patient and clinician ethical perspectives on the 2006 Centers for Disease Control and prevention HIV testing methods. Public Health Rep 127: 318–329.
35. Schnall R, Clark S, Olender S, Sperling JD (2013) Providers' perceptions of the factors influencing the implementation of the New York State mandatory HIV testing law in two Urban academic emergency departments. Acad Emerg Med Off J Soc Acad Emerg Med 20: 279–286. doi: 10.1111/acem.12084.
36. Awad GH, Sagrestano LM, Kittleson MJ, Sarvela PD (2004) Development of a measure of barriers to HIV testing among individuals at high risk. AIDS Educ Prev Off Publ Int Soc AIDS Educ 16: 115–125.
37. Hoxhaj S, Davila JA, Modi P, Kachalia N, Malone K, et al. (2011) Using nonrapid HIV technology for routine, opt-out HIV screening in a high-volume urban emergency department. Ann Emerg Med 58: S79–84. doi: 10.1016/j.annemergmed.2011.03.030.
38. Chen JC, Goetz MB, Feld JE, Taylor A, Anaya H, et al. (2011)A provider participatory implementation model for HIV testing in an ED.Am J Emerg Med 29: 418–426. doi: 10.1016/j.ajem.2009.11.016.
39. Korthuis PT, Berkenblit GV, Sullivan LE, Cofrancesco J Jr, Cook RL, et al. (2011) General internists' beliefs, behaviors, and perceived barriers to routine HIV screening in primary care. AIDS Educ Prev Off Publ Int Soc AIDS Educ 23: 70–83. doi: 10.1521/aeap.2011.23.3_supp.70.
40. Brown J, Kuo I, Bellows J, Barry R, Bui P, et al. (2008) Patient perceptions and acceptance of routine emergency department HIV testing. Public Health Rep 123 Suppl 3: 21–26.
41. Ubhayakar ND, Lindsell CJ, Raab DL, Ruffner AH, Trott AT, et al. (2011) Risk, reasons for refusal, and impact of counseling on consent among ED patients declining HIV screening. Am J Emerg Med 29: 367–372. doi: 10.1016/j.ajem.2009.10.005.
42. Wing C (2009) Effects of written informed consent requirements on HIV testing rates: evidence from a natural experiment. Am J Public Health 99: 1087–1092. doi: 10.2105/AJPH.2008.141069.
43. Zetola NM, Grijalva CG, Gertler S, Hare CB, Kaplan B, et al. (2008) Simplifying consent for HIV testing is associated with an increase in HIV testing and case detection in highest risk groups, San Francisco January 2003-June 2007. PLOS One 3: e2591. doi: 10.1371/journal.pone.0002591.
44. Nayak SU, Welch ML, Kan VL (2012) Greater HIV testing after Veterans Health Administration policy change: the experience from a VA Medical Center in a high HIV prevalence area. J Acquir Immune Defic Syndr 1999 60: 165–168. doi: 10.1097/QAI.0b013e318251aefe.

HIV-1 Subtype C Unproductively Infects Human Cardiomyocytes *In Vitro* and Induces Apoptosis Mitigated by an Anti-Gp120 Aptamer

Walter R. Lopes de Campos[1], Nthato Chirwa[1], Grace London[1], Lia S. Rotherham[1], Lynn Morris[2], Bongani M. Mayosi[3], Makobetsa Khati[1,3]*

1 Emerging Health Technologies Competency Area, Biosciences Unit, Council for Scientific and Industrial Research, Pretoria, South Africa, **2** National Institute for Communicable Diseases, Sandringham, South Africa, **3** Department of Medicine, Groote Schuur Hospital and University of Cape Town, Cape Town, South Africa

Abstract

HIV-associated cardiomyopathy (HIVCM) is of clinical concern in developing countries because of a high HIV-1 prevalence, especially subtype C, and limited access to highly active antiretroviral therapy (HAART). For these reasons, we investigated the direct and indirect effects of HIV-1 subtype C infection of cultured human cardiomyocytes and the mechanisms leading to cardiomyocytes damage; as well as a way to mitigate the damage. We evaluated a novel approach to mitigate HIVCM using a previously reported gp120 binding and HIV-1 neutralizing aptamer called UCLA1. We established a cell-based model of HIVCM by infecting human cardiomyocytes with cell-free HIV-1 or co-culturing human cardiomyocytes with HIV-infected monocyte derived macrophages (MDM). We discovered that HIV-1 subtype C unproductively (i.e. its life cycle is arrested after reverse transcription) infects cardiomyocytes. Furthermore, we found that HIV-1 initiates apoptosis of cardiomyocytes through caspase-9 activation, preferentially via the intrinsic or mitochondrial initiated pathway. CXCR4 receptor-using viruses were stronger inducers of apoptosis than CCR5 utilizing variants. Importantly, we discovered that HIV-1 induced apoptosis of cardiomyocytes was mitigated by UCLA1. However, UCLA1 had no protective effective on cardiomyocytes when apoptosis was triggered by HIV-infected MDM. When HIV-1 was treated with UCLA1 prior to infection of MDM, it failed to induce apoptosis of cardiomyocytes. These data suggest that HIV-1 causes a mitochondrial initiated apoptotic cascade, which signal through caspase-9, whereas HIV-1 infected MDM causes apoptosis predominantly via the death-receptor pathway, mediated by caspase-8. Furthermore the data suggest that UCLA1 protects cardiomyocytes from caspase-mediated apoptosis, directly by binding to HIV-1 and indirectly by preventing infection of MDM.

Editor: Andrew D. Badley, Mayo Clinic, United States of America

Funding: This work was supported by Department of Science and Technology (http://www.dst.gov.za/). The funders had no role in study design, data collection and analysis, decision to publish, or preparation of the manuscript.

Competing Interests: The authors have declared that no competing interests exist.

* Email: Mkhati@csir.co.za

Introduction

South Africa has the highest HIV-1 prevalence that is almost exclusively subtype C [4]. Chronic HIV-1 infection causes a broad range of clinical complications, some of which remain poorly elucidated. One such disease is HIV-associated cardiomyopathy (HIVCM). HIVCM is characterized by the loss of cardiomyocytes and their replacement by fibrous tissue due to chronic HIV-1 infection. The pathogenesis of HIVCM remains incompletely understood, although direct and indirect effects of HIV infection are thought to play a role [1,2,3].

There is increasing clinical and experimental data that point to a direct role of HIV-1 and its associated proteins as important causes of HIVCM [4,5,6,7,8]. HIV-1 infection of human cardiomyocytes has been observed in cardiac biopsies of HIV positive patients [9,10,11], although its role in the pathogenesis of the disease is controversial. More clear is the role played by its structural, surface envelope glycoprotein called gp120, which has been reported to cause apoptosis of rodent cardiomyocytes [4,5,6,7,8]. The cardio toxic effects are believed to be triggered in a caspase-dependent, mitochondria-initiated fashion, when gp120 interacts with the CXCR4 receptor on the surface of cardiomyocytes [12]. This in turn results in the induction of a negative ionotropic effect through increase in nitric oxide (NO) production via p38 mitogen activated protein kinase (p38 MAPK)-iPLA2-troponin I initiated NF-κB activation [6,7,8]. The end result of NO production is free-radical insult through the formation of reactive oxygen species (ROS), leading to the loss of mitochondrial membrane potential and membrane permeabilization, in a Bcl-2-inhibitable manner [13,14]. The exact pathway is not fully understood but leakage of cytochrome *c* into the cell cytosol following permeabilization of the mitochondrial membrane triggers the activation of the caspase 9/3 complex eventually culminating in nuclear DNA fragmentation [15].

The apoptotic signal is not restricted to host cell interaction with viral proteins. Cytokines secreted by HIV-infected cells, primarily infiltrating macrophages, also play a role in the development of HIVCM. Tumor necrosis factor (TNF) has been suggested to be the main cause in murine cells [16,17]. It interacts with its respective death receptor, TNF-R1, leading to extrinsic or death-receptor mediated apoptosis [16,17]. However, *in vitro* apoptosis triggered by gp120 is initiated preferentially through the CXCR4 receptor than the death-receptor. Analysis of cardiac biopsies revealed strong expression of both caspase 9 and TNF, which was detected in infiltrating inflammatory cells of HIVCM patients, but not in HIV-infected patients without HICVM, making a strong argument towards death-receptor initiated apoptosis *in vivo* [4]. These suggest that both pathways are at play, but why and under which conditions each pathway is favored remains unclear.

In this paper, we report the HIV-1 infection kinetics of well characterized human cord-blood stem cell-derived cardiomyocytes as well as the associated apoptotic pathways and receptors involved during HIV-cardiomyocyte interaction. Importantly, we also show that a shortened and synthetic derivative of gp120 binding and HIV-1 broadly neutralizing aptamer called UCLA1 [18] mitigated HIV-initiated apoptosis in the cardiomyocytes.

Results

Phenotyping human cardiomyocytes

To confirm the phenotype of the human cord-blood stem cell-derived cardiomyocytes, we stained the cells with antibodies for known cardiac cell markers. The cells stained positive for canonical cardiac specific markers such as α-MHC, Cx43 and cTnT, respectively (Figure 1A–C).

HIV-1 entry into cardiomyocytes is co-receptor independent and abortive

To establish the cell-based HIVCM model and investigate the effect of HIV-1 on human cardiomyocytes, we first evaluated if different HIV-1 subtype C strains, as defined by co-receptor usage, can productively infect human cardiomyocytes. Cultured human cardiomyocytes were infected by all the R5, X4 and R5/X4 subtype C HIV-1 isolates tested in the presence or absence of respective co-receptor inhibitors as evidenced by the presence of proviral DNA (Table 1). While all the tested subtype C HIV-1 isolates also infected PBMC, we observed successful inhibition of infection of PBMC in the presence of specific inhibitors of the relevant co-receptors (Table 1). In HIV-1_{CM9} infected cardiomyocytes, we observed time-dependent peak in pro-viral DNA 2 hours post infection and subsequent decrease to almost undetectable levels after 24 hours and complete absence after 6 days (Figure 2A). This contrasted with the infection kinetics observed in PBMC in which there was a time-associated increase of pro-viral DNA (Figure 2A). Synthesis of pro-viral DNA in cardiomyocytes was inhibited by zidovudine (AZT) in a dose-dependent manner (Figure 2B). The absence of p24 viral capsid protein in cardiomyocytes, measured daily over 7 days, suggested that HIV-1 cannot replicate inside cardiomyocytes; as opposed to replication in PHA-treated, IL-2 stimulated primary PBMC as measured by an increase in p24 viral protein (Figure 2C). Taken together, the data suggest that while HIV-1 infects cardiomyocytes, the virus does not enter using the classic co-receptors and the infection is non-productive.

Apoptosis of cardiomyocytes is predominantly triggered by X4 viruses and is down regulated by AMD3100 and UCLA1

After establishing that all R5, X4 and R5X4 HIV-1 subtype C isolates tested unproductively infected cardiomyocytes, we next investigated whether or not they induce apoptosis of cardiomyocytes to further probe HIV-cardiomyocyte interaction in our cellular model. Induction of apoptosis in cardiomyocytes by X4 viruses was on average 3 times higher than that of R5 viruses– 54%±6.6% TUNEL positive for X4 viruses vs. 18%±5.3% for R5 viruses (Figure 3). Dual-tropic (R5X4) viruses also induced considerably more apoptosis in cardiomyocytes than R5-tropic viruses; by a magnitude of 2.7 (Figure 3). When R5 viruses were pre-incubated with UCLA1 before infecting cardiomyocytes, apoptosis was reduced from an average of 18%±5.3% to background or mock infected levels (Figure 3). AMD3100 also reduced apoptosis of R5 infected cardiomyocytes from 18%±5.3% to about mock infected levels (Figure 3). Reduction in apoptosis was stronger in cardiomyocytes infected with X4 and R5/X4 viruses, respectively, where on average the TUNEL positive population decreased from 52%±6% to 5%±3% ($P<0.001$) in the presence of AMD3100 (Figure 2). The UCLA1 aptamer did not show a strong protective effect as AMD3100 but the percentage of TUNEL positive cardiomyocyte decreased from 52%±6% to 13%±6% ($P<0.001$) when compared to untreated but HIV-1 infected cardiomyocyte (Figure 3). On the other hand, RANTES, the physiological ligand for the CCR5 chemokine receptor, had no statistically significant effect in protecting cardiomyocytes from HIV-1 associated apoptosis when compared to untreated but HIV-1 infected cardiomyocytes (Figure 3). Collectively, these data suggest that apoptosis of cardiomyocytes is triggered through the CXCR4 receptor, predominantly by X4 viruses and is down regulated by AMD3100 and UCLA1.

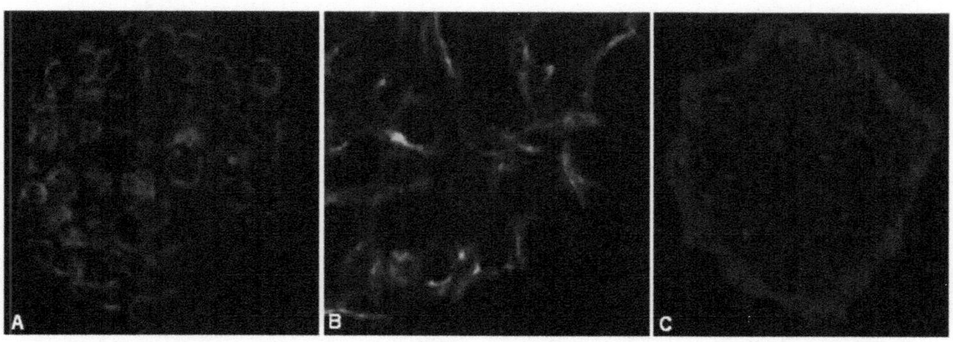

Figure 1. Phenotyping cultured human cardiomyocytes. Human cardiomyocytes cultured on microscope cover slips where phenotyped using cardiac markers (A) α-MHC (63× magnification) (AF546-labeled secondary antibody [red]) (B) Cx43 (x40) (AF488-labeled primary antibody [green]) and (C) cTnT (40× magnification) (AF546-labeled secondary antibody [red]). Cardiomyocytes where imaged on a Zeiss 780 immunofluorescent confocal microscope.

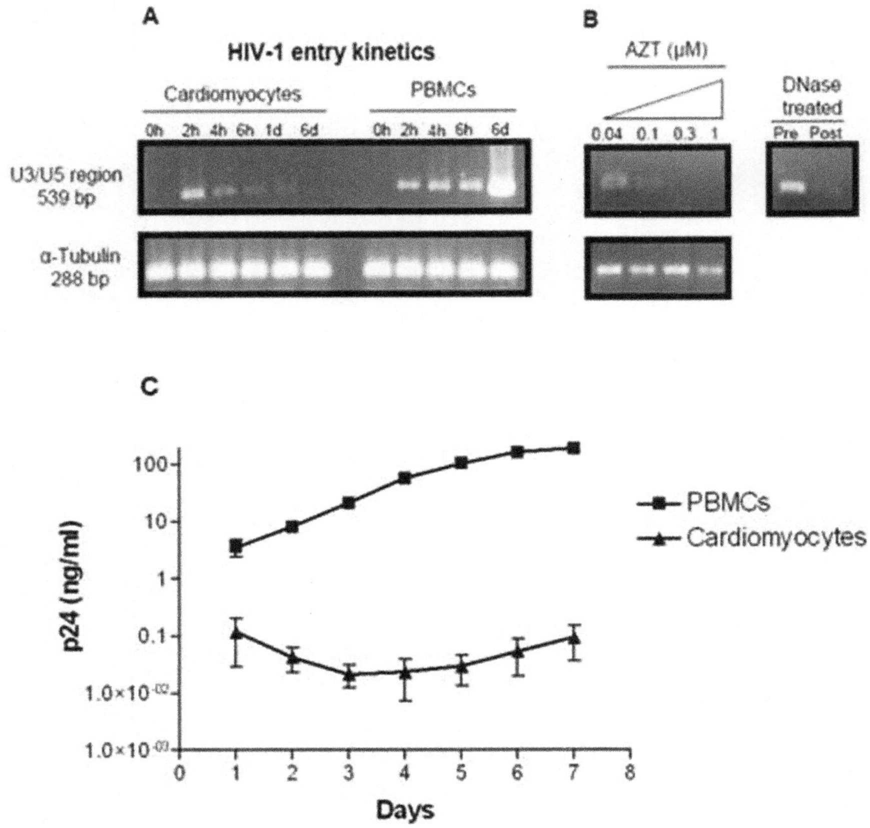

Figure 2. Kinetics of HIV-1 infection of CM and PBMC. (A) Agarose-gel electrophoresis of the PCR-amplified U3/U5 region of a dual tropic (R5X4) HIV-1 subtype C isolate called HIV-1_{CM9} infected culture lysates at different times after infection. The 539 bp fragment indicates the presence of proviral DNA. A 288 bp region of the gene coding for α-tubulin is a control ensuring equal loading of the wells. (B) Proviral DNA in CM exposed to serial dilutions of AZT. (Insert) Agarose-gel electrophoresis of cell-free HIV-1_{CM9} culture digested with DNaseI for 1 h prior to infection. (C) Detection of replication of HIV-1_{CM9} in CM and PBMC using p24 ELISA.

HIV-1 initiates apoptosis of cardiomyocytes preferentially through the intrinsic or mitochondrion-initiated pathway mediated by caspase 9 activation

Cytochrome *c* leakage from the mitochondria as well as caspase 9 activation are markers of the intrinsic mitochondrial-initiated pathway and caspase 8 activation is the canonical caspase of the extrinsic apoptotic pathway. In this experiment we investigated the preferred apoptotic pathways in cardiomyocytes directly infected by HIV-1. We found that in the untreated control cardiomyocytes, only 2.4%±0.7% cells stained positive for cytochrome *c* release (Figure 4A). On the other hand, 41.77%±3.0% of HIV-infected cardiomyocytes stained positive for cytochrome c release (Figure 4B). The preferential caspase 8 inhibitor reduced cytochrome c release in HIV-1 infected cardiomyocytes to 32.2%±5.3% (Figure 4C). The preferential caspase 9 inhibitor significantly reduced cytochrome c release in HIV-1 infected cardiomyocytes to 14.3%±3.6% (Figure 4D). UCLA1 also significantly reduced cytochrome c release in HIV-1 infected cardiomyocytes to 22.4%±4.4% (Figure 4E).

There was an inversely proportional link between total cellular ATP, which was used as marker of enhanced oxidative stress and hence a surrogate measure of cellular viability, and caspase 9 activation during HIV-1 infection of cardiomyocytes (Figure 5). A drop in ATP levels was observed 1 day after peak caspase 9 activity and subsequent recovery at day 5 correlated with a decrease in caspase 9 levels. Both caspase 9i and UCLA1 protected HIV-1 infected cardiomyocytes from cell death as indicated by an exponential increase in cellular ATP from day 3 to 7 (Figure 5A).

Caspase 8 activation in HIV-1 infected cardiomyocytes was not significantly higher from the untreated control cells or any other test condition (Figure 5B). Furthermore, there was no statistical difference ($P=0.5$) between cells treated with caspase 8i or UCLA1 and untreated, infected cells up to day 3 (Figure 5B). There was however an exponential increase in enzyme activity levels in infected, UCLA1 treated cells, very similar to untreated controls from day 3 to 7 (Figure 5B). The opposite was observed with caspase 8i treated cells, where there was a decline in enzyme activity up to day 4 followed by an increase up to day 7 (Figure 5B).

Peak caspase 9 enzyme activity was observed two days post-exposure to HIV-1, resulting in a 9.3 fold increase in enzyme levels, when compared to the untreated controls (Figure 5C). This was followed by a sharp decrease in enzyme activity relative to control cells. The preferential caspase 9 inhibitor significantly reduced the enzyme activity in the presence of HIV-1 at days 1–2 of treatment (Figure 5C). UCLA1 also had a modulatory effect in caspase 9 activity during HIV-infection infection (RLU =2410, $P=0.001$), albeit weaker than that of casp9i (RLU =1515, $P=0.02$). All other test conditions did not significantly affect caspase 9 levels ($P>0.07$) during the entire duration of the experiment (Figure 5C). Taken together, the data suggest that both intrinsic and extrinsic apoptosis are perhaps triggered by

Table 1. HIV-1 infection of cultured human cardiomyocytes (CM) and peripheral blood mononuclear cells (PBMCs), activated with phytohemagglutinin (PHA) and treated with interleukin-2 (IL-2)) in the presence of inhibitors.

		Entry Inhibitors							
		No inhibitors		AMD3100 (500 nM)		RANTES (100 nM)		UCLA1 (100 nM)	
HIV Strain	Tropism	CM	PBMC	CM	PBMC	CM	PBMC	CM	PBMC
SW2	R 5	+	+	+	+	+	–	+	–
SW4	R 5	+	+	+	+	+	–	+	–
SW12	X4	+	+	+	–	+	+	+	–
TM46b	X4	+	+	+	–	+	+	+	–
CM9	R5X4	+	+	+	–	+	+	+	–
DU179-99	R5X4	+	+	+	+	+	+	+	–
RP1	R5X4	+	+	+	+	+	+	+	–

The presence of pro-viral DNA as indicated by the presence of a 539 bp fragment amplified from the U3/U5 region was indicative of viral entry and is shown as +. PCR negative samples were considered entry negative and are shown as –. This study was done in triplicates and repeated twice.

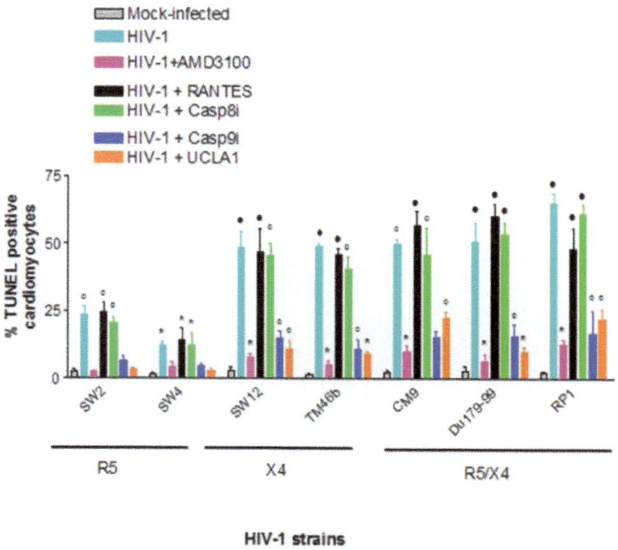

Figure 3. Quantification of the relationship between HIV-1 tropism and induction of CM apoptosis using TUNEL assay. Statistically significant TUNEL positive results compared to mock-infected control cells were determined by the student *t*-test and are marked as: *, $P<0.05$; ·, $P<0.005$; °, $P<0.0005$ (n = 3± SEM).

HIV-1 in cardiomyocytes, however the intrinsic or mitochondrion initiated pathway is probably dominant as indicated by cytochrome c release and the high levels of caspase 9 activity in HIV-1 infected cardiomyocytes. Thus caspase 9 is possibly a key player in apoptosis of HIV-1 infected cardiomyocytes since its inhibition resulted in significant reduction of cytochrome c release and almost completes abrogation of apoptosis in HIV-1 infected cardiomyocytes, while inhibition of caspase 8 had a much less pronounced effect.

HIV-1 infected macrophages preferentially trigger extrinsic or death receptor apoptotic pathway in cardiomyocytes

There is evidence suggesting that infiltrating HIV-1 infected macrophages in cardiac tissue are strongly associated with caspase-dependent cardiomyocyte apoptosis. Therefore, to mimic the *in vivo* environment and to help further establish the HIVCM cellular model, we investigated if MDM experimentally infected with HIV-1 can induce apoptosis of cardiomyocytes-MDM co-cultures. MDM infected with R5 and R5X4 viruses significantly induced apoptosis of cardiomyocytes-MDM co-cultures compared to mock-infected MDM (Figure 6). AMD3100 ($P>0.09$) and UCLA1 ($P>0.07$) did not significantly protect cardiomyocytes from apoptosis induced by HIV-1 infected MDM (Figure 6). However, significant protection against apoptosis was achieved in the presence of TNF-R1 ($P<0.02$) and casp8i ($P<0.02$), which are both key components of the extrinsic apoptotic pathway (Figure 6). Thus, the data suggest that HIV-1 infected MDM induce apoptosis in uninfected cardiomyocytes-MDM co-cultures via the extrinsic or death receptor pathway.

Discussion

In this study, we have showed for the first time that UCLA1 [18], a synthetic derivative of gp120 binding aptamer called B40 [19,20,21,22], mitigated HIV-1 subtype C induced apoptosis of human cord-blood stem cell-derived cardiomyocytes. We showed

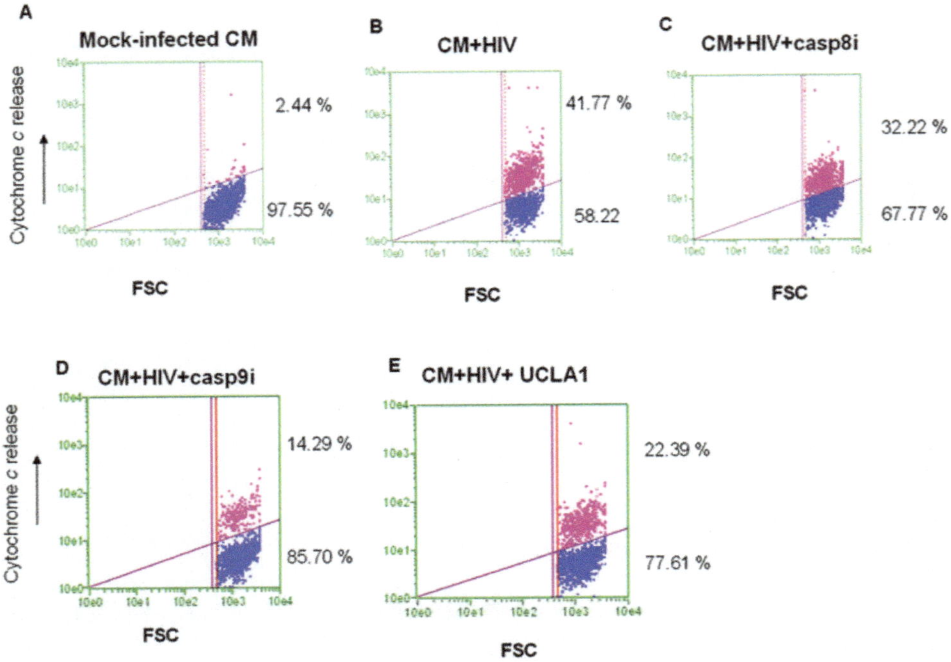

Figure 4. Cytochrome *c* release in HIV-1$_{CM9}$-infected CM. CM were either (A) mock infected; (B) HIV-1 infected; (C) infected in the presence of casp8i; (D) infected in the presence of casp9i and (E) infected with virus pre-incubated with UCLA1. Data were presented in dot plots relating fluorescent intensity as a measure of cytochrome *c* release against forward scatter.

that these stem cell-derived human cardiomyocytes expressed Tropic T, Connexin 43 and α-MHC cardiac specific canonical markers in addition to the Troponin 1 marker, which we showed that they also express in our recent publication [21]. Thus, these

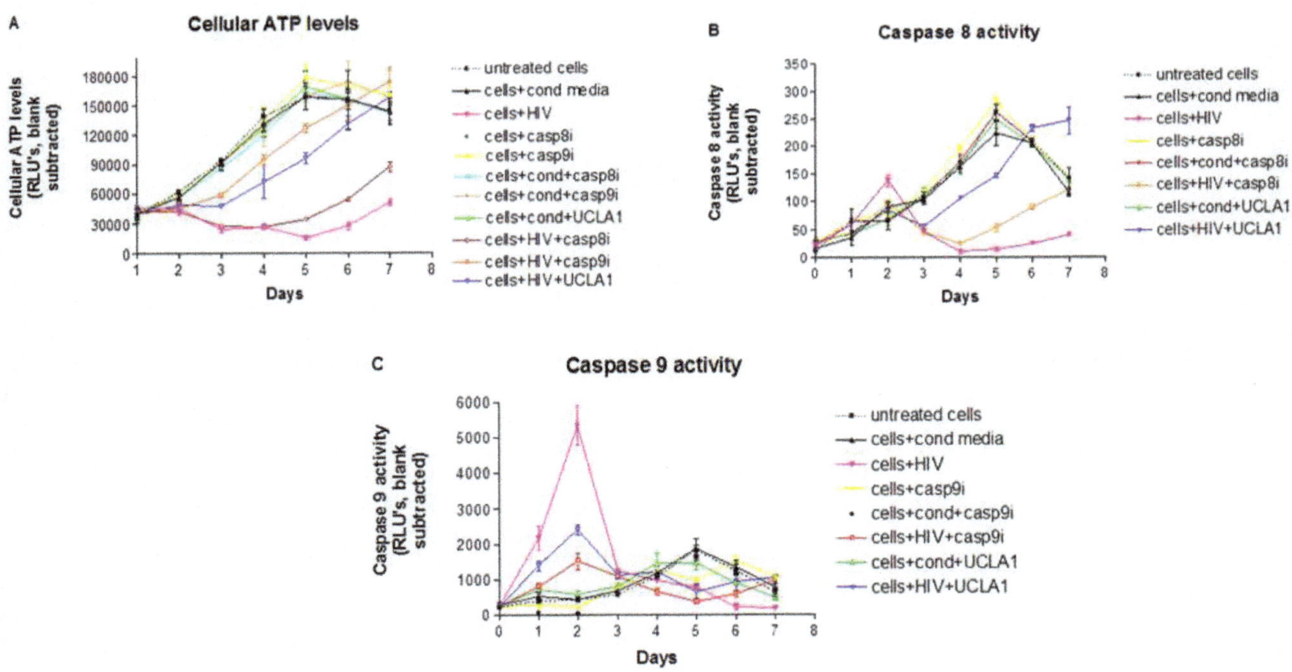

Figure 5. Caspase 8 and 9 activities in CM infected with HIV-1. CM were exposed to: media alone; conditioned media containing virus; HIV; 100 μM of casp8i; 100 μM of casp9i; conditioned media and 100 μM of casp8i; conditioned media and 100 μM of casp9i; conditioned media and 100 nM UCLA1 aptamer; HIV and 100 μM of casp8i; HIV and 100 μM of casp9i; HIV pre-incubated for 1 h with 100 nM of UCLA1 aptamer. Cells were harvested daily for 7 days. (A) ATP levels were measured as a correlate of cell viability; (B) caspase 8 and (C) caspase 9 activities were measured as indicators of extrinsic and intrinsic apoptosis, respectively. All assays were luminescence-based and presented as graphs relating RLU to number of days (n = 3± SEM).

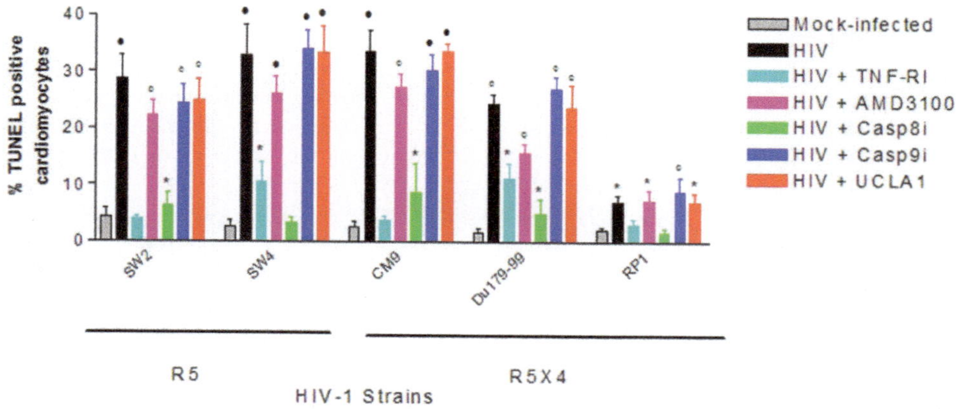

Figure 6. CM apoptosis in a co-culture model with HIV-infected MDM. MDM were infected with the R5-tropic viruses SW2, SW4 or the dual tropic viruses CM9, DU179-99 and RP1 for 24 h. Uninfected CM were added and the co-cultures were then incubated for a further 24 h. Following incubation, the cell monolayers were stained for TUNEL detection. Statistically significant TUNEL positive results compared to mock-infected control cells were determined by the student *t*-test and are marked as: *, $P<0.05$; ·, $P<0.005$; °, $P<0.0005$ (n = 3± SEM).

data extend earlier findings that these cells expressed Nkx2.5, GATA-4, MEF2C, SERCA2a, α-MHC, α-sarcomeric actin [23] and Troponin I [21,23]. In addition to being positive for the immunological cardiomyocytes markers, these cells were shown to be capable of synchronized contraction [23]. These human cord-blood stem cell-derived cardiomyocytes used in this study, are similar to recently reported human embryonic stem cell-derived cardiomyocytes, which are also capable of spontaneous beating [24].

Furthermore, we also showed that while HIV-1 subtype C infects the human cardiomyocytes, it does not necessarily enter using the classic CCR5 or CXCR4 co-receptors. These data indirectly confirm and extend previous studies using rat heart cells, where it was shown that HIV-1 subtype B entered cultured neonatal rat ventricular myocytes by macropinocytosis but did not replicate [4,5]. We also observed that despite entering human cardiomyocytes, a dual tropic (R5X4) HIV-1 subtype C isolate called HIV-1_{CM9} was unable to complete its life cycle, as indicated by the time-dependent decrease in pro-viral DNA upon infection as well as by the absence of p24 antigen in culture supernatants of HIV-1 infected human cardiomyocytes, further extending earlier findings by others [4,5]. It is likely that the pro-viral pre-integration, nuclear-localization complex is never formed resulting in a time-dependent degradation of the pro-viral DNA in the cytoplasm. In addition to HIV-1 previously shown to infect rat ventricular myocytes [4,5], there is also *in vivo* clinical evidence suggesting direct infection of cardiomyocyte in AIDS patients [10,11] but these studies were limited to detecting viral nucleic acid and proteins in cardiac biopsies, which is a mixture of different cells including macrophages. Thus, our study does not only confirm and extend earlier findings by others [4,5] but it is the first to investigate whether or not HIV-1 in general and subtype C in particular, could directly infect cultured human cardiomyocytes. Our study is also the first to show that monocyte derived macrophages infected with HIV-1 could cause apoptosis of cultured human cardiomyocytes.

Our data have also revealed that although HIV-1 subtype C did not complete its life cycle in human cardiomyocytes, it was still capable of inducing significant caspase-dependent apoptosis. Furthermore, entry was not required for apoptosis since the apoptotic signal is probably initiated by interaction with the cell-surface receptors, the CXCR4 chemokine receptor and the TNF-R1 death receptor. The predominant apoptotic pathway varied from CXCR4-triggered, mitochondrion-initiated to CD95/Fas-ligand initiated, depending on the culture conditions as previously reported in T cells [25,26]. In the absence of monocyte derived macrophages, cell free HIV-1 possibly interacts directly with the CXCR4 chemokine receptor on cardiomyocytes [12], resulting in cell death. This death-inducing signaling however was significantly stronger using X4 and dual tropic (R5X4) viruses, possibly because these viruses interact with higher affinity with the CXCR4 receptor than R5 tropic viruses. The UCLA1 binding site maps to the co-receptor binding region of gp120 on HIV-1 [18,20,22,27], which may explain its strong anti-apoptotic properties, very similar to that brought about by the highly selective CXCR4 receptor ligand AMD3100. This observation, together with cytochrome *c* leakage into the cell cytosol points to a CXCR4/HIV-1 interaction as the key apoptosis trigger as recently reported in murine cardiomyocytes [12] and earlier in primary human macrophages [28], resulting in mitochondrial initiated apoptosis [4,25] independent of death-receptor mediated signaling [29]. It has been reported that the CXCR4 receptor is involved in both caspase-dependent and caspase-independent apoptosis induction [12]. There is however some controversy regarding the circumstances under which each pathway is favored. Some groups have reported that caspase-dependent apoptosis requires interaction with both CD4 and CXCR4 receptors, and in the absence of CD4, the apoptotic signal initiated by CXCR4 is caspase-independent [26,30,31]. On the other hand, another study conducted by Roggero and co-workers revealed that CXCR4 cooperation with a CD4 signal was not required for the induction of mitochondrial-mediated apoptosis [25]. Furthermore, it was previously shown that deletion of the cytoplasmic tail of CD4 in cells co-transfected with both CD4 and CXCR4 did not shift the apopotic pathway from caspase-dependent to caspase-independent [32,33].

In this study, we also observed that both apoptotic pathways were intimately related with caspase activity, an observation that is not supported by others who used gp120 and T-cells [31]. This discrepancy could be explained by the fact that we used fully infectious HIV-1 subtype C primary isolates with trimeric envelope and macrophage-cardiomyocyte co-cultures instead of recombinant monomeric gp120 and T-cells. Notwithstanding, the 9-fold increase in cellular caspase 9 levels, and the improved cell survival brought about by its inhibition, further strengthens the argument for a caspase-dependent apoptotic pathway.

In addition, we observed a second, caspase-dependent apoptotic pathway, initiated at the TNF-R1 death receptor in the presence of HIV-1. Although the peak in caspase 8 activity was not statistically significant, there was a significant degree of cellular protection when HIV-infected cardiomyocytes were treated with the preferential caspase 8 inhibitor Z-IETD-FMK. Caspase 8 is regarded as a key initiator of death receptor mediated apoptosis and under physiological conditions, it is primed by the TNF superfamily member of related apoptosis triggers [34,35]. Our case for extrinsic apoptosis rests on the merit of its inhibition rather than on up-regulation of its downstream effector caspase.

The macrophage-cardiomyocyte co-culture model shows a drastic shift in the preferential apoptotic trigger, towards the extrinsic pathway, which is likely initiated by interaction with TNF-R1 secreted by death-signaling molecules produced by HIV-1 infected monocyte derived macrophages. Under these conditions apoptosis progressed with much more rapid kinetics, measured in hours as opposed to days when initiated by the CXCR4 receptor. The almost complete abrogation of apoptosis in the presence of TNF-R1 as well as casp8i sheds further light into preferential apoptotic pathways and receptor trigger during HIV-1 infection of cardiomyocyte. In this scenario, the UCLA1 had no impact in apoptosis modulation, which was expected since the extrinsic or death-receptor initiated apoptosis was most likely triggered by monocyte derived macrophages, rather than viral factors. Nonetheless, by preventing macrophage infection, UCLA1 can strongly modulate both apoptotic pathways. A further advantage of UCLA1 over conventional anti-retrovirals is that it probably neutralizes the deleterious effects of cell-free virus by binding to gp120 envelope protein and preventing it from interacting with the CXCR4 chemokine receptor and thereby preventing or reducing apoptosis. This reasoning is consistent with the observation that protease inhibitors used in anti-retroviral therapy give rise to non-infectious virions with fully functional envelope glycoproteins that have been observed to lead to apoptosis of non-infected $CD4^{+}$ and $CD8^{+}$ T-cells [36]. Since the ratio of circulating non-infectious to infectious virions is exponentially greater [37,38], the role played by these non-infectious virus particles in the progression to cardiovascular disease cannot be ignored, particularly in cell expressing the CXCR4 chemokine receptor. Therefore, it is perhaps erroneous to assume that because these viral particles are not capable of productive infection, that they play no role in HIV-1 pathogenesis, which includes HIV-associated cardiomyopathy.

In summary, this study demonstrated that HIV-1 subtype C unproductively infects human cord-blood stem cell-derived cardiomyocytes and, while the virus did not replicate in the human cardiomyocytes, it directly (cell free virus) and indirectly (macrophage-associated virus) induced apoptosis, which could be mitigated by UCLA1 in culture. The limitation of this study is the use of human cord-blood stem cell-derived cardiomyocytes, which formed clumps in culture and hence seemed not to exhibit a distinct morphology and antibody staining pattern usually observed in primary cardiomyocytes. The future research challenge will be to extend this proof-in-principle observation that UCLA1 can protect human cardiomyocytes from both direct and indirect effects of HIV-1 in human heart tissue samples and in an advanced model of HIV-1 associated cardiomyopathy.

Materials and Methods

Ethics statement

The human cord-blood stem cell-derived cardiomyocytes were purchased from Celprogen Inc. (USA) and human buffy coats, which are the residual material after plasma, platelets, and red cell separation for patient use, were supplied by the South African National Blood Services. The investigation with human cells conformed to the principles outlined in the Declaration of Helsinki [39] and approval was granted by the human research ethics committee of the University of Witwatersrand (protocol number M071031).

Cell cultures

The human cord-blood stem cell-derived cardiomyocytes were cultured as previously described [21,23].

Peripheral-blood mononuclear cells (PBMC) and monocyte derived macrophages (MDM) were isolated from heparinized human buffy coats of normal, HIV-negative donors and cultured as previously described [27].

Phenotyping the cardiomyocyte

To confirm the cardiac phenotype of the human cord-blood stem cell-derived cardiomyocytes, we stained the cells with antibodies for known cardiac specific markers. Cardiomyocytes were seeded on cover slips obtained from Celprogen (Celprogen Inc, USA) and fixed with ice-cold methanol for 30 min. Primary antibodies diluted 1:100 with blocking buffer (PBS containing 1% bovine serum albumin (BSA) were applied on cover slips for 1 h at room temperature. Primary monoclonal antibodies included mouse anti-alpha myosin heavy chain (α-MHC) (Abcam plc, UK), mouse anti-connexin43 (Cx43) Alexa Fluor 488 conjugated (Invitrogen, USA), and goat polyclonal anti-Troponin T (cTnT) (Santa Cruz Biotechnology, USA). Cardiomyocytes were washed four times with ice-cold PBS, then incubated with 1:200 dilution of labelled secondary partner antibodies, which included donkey anti-goat Alexa Fluor 546 conjugate (Invitrogen, USA) and goat anti-mouse Alexa Fluor 546 conjugate (Invitrogen, USA). The cardiomyocyte monolayer was covered with a standard glass slide in the presence of mounting medium containing 4′-6-Diamidino-2-phenylindole (DAPI) nuclear stain (Santa Cruz Biotechnology, USA) and imaged using an immunofluorescent confocal microscope (Zeiss LSM780, Germany).

HIV-1 isolates and virus conditioned media

A panel of 7 previously reported [40,41] clinical isolates of HIV-1 subtype C were used. This included two R5 viruses (SW2, SW4), two X4 viruses (SW12 and TM46b) and three R5X4 viruses (CM9, Du179-99 and RP1).

Virus conditioned media was prepared from day 5 culture supernatants of HIV-infected phytohemagglutinin (PHA)-stimulated IL-2 treated PBMC. Virus was separated from the supernatants by size-exclusion centrifugation using a 200 KDa NWM filter (Millipore, USA). This allowed for the separation of cell-free virions from cellular debris and viral proteins.

Anti-HIV-1 molecules and aptamer

Zidovudine (AZT), AMD3100 and RANTES (regulated upon activation, normal T-cell expressed, and secreted) were obtained through the AIDS Research and Reference Reagent Program, Division of AIDS, NIAID, NIH, USA. A fully characterized UCLA1 aptamer, previously reported [18] was donated by William James, University of Oxford, United Kingdom. Briefly, UCLA1 is a shortened and synthetic derivative of gp120 binding and HIV-1 neutralizing aptamer called B40 [19,20,21,22].

Infection of cells with HIV-1 and PCR detection of proviral DNA

A total of 5×10^4 cardiomyocytes or PBMC cultured in 96-well plates (Corning, USA) were infected with HIV-1 at a concentration of 200 ng/ml p24 in the absence or presence of 500 nM of the entry inhibitor AMD3100, 100 nM RANTES or 100 nM of UCLA1 aptamer. Following incubation for different time intervals, protein digestion and inactivation of proteinase K (10 min at 95°C) the cell lysate was subjected to PCR amplification as previously described [42].

Detection and modulation of HIV-1 initiated apoptosis in cardiomyocytes by TUNEL assay

Cardiomyocytes seeded at a density of 2×10^4 cells/well were treated either with culture medium (mock-treatment), 500 nM of AMD3100, 100 nM RANTES, 100 nM of Z-IETD-FMK, a preferential caspase 8 inhibitor-casp8i (Promega, USA), 100 nM Z-LEHD-FMK, a preferential caspase 9 inhibitor-casp9i (Promega, USA) for 1 hour at 37°C in the CO_2 incubator. For UCLA1 inhibition, 100 nM of the aptamer was incubated with HIV-1 for 1 hour prior to infection. Cells were then exposed to HIV-1 subtype C clinical isolates at 30 ng/ml p24. After 3 days of incubation, the cell monolayers cultured in flat-bottom 96-well plates (Corning, USA) were fixed in 1% (w/v) paraformaldehyde and washed twice with 200 µl of a proprietary wash buffer (Guava Technologies, USA). The cells were then resuspended in 25 µl of a Brd-UTP labelling mix (Guava Technologies, USA) and incubated for 60 min at 37°C and stained with anti-BrdU-TRITC according to the manufacturer's instruction (Guava Technologies, USA). Data was analysed using the TUNEL assay program in the Cytosoft data acquisition and analysis software, Version 5.2 (Guava Technologies, USA). A total of 2000 events were acquired at a time and each well was acquired in triplicate. The results were displayed in a dot plot relating forward scatter (FSC) over fluorescence intensity (PM1) as well as a histogram (PM1 fluorescence intensity vs. number of events). The general apoptosis inducer staurosporin (Sigma-Aldrich, USA) was used as a positive control for terminal deoxynucleotidyl transferase dUTP nick end label (TUNEL) staining.

Indirect immuno-fluorescence for Cytochrome c release detection

Cardiomyocytes were either mock-infected or infected with the HIV-1_{CM9} dual tropic strain for 2 days in the presence of either 100 nM of casp8i; 100 nM of casp9i or 100 nM of UCLA1. For all casp8i and casp9i, the inhibitors were added to the cell monolayer 2 hours prior to infection. The UCLA1 aptamer was first incubated with the virus for 1 hour before infection. Following 2 days of incubation the cells were harvested, fixed, stored and washed as above. A total of 2×10^4 cells/well in 96-well, U-bottom plates, were treated with 5 µg/ml of mouse-anti human cytochrome *c* monoclonal antibody (Santa Cruz Biotechnology, Inc., USA) in 20 µl for 1 h at 37°C. The cells were then harvested by centrifugation, washed twice in an equal volume of PBS and counter stained with 1 µg/ml of Alexa Fluor 514 goat anti-mouse polyclonal antibody (Invitrogen, USA) for 30 min at room temperature. At the end of the incubation, rinsing buffer was added up to 200 µl and the cells were analyzed in the Guava EasyCyte Plus flow cytometer (Guava Technologies, USA).

Caspase 8 and 9 enzyme activity and cell viability

Cardiomyocytes were seeded in 96-well tissue culture plates as previously described [21]. The cells were then exposed to eleven different conditions, namely 1 – media alone, 2 – conditioned media, 3 – HIV-1, 4 –100 µM of preferential caspase 8 inhibitor Z-IETD-FMK (casp8i) (Promega, USA), 5 –100 µM of preferential caspase 9 inhibitor Z-LEHD-FMK (casp9i) (Promega, USA), 6 – conditioned media and 100 µM Z-LEHD-FMK, 7 – conditioned media and 100 µM Z-IETD-FMK, 8 – conditioned media and 100 nM UCLA1 aptamer, 9 – HIV pre-incubated for 1 h with 100 nM of UCLA1 aptamer, 10 – HIV and 100 µM Z-LEHD-FMK, 11 – HIV-1 and 100 µM Z-IETD-FMK. The cells were harvested daily for 7 days followed by quantification of the caspases and cellular ATP levels, using the Caspase-Glo8, Caspase-Glo9 and the CellTiter-Glo luminescence-based detection kits as instructed by the supplier (Promega, USA). Wells containing media alone were used as controls for background luminescence and subtracted from the test values. The results were expressed as relative light units (RLUs) and plotted in a graph relating RLU to number of days.

Cardiomyocytes apoptosis in HIV-infected macrophage co-cultures

Day 7 monocyte derived macrophages (MDM) seeded at a density of 2×10^4 cells/well in a 24 well tissue culture plate (Corning, USA) were infected with R5 and dual-tropic viruses (30 ng/ml, p24) for 24 h in 200 µl of X-VIVO 10 medium (BioWhittaker) supplemented with 2% autologous serum. The cells were then washed 3 times with an equal volume of PBS followed by the addition of 2×10^4 uninfected cardiomyocytes. To investigate apoptotic modulators, cells were cultured in the presence or absence of a TNF inhibitor (TNF-Ra, R&D Systems, USA), AMD3100, casp8i and casp9i. UCLA1 was pre-incubated with virus for 1 hour prior to infection. Controls included mock-infected cardiomyocyte-macrophage co-cultures. Following two days of exposure the cell monolayer was washed twice with warm PBS prior to trypsin (Lonza, USA) treatment. The strong adhesion properties of MDM were exploited to recover the less adherent cardiomyocytes. A 2 min trypsin treatment at 37°C was enough to recover over 95% of the cardiomyocytes but less than 3% of the macrophages, thereby minimizing cross-contamination. Purity of cardiomyocytes cultures and contamination by MDM was determined by flow cytometry using a 1:200 dilution of a FITC-conjugated antibody directed against the CD4 cell surface receptor, which is absent on cardiomyocytes. Cardiomyocytes were then stained for TUNEL detection as described above.

Acknowledgments

We thank the generous donation of UCLA1 aptamer by William James, Ian McGowan and Brian Sproat under the NIH Aptamer Microbicide Program, grant number 5U01AI066734-03. We also thank the AIDS Research and Reference Reagent Program, Division of AIDS, NIAID, NIH, USA for providing AZT.

Author Contributions

Conceived and designed the experiments: WRL MK. Performed the experiments: WRL NC GL LSR. Analyzed the data: WRL NC GL MK. Contributed reagents/materials/analysis tools: LM BMM. Wrote the paper: WRL NC LM BMM MK. Obtained permission for use of cell lines: MK.

References

1. Ntsekhe M, Hakim J (2005) Impact of human immunodeficiency virus infection on cardiovascular disease in Africa. Circulation 112: 3602–3607.
2. Ntsekhe M, Mayosi BM (2009) Cardiac manifestations of HIV infection: an African perspective. Nat Clin Pract Cardiovasc Med 6: 120–127.
3. Magula NP, Mayosi BM (2003) Cardiac involvement in HIV-infected people living in Africa: a review. Cardiovasc J S Afr 14: 231–237.
4. Twu C, Liu NQ, Popik W, Bukrinsky M, Sayre J, et al. (2002) Cardiomyocytes undergo apoptosis in human immunodeficiency virus cardiomyopathy through mitochondrion- and death receptor-controlled pathways. Proc Natl Acad Sci U S A 99: 14386–14391.
5. Fiala M, Popik W, Qiao JH, Lossinsky AS, Alce T, et al. (2004) HIV-1 induces cardiomyopathyby cardiomyocyte invasion and gp120, Tat, and cytokine apoptotic signaling. Cardiovasc Toxicol 4: 97–107.
6. Kan H, Xie Z, Finkel MS (2000) HIV gp120 enhances NO production by cardiac myocytes through p38 MAP kinase-mediated NF-kappaB activation. Am J Physiol Heart Circ Physiol 279: H3138–3143.
7. Kan H, Birkle D, Jain AC, Failinger C, Xie S, et al. (2005) p38 MAP kinase inhibitor reverses stress-induced cardiac myocyte dysfunction. J Appl Physiol 98: 77–82.
8. Kan H, Xie Z, Finkel MS (2006) iPLA2 inhibitor blocks negative inotropic effect of HIV gp120 on cardiac myocytes. J Mol Cell Cardiol 40: 131–137.
9. Lipshultz SE, Fox CH, Perez-Atayde AR, Sanders SP, Colan SD, et al. (1990) Identification of human immunodeficiency virus-1 RNA and DNA in the heart of a child with cardiovascular abnormalities and congenital acquired immune deficiency syndrome. Am J Cardiol 66: 246–250.
10. Herskowitz A, Wu TC, Willoughby SB, Vlahov D, Ansari AA, et al. (1994) Myocarditis and cardiotropic viral infection associated with severe left ventricular dysfunction in late-stage infection with human immunodeficiency virus. J Am Coll Cardiol 24: 1025–1032.
11. Grody WW, Cheng L, Lewis W (1990) Infection of the heart by the human immunodeficiency virus. Am J Cardiol 66: 203–206.
12. Yuan Y, Kan H, Fang Q, Chen F, Finkel MS (2008) CXCR4 receptor antagonist blocks cardiac myocyte p38 MAP kinase phosphorylation by HIV gp120. Cardiovasc Toxicol 8: 173–180.
13. Kroemer G, Dallaporta B, Resche-Rigon M (1998) The mitochondrial death/life regulator in apoptosis and necrosis. Annu Rev Physiol 60: 619–642.
14. Green DR, Reed JC (1998) Mitochondria and apoptosis. Science 281: 1309–1312.
15. Budihardjo I, Oliver H, Lutter M, Luo X, Wang X (1999) Biochemical pathways of caspase activation during apoptosis. Annu Rev Cell Dev Biol 15: 269–290.
16. Finkel MS, Oddis CV, Jacob TD, Watkins SC, Hattler BG, et al. (1992) Negative inotropic effects of cytokines on the heart mediated by nitric oxide. Science 257: 387–389.
17. Monsuez JJ, Escaut L, Teicher E, Charniot JC, Vittecoq D (2007) Cytokines in HIV-associated cardiomyopathy. Int J Cardiol 120: 150–157.
18. Cohen C, Forzan M, Sproat B, Pantophlet R, McGowan I, et al. (2008) An aptamer that neutralizes R5 strains of HIV-1 binds to core residues of gp120 in the CCR5 binding site. Virology 381: 46–54.
19. Dey AK, Griffiths C, Lea SM, James W (2005) Structural characterization of an anti-gp120 RNA aptamer that neutralizes R5 strains of HIV-1. Rna 11: 873–884.
20. Dey AK, Khati M, Tang M, Wyatt R, Lea SM, et al. (2005) An aptamer that neutralizes R5 strains of human immunodeficiency virus type 1 blocks gp120-CCR5 interaction. J Virol 79: 13806–13810.
21. Lopes de Campos WR, Coopusamy D, Morris L, Mayosi BM, Khati M (2009) Cytotoxicological analysis of a gp120 binding aptamer with cross-clade human immunodeficiency virus type 1 entry inhibition properties: comparison to conventional antiretrovirals. Antimicrob Agents Chemother 53: 3056–3064.
22. Joubert MK, Kinsley N, Capovilla A, Sewell BT, Jaffer MA, et al. (2010) A modeled structure of an aptamer-gp120 complex provides insight into the mechanism of HIV-1 neutralization. Biochemistry 49: 5880–5890.
23. Perez R, Michael VR, Sharma R, Punzalan R, Shaleekha K, et al. (2006) Synchronized contracting cardiomyocytes in culture from human cord blood-derived stem cells as a potential source of cardiomyocyte-based therapeutics and alternative to heart transplantation. Stem Cell Research and Therapeutics Conference, March 2–3. Available: http://www.celprogen.com/publications/StemCellCardiomyocytes.pdf.
24. Fernandes S, Naumova AV, Zhu WZ, Laflamme MA, Gold J, et al. (2010) Human embryonic stem cell-derived cardiomyocytes engraft but do not alter cardiac remodeling after chronic infarction in rats. J Mol Cell Cardiol 49: 941–949.
25. Roggero R, Robert-Hebmann V, Harrington S, Roland J, Vergne L, et al. (2001) Binding of human immunodeficiency virus type 1 gp120 to CXCR4 induces mitochondrial transmembrane depolarization and cytochrome c-mediated apoptosis independently of Fas signaling. J Virol 75: 7637–7650.
26. Bottarel F, Feito MJ, Bragardo M, Bonissoni S, Buonfiglio D, et al. (1999) The cell death-inducing ability of glycoprotein 120 from different HIV strains correlates with their ability to induce CD4 lateral association with CD95 on CD4+ T cells. AIDS Res Hum Retroviruses 15: 1255–1263.
27. Khati M, Schuman M, Ibrahim J, Sattentau Q, Gordon S, et al. (2003) Neutralization of infectivity of diverse R5 clinical isolates of human immunodeficiency virus type 1 by gp120-binding 2′F-RNA aptamers. J Virol 77: 12692–12698.
28. Herbein G, Mahlknecht U, Batliwalla F, Gregersen P, Pappas T, et al. (1998) Apoptosis of CD8+ T cells is mediated by macrophages through interaction of HIV gp120 with chemokine receptor CXCR4. Nature 395: 189–194.
29. Adachi S, Gottlieb RA, Babior BM (1998) Lack of release of cytochrome C from mitochondria into cytosol early in the course of Fas-mediated apoptosis of Jurkat cells. J Biol Chem 273: 19892–19894.
30. Nardelli B, Gonzalez CJ, Schechter M, Valentine FT (1995) CD4+ blood lymphocytes are rapidly killed in vitro by contact with autologous human immunodeficiency virus-infected cells. Proc Natl Acad Sci U S A 92: 7312–7316.
31. Vlahakis SR, Algeciras-Schimnich A, Bou G, Heppelmann CJ, Villasis-Keever A, et al. (2001) Chemokine-receptor activation by env determines the mechanism of death in HIV-infected and uninfected T lymphocytes. J Clin Invest 107: 207–215.
32. Jacotot E, Krust B, Callebaut C, Laurent-Crawford AG, Blanco J, et al. (1997) HIV-1 envelope glycoproteins-mediated apoptosis is regulated by CD4 dependent and independent mechanisms. Apoptosis 2: 47–60.
33. Biard-Piechaczyk M, Robert-Hebmann V, Richard V, Roland J, Hipskind RA, et al. (2000) Caspase-dependent apoptosis of cells expressing the chemokine receptor CXCR4 is induced by cell membrane-associated human immunodeficiency virus type 1 envelope glycoprotein (gp120). Virology 268: 329–344.
34. Boldin MP, Goncharov TM, Goltsev YV, Wallach D (1996) Involvement of MACH, a novel MORT1/FADD-interacting protease, in Fas/APO-1- and TNF receptor-induced cell death. Cell 85: 803–815.
35. Muzio M, Chinnaiyan AM, Kischkel FC, O'Rourke K, Shevchenko A, et al. (1996) FLICE, a novel FADD-homologous ICE/CED-3-like protease, is recruited to the CD95 (Fas/APO-1) death – inducing signaling complex. Cell 85: 817–827.
36. Esser MT, Bess JW Jr, Suryanarayana K, Chertova E, Marti D, et al. (2001) Partial activation and induction of apoptosis in CD4(+) and CD8(+) T lymphocytes by conformationally authentic noninfectious human immunodeficiency virus type 1. J Virol 75: 1152–1164.
37. Dimitrov DS, Willey RL, Sato H, Chang LJ, Blumenthal R, et al. (1993) Quantitation of human immunodeficiency virus type 1 infection kinetics. J Virol 67: 2182–2190.
38. Piatak M Jr, Saag MS, Yang LC, Clark SJ, Kappes JC, et al. (1993) High levels of HIV-1 in plasma during all stages of infection determined by competitive PCR. Science 259: 1749–1754.
39. World Medical Association Declaration of Helsinki (1997) Recommendations guiding physicians in biomedical research involving human subjects. Cardiovasc Res 35: 2–3.
40. Cilliers T, Willey S, Sullivan WM, Patience T, Pugach P, et al. (2005) Use of alternate coreceptors on primary cells by two HIV-1 isolates. Virology 339: 136–144.
41. Coetzer M, Cilliers T, Ping LH, Swanstrom R, Morris L (2006) Genetic characteristics of the V3 region associated with CXCR4 usage in HIV-1 subtype C isolates. Virology 356: 95–105.
42. Schmidtmayerova H, Alfano M, Nuovo G, Bukrinsky M (1998) Human immunodeficiency virus type 1 T-lymphotropic strains enter macrophages via a CD4- and CXCR4-mediated pathway: replication is restricted at a postentry level. J Virol 72: 4633–4642.

16

Community-Based Evaluation of PMTCT Uptake in Nyanza Province, Kenya

Pamela K. Kohler[1]*, John Okanda[2], John Kinuthia[3], Lisa A. Mills[4], George Olilo[2], Frank Odhiambo[2], Kayla F. Laserson[4], Brenda Zierler[5], Joachim Voss[5], Grace John-Stewart[6]

1 Global Health and Psychosocial & Community Health, University of Washington, Seattle, Washington, United States of America, **2** Center for Global Health Research, Kenya Medical Research Institute, Kisumu, Kenya, **3** Kenyatta National Hospital/University of Nairobi, Nairobi, Kenya, **4** Kenya Medical Research Institute/Centers for Disease Control and Prevention (KEMRI/CDC) Research and Public Health Collaboration, Kisumu, Kenya; and Division of HIV/AIDS Prevention, CDC, Atlanta, Georgia, United States of America, **5** Biobehavioral Nursing & Health Systems, University of Washington, Seattle, Washington, United States of America, **6** Global Health, Medicine, Pediatrics, and Epidemiology, University of Washington, Seattle, Washington, United States of America

Abstract

Introduction: Facility-based assessments of prevention of mother-to-child HIV transmission (PMTCT) programs may overestimate population coverage. There are few community-based studies that evaluate PMTCT coverage and uptake.

Methods: During 2011, a cross-sectional community survey among women who gave birth in the prior year was performed using the KEMRI-CDC Health and Demographic Surveillance System in Western Kenya. A random sample (n = 405) and a sample of women known to be HIV-positive through previous home-based testing (n = 247) were enrolled. Rates and correlates of uptake of antenatal care (ANC), HIV-testing, and antiretrovirals (ARVs) were determined.

Results: Among 405 women in the random sample, 379 (94%) reported accessing ANC, most of whom (87%) were HIV tested. Uptake of HIV testing was associated with employment, higher socioeconomic status, and partner HIV testing. Among 247 known HIV-positive women, 173 (70%) self-disclosed their HIV status. Among 216 self-reported HIV-positive women (including 43 from the random sample), 82% took PMTCT ARVs, with 54% completing the full antenatal, peripartum, and postpartum course. Maternal ARV use was associated with more ANC visits and having an HIV tested partner. ARV use during delivery was lowest (62%) and associated with facility delivery. Eighty percent of HIV infected women reported having their infant HIV tested, 11% of whom reported their child was HIV infected, 76% uninfected, 6% declined to say, 7% did not recall; 79% of infected children were reportedly receiving HIV care and treatment.

Conclusions: Community-based assessments provide data that complements clinic-based PMTCT evaluations. In this survey, antenatal HIV test uptake was high; most HIV infected women received ARVs, though many women did not self-disclose HIV status to field team. Community-driven strategies that encourage early ANC, partner involvement, and skilled delivery, and provide PMTCT education, may facilitate further reductions in vertical transmission.

Editor: Claire Thorne, UCL Institute of Child Health, University College London, United Kingdom

Funding: This study was funded by the National Institutes of Health (www.nih.gov): A Kenya Free of AIDS (R24 HD056799); and received assistance from the University of Washington Center for AIDS Research (P30 AI027757 and K24 HD054314). The funders had no role in study design, data collection and analysis, decision to publish, or preparation of the manuscript.

Competing Interests: The authors have declared that no competing interests exist.

* Email: pkohler2@uw.edu

Introduction

Global elimination of mother-to-child HIV transmission (MTCT) is targeted for 2015 and is an initiative which will require strategic improvements in service delivery. [1] As PMTCT interventions have expanded globally, challenges in delivery and uptake of services have persisted. The World Health Organization (WHO) estimated that in 2010, in low and middle income countries, only 35% of pregnant women received HIV testing, and less than half of HIV infected women tested accessed antiretrovirals (ARVs) for PMTCT. [2] By 2012, the 21 Global Plan for Elimination of Pediatric HIV priority countries reported 64% coverage, however the pace of decline in the number of newly infected children has been slow in some countries. [3] To meet elimination (eMTCT) goals, a focus in sub-Saharan Africa is critical given the high HIV prevalence among women of childbearing age in this region.

PMTCT programs involve a cascade of interventions, which begins with HIV counseling and testing of pregnant women at initiation of antenatal care (ANC), and provision of ARVs throughout pregnancy, peripartum, and in the postpartum period to prevent vertical HIV transmission. [4] Modeling suggests that improving PMTCT coverage throughout the cascade would decrease infant HIV more than improving maternal antiretroviral regimens. [5] The Kenya Ministry of Health has made great strides to increase PMTCT coverage, with provision of ARVs to HIV-infected pregnant women increasing from 20% uptake in 2005 [6] to 69% in 2011. [7] As a result, new child HIV infections in Kenya have decreased, averting 46,000 new infections since the introduction of PMTCT. [7] However, the number of newly infected children per year remain high (13,000 in 2012), [3] and recent estimates of MTCT rates, while ≤5% in clinical trial settings, [8–11] range from 8 - 27% in Kenyan surveys [7,12–14].

Most PMTCT assessments are clinic-based, and few studies sample a broader population of mothers which includes those who never accessed clinics. While clinic-based assessment is informative, this can exclude vulnerable and underserved women, overestimating PMTCT coverage and failing to adequately capture barriers to accessing PMTCT. A study from Uganda noted markedly lower estimates of antenatal HIV testing in community-based assessment than in clinic-based assessment. [15] Another recent study in Cameroon, Cote D'Ivoire, South Africa, and Zambia similarly found that facility-based estimates of PMTCT coverage exceeded coverage estimates observed in the community [16].

Expansion of PMTCT coverage in Kenya faces persistent barriers due to social, cultural, programmatic, logistical, and policy challenges also seen in other sub-Saharan countries. [17–23] To complement a clinic-based assessment conducted in 2009, [24] this survey aimed to assess PMTCT coverage and barriers to access to PMTCT from a community perspective.

Methods

Study Design

A cross-sectional community-level survey assessing knowledge and uptake of PMTCT services among women of child-bearing age was performed March – June, 2011 in the Kenya Medical Research Institute (KEMRI) and US Centers for Disease Control (CDC) Health and Demographic Surveillance System (HDSS) area in Nyanza Province, Kenya.

Study Location

The HDSS covers 385 villages with a population of approximately 220,000. Three regions situated in Siaya County make up this area: Karemo, Gem and Asembo. [25] All three regions are rural. The HDSS was launched in September 2001 by the US Centers for Disease Control and Prevention (CDC) in collaboration with the Kenya Medical Research Institute (KEMRI) and serves as a community-based platform. The HDSS provides demographic and health information as well as disease- or intervention-specific information. Since its inception, the HDSS has collected 13 years of population-level data. Home-based HIV counseling and testing (HBCT) of the HDSS population has been conducted since 2008, but had not been implemented in all areas at the time of the study. The HDSS area includes 41 health facilities that provide care to pregnant women.

Study Population

Women, maternal age 14 years and older (mothers 14–17 are considered emancipated minors), who were residents in the HDSS area, and had delivered a baby within the previous year (January to December 2010) were recruited. Residency was defined as having lived in the area for at least 4 consecutive months. We leveraged existing HDSS program data to identify and recruit two groups representing two target populations for prevention services: a random community sample to assess factors influencing uptake of general services (access to ANC and maternal HIV testing); and a second sample of HIV infected women, known via previous home-based testing and counseling in the region, to assess factors influencing uptake of HIV-specific services (use of ARVs and infant HIV testing). The same inclusion criteria applied to both general community and HIV-positive groups, with the addition that women in the HIV-positive group must have completed HIV-testing prior to the delivery of the infant.

Sampling

Sampling was limited by the number of women meeting recruitment criteria in the HDSS database. We were able to generate a random list of 523 women from non-HBCT areas to represent a general community assessment of ANC and HIV-testing uptake. In HBCT areas, only 275 women were HIV positive, thus all HIV positive mothers who were diagnosed prior to delivery were approached.

Data Collection

Trained fieldworkers were assigned a list of names and locations for all selected participants. Village reporters assisted fieldworkers to locate the mother participant and introduce the study. Fieldworkers administered surveys and recorded GPS location on hand-held PDAs using electronic forms (Pendragon Software Corporation, Buffalo Grove, IL); paper forms were used as a back-up. Mothers' surveys were adapted from clinic-based surveys used previously in this region [24]. Women were surveyed regarding their knowledge, opinions and use of ANC and PMTCT services at last pregnancy.

Outcomes of interest included self-report of uptake of ANC, HIV testing, maternal ARVs for PMTCT, infant testing, and infant ARVs. Potential cofactors assessed included demographics, educational achievement, and marital status, as well as knowledge about HIV and disease transmission. Due to limitations in determining income through household surveys, asset-based indicators (ownership of goods, including mobile phones, cattle, television or refrigerator, and roof type) were used as measures of socioeconomic status. [26,27] Fieldworkers were not informed of HIV status of participants, thus participant self-reported HIV status was used. In 2010, Kenya national PMTCT guidelines adopted WHO PMTCT Option A (zidovudine during pregnancy with infant nevirapine during breastfeeding for women without advanced HIV, or triple-drug antiretroviral therapy for women with advanced disease) with a provision to implement Option B (triple-drug antiretroviral therapy for all women, stopping after breastfeeding for those without advanced disease) in higher resource systems. As national adoption of new guidelines was slow, and only half of national facilities offered PMTCT, [12] we chose to assess self-report of any maternal ARV uptake at each of three time-points: antenatal, perinatal, and postpartum.

Data Analysis

Descriptive proportions of those accessing services in the PMTCT cascade were generated. Data analysis utilized chi-square analyses with Fisher's exact tests for comparison of proportions using STATA SE version 11 (STATACorp, College Station, Texas). Wilcoxon Mann-Whitney tests were used for comparisons where continuous data were not normally distributed. Multivariate analysis using generalized linear models further assessed adjusted prevalence ratios of uptake. A priori covariates of age and education level were included in the model with correlates identified in univariate analyses. Variables were retained in the model if they were significantly associated with the outcome and/or if their inclusion substantially changed the estimates by 10%.

Analysis was modeled to assess key steps in the PMTCT cascade: correlates of ANC attendance were assessed among women in the community sample (n = 405); correlates of HIV testing were assessed among women attending ANC with unknown or previously negative HIV status (n = 362); and correlates of maternal and infant ARV uptake were assessed among self-identified HIV-positive women (n = 216).

Ethical Considerations

Prior to study start, community engagement activities were held targeting the area senior health officials, the local community advisory board, the village reporters, chiefs and assistant chiefs. Written informed consent was obtained from all study participants, both to be interviewed and also to have their data from these surveys linked to their HDSS record. In Kenya, women with pregnancy are considered emancipated and were therefore able to consent to study participation without parental assent. All study procedures, including enrollment of emancipated minors, were approved by the University of Washington Institutional Review Board (#36022) and the Kenya Medical Research Institute Ethical Review Committee (#1714). Written permission was also received from provincial medical and public health offices.

Results

Enrollment

A random sample of 523 women who delivered in the previous year was identified, 437 (83.6%) were located, and 405 (92.7% of those located) agreed to participate (Figure 1). Among 275 women known to be HIV infected through prior HBCT, 247 (89.8%) consented to participate. However, only 173 (70%) of those enrolled reported to fieldworkers that they were HIV-positive and subsequently answered questions about PMTCT. Thus, the HIV-infected sample includes 43 women from the random community sample and 173 women from the HBCT sample to total 216 women.

Population Characteristics

Among the 405 women in the general community sample, most were married (79% monogamous and 15% polygamous) (Table 1). The majority were of poor socioeconomic status; 42% held any job or small-business (less than 2% were salaried workers), and less than half of the women had completed a primary education. The median number of mobile phones per household was 1 (IQR 0-2), with 71% of women reporting one or more phones in the household. Under half of households reported cattle ownership (median 0, IQR 0-2), and >90% of households did not own a television or refrigerator. Approximately one third (29%) had better than a grass roof (a marker of higher socioeconomic status), and all but one of these were iron sheet.

Women reported a median of 4 (IQR 3-6) pregnancies. Although uptake of ANC was high (94%), most women started ANC late (median 5 months gestation at first ANC visit, IQR 4-6) and completed fewer than the recommended 4 ANC visits (median 3 visits, IQR 2-4). Uptake of skilled delivery, defined as a doctor, nurse or midwife, was 44%, with 20% reporting no assistance at all. Less than half of women reported delivering in a health facility (n = 170, 42.0%); 210 (52%) delivered at home and 14 (3.5%) delivered on the roadside while attempting to reach a health facility.

PMTCT Cascade

Most (94%) women from the random community sample reported attending ANC during the last pregnancy, among whom 89% reported that they were offered HIV testing and 87% reported being tested. Among women in the random sample, regardless of ANC attendance, 324 (80%) reported uptake of HIV testing, 4% were known positive, and 16% did not accept testing during the last pregnancy (Figure 2). Among women in the random sample who ever agreed to HIV testing, prevalence of HIV by self-report was 11% positive, 85% negative and 4% declined to answer.

Among 216 HIV-positive women, 82% reported receipt of maternal ARVs at any time-point (prenatal, labor and delivery, or postpartum), however uptake at all three time-points was considerably lower (54%). This was primarily driven by lower uptake during labor/delivery time-points (62% compared to 72% antenatal and 72% postpartum).

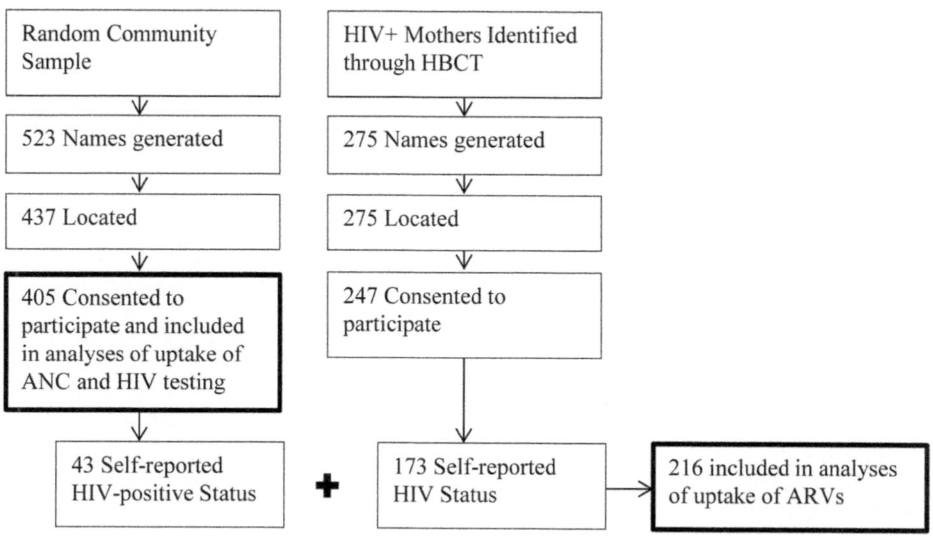

Figure 1. Sampling and Enrollment.

Table 1. Population and Sample.

Participant Characteristic	Community Sample	HIV+ Mothers*
	(n = 405)	(n = 216)
	n(%) or median (IQR)	**n(%) or median (IQR)**
Demographic Information		
Age	25 (22–30)	29 (25–32)
Years of residence in village	7.2 (3.5–12)	9.5 (5–14)
Marital status		
Married monogamous	318 (78.5)	159 (73.6)
Married polygamous	60 (14.8)	35 (16.2)
Single	17 (4.2)	7 (3.2)
Widowed	10 (2.5)	15 (6.9)
Occupation		
Unemployed	71 (17.5)	39 (18.1)
Housewife	163 (40.3)	98 (45.4)
Salaried job or small business	170 (42.0)	77 (35.7)
Completed primary education	184 (45.4)	112 (51.9)
Cattle ownership (≥in household)	192 (47.4)	89 (41.2)
Mobile phone ownership (≥in household)	289 (71.4)	152 (70.4)
Roof type		
Grass	288 (71.1)	120 (55.6)
Corrugated iron sheet or better	116 (28.6)	96 (44.4)
Pregnancy Information		
Number of times pregnant	4 (3–6)	4 (3–6)
Any antenatal care last pregnancy	379 (93.6)	209 (96.8)
Number of ANC visits	3 (2–4)	3 (3–4)
Timing of first ANC visit (months pregnant)	5 (4–6)	5 (4–6)
Transport time to ANC (hours)	1 (0.5–1.5)	1 (0.5–1.5)
HIV Testing		
HIV tested last pregnancy	340 (84.0)	–
HIV test at first ANC visit (among those tested)	304 (89.4)	–
Tested at government facility (among those tested)	(86.2)	–
Delivery Care		
Delivery care		
Skilled attendant (nurse, doctor or midwife)	176 (43.5)	101 (46.8)
Unskilled attendant (family member or traditional birth attendant)	145 (35.8)	67 (31.0)
No assistance	45 (20.0)	45 (20.8)
Vaginal delivery (no instruments)	383 (95.3)	203 (94.0)
Knowledge and Beliefs		
Is there any way to prevent HIV (yes)	298 (73.6)	192 (88.9)
Can pregnant women give HIV to baby (yes)	261 (64.4)	172 (79.6)
Can ARVs prevent MTCT of HIV (yes)	210 (51.9)	158 (73.2)

*Includes 43 mothers from community sample and 173 mothers from HBTC.
Women who delivered an infant in the previous year and resided in the Demographic Health and Surveillance System Area, Nyanza Province, Kenya (2011).

Seventy-nine percent of HIV-positive women reported administering infant ARVs for prevention of HIV transmission. Among the 81% (176/216) of infants tested for HIV, 11% of mothers reported that their infant was HIV-positive and 76% reported that the infant tested negative, 6% declined to report their child's HIV status, and 7% stated that they did not remember the test results. Timing of infant HIV diagnosis was not reported, though a national early infant diagnosis program with testing recommendations at six weeks was initiated in the previous year, December 2009. Among the 19 positive infants, 15 (79%) were reported to be receiving care and treatment for HIV, 1 child died prior to receiving treatment, and another 3 did not receive treatment because of fear of others finding out (n = 1), denial (n = 1), and being unaware of treatment (n = 2).

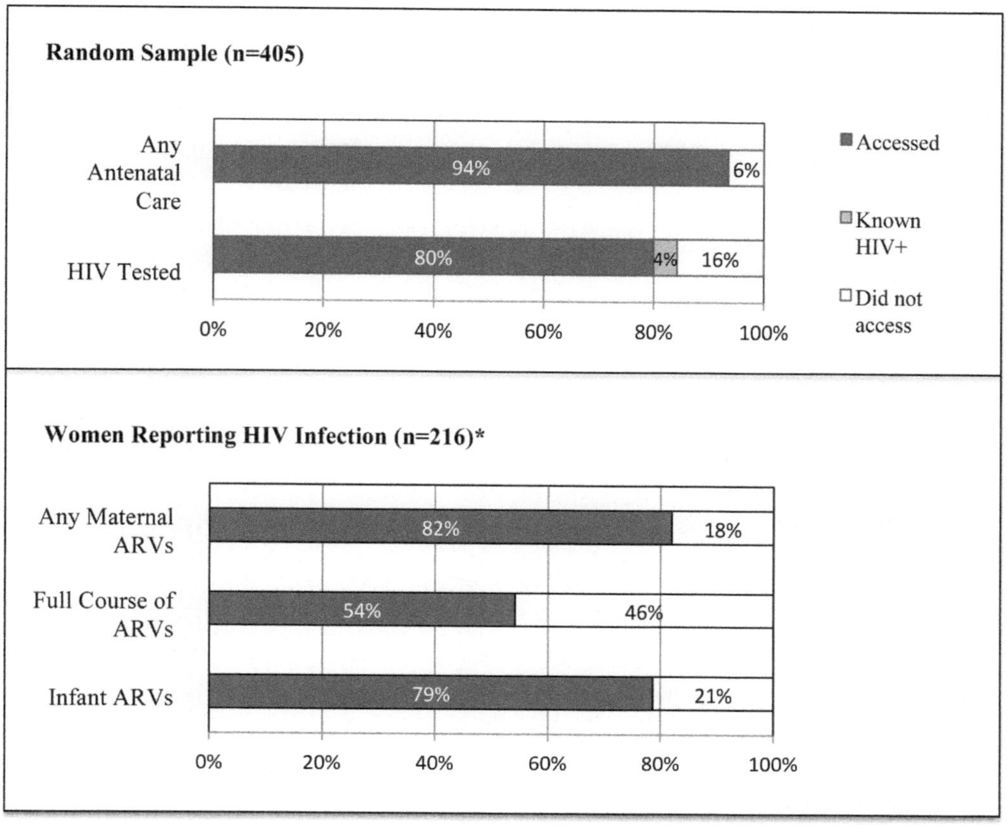

Figure 2. Uptake throughout cascade of PMTCT Services among Women in the Demographic Health Surveillance System Area, Nyanza Province, Kenya (2011). *Includes HIV+ oversample and does not reflect population HIV prevalence.

Correlates of ANC Uptake in the Random Community Sample

Factors associated with report of ANC uptake at most recent pregnancy among women in the community sample are detailed in Table 2. In bivariate analyses, completion of primary education was associated with uptake of ANC. Among women who did not access ANC, 12% had completed primary education compared to 48% of women who accessed ANC (p<0.001) [Adjusted Prevalence Ratio (aPR):1.09; 95% Confidence Interval (CI): 1.04–1.15]. Women who did not access ANC reported a higher number of pregnancies than those who accessed ANC (median 5 vs. 4, p<0.001) (aPR: 0.94; 95%CI: 0.89–0.99).

Correlates of HIV Testing

Of 362 women attending ANC whose prior HIV status was negative or unknown, 87% reported being tested for HIV, and most HIV testing (89%) occurred at the first ANC visit (Table 2). Cofactors associated with HIV testing were occupation (31% versus 15% of those not accessing vs. accessing ANC, p = 0.03), mobile phone at home (50% vs. 75% of those not accessing vs. accessing ANC, p<0.001), partner having been tested for HIV (36% vs. 60% of those not accessing vs. accessing ANC, p = 0.003), and knowledge of PMTCT (34% vs. 55% of those not accessing vs. accessing ANC, p = 0.01). In adjusted models, socioeconomic indicators (cattle, phone ownership, and roof type) and report of partner HIV testing were significantly associated with an increased likelihood of acceptance of HIV testing.

Correlates of Maternal ARV Uptake

Factors associated with uptake of maternal ARVs are described in Table 3. Women who did not access any ARVs reported fewer ANC visits than those who used ARVs (median 2 vs. 4, p = 0.002), and they were less likely to have a partner who was tested for HIV (53% vs. 76% of those without vs. with ARV uptake). Among those who knew their partner's HIV status, having an HIV-positive partner was associated with uptake of maternal ARVs. Correlates of uptake of a complete course of maternal ARVs included more education (41% vs. 61% of those who had an incomplete vs. complete ARV course had finished primary school, p = 0.006). Women who accessed a skilled provider at delivery had increased uptake of ARVs specifically during the labor/delivery time point (p = 0.02). In multivariate analyses, adjusted for number of ANC visits, partner HIV testing, and access to a skilled provider at delivery, older age and a higher number of ANC visits during the last pregnancy were associated with uptake of any antiretrovirals for PMTCT. A full course of PMTCT was associated with completion of primary education. Adjusted prevalence ratios for each of the primary outcomes are detailed in Table 4.

Correlates of Infant ARV

Administration of infant ARVs for PMTCT was highly correlated with maternal ARV uptake. While 160 of 174 (92%) women who took ARVs also administered them to their infant, 10 out of 39 (26%) women who did not take ARVs gave their infants ARVs (p<0.001).

Table 2. Reported uptake of antenatal care and HIV-testing in the random community sample.

Population	*Random community sample*			*Those who accessed ANC with negative or unknown HIV status*		
	(n = 405)			*(n = 362)*		
Uptake of Service	*No ANC*	*ANC*		*No HIV Test*	*HIV Tested*	
	n(%) or med (IQR)	*n(%) or med (IQR)*	*p-value*	*n(%) or med (IQR)*	*n(%) or med (IQR)*	*p-value*
	26 (6.4)	*379 (93.6)*		*48 (13.3)*	*314 (86.7)*	
Demographic Information						
Age	27 (23–32)	25 (22–30)	0.17	24.5 (22–28)	25 (22–30)	0.62
Years of residence in village	9 (4–13)	7 (3.5–11.3)	0.34	7 (3.5–10.3)	7 (3.3–11.5)	0.91
Marital status			0.63			0.23
Married monogamous	22 (84.6)	296 (78.1)		34 (70.8)	250 (79.6)	
Married polygamous	3 (11.5)	57 (15.0)		12 (25.0)	43 (13.7)	
Single	0 (0.0)	17 (4.5)		2 (4.2)	15 (4.8)	
Widowed	1 (3.9)	9 (2.4)		0 (0.0)	6 (1.9)	
Occupation			0.62			0.03
Unemployed	6 (23.1)	65 (17.2)		15 (31.3)	47 (15.0)	
Housewife	11 (42.3)	152 (40.2)		17 (35.4)	129 (41.2)	
Employed	9 (34.6)	161 (42.6)		16 (33.3)	137 (43.8)	
Completed primary education	3 (12.0)	181 (47.9)	<0.001	19 (39.6)	154 (49.2)	0.28
Cattle ownership (≥1 in household)	13 (50.0)	179 (47.5)	0.84	16 (33.3)	154 (49.4)	0.04
Mobile phone (≥1 in household)	15 (57.7)	274 (72.5)	0.12	24 (50.0)	236 (75.4)	<0.001
Roof type			1.00			0.06
Grass	19 (73.1)	269 (71.2)		40 (83.3)	217 (69.3)	
Corrugated iron sheet or better	7 (26.9)	109 (28.8)		8 (16.7)	96 (30.7)	
Pregnancy Information						
Number of times pregnant	5 (4–7)	4 (3–6)	0.001	3 (3–4.5)	4 (3–6)	0.23
HIV Testing						
Partner tested for HIV	–	–		16 (36.4)	179 (60.3)	0.003
Partner HIV positive (among tested)	–	–		1 (6.7)	19 (11.0)	1.00
Knowledge and Beliefs*						
Is there any way to prevent HIV	15 (60.0)	283 (75.1)	0.10	29 (61.7)	240 (76.7)	0.03
Pregnant women can give HIV to baby	14 (56.0)	247 (65.3)	0.39	28 (59.6)	205 (65.3)	0.51
Can prevent MTCT of HIV	10 (71.4)	200 (81.3)	0.48	16 (34.0)	171 (54.6)	0.01

* % women answering agree/yes to knowledge questions.
Women who delivered an infant in the previous year and reside in the Demographic Health and Surveillance System Area, Nyanza Province, Kenya (2011).

Sensitivity Analyses

Among women known to be HIV infected through previous home-based counseling and testing, 14 (5.7%) declined to answer questions about their HIV status and 60 (24.3%) reported to our field workers that they were HIV-negative. In a sensitivity analysis attempting to account for the low self-report among known HIV-positive women, in which we considered the most liberal (that all known HIV-positive women who did not self-report HIV-positive status *accessed* PMTCT services) and conservative (that all known HIV-positive women who did not self-report HIV-positive status *did not access* PMTCT) estimates, the expected range of any PMTCT ARV uptake was 61–87%, ARVs at all three time points was 35–66%, and infant ARV administration was 59–84%. In the HBCT sample, we further compared characteristics of women who reported or denied HIV-positive status in both univariate and multivariate models, and did not find differences in education, marital status, economic indicators, delivery provider, or HIV knowledge. HIV-positive women who did not report their status were younger than those who did (median 25.5 vs. 29 years) (Table 5).

Discussion

In this community-based study of women in western Kenya with a pregnancy during the prior calendar year, we observed high rates of accessing antenatal care at least once, with most reporting HIV testing offered at the first ANC visit. Using a community lens, our study suggests that facilities in this region serve almost all pregnant women at some point, and almost 90% of women with previously unknown HIV status reported receiving HIV testing during their pregnancy. Most (>80%) HIV infected women reported using ARVs for PMTCT. Because a large proportion of HIV infected women did not disclose their status to the field workers, complete ascertainment of ARV use was not possible.

Table 3. Reported uptake of maternal antiretrovirals among HIV-positive women.

Uptake of Maternal Antiretrovirals	*None*	*Any*		*No or Some*	*Full Course**	
	n(%) or med (IQR)	*n(%) or med (IQR)*	*p-value*	*n(%) or med (IQR)*	*n(%) or med (IQR)*	*p-value*
	39 (18.1)	*177 (81.9)*		*99 (45.8%)*	*117 (54.2%)*	
Demographic Information						
Age	26 (23–33)	29 (25–32)	0.06	28 (25–32)	29 (25–32)	0.62
Marital status			0.71			0.86
Married monogamous	27 (69.2)	132 (74.6)		71 (71.7)	88 (75.2)	
Married polygamous	7 (18.0)	28 (15.8)		16 (16.2)	19 (16.2)	
Single	2 (5.1)	5 (2.8)		4 (4.0)	3 (2.6)	
Widowed	3 (7.7)	12 (6.8)		8 (8.1)	7 (6.0)	
Occupation			0.27			0.07
Unemployed	7 (18.0)	32 (18.3)		17 (17.4)	22 (19.0)	
Housewife	22 (56.4)	76 (43.4)		53 (54.1)	45 (38.8)	
Employed	10 (25.6)	67 (38.3)		28 (28.6)	49 (42.2)	
Completed primary education	16 (41.0)	96 (54.2)	0.16	41 (41.4)	71 (60.7)	0.006
Cattle ownership (≥1 in household)	19 (48.7)	70 (39.6)	0.37	40 (40.4)	49 (41.9)	0.89
Mobile phone (≥1 in household)	27 (69.2)	125 (70.6)	0.85	64 (64.7)	88 (75.2)	0.10
Roof type			0.72			0.89
Grass	23 (59.0)	97 (54.8)		56 (56.6)	64 (54.7)	
Corrugated iron sheet or better	16 (41.0)	80 (45.2)		43 (43.4)	53 (45.3)	
Pregnancy Information						
Number of times pregnant	4 (3–6)	4 (3–6)	0.33	4 (3–6)	4 (3–6)	0.66
ANC during last pregnancy	36 (92.3)	173 (97.7)	0.11	94 (95.0)	115 (98.3)	0.25
Timing of first ANC (months pregnant)	6 (5–7)	5 (4–6)	0.18	5 (4–6)	5 (4–6)	0.25
Number of ANC visits	3 (2–4)	4 (3–4)	0.002	3 (2–4)	4 (3–4)	0.23
HIV Testing						
First HIV test before learned was pregnant	11 (28.2)	79 (44.6)	0.07	37 (37.4)	53 (45.3)	0.27
Partner tested for HIV	18 (52.9)	117 (75.5)	0.01	59 (67.8)	76 (74.5)	0.33
Partner HIV-positive (among tested)	8 (44.4)	84 (75.7)	0.01	37 (63.8)	55 (77.5)	0.12
Delivery Care						
Skilled provider at delivery	13 (33.3)	88 (50.6)	0.08	40 (40.8)	61 (53.0)	0.10
Knowledge and Beliefs						
Is there any way to prevent HIV	31 (81.6)	161 (91.0)	0.14	80 (81.6)	112 (95.7)	0.001
Pregnant can women give HIV to baby	29 (74.4)	143 (81.3)	0.38	74 (75.5)	98 (83.8)	0.17
Can prevent MTCT of HIV	26 (66.7)	132 (75.4)	0.31	66 (67.4)	92 (79.3)	0.06

*Defined as uptake at antenatal, peripartum, and postpartum time points.
All women reporting HIV-positive status: including 43 from random sample and 173 from HBCT sample, Nyanza Province, Kenya (2011).

The denial of HIV status by some women to interviewers was unexpected and posed a challenge to complete ascertainment of ARV use in this community survey. It also suggests that acceptance of HIV testing in the home may not readily translate to subsequent disclosure of HIV status and access to HIV services. To account for this possibility, we presented the ranges of uptake in sensitivity analyses to compensate for women who did not self-disclose their HIV status. With the most conservative scenario assuming that none of these women accessed PMTCT, at least 60% of HIV-infected women would have received some pregnancy ARVs.

Although we noted excellent PMTCT coverage, there were several key opportunities for improvement. For example, entry into ANC, was often late, and uptake of a complete course of ARVs for PMTCT was low (54%). These numbers may be even lower considering the high number of known HIV-positive women who declined to reveal their status. This highlights challenges in engagement throughout the cascade, which are especially important since late uptake of ARVs for PMTCT is associated with a higher risk of transmission. [28] As maternal ARV uptake is correlated with infant ARV uptake, and skilled delivery is associated with maternal survival as well as uptake of ARVs, an emphasis on encouraging early uptake of ANC, access to skilled delivery, and ARVs for personal health, may dually promote maternal and infant well-being and survival.

Knowledge of HIV prevention and PMTCT were associated with uptake of HIV testing and maternal ARVs. Given the cross-sectional study design, it is impossible to know whether the

Table 4. Summary of Adjusted Prevalence Ratios (PR) for Accessing Steps of PMTCT Care.

	ANC	*HIV Testing*	*Maternal ARVs*	*Full Course Maternal ARVs*
	PR (95%CI)	*PR (95%CI)*	*PR (95%CI)*	*PR (95%CI)*
Demographic Information				
Age*			1.02 (1.00–1.03)†	
Occupation				
Unemployed		Ref		
Housewife		1.16 (1.00–1.35)		
Employed		2.73 (1.00–1.22)		
Completed primary education	1.09 (1.04–1.15)¥			1.37 (1.06–1.79)†
Cattle ownership (one or> in household)		1.08 (1.01–1.17)†		
Mobile phone ownership (one or> in household)		1.13 (1.00–1.26)†		1.19 (0.88–1.62)
Roof type				
Grass		Ref		
Corrugated iron sheet or better		1.12 (1.04–1.20)‡		
Pregnancy Information				
Number of times pregnant*	0.94 (0.89–0.99)†			
Number of ANC visits*			1.08 (1.03–1.13)‡	
HIV Testing				
Partner tested for HIV		1.13 (1.03–1.24)‡	1.16 (0.97–1.39)	
Delivery Care				
Skilled provider at delivery			1.10 (0.96–1.26)	1.16 (0.94–1.49)

Samples for each column described in previous tables; all variables in final adjusted models presented.
*Prevalence ratios for continuous and ordinal variables are for each one unit change in the variable.
†p<0.05, ‡p<0.01, ¥p<0.001.

knowledge or uptake came first. In our survey, only 52% of women reported that they thought MTCT of HIV could be prevented. Among HIV infected women, PMTCT knowledge was higher at 73%. Women who knew that ARVs could decrease MTCT were more likely to report having taken a complete ARV course than those who did not. This suggests that investing more in early counseling regarding PMTCT ARVs in clinics will be useful to support sustained adherence to ARVs. Community-based activities that stress the effectiveness of PMTCT in preventing new infections will be important to fully realize benefits of PMTCT.

Socioeconomic indicators correlated with uptake of interventions throughout the PMTCT cascade. Maternal education was associated with ANC attendance and maternal ARVs; and higher socioeconomic status also correlated with uptake of HIV testing and ARVs. These associations may reflect easier access to care among women with higher socioeconomic status, or a better understanding of the benefit of HIV testing or ARVs. Approximately 70% of women reported having mobile phone availability, the majority of which were shared within the household. Mobile phones are being assessed as a tool (*m*Health) to improve PMTCT. [29–31] Although assessed as a measure of socioeconomic status, our observation that women without mobile phones were less likely to have HIV testing or to take ARVs suggests that these women may need specialized attention. *mHealth* interventions, while a very promising approach to improving engagement in care, may need to supply phones to these higher risk mothers to facilitate uptake of PMTCT and other health services.

The association between awareness of partner HIV testing and uptake of maternal HIV testing and ARVs in our study is consistent with previous studies, which have noted associations between partner disclosure, [32] social support from a spouse, [33] partner attendance at antenatal HIV counseling and testing, [34] and uptake of or adherence to PMTCT. These studies have generated enthusiasm for partner involvement. However, it is possible that these strategies may inadvertently marginalize women without supportive partners, or increase risk for gender-based violence. For example, a requirement that male partners attend ANC in Uganda resulted in women paying men (often not their partners) to attend clinic with them. [35] Male partner involvement may be simply a proxy for maternal self-efficacy, partner support, and communication that fosters access to care. Further studies are needed to discern the impact of male partner interventions on PMTCT, including unintended consequences.

Consistent with other national surveys, fewer than half of the women in this survey accessed a skilled provider for assistance during delivery. [36] The delivery time-point also had the lowest level of ARV uptake. Efforts to improve access to skilled care during delivery may provide multiplicative benefit to maternal and neonatal morbidity and mortality, as well as PMTCT. Community-based efforts to enhance the ability of unskilled providers to refer and educate about PMTCT services could be considered in order to reach the large proportion of women who deliver outside of formal health facilities. [37] Movement towards Option B+, which provides lifelong therapy to all pregnant women, may further improve uptake at delivery.

This analysis had several strengths in that it utilized a community-based approach to assess uptake of health services. Regional home-based counseling and testing in the HDSS further

Table 5. Sensitivity Analyses.

	Admitted HIV Positive Status	*Reported HIV Negative Status*		*Prevalence Ratio*
	n (%) or med (IQR)	*n (%) or med (IQR)*	*p-value*	*PR (95% Confidence Interval)*
	n = 173	*n = 60*		
Age (years)	29 (25–33)	25.5 (23–29.5)	0.003	
Age category (years)			0.01	0.53 (0.32–0.86)
15–20	7 (4.1)	9 (15.0)		
21–34	137 (79.2)	45 (75.0)		
35–46	29 (16.8)	6 (10.0)		
Marital status			0.24	
Married monogamous	128 (74.0)	44 (73.3)		
Married polygamous	28 (16.2)	9 (15.0)		
Single	7 (4.1)	6 (10.0)		
Widowed	10 (5.8)	1 (1.7)		
Occupation			0.59	
Unemployed	30 (17.5)	7 (11.9)		
Housewife	80 (46.8)	31 (52.5)		
Employed	61 (35.7)	21 (35.6)		
Completed primary education	95 (54.9)	30 (50.0)	0.55	
Skilled provider at delivery	71 (41.5)	23 (38.3)	0.76	
Is there any way to prevent HIV	155 (89.6)	51 (85.0)	0.35	
Pregnant can women give HIV to baby	138 (79.8)	47 (78.3)	0.85	
Can prevent MTCT of HIV	128 (74.0)	42 (71.2)	0.73	

Comparison of characteristics of women known to be HIV infected who disclosed or denied HIV status to field interviewers.

allowed for increased sampling of HIV-positive women and verification of self-reported status.

Community based approaches, such as the existing HDSS household annual surveys, provide a tool to efficiently assess interventions received by women during their most recent pregnancy and sample women attending a variety of clinics or not accessing any clinical services. In demographic surveys that include routine HIV surveillance, it is possible to rapidly sample women who should have received PMTCT ARVs to understand whether women access PMTCT programs and systems are effectively providing PMTCT services.

In contrast to studies from Uganda and a multi-national study (Cameroon, Cote d'Ivoire, Zambia), [16] our community PMTCT coverage estimate did not appear to differ markedly from national facility-based estimates. [7] However, while able to access a broader sample of women than a clinic-based approach, our approach had limitations in using self-report in the absence of biological samples. In our case, many women who were recorded as HIV infected in the HBCT database did not report HIV-positive status to the interviewer in this home-based survey, despite recent acceptance of home-based testing and identification of interviewers as being from the same program. This suggests that either women did not want to reveal their status a new interviewer but may have actually accepted PMTCT, or that women may not have accepted PMTCT because of unwillingness to acknowledge or misunderstanding of their HIV-positive status at health facilities, similarly to during home interviews. Respecting the confidentiality of the participant and her right to not disclose to the interviewer was an important ethical consideration which would be present in any community-based survey. Despite these limitations, our coverage findings are remarkably similar to the 2012 Kenya AIDS Indicator Survey (KAIS) (87% uptake of HIV-testing; 72% antepartum prophylaxis; 69% peripartum prophylaxis; 75% postpartum prophylaxis; and 15% infant HIV infection).

Each of the possible approaches for assessing population-level uptake and health impact of HIV prevention services poses methodological challenges. Facility-based surveys may fail to assess outcomes of women who never access clinic-based services, while community-based approaches may fail to reach women who deny HIV status or decline HIV testing. Even with biological testing, 15% of respondents in the KAIS PMTCT surveys refused HIV testing. Furthermore, program indicators of uptake, while important in understanding issues related to engagement in care, are not equivalent to measures of program effectiveness. Findings from the PEARL Study demonstrated that program data in Cote D'Ivoire suggested markedly different rates of reported uptake of nevirapine (41%) compared to presence of nevirapine cord-blood samples collected from infants (16%). [38] Often this is a result of challenges in monitoring program data, but it also may reflect adherence challenges throughout the complete course of ARVs. Future larger-scale studies with biological markers of HIV status and antiretroviral coverage, and with approaches that better protect participant privacy such as computer-assisted self-interview tools, are indicated to more rigorously assess engagement in and coverage of PMTCT services.

Conclusions

This household-based survey complements Kenyan facility-based assessments and observed similarly high PMTCT coverage estimates. However, although most HIV infected women received ARVs, fewer received a complete course, many started ANC late, and a surprising number of women declined to reveal their status. Involving partners or utilizing mobile phones may enhance PMTCT delivery, though care should be taken to avoid marginalization of women without supportive partners or access to mobile phone technology. Efforts specifically targeting stigma reduction around disclosure of HIV status and provision of ARVs during the labor and delivery period are necessary. Community driven strategies that encourage early uptake of ANC and skilled attendance at delivery, and that emphasize education about the effectiveness of PMTCT, may facilitate completion of ARVs and subsequent reductions in perinatal HIV transmission.

Acknowledgments

Authors gratefully acknowledge the support of Dr. Martina Morris, Dr. Barbara Richardson, Dr. Nancy Woods, and Dr. Lisa Manhart; the UW Center for Integrated Health of Women, Adolescents, and Children (Global WACh); and the Kenya Health Demographic Surveillance System team.

Disclaimer

Published with the approval of the Director, Kenya Medical Research Institute. The findings and conclusions in this report are those of the authors, and do not necessarily represent the views of their institutions, including the Centers for Diseases Control and Prevention and Kenya Medical Research Institute.

Meetings

Findings were presented at the XIX International AIDS Conference, July 22–27, 2012 in Washington DC, USA.

Author Contributions

Conceived and designed the experiments: PKK GJS JK LAM FO KFL. Performed the experiments: PKK JK JO GO FO. Analyzed the data: PKK GO. Contributed reagents/materials/analysis tools: PKK GJS JK LAM FO KFL. Wrote the paper: PKK LAM JK JO FO KFL BZ JV GJS.

References

1. Joint United Nations Programme on HIV/AIDS (UNAIDS) (2011) Countdown to zero: Global Plan towards the Elimination of New HIV Infections among Children by 2015 and Keeping their Mothers Alive. Geneva.
2. World Health Organization (2011) Global HIV/AIDS Response: Epidemic update and health section progress towards Universal Access: progress report 2011.
3. Joint United Nations Programme on HIV/AIDS (UNAIDS) (2013) 2013 Progress Report on the Global Plan towards the elimination of new HIV infections among children by 2015 and keeping their mothers alive.
4. Stringer EM, Chi BH, Chintu N, Creek TL, Ekouevi DK, et al. (2008) Monitoring effectiveness of programmes to prevent mother-to-child HIV transmission in lower-income countries. Bull World Health Organ 86: 57–62.
5. Barker PM, Mphatswe W, Rollins N (2011) Antiretroviral drugs in the cupboard are not enough: the impact of health systems' performance on mother-to-child transmission of HIV. J Acquir Immune Defic Syndr 56: e45–48.
6. UNICEF (2008) Children and AIDS: Second Stocktaking Report.
7. NACC NASCOP (2012) Kenya AIDS Epidemic update 2011. Nairobi, Kenya.
8. Marazzi MC, Nielsen-Saines K, Buonomo E, Scarcella P, Germano P, et al. (2009) Increased infant human immunodeficiency virus-type one free survival at one year of age in sub-saharan Africa with maternal use of highly active antiretroviral therapy during breast-feeding. Pediatr Infect Dis J 28: 483–487.
9. Shapiro RL, Hughes MD, Ogwu A, Kitch D, Lockman S, et al. (2010) Antiretroviral regimens in pregnancy and breast-feeding in Botswana. N Engl J Med 362: 2282–2294.
10. de Vincenzi I, Group KBS (2011) Triple antiretroviral compared with zidovudine and single-dose nevirapine prophylaxis during pregnancy and breastfeeding for prevention of mother-to-child transmission of HIV-1 (Kesho Bora study): a randomised controlled trial. Lancet Infect Dis 11: 171–180.
11. Kilewo C, Karlsson K, Ngarina M, Massawe A, Lyamuya E, et al. (2009) Prevention of mother-to-child transmission of HIV-1 through breastfeeding by treating mothers with triple antiretroviral therapy in Dar es Salaam, Tanzania: the Mitra Plus study. J Acquir Immune Defic Syndr 52: 406–416.
12. National AIDS Control Council (2010) United Nations General Assembly Special Session on HIV and AIDS, Country Report – Kenya.
13. Kiarie J (2012) National Evaluation of PMTCT Services: Kenya. 19th Conference on Retroviruses and Opportunistic Infections. Seattle, USA.
14. Sirengo M, Muthoni L, Kellogg TA, Kim AA, Katana A, et al. (2014) Mother-to-child transmission of HIV in Kenya: results from a nationally representative study. J Acquir Immune Defic Syndr 66 Suppl 1: S66–74.
15. Larsson EC, Waiswa P, Thorson A, Tomson G, Peterson S, et al. (2009) Low uptake of HIV testing during antenatal care: a population-based study from eastern Uganda. Aids 23: 1924–1926.
16. Stringer JS, Stinson K, Tih PM, Giganti MJ, Ekouevi DK, et al. (2013) Measuring coverage in MNCH: population HIV-free survival among children under two years of age in four African countries. PLoS Med 10: e1001424.
17. Peltzer K, Mosala T, Shisana O, Nqueko A, Mngqundaniso N (2007) Barriers to prevention of HIV transmission from mother to child (PMTCT) in a resource poor setting in the Eastern Cape, South Africa. Afr J Reprod Health 11: 57–66.
18. Nguyen TA, Oosterhoff P, Ngoc YP, Wright P, Hardon A (2008) Barriers to access prevention of mother-to-child transmission for HIV positive women in a well-resourced setting in Vietnam. AIDS Res Ther 5: 7.
19. Kiarie JN, Farquhar C, Richardson BA, Kabura MN, John FN, et al. (2006) Domestic violence and prevention of mother-to-child transmission of HIV-1. AIDS 20: 1763–1769.
20. Chamla DD, Olu O, Wanyana J, Natseri N, Mukooyo E, et al. (2007) Geographical information system and access to HIV testing, treatment and prevention of mother-to-child transmission in conflict affected Northern Uganda. Confl Health 1: 12.
21. Kinuthia J, Kiarie J, Farquhar C, Richardson B, Nduati R, et al. (2010) Missed Opportunities in Uptake of PMTCT of HIV Interventions: Are Health Systems Failing HIV-infected Mothers? [Abstract]. 17th Conference on Retroviruses and Opportunistic Infections. San Francisco, CA.
22. Mbonye AK, Hansen KS, Wamono F, Magnussen P (2010) Barriers to prevention of mother-to-child transmission of HIV services in Uganda. J Biosoc Sci 42: 271–283.
23. Otieno PA, Kohler PK, Bosire RK, Brown ER, Macharia SW, et al. (2010) Determinants of failure to access care in mothers referred to HIV treatment programs in Nairobi, Kenya. AIDS Care: 1–8.
24. Kinuthia J, Kiarie JN, Farquhar C, Richardson BA, Nduati R, et al. (2011) Uptake of prevention of mother to child transmission interventions in Kenya: health systems are more influential than stigma. J Int AIDS Soc 14: 61.
25. Odhiambo FO, Laserson KF, Sewe M, Hamel MJ, Feikin DR, et al. (2012) Profile: the KEMRI/CDC Health and Demographic Surveillance System—Western Kenya. Int J Epidemiol 41: 977–987.
26. Jehu-Appiah C, Aryeetey G, Spaan E, Agyepong I, Baltussen R (2010) Efficiency, equity and feasibility of strategies to identify the poor: an application to premium exemptions under National Health Insurance in Ghana. Health Policy 95: 166–173.
27. Filmer D, Scott K (2012) Assessing asset indices. Demography 49: 359–392.
28. Chibwesha CJ, Giganti MJ, Putta N, Chintu N, Mulindwa J, et al. (2011) Optimal time on HAART for prevention of mother-to-child transmission of HIV. J Acquir Immune Defic Syndr 58: 224–228.
29. Lester RT, Ritvo P, Mills EJ, Kariri A, Karanja S, et al. (2010) Effects of a mobile phone short message service on antiretroviral treatment adherence in Kenya (WelTel Kenya1): a randomised trial. Lancet 376: 1838–1845.
30. Chiasson MA, Hirshfield S, Rietmeijer C (2010) HIV prevention and care in the digital age. J Acquir Immune Defic Syndr 55 Suppl 2: S94–97.
31. Karanja S, Mbuagbaw L, Ritvo P, Law J, Kyobutungi C, et al. (2011) A workshop report on HIV mHealth synergy and strategy meeting to review emerging evidence-based mHealth interventions and develop a framework for scale-up of these interventions. Pan Afr Med J 10: 37.
32. Jasseron C, Mandelbrot L, Dollfus C, Trocmé N, Tubiana R, et al. (2011) Non-Disclosure of a Pregnant Woman's HIV Status to Her Partner is Associated with Non-Optimal Prevention of Mother-to-Child Transmission. AIDS Behav.
33. Nassali M, Nakanjako D, Kyabayinze D, Beyeza J, Okoth A, et al. (2009) Access to HIV/AIDS care for mothers and children in sub-Saharan Africa: adherence to the postnatal PMTCT program. AIDS Care 21: 1124–1131.
34. Msuya SE, Mbizvo EM, Hussain A, Uriyo J, Sam NE, et al. (2008) Low male partner participation in antenatal HIV counselling and testing in northern Tanzania: implications for preventive programs. AIDS Care 20: 700-709.
35. Otim R (2012) Soroti women pay men Shs5,000 to go with them for antenatals. Daily Monitor. Uganda.
36. Kenya National Bureau of Statistics (KNBS) and ICF Macro (2010) Kenya Demographic and Health Survey 2008-09. Calverton, Maryland.
37. Mbuagbaw LC, Gofin R (2011) A new measurement for optimal antenatal care: determinants and outcomes in Cameroon. Matern Child Health J 15: 1427–1434.
38. Stringer EM, Ekouevi DK, Coetzee D, Tih PM, Creek TL, et al. (2010) Coverage of nevirapine-based services to prevent mother-to-child HIV transmission in 4 African countries. Jama 304: 293–302.

17

Incidence of HIV-Associated Tuberculosis among Individuals Taking Combination Antiretroviral Therapy: A Systematic Review and Meta-Analysis

Tendesayi Kufa[1,2]*, Tonderai Mabuto[1]*, Evans Muchiri[1], Salome Charalambous[1,2], Dominique Rosillon[3], Gavin Churchyard[1,2], Rebecca C. Harris[4]

1 The Aurum Institute, Johannesburg, South Africa, **2** The School of Public Health, University of the Witwatersrand, Johannesburg, South Africa, **3** GlaxoSmithKline Vaccines, Wavre, Belgium, **4** CROMSOURCE on behalf of GlaxoSmithKline Vaccines, Wavre, Belgium

Abstract

Background: Knowledge of tuberculosis incidence and associated factors is required for the development and evaluation of strategies to reduce the burden of HIV-associated tuberculosis.

Methods: Systematic literature review and meta-analysis of tuberculosis incidence rates among HIV-infected individuals taking combination antiretroviral therapy.

Results: From PubMed, EMBASE and Global Index Medicus databases, 42 papers describing 43 cohorts (32 from high/intermediate and 11 from low tuberculosis burden settings) were included in the qualitative review and 33 in the quantitative review. Cohorts from high/intermediate burden settings were smaller in size, had lower median CD4 cell counts at study entry and fewer person-years of follow up. Tuberculosis incidence rates were higher in studies from Sub-Saharan Africa and from World Bank low/middle income countries. Tuberculosis incidence rates decreased with increasing CD4 count at study entry and duration on combination antiretroviral therapy. Summary estimates of tuberculosis incidence among individuals on combination antiretroviral therapy were higher for cohorts from high/intermediate burden settings compared to those from the low tuberculosis burden settings (4.17 per 100 person-years [95% Confidence Interval (CI) 3.39–5.14 per 100 person-years] vs. 0.4 per 100 person-years [95% CI 0.23–0.69 per 100 person-years]) with significant heterogeneity observed between the studies.

Conclusions: Tuberculosis incidence rates were high among individuals on combination antiretroviral therapy in high/intermediate burden settings. Interventions to prevent tuberculosis in this population should address geographical, socioeconomic and individual factors such as low CD4 counts and prior history of tuberculosis.

Editor: Robert J. Wilkinson, Institute of Infectious Diseases and Molecular Medicine, South Africa

Funding: GlaxoSmithKline Biologicals S.A. funded the work disclosed in this manuscript (for data collection for the reported study). Co-author Dominique Rosillon is employed by GlaxoSmithKline Vaccines and co-author Rebecca C. Harris was employed by CROMsource during the course of the study. GlaxoSmithKline provided support in the form of salary for author DR, but did not have any additional role in the study design, data collection and analysis, decision to publish, or preparation of the manuscript. The specific roles of this author is articulated in the 'author contributions' section. CROMsource provided support in the form of salary for author RCH, but did not have any additional role in the study design, data collection and analysis, decision to publish, or preparation of the manuscript.

Competing Interests: The authors have read the journal's policy and have the following conflicts: DR is employed by GlaxoSmithKline Vaccines and has stock ownership in the GlaxoSmithKline Group of Companies. RH was an employee of CROM source working on behalf of GlaxoSmithKline Vaccines. All other authors declare no conflicts of interest. This does not alter the authors' adherence to PLOS ONE policies on sharing data and materials.

* Email: tkufa@auruminstitute.org (TK); tmabuto@auruminstitute.org (TM)

Introduction

Human immune deficiency virus (HIV)-associated tuberculosis (TB) is an important public health problem particularly in high HIV prevalence settings. In 2012, the World Health Organisation (WHO) estimated that up to 1.1 million reported TB cases and 320 000 deaths from TB occurred in people living with HIV [1]. In the same year, up to 75% of all HIV-associated TB cases occurred in Sub-Saharan Africa [1]. Combination antiretroviral therapy (cART) or highly active antiretroviral therapy (HAART) reduces the risk of TB by 67% (95% CI 61–73%) among people living with HIV [2]. The risk of TB declines in proportion to the increases in CD4 counts after cART initiation [3]. In the high burden setting of Cape Town, South Africa, the risk of TB while on cART with a CD4 count of >700 cells/ml^3 remained four fold higher than in HIV-uninfected persons from the same community [4]. Because cART alone is not sufficient to prevent HIV-associated TB, additional strategies are required. In order to develop additional strategies for preventing HIV-associated TB in people taking cART such as novel TB vaccines, an understanding of the incidence of and risk factors for HIV-associated TB in high/intermediate and low TB burden settings is required. We conducted a systematic review and meta-analysis to summarise and describe trends in the incidence of TB among adults taking

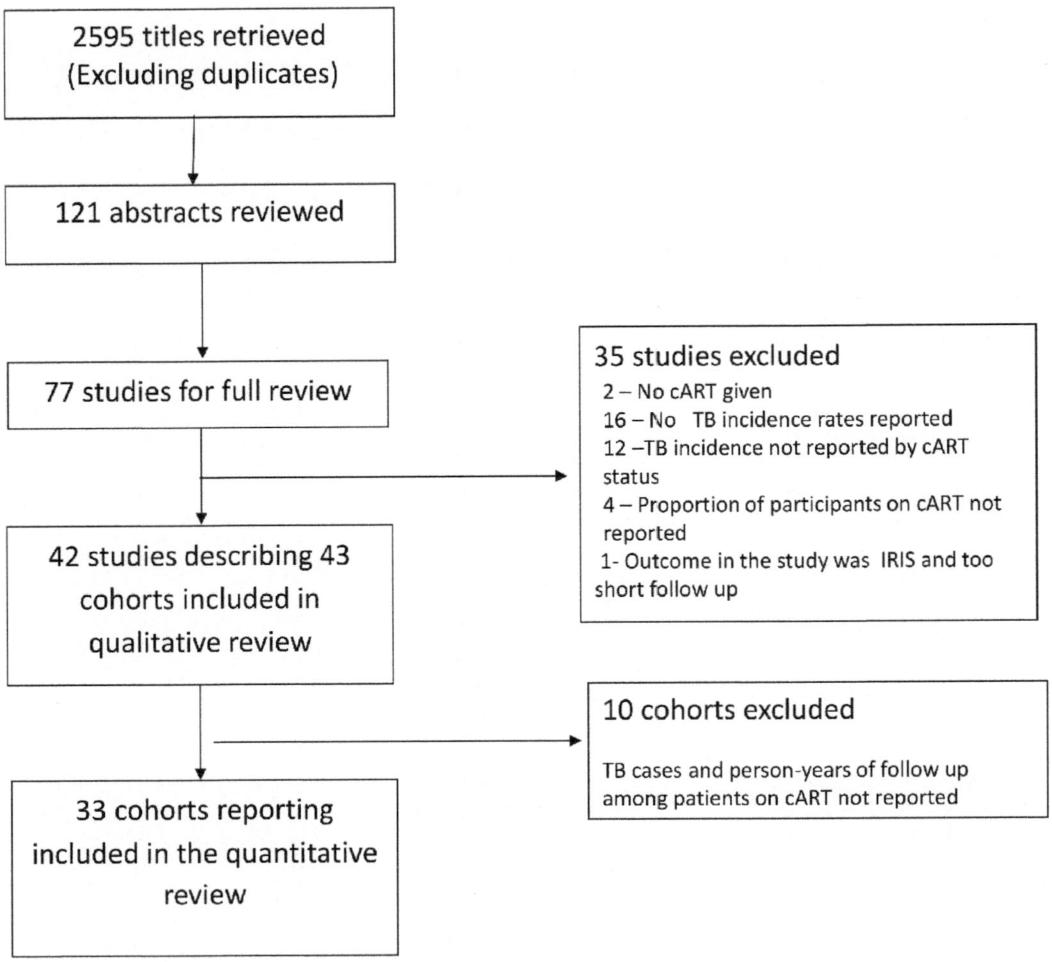

Figure 1. Summary of search findings.

cART in high/intermediate and low TB burden settings, stratified by geographical region, CD4 count, previous history of TB and duration on cART. We highlight the disparities in TB incidence rates between high and low TB burden settings and discuss the implications for interventions to further reduce the risk of HIV-associated TB among individuals on cART.

Methods

Search strategy and selection of papers

PubMed, EMBASE and Global Index Medicus databases were searched in parallel using search strings adapted to the requirements of each database (Table S1). For the PubMed search we conducted two separate searches using MeSH terms i) *"tuberculosis"* AND *"incidence"* ii) "tuberculosis" AND "HAART" with all the available qualifiers. Both PubMed searches were limited to papers describing studies in humans, published in English between 1st January 2000 and 31st March 2012. For the EMBASE search we used EMTREE terms "tuberculosis" AND "incidence" OR "HAART" with all the available qualifiers and limited the search to papers describing studies in humans, published in English between 1st January 2000 and 31st March 2012. For the Global Index Medicus search, we searched all indexes and all sources (which include AIM, LILACS, IMEMR, IMSEAR, WPRIM, WHOLIS and Medline) using the keywords *"tuberculosis" "incidence" "HAART"* and limited the search to studies written in the English language. No other limits applied.

The search outputs were imported into a combined file in reference management software and duplicates removed. Two independent reviewers (TM and TK) screened all titles and abstracts to identify papers for full text review. Full texts were then screened by the same reviewers and eligibility criteria applied. Eligibility for inclusion required reporting a TB incidence rate for a cohort of individuals on cART and more than 100 participants included in the cohort. Review papers, papers exclusively reporting multi-drug or extensively drug resistant (MDR/XDR) TB as outcomes, and papers reporting exclusively on children younger than 15 years of age were not eligible. Where discordance occurred in the independent review of papers, the papers were discussed and consensus achieved. References lists included in the eligible papers were hand searched in order to identify additional eligible papers. The search criteria and other methods used in the review were included in a protocol outline agreed upon by the authors before data collection commenced. This protocol outline can be found in the supplementary information (Table S2).

Abstraction of data from eligible papers

Data on study characteristics (including but not limited to: author, date of publication, location, sample size, cohort characteristics and TB incidence rates) were abstracted using a

Table 1. Characteristics of study cohorts from high burden settings and from low burden settings.

Characteristic	High/intermediate burden (N = 32)		Low burden (N = 11)	
	number of cohorts		number of cohorts	
Prospective study design (n, %)	32	16 (50)	11	2 (18.2)
Cohort size (range)	32	101–19325	11	1824–72850
Cohorts from clinical care settings (n, %)	32	24 (75)	11	11 (100)
% males in the cohort, (range)	31	21–91	10	67–77
Median/mean age of cohort, (range)	28	31–38	10	33–41
% of cohort with prior history of TB, (range)	20	0–100	3	0–13.9
% of cohort who were MSM, (range)	4	18.7–59	6	17.3–58.7
% of cohort who were IDU, (range)	3	1.6–14	6	4.8–59
% of cohort on cART at baseline/by end of study, (range)	32	5.7–100	11	10.2–100
Cohort with 100% of participants on cART, (n, %)	32	22 (68.8)	11	5 (45.5)
% of cohort on NNRTI-based treatment, (range)	10	35–100	2	26.3–33
% of cohort on PI- based treatment, (range)	5	3.2–73	2	56–63
Median CD4 count at cohort entry, cells/μl), (range)	27	37–444	10	207–422
Median CD4 count at cART initiation(cells/μl), (range)	20	97–252	5	207–297
Median duration of follow up in months, (range)	24	8–73	4	15.8–56.4
Person-years of follow up, (range)	27	159–18162	10	14711–427957
Person-years of follow up on cART,(range)	25	65.1–18162	8	11248–313807
Availability of mycobacterial culture, (n, %)	29	19 (65.3)	10	10 (100%)

N is total number of cohorts, n is number of cohorts with the characteristic, IQR – interquartile range, MSM- men who have sex with men, IDU- intravenous drug user, NNRTI – non-nucleoside reverse transcriptase inhibitors, PI – protease inhibitors, cART- combination antiretroviral therapy.

standardized form (Table S3). If a study described two or more distinct cohorts, data was abstracted for each of the cohorts meeting the criteria for inclusion in the review.

Estimates of national TB incidence rates, national adult HIV prevalence rates and World Bank income classification for the country and year each study was published were obtained from the WHO database of TB burden [5], UNAIDS Global HIV estimates [6,7] and the World Bank classifications respectively [8]. We used the estimates of national HIV prevalence rates last updated in 2009, and the estimates of national TB incidence rates last updated in 2010. Therefore, the HIV estimates from 2009 were used for studies published after 2009 and, the 2010 estimates of national TB incidence were used for studies published after 2010. For multi-country studies, the data on national TB incidence and HIV prevalence rates were not abstracted but were assigned to low or high burden depending on the average national TB incidence rate in the countries the cohorts were from. Cohorts described in the studies were classified as high/intermediate burden if the estimated national TB incidence rate for the country and year were ≥25 per 100 000 population per year, and as low burden if the TB incidence rates were below this threshold. Cohorts were also classified as being from low, middle or high income settings according to the World Bank income classification.

Assessment of study quality

Study quality was assessed using a standardized tool (see Table S4) adapted from the Newcastle-Ottawa Scale (NOS) for cohort studies [9]. The tool was used to assess the following study characteristics: sampling methods, presence of sampling bias, exclusion of TB at cohort entry, outcomes ascertainment during follow up, duration of follow up and loss to follow up rates. Each of these criteria was assigned a score as shown in Box 1 (Table S4). The highest possible score was 6 and studies with scores ≥4 were considered to be of good quality. No studies were excluded from the reviews on the basis of their quality scores.

Data analysis and presentation

In the qualitative part of the review, all eligible cohorts reporting a TB incidence rate among individuals on cART were classified into high/intermediate and low burden settings and described with respect to cohort characteristics. TB incidence rates were summarized according to CD4 cell count strata, duration on cART and by prior history of TB. Where studies only reported number of TB cases and person-years of follow up for the different strata in the cohort, the incidence rates and confidence intervals were computed in Stata 12 (Stata Corporation, College Station, Texas, USA).

Meta-analysis

Meta-analyses (quantitative reviews) were conducted to determine summary estimates of the TB incidence rates among HIV-infected individuals on cART overall and point estimates across different categories or strata of study quality, study designs, national HIV prevalence rates, national TB incidence rates, CD4 count, durations on cART and prior history of TB. To be eligible for inclusion in meta-analyses, studies were required to report both the number of TB cases and person-years of follow up by the different categories listed. These fields were required to enable estimation of incidence rates of TB and associated standard errors using the random effects model. These data were recorded onto the abstraction forms and entered into an Excel 2007 sheet (Microsoft Corporation, Washington, USA) and exported into

Table 2. Summary of study quality.

Criteria	high burden (N = 32)		low burden(N = 11)	
	n (%)	studies	n (%)	studies
1. *Sampling method*				
Reported sampling method used	32 (100)	all studies	11 (100)	all studies
2. *Sampling bias*				
Assessed and reported on sampling bias	18 (56.3)	4,11, 14, 17, 19, 20, 22, 24, 30, 31, 33, 34, 36,37, 38, 39, 43,47	2 (18.2)	29, 32
3. *Screening of TB at study commencement*				
Reported screening/exclusion of TB at cohort entry	32 (100)	all studies	11 (100)	all studies
4. *Ascertainment of outcomes*				
Smear + culture + clinical + chest radiograph	21 (62.5)	4, 14, 17, 19, 20, 21, 24, 27, 28, 30, 31, 33,34, 35, 36, 37, 42, 43,46, 47, 49	7 (63.6)	12, 15, 26, 32, 35, 48, 49
Smear + clinical + chest radiograph (no culture)	7 (21.2)	10, 11, 25,38, 39, 41, 50		
Clinical + chest radiograph (no smear or culture)	1 (3.0)	30	0 (0)	
Treatment initiation records only	2 (6.1)	22, 23,	1 (9.1)	18
Not specified	2 (6.1)	40, 45	3 (27.2)	16, 29, 44
5. *Median duration of follow up*				
Median follow-up <9 months	1 (3)	41	0 (0)	
Median follow-up ≥9 months	23 (72.7)	4, 14, 17, 19, 20, 21, 22, 23, 24, 25 28, 30, 31, 33, 34, 36, 37,39, 42, 43, 45, 46, 47	5 (45.4)	15, 18, 29, 32,44
Median follow up not reported	8 (24.2)	10, 11, 27, 35, 38, 40, 49, 50	6 (55.5)	12, 13, 16, 26, 48, 49
6. *Loss to follow up*				
<20% of participants lost to follow-up	15 (45.5)	11,14, 17, 19, 20, 21, 22, 23, 24, 27 28, 31, 36, 39, 40	1 (9.1)	29
>20% of participants lost to follow-up	1 (3.0)	4	0	
Loss to follow up not reported	16 (48.5)	10, 25, 30, 33, 34, 35, 37, 38, 41, 42, 43, 45, 46, 47, 49, 50	10 (90.9)	12, 13, 15, 16, 18, 26, 32, 44, 48, 49
Overall study quality score (median, range)	5 (2–6)		3 (2–5)	
Studies with quality score ≥4	24 (72.7)	4, 11, 14, 17, 19, 20, 21, 22, 23, 24, 27, 28, 30, 31, 33, 34, 36, 37,38, 39, 42, 43, 46, 47,	3 (27.3)	15, 29, 32

n = number of studies with characteristic.

Stata 12 for analysis. I-squared estimates were used to determine heterogeneity between studies.

Results

Summary of studies

From 2945 unique study titles retrieved, 121 titles were eligible for abstract review and 77 for full text review. From the full texts reviewed, 42 studies [4,10–50] describing 43 cohorts were eligible for inclusion in the qualitative review and a subset of 33 cohorts for inclusion in the quantitative review (meta-analysis - Figure 1). Of the 43 cohorts, 32 (74%) were from high/intermediate burden settings with national TB incidence rates ranging from of 46 to 981 per 100 000 and national HIV prevalence rate ranging from 0.3% to 18.2%. Eleven cohorts (26%) were from low burden settings with national TB incidence rates ranging from 4.1 to 17 per 100 000 population per year and national HIV prevalence rate of 0.2% to 0.6%. The full list and characteristics of papers included in the review are presented in Table S5.

Characteristics of cohorts from high/intermediate and low burden settings are presented in Table 1. When compared to cohorts from low burden settings, cohorts from high/intermediate burden were smaller in size, had lower median CD4 cell counts at study entry and had fewer person-years follow up. TST positivity was reported for a few cohorts in both settings (five cohorts (15.6%) from high/intermediate burden settings and five (45.5%) cohorts from low burden settings).

Study quality

Table 2 describes the findings of the study quality assessment. The overall quality scores ranged from 2–6 with the majority of the papers (27 of 42 studies, 64%) being considered to be of acceptable quality (score ≥4).

Table 3. TB cases characteristics and incidence rates reported in high burden cohorts and in low burden cohorts.

Cohort characteristics	High/intermediate TB burden (N = 32) Number of cohorts reporting		Low TB burden (N = 11) Number of cohorts reporting	
Proportion (%) of TB cases with pulmonary TB (range)	16	43–81	6	44–65
Proportion (%) of TB cases who are male (range)	5	33.2–67.6	4	63.3–91
Median CD4 count of TB cases at study entry, cells/μl (range)	8	75–197	3	80–179
TB incidence rate among those on cART, cases/100person-years, (range)	32	0.6–10.5	11	0.02–1.5
TB incidences across baseline CD4 count strata cases/100person-years, (range)				
<100	6	0.6–6.8	1	0.84
101–200	2	1.7–4.8	0	.
201–350	3	1.7–3.7	1	0.47
351–500	3	1.8–3	1	0.19
>500	1	2	1	0.17
TB incidences across current CD4 count strata, cases/100person-years,(range)				
<100	4	8.9–25.5	3	0.11–0.83
101–200	4	3.6–11.2	1	0.09
201–350	3	1.8–7.8	2	0.08–0.26
351–500	3	0.7–5.0	3	0.04–0.21
>500	2	1.5–4.1	2	0.06–0.1
TB incidences with increasing duration on cART cases/100person-years,(range)				
0–3months	14	3.4–23	5	0.22–1.7
3–6months	10	2.2–10.7	4	0.15–1
6–12months	10	1.2–7.0	5	0.07–0.62
12–24 months	13	1.3–6.7	3	0.07–0.33
24–36 months	7	1.4–7.4	3	0.09–0.18
>36 months	4	0.4–5.8	1	0.05
TB incidence among those with prior history of TB, cases/100person-years, (range)	6	1.9–11.9	1	1.19
TB incidence among those with no prior history of TB cases/100person-years, (range)	6	1.8–8.1	1	1.83

N is total number of cohorts, n is number of cohorts with the characteristic, IQR – interquartile range, cART- combination antiretroviral therapy.

Qualitative review of TB incidence rates

Table 3 summarises the characteristics of TB cases and the TB incidence rates reported across different CD4 count and duration on cART strata, for both high/intermediate and low burden cohorts. The proportion of TB cases with pulmonary TB was higher in cohorts from high/intermediate burden settings compared to those from low burden settings. The median CD4 counts at study entry among individuals who subsequently developed TB were similar between high/intermediate and low burden cohorts. The TB incidence rates reported among individuals on cART were seven to 30 times higher in cohorts from high/intermediate burden settings compared to those from low TB burden settings.

In cohorts from high/intermediate and low burden settings, TB incidence rates generally increased with decreasing current CD4 counts and CD4 count at cART initiation, more so with CD4 counts less than 200 cells/μl (Table 3). TB incidence rates also increased with durations on cART less than six months. In six cohorts from high/intermediate burden settings, TB incidence rates were higher among those with prior history of TB compared to those with no prior history of TB (1.9–11.9 per 100 person-years compared to 1.8–8.1 per 100 person-years).

TB incidence rates among individuals on cART also varied with geographical location with highest incidence rates found in cohorts from Sub-Saharan Africa (range 0.9–7.82 per 100 person-years, n = 23), followed by those in Asia (range 1.32–2.83 per 100 person-years, n = 2), in South America (0.2–2.6 per 100 person-years, n = 4), and in Europe and North America (range 0.02–1.9 per 100 person-years, n = 9). Rates were much higher among cohorts from low income countries (range 0.9–8.6 per 100 person-years, n = 16) and middle income countries (0.6–10.5 per 100 person-years,

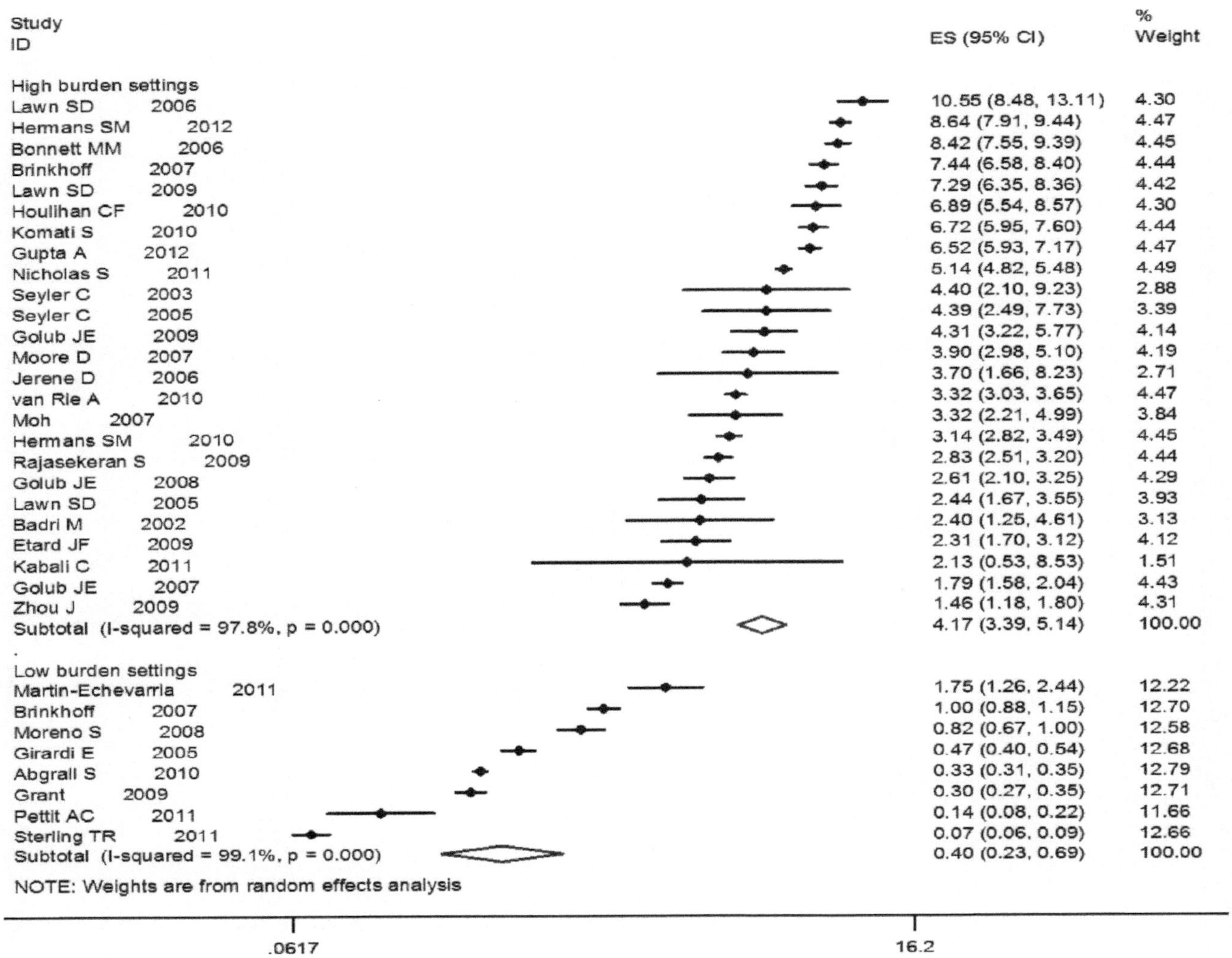

Figure 2. Forest plot showing summary estimates of TB incidence rates among individuals on cART comparing cohorts from high TB burden settings to low TB burden settings.

n = 16); compared to those from high income countries (0.02–1.9 per 100 person-years, n = 9).

Meta-analysis of TB incidence among HIV-infected adults on cART

Thirty-three cohorts were eligible for inclusion in the meta-analysis. (See Figure 2). Heterogeneity was computed separately for high/intermediate ($I^2 = 98\%$, p-value <0.001) and low ($I^2 = 99.1\%$, p-value <0.001) burden settings and was large in both settings. As expected, the summary estimate of TB incidence among those on cART was higher for cohorts from high/intermediate burden settings compared to those from the low burden settings–4.17 per 100 person-years (95% CI 3.39–5.14 per 100 person-years) vs. 0.4 per 100 person-years (95% CI 0.23–0.69 per 100 person-years, (Figure 2). In the analyses stratifying summary estimates of TB incidence rates by study quality, study design (retrospective or prospective studies), national TB incidence rates and national HIV prevalence rates (see Table 4), heterogeneity remained high. This implied that these variables did not explain most of the heterogeneity observed in the TB incidence rates.

Meta-analysis of TB incidence among HIV-infected adults on cART stratified by CD4 counts, duration on cART and prior history of TB

Summary estimates of TB incidence rates stratified by CD4 counts at entry, duration on cART and prior history of TB are shown in Table 5. The summary estimates of the TB incidence rates were higher in cohorts from high/intermediate burden settings compared to those from low burden settings across all baseline CD4 count strata, duration on cART and prior history of TB strata, although inference was limited by number of cohorts. Among cohorts from high/intermediate burden settings, TB incidence rates were higher in the baseline CD4 count <200 cells/μl stratum compared to those in 200–350 cells/μl or >350 cells/μl strata. There was significant heterogeneity in the TB incidence rates across the different strata in the meta-analysis.

Discussion

This review summarises and describes trends in TB incidence rates among HIV-infected adults on cART, comparing cohorts from high/intermediate burden settings with those from low burden settings. In the qualitative review, the incidence rates in cohorts from high/intermediate burden settings were seven to 30

Table 4. Summary estimates from meta-analysis of TB incidence rates stratified study level variables.

Variable	High/intermediate burden				Low burden			
	N Studies	Summary estimate (per 100 person-years)	$I^{2¥}$	p^*	N studies	Summary estimate (per 100 person-years)	I^2	p^*
Study quality								
low	10	3.7 (2.3–5.6)	98.8%	<0.001	6	0.37 (0.18–0.77)	93.3%	<0.001
high	14	4.5 (3.6–5.5)	95.5%	<0.001	2	0.50 (0.19–1.31)	98.4%	<0.001
Study Design								
Retrospective	13	3.7 (2.7–5.3)	98.7%	<0.001	6	0.40 (0.16–1.04)	99.3%	<0.01
Prospective	12	4.6 (3.6–6.0)	95.2%	<0.001	2	0.39 (0.28–0.55)	943%	<0.01
National TB incidence rates (per 100 000 population)								
<25					6	0.34 (0.18–0.64)	99%	<0.001
25–200	7	2.8 (2.1–3.6)	83.7%	<0.001				
201–800	6	3.7 (2.1–6.4)	98%	<0.001				
>800	8	5.6 (4.2–7.4)	96.7%	<0.001				
National HIV prevalence rates								
<1%	4	2.3 (1.8–3.0)	88.8%	<0.001	6	0.34 (0.18–0.64)	99%	<0.001
1–4.9%	3	3.7 (2.7–4.9)	0	0.735				
5–10%	5	4.3 (2.3–8.1)	98.1%	<0.001				
>10%	9	5.2 (3.9–6.9)	96.3%	<0.001				

*¥I^2- Amount of heterogeneity not explained by the variable, *p-value for heterogeneity not explained by the variable, N – number of cohorts.*

Table 5. Summary estimates from meta-analysis of TB incidence rates stratified by baseline CD4 count, duration on cART and previous history of TB.

Variable	High/intermediate burden				Low burden			
	N Studies	Summary estimate (per 100 person-years)	$I^{2¥}$	p^*	N Studies	Summary estimate (per 100 person-years)	I^2	p^*
Baseline CD4 count								
<200	5	4.47 (3.55–5.63)	89.6%	<0.001	1	0.84 (0.31–1.62)	-	-
200–350	3	2.32 (1.54–3.51)	42.3%	0.177	1	0.46 (0.35–0.60)	-	-
>350	3	2.34 (1.78–3.08)	0.00%	0.877	1	0.23 (0.16–0.34)	-	-
Duration on cART								
<3months	6	13.67 (10.62–17.60)	86.9%	<0.001	3	0.73 (0.27–1.99)	96.3%	<0.01
3–6 months	6	6.11 (4.62–8.09)	76.4%	0.001	3	0.46 (0.18–1.19)	93.6%	<0.01
6–12 months	6	3.14 (2.20–4.48)	83.9%	<0.001	3	0.29 (0.12–0.74)	94.5%	<0.01
12–24 months	4	3.94 (1.97–7.88)	94.5%	<0.001	3	0.19 (0.08–0.47)	94.8%	<0.01
>24 months	1	5.87(5.15–6.68)	-	-	2	0.09(0.03–0.23)	91.3%	<0.01
Previous History TB								
Yes	4	4.74 (2.10–10.73)	93.1%	<0.001	1	1.20 (0.39–3.71)	-	-
No	4	2.78 (1.36–5.68)	97.1%	<0.001	1	1.83 (1.30–2.59)	-	-

*¥I^2- Amount of heterogeneity not explained by the variable, *p-value for heterogeneity not explained by the variable, N – number of cohorts.*

times higher than rates in cohorts those from low burden settings. In the quantitative review the rates in high/intermediate burden settings were 10 times higher than those from low burden settings. Rates were highest in cohorts from low/middle income countries, from Sub-Saharan Africa, especially among individuals with baseline and current CD4 counts less than 200 cells/μl and among those on cART for less than six months.

Geographic and socio-economic factors

Our review suggests that background socio-economic conditions as measured by the World Bank classification may be associated with increased TB incidence among individuals on cART. In a 2009 study, Dye *et al* found that improvements in sanitation, lower child mortality and a higher human development index were associated with declines in national TB notification rates among 134 countries studied [51]. In this review, Sub-Saharan Africa, a region largely consisting of low income countries had the highest TB incidence rates among HIV-infected individuals on cART and should be a priority region for implementation of public health interventions which address social determinants of TB.

Individual level factors

The high rates of TB among HIV-infected adults on cART in this review, particularly in cohorts from high burden settings confirm that cART alone is not sufficient to prevent TB in populations with HIV [2]. Results reported here indicate that additional strategies at individual level are required to prevent HIV-associated TB particularly for individuals who have low CD4 counts, previous history of TB disease or recently initiated cART. Low CD4 counts during treatment with cART may be a result of i) late presentation for cART initiation, ii) sub-optimal immune reconstitution, or iii) treatment failure on cART [52,53]. Concerted efforts should be made to ensure initiation of cART at higher CD4 counts, better adherence to cART and better retention in HIV care. The high rates of TB in the first six months after cART initiation observed in this review may be attributed to inadequate TB screening at start of cART [52], or to unmasking of subclinical TB due to restoration of TB specific immune responses or paradoxical immune reconstitution syndrome (IRIS). [52–54] IRIS has been associated with low CD4 counts at cART initiation and could be avoided by initiating cART at higher CD4 counts, [52–54] or by adequately excluding and treating TB before initiating cART. In settings with both high HIV prevalence and high TB transmission, TB in individuals with HIV can be also prevented through the scaling up of TB preventive therapy and strengthening TB infection control measures at facility and community levels as repeated TB episodes among those on cART have been linked to re-infection [55].

Implications for further research

The findings of this review can inform the development of additional tools - such as new TB vaccines and drug regimens for TB preventive therapy - to prevent TB in HIV-infected populations. Should a vaccine candidate or preventive therapy regimen progress to phase IIb or III trials including HIV-infected subjects and measuring TB disease as an endpoint, large numbers of subjects will be needed to obtain a sufficient number of endpoints in the trials. High/intermediate burden settings should be priority locations for the conduct of such trials to help minimise the required sample size. However, with cART initiation occurring at increasingly higher CD4 count thresholds and use of isoniazid preventive therapy (IPT) being scaled up in most settings, the expected number of endpoints in such HIV-infected populations may be smaller and such trials may become infeasible even in high/intermediate burden settings. Prioritising enrolments of participants with prior history of TB may increase the number of endpoints in such trials.

Strengths and limitations

Summarising the TB incidence rates among individuals taking cART emphasises the magnitude of the TB burden especially in high TB and HIV burden settings. Such data highlight the limitations of cART as a tool for TB prevention in such settings, with challenges remaining due to ongoing transmission, late presentation into care or sub-optimal immune restoration in cART care. This review included 42 studies, the majority of which were of good quality. However this review also had some important limitations. We restricted our search to literature published in English as we did not have resources for translation. We did not search conference abstracts as these were likely to have incomplete follow up data. Twenty-three percent of the cohorts included in the qualitative review were not eligible for inclusion in the meta-analysis because they did not report number of TB cases, or the person – years of follow up stratified by use of cART. There was limited duration of follow up of participants especially in studies from high/intermediate burden settings. The association of longer duration of follow up in the cohort with reduction in TB incidence was evident in the reported rates and from the meta-analysis. This may have contributed to higher rates of TB observed in the cohorts from high/intermediate TB burden settings. There was large heterogeneity in the TB incidence rates in both high/intermediate burden and low TB burden settings which was not fully explained by study variables in stratified analyses. Conducting univariable or multivariable meta-regression analyses would have allowed us to better the determine factors accounting for the heterogeneity observed but the limited number of studies particularly from low TB burden settings precluded this. TB incidence rates in individuals on cART are likely influenced by local TB transmission and the rates of reactivation of latent infection. Data on TST positivity were not available for most studies and any heterogeneity as a result of these two variables could not be accounted for. Another limitation was that the review and meta-analysis included data collected at the individual level in the studies which were then aggregated to give study level variables. This made the review prone to aggregation bias.

Despite these limitations, the study provides valuable information for the evaluation, planning and implementation of preventive strategies for HIV-associated TB. Strategies to further reduce the risk of TB among individuals on cART such as the use of TB preventive therapy regimens, early initiation of cART, better TB screening at initiation of and during cART, and TB infection control can be appropriately targeted based on these data.

Acknowledgments

The authors thank Edith Roset-Bahmanyar for her contribution to the design of the systematic literature review, and Sofia Dos Santos Mendes (XPE Pharma&Science on behalf of GlaxoSmithKline Vaccines) for editorial assistance.

Author Contributions

Conceived and designed the experiments: TK SC GC RCH. Performed the experiments: TK TM. Analyzed the data: TK TM EM SC DR GC RCH. Contributed reagents/materials/analysis tools: TK TM EM SC DR GC RCH. Wrote the paper: TK. Reviewed iterative versions of the manuscript: TM EM SC DR GC RCH. Conducted the literature search and came up with a list of studies of studies for inclusion in the review: TK TM.

References

1. World Health Organisation (2013) Global Tuberculosis Report 2013. Geneva, Switzerland. Available: http://apps.who.int/iris/bitstream/10665/91355/1/9789241564656_eng.pdf. Accessed 2014 Jan 16.
2. Lawn SD, Wood R, De Cock KM, Kranzer K, Lewis JJ, et al. (2010) Antiretrovirals and isoniazid preventive therapy in the prevention of HIV-associated tuberculosis in settings with limited health-care resources. Lancet Infect Dis 10: 489–498.
3. Suthar AB, Lawn SD, Del Amo J, Getahun H, Dye C, et al. (2012) Antiretroviral Therapy for Prevention of Tuberculosis in Adults with HIV: A Systematic Review and Meta-Analysis. PLoS Med 9: e1001270.
4. Gupta A, Wood R, Kaplan R, Bekker LG, Lawn SD (2012) Tuberculosis Incidence Rates during 8 Years of Follow-Up of an Antiretroviral Treatment Cohort in South Africa: Comparison with Rates in the Community. PLoS One 7: e34156.
5. World Health Organisation(2010) Tuberculosis Country Profiles. Available: http://www.who.int/tb/country/data/download/en/index.html. Accessed 2012 May 10.
6. UNAIDS (2010) HIV estimates with uncertainity bounds 2009. Availble: http://www.unaids.org/globalreport/documents/HIV_Estimates_GR2010_2009_en.xls. Accessed 2012 May 10.
7. UNAIDS (2012) Adult (15–49) HIV prevalence percent by country, 1990–2007. Available: data.unaids.org/pub/.../20080813_gr08_prev1549_1990_2007. Accessed 2012 May 10.
8. World Bank (2012) World Bank Analytical Classifications 1987–2010. Available: http://data.worldbank.org/about/country-classifications. Accessed 2012 Jul 1.
9. Wells GA SB, O'Connell D, Peterson J, Welch V, Losos M, et al. (n.d.) The Newcastle-Ottawa Scale (NOS) for assessing the quality of nonrandomised studies in meta-analyses. Ottawa Hospital Research Institute. Available: http://www.medicine.mcgill.ca/rtamblyn/Readings/The%20Newcastle%20-%20Scale%20for%20assessing%20the%20quality%20of%20nonrandomised%20studies%20in%20meta-analyses.pdf. Accessed 2012 May 11.
10. Hermans S, van Leth F, Manabe Y, Hoepelman A, Lange J, et al. (2012) Earlier initiation of antiretroviral therapy, increased tuberculosis case finding and reduced mortality in a setting of improved HIV care: a retrospective cohort study. HIV Med.
11. Worodria W, Massinga-Loembe M, Mayanja-Kizza H, Namaganda J, Kambugu A, et al. (2011) Antiretroviral treatment-associated tuberculosis in a prospective cohort of HIV-infected patients starting ART. Clin Dev Immunol 2011: 758350.
12. Taarnhoj GA, Engsig FN, Ravn P, Johansen IS, Larsen CS, et al. (2011) Incidence, risk factors and mortality of tuberculosis in Danish HIV patients 1995–2007. BMC Pulm Med 11: 26.
13. Pettit AC, Jenkins CA, Stinnette SE, Rebeiro PF, Blackwell RB, et al. (2011) Tuberculosis risk before and after highly active antiretroviral therapy initiation: does HAART increase the short-term TB risk in a low incidence TB setting? J Acquir Immune Defic Syndr 57: 305–310.
14. Nicholas S, Sabapathy K, Ferreyra C, Varaine F, Pujades-Rodriguez M (2011) Incidence of tuberculosis in HIV-infected patients before and after starting combined antiretroviral therapy in 8 sub-Saharan African HIV programs. J Acquir Immune Defic Syndr 57: 311–318.
15. Martin-Echevarria E, Rodriguez-Zapata M, Torralba M, Fernandez JM, Moreno A, et al. (2011) Incidence of tuberculosis in HIV-infected patients receiving HAART: interaction between TST and CD4 count. Int J Tuberc Lung Dis 15: 1347–1352.
16. Kruk A, Bannister W, Podlekareva DN, Chentsova NP, Rakhmanova AG, et al. (2011) Tuberculosis among HIV-positive patients across Europe: changes over time and risk factors. AIDS 25: 1505–1513.
17. Kabali C, von Reyn CF, Brooks DR, Waddell R, Mtei L, et al. (2011) Completion of isoniazid preventive therapy and survival in HIV-infected, TST-positive adults in Tanzania. Int J Tuberc Lung Dis 15: 1515–1521, i..
18. Sterling TR, Lau B, Zhang J, Freeman A, Bosch RJ, et al. (2011) Risk factors for tuberculosis after highly active antiretroviral therapy initiation in the United States and Canada: implications for tuberculosis screening. J Infect Dis 204: 893–901.
19. Van Rie A, Westreich D, Sanne I (2011) Tuberculosis in patients receiving antiretroviral treatment: incidence, risk factors, and prevention strategies. J Acquir Immune Defic Syndr 56: 349–355.
20. Lawn SD, Kranzer K, Edwards DJ, McNally M, Bekker LG, et al. (2010) Tuberculosis during the first year of antiretroviral therapy in a South African cohort using an intensive pretreatment screening strategy. AIDS 24: 1323–1328.
21. Komati S, Shaw PA, Stubbs N, Mathibedi MJ, Malan L, et al. (2010) Tuberculosis risk factors and mortality for HIV-infected persons receiving antiretroviral therapy in South Africa. AIDS 24: 1849–1855.
22. Houlihan CF, Mutevedzi PC, Lessells RJ, Cooke GS, Tanser FC, et al. (2010) The tuberculosis challenge in a rural South African HIV programme. BMC Infect Dis 10: 23.
23. Hermans SM, Kiragga AN, Schaefer P, Kambugu A, Hoepelman AI, et al. (2010) Incident tuberculosis during antiretroviral therapy contributes to suboptimal immune reconstitution in a large urban HIV clinic in sub-Saharan Africa. PLoS One 5: e10527.
24. Hanrahan CF, Golub JE, Mohapi L, Tshabangu N, Modisenyane T, et al. (2010) Body mass index and risk of tuberculosis and death. AIDS 24: 1501–1508.
25. Dembele M, Saleri N, Carvalho AC, Saouadogo T, Hien AD, et al. (2010) Incidence of tuberculosis after HAART initiation in a cohort of HIV-positive patients in Burkina Faso. Int J Tuberc Lung Dis 14: 318–323.
26. Abgrall S, Del Giudice P, Melica G, Costagliola D (2010) HIV-associated tuberculosis and immigration in a high-income country: incidence trends and risk factors in recent years. AIDS 24: 763–771.
27. Zhou J, Elliott J, Li PC, Lim PL, Kiertiburanakul S, et al. (2009) Risk and prognostic significance of tuberculosis in patients from The TREAT Asia HIV Observational Database. BMC Infect Dis 9: 46.
28. Lawn SD, Myer L, Edwards D, Bekker LG, Wood R (2009) Short-term and long-term risk of tuberculosis associated with CD4 cell recovery during antiretroviral therapy in South Africa. AIDS 23: 1717–1725.
29. Grant AD, Bansi L, Ainsworth J, Anderson J, Delpech V, et al. (2009) Tuberculosis among people with HIV infection in the United Kingdom: opportunities for prevention? AIDS 23: 2507–2515.
30. Golub JE, Pronyk P, Mohapi L, Thsabangu N, Moshabela M, et al. (2009) Isoniazid preventive therapy, HAART and tuberculosis risk in HIV-infected adults in South Africa: a prospective cohort. AIDS 23: 631–636.
31. Etard JF, Diouf A, De Beaudrap P, Akoi K, Ngom-Gueye NF, et al. (2009) Short and Long-Term Incidence of Tuberculosis and CD4-Cell Count Dynamic on HAART in Senegal. Open AIDS J 3: 63–70.
32. Moreno S, Jarrin I, Iribarren JA, Perez-Elias MJ, Viciana P, et al. (2008) Incidence and risk factors for tuberculosis in HIV-positive subjects by HAART status. Int J Tuberc Lung Dis 12: 1393–1400.
33. Lannoy LH, Cortez-Escalante JJ, Evangelista Mdo S, Romero GA (2008) Tuberculosis incidence and risk factors among patients living with HIV/AIDS in public health service institutions in Brasilia, Federal District. Rev Soc Bras Med Trop 41: 549–555.
34. Golub JE, Durovni B, King BS, Cavalacante SC, Pacheco AG, et al. (2008) Recurrent tuberculosis in HIV-infected patients in Rio de Janeiro, Brazil. AIDS 22: 2527–2533.
35. Moore D, Liechty C, Ekwaru P, Were W, Mwima G, et al. (2007) Prevalence, incidence and mortality associated with tuberculosis in HIV-infected patients initiating antiretroviral therapy in rural Uganda. AIDS 21: 713–719.
36. Moh R, Danel C, Messou E, Ouassa T, Gabillard D, et al. (2007) Incidence and determinants of mortality and morbidity following early antiretroviral therapy initiation in HIV-infected adults in West Africa. AIDS 21: 2483–2491.
37. Miranda A, Morgan M, Jamal L, Laserson K, Barreira D, et al. (2007) Impact of antiretroviral therapy on the incidence of tuberculosis: the Brazilian experience, 1995–2001. PLoS One 2: e826.
38. Golub JE, Saraceni V, Cavalcante SC, Pacheco AG, Moulton LH, et al. (2007) The impact of antiretroviral therapy and isoniazid preventive therapy on tuberculosis incidence in HIV-infected patients in Rio de Janeiro, Brazil. AIDS 21: 1441–1448.
39. Lawn SD, Myer L, Bekker LG, Wood R (2006) Burden of tuberculosis in an antiretroviral treatment programme in sub-Saharan Africa: impact on treatment outcomes and implications for tuberculosis control. AIDS 20: 1605–1612.
40. Jerene D, Naess A, Lindtjorn B (2006) Antiretroviral therapy at a district hospital in Ethiopia prevents death and tuberculosis in a cohort of HIV patients. AIDS Res Ther 3: 10.
41. Bonnet MM, Pinoges LL, Varaine FF, Oberhauser BB, O'Brien DD, et al. (2006) Tuberculosis after HAART initiation in HIV-positive patients from five countries with a high tuberculosis burden. AIDS 20: 1275–1279.
42. Seyler C, Toure S, Messou E, Bonard D, Gabillard D, et al. (2005) Risk factors for active tuberculosis after antiretroviral treatment initiation in Abidjan. Am J Respir Crit Care Med 172: 123–127.

43. Lawn SD, Badri M, Wood R (2005) Tuberculosis among HIV-infected patients receiving HAART: long term incidence and risk factors in a South African cohort. AIDS 19: 2109–2116.
44. Girardi E, Sabin CA, d'Arminio Monforte A, Hogg B, Phillips AN, et al. (2005) Incidence of Tuberculosis among HIV-infected patients receiving highly active antiretroviral therapy in Europe and North America. Clin Infect Dis 41: 1772–1782.
45. Seyler C, Anglaret X, Dakoury-Dogbo N, Messou E, Toure S, et al. (2003) Medium-term survival, morbidity and immunovirological evolution in HIV-infected adults receiving antiretroviral therapy, Abidjan, Cote d'Ivoire. Antivir Ther 8: 385–393.
46. Hung CC, Hsiao CF (2003) Recurrence of tuberculosis in HIV-1-infected adults treated after rifamycin-based treatment and highly active antiretroviral therapy. J Acquir Immune Defic Syndr 34: 437–439.
47. Badri M, Wilson D, Wood R (2002) Effect of highly active antiretroviral therapy on incidence of tuberculosis in South Africa: a cohort study. Lancet 359: 2059–2064.
48. Jones JL, Hanson DL, Dworkin MS, DeCock KM (2000) HIV-associated tuberculosis in the era of highly active antiretroviral therapy. The Adult/Adolescent Spectrum of HIV Disease Group. Int J Tuberc Lung Dis 4: 1026–1031.
49. Brinkhof MW, Egger M, Boulle A, May M, Hosseinipour M, et al. (2007) Tuberculosis after initiation of antiretroviral therapy in low-income and high-income countries. Clin Infect Dis 45: 1518–1521.
50. Rajasekaran S, Raja K, Jeyaseelan L, Vijila S, Priya K, et al. (2009) Post-HAART tuberculosis in adults and adolescents with HIV in India: Incidence, clinical and immunological profile. Indian Journal of Tuberculosis 69–76.
51. Dye C, Lonnroth K, Jaramillo E, Williams BG, Raviglione M (2009) Trends in tuberculosis incidence and their determinants in 134 countries. Bull World Health Organ 87: 683–691.
52. Lawn SD, Wood R (2011) Tuberculosis in antiretroviral treatment services in resource-limited settings: addressing the challenges of screening and diagnosis. J Infect Dis 204 Suppl 4: S1159–1167.
53. Laureillard D, Marcy O, Madec Y, Chea S, Chan S, et al. (2013) Paradoxical tuberculosis-associated immune reconstitution inflammatory syndrome after early initiation of antiretroviral therapy in a randomized clinical trial. AIDS 27: 2577–2586.
54. Manabe YC, Breen R, Perti T, Girardi E, Sterling TR (2009) Unmasked tuberculosis and tuberculosis immune reconstitution inflammatory disease: a disease spectrum after initiation of antiretroviral therapy. J Infect Dis 199: 437–444.
55. Middelkoop K, Bekker LG, Shashkina E, Kreiswirth B, Wood R (2012) Retreatment tuberculosis in a South African community: the role of re-infection, HIV and antiretroviral treatment. Int J Tuberc Lung Dis 16: 1510–1516.

18

detectIR: A Novel Program for Detecting Perfect and Imperfect Inverted Repeats Using Complex Numbers and Vector Calculation

Congting Ye[1,2], Guoli Ji[1,3]*, Lei Li[1,2], Chun Liang[2,4]*

1 Department of Automation, Xiamen University, Xiamen, Fujian 361005, China, **2** Department of Biology, Miami University, Oxford, Ohio 45056, United States of America, **3** Innovation Center for Cell Biology, Xiamen University, Xiamen, Fujian 361005, China, **4** State Key Laboratory for Biology of Plant Diseases and Insect Pests, Institute of Plant Protection, Chinese Academy of Agricultural Sciences, Beijing 100193, China

Abstract

Inverted repeats are present in abundance in both prokaryotic and eukaryotic genomes and can form DNA secondary structures – hairpins and cruciforms that are involved in many important biological processes. Bioinformatics tools for efficient and accurate detection of inverted repeats are desirable, because existing tools are often less accurate and time consuming, sometimes incapable of dealing with genome-scale input data. Here, we present a MATLAB-based program called *detectIR* for the perfect and imperfect inverted repeat detection that utilizes complex numbers and vector calculation and allows genome-scale data inputs. A novel algorithm is adopted in *detectIR* to convert the conventional sequence string comparison in inverted repeat detection into vector calculation of complex numbers, allowing non-complementary pairs (mismatches) in the pairing stem and a non-palindromic spacer (loop or gaps) in the middle of inverted repeats. Compared with existing popular tools, our program performs with significantly higher accuracy and efficiency. Using genome sequence data from HIV-1, *Arabidopsis thaliana, Homo sapiens* and *Zea mays* for comparison, *detectIR* can find lots of inverted repeats missed by existing tools whose outputs often contain many invalid cases. *detectIR* is open source and its source code is freely available at: https://sourceforge.net/projects/detectir.

Editor: Silvio C. E. Tosatto, Universita' di Padova, Italy

Funding: This work was supported partially by National Institutes of Health National Institute of General Medical Sciences grant (1R15GM94732-1 A1 to CL), the National Natural Science Foundation of China (61174161, 61375077 and 61201358), the Natural Science Foundation of Fujian Province of China (2012J01154), the specialized Research Fund for the Doctoral Program of Higher Education of China (20130121130004 and 20120121120038), and the Fundamental Research Funds for the Central Universities in China (2013121025, 201412G009 and CBX2014007). The funders had no role in study design, data collection and analysis, decision to publish, or preparation of the manuscript.

Competing Interests: The authors have declared that no competing interests exist.

* Email: liangc@miamioh.edu (CL); glji@xmu.edu.cn (GJ)

Introduction

An inverted repeat is a nucleotide sequence fragment that can form self-complementary pairing between its two halves. The perfect inverted repeats are also known as palindrome where one of these two halves is exactly the reverse complement of the other; in contrast, imperfect inverted repeats contain nucleotide pairs that are not reversely complementary (*i.e.*, mismatched), often with a non-palindromic spacer (loop or gaps) in the middle [1] [2] [3]. Abundant inverted repeats are present in both prokaryotic and eukaryotic genomes with nonrandom distributions, and they are involved in many biological processes including DNA replication [4], DNA transition [5] and DNA methylation [6]. In yeast, long inverted repeats were demonstrated to be mitotic recombination hotspots, and quasipalindromes (imperfect inverted repeats) underwent deletion more frequently [7]. In mouse embryonic stem cells, inverted repeats get involved in the generation of unstable chromosomal rearrangements [8]. Inverted repeats of >=6 complementary nucleotides, either perfect or imperfect, can form secondary structures – cruciforms in double stranded DNA [9]. Some DNA-binding proteins have their two binding sites arranged as in an inverted repeat [3] [4] [10]. Using atomic force microscopy images, the DNA-binding protein PARP-1 was shown to bind the cruciform structure generated by a 106-*nt* inverted repeat within an *E. coli* plasmid [5]. PARP-1 was found to participate in chromatin structure coordination and gene expression regulation [11], and it did show a binding preference to cruciform structures than loops or linear DNAs [9]. In humans, a 14-*nt* imperfect inverted repeat sequence located in distal promoter region of human HFE gene can form a cruciform structure that binds PARP-1 protein to repress HFE transcription, and increased ion level can trigger PARP-1 breakdown to release such transcriptional repression [12]. Interestingly, using 2D electrophoretic analysis of DNA replication intermediates, single-stranded hairpins formed by imperfect inverted repeats with a central non-palindromic spacer, rather than double-stranded cruciforms, proved to be responsible for replication stalling that induces genome instability [13]. On the other hand, as a part of gene expression production, hairpin is a common and important secondary structural element in RNA transcripts, and its single-stranded template DNA must have a relevant inverted repeat [3], suggesting that inverted repeats in transcribed DNAs might play a potential regulatory role in resultant RNA transcripts. For instance, in yeast and mammalian pre-mRNAs, inverted repeats located in introns were shown to affect alternative splicing [14] [15] [16]. Moreover, inverted repeats have been utilized for gene silencing in fungi and plants for many years [17] [18] [19]. They also delineate transposon element boundaries. For instance, miniature inverted repeat transposable elements (MITEs) are characterized by their terminal inverted repeats [20]. Genes away from MITEs show higher expression than those that contain or are close to MITEs [21]. Clearly, the role of inverted repeats in gene expression regulation is worthy of further wet-lab experimental investigation and validation. The identification and characterization of inverted repeats at genome-wide scale will offer an important glimpse and survey that will facilitate our understanding of inverted repeats and their biological functions.

Lu et al. examined the distribution of perfect inverted repeats (palindromes) in human genome [22]. They found that palindromes show higher abundance in introns than exons while upstream regions (*i.e.*, 2,000 bp upstream from translational start site) also contain rich palindromes that can serve as binding sites for transcription factors. Interestingly, they also scanned the human genome for imperfect inverted repeats (*i.e.*, near-perfect palindromes of $< = 4$ mismatches between two halves, with a short spacer in the middle) and found a similar distribution pattern as perfect inverted repeats [22]. In yeast *Saccharomyces cerevisiae* genome, both palindromes and imperfect inverted repeats (*i.e.*, the pairing stem length >6 *nt* and the spacer length less than 77 *nt*) were significantly richer than randomized genome [3]. In particular, imperfect inverted repeats with short spacers, which have a greater susceptibility to cruciform extrusion than long spacers, were significantly enriched in intergenic regions near 3′ gene ends than near 5′ gene ends [3]. Using yeast relatives *S. paradoxus*, *S. mikatae* and *S. bayanus*, Humphey-Dixon and coworkers studied the conservation of both perfect and imperfect inverted repeats in yeast *S. cerevisiae* genome, and they found that both conserved inverted repeats in promoters and inverted repeats in the promoters of highly expressed genes are most frequently located near the transcriptional start sites, indicating their potential function in transcriptional regulation [23]. As more and more genome sequences are available for different species, it is important for us to conduct genome-wide comparative study to determine the distributions, properties, and conservation of inverted repeats among different species, either distantly or closely related, in order to deepen our understanding of inverted repeats and their biological importance.

To better understand the roles of inverted repeats in genome organization and evolution, developing efficient programs to conduct genome-wide detection of inverted repeats is particularly important. Recently, a MATLAB-based tool *findIR* [24] was created for detecting perfect inverted repeats. In comparison with the existing similar tools that adopt conventional string comparison algorithms, *findIR* deployed a novel algorithm that uses prime number scoring system and turns sequence search into the calculation, search and comparison of numbers. Consequently, *findIR* proved to have obviously higher accuracy in detecting perfect inverted repeats than several popular tools, and it was capable of processing genome-scale inputs. Unfortunately, it is difficult to use prime numbers to represent imperfect inverted repeats that contain non-complementary pairs in the pairing stem (*i.e.*, two halves) and a central non-palindromic spacer. The search and validation strategy of *findIR* is not designed for detecting imperfect inverted repeats. Moreover, *findIR* is limited to detect perfect inverted repeats of length shorter than 1,000 *nt* and the robust vector calculation power of MATLAB has not been utilized at all by *findIR* to enhance the program efficiency.

Here, we developed a novel program *detectIR* that also turns sequence search into numerical calculation and manipulation using complex numbers, which can represent both perfect and imperfect IRs accurately and efficiently. In comparison with *findIR*, the novelty of *detectIR* lies in a novel mapping schema that utilizes complex numbers, a distinctive and effective strategy of search and validation to evaluate candidates of both perfect and imperfect inverted repeats, and the utilization of MATLAB built-in vector calculation power that enables simultaneous detection of inverted repeats of same length to improve the program efficiency significantly.

Design and Implementation

Most existing bioinformatics tools in inverted repeat detection rely on string comparison that is often computational resource demanding and less accurate. Using a novel algorithm that employs prime number scoring system and numerical calculation and search to detect perfect inverted repeats (or palindromes), *findIR* was demonstrated to have much higher accuracy than BioPHP (http://www.biophp.org/minitools/find_palindromes), MATLAB built-in *palindromes* function and EMBOSS *palindrome* tool [25] in detecting perfect inverted repeats. However, both EMBOSS *palindrome* tool and MATLAB built-in *palindromes* function can detect imperfect inverted repeats that contain a central non-palindromic spacer (loop) and/or non-complementary pairs in the pairing stem. In the core algorithm of *findIR*, nucleotide bases are first mapped to a prime number scoring system in which scores of reversely complementary bases can cancel each other out, and a cumulative score is computed for each base along the whole target sequence. Then, *findIR* searches all the pairs of positions whose cumulative scores are the same to construct candidates of perfect inverted repeats. *findIR* finally validates the candidate based on the principle that if a subsequence is a valid perfect inverted repeat, the number of nested perfect inverted repeats within the subsequence, all of which share the same center, should be equal to the half-length of the subsequence. This search and validation strategy makes *findIR* impossible to detect imperfect inverted repeats. Moreover, the prime number scoring system has its innate difficulty to represent imperfect inverted repeats that often contains a central non-palindromic spacer and/or non-complementary pairs in the pairing stem. In addition, *findIR* is limited to detect perfect inverted repeats of length shorter than 1,000 *nt*, presenting a size constraint for large genomes where longer inverted repeats may exist. Here, we developed a novel program called *detectIR* that maps the nucleotide sequence to a complex number vector so that both perfect and imperfect inverted repeats can be searched (see examples in Figure 1). Compared with *findIR*, *detectIR* adopted a totally different algorithm in perfect inverted repeat detection, which had been modified and extended to search for imperfect inverted repeats. In particular, for both perfect and imperfect inverted repeat detection, we have taken advantage of MATLAB built-in vector calculation to search and validate inverted repeats candidates of the same size simultaneously. Our program proves to be much faster and more accurate in detecting both perfect and imperfect inverted repeats than the previously mentioned tools. Moreover, our program can accept a large genome input like chromosome 1 of *Homo sapiens* and *Zea mays* that can often result in an execution crash in other tools.

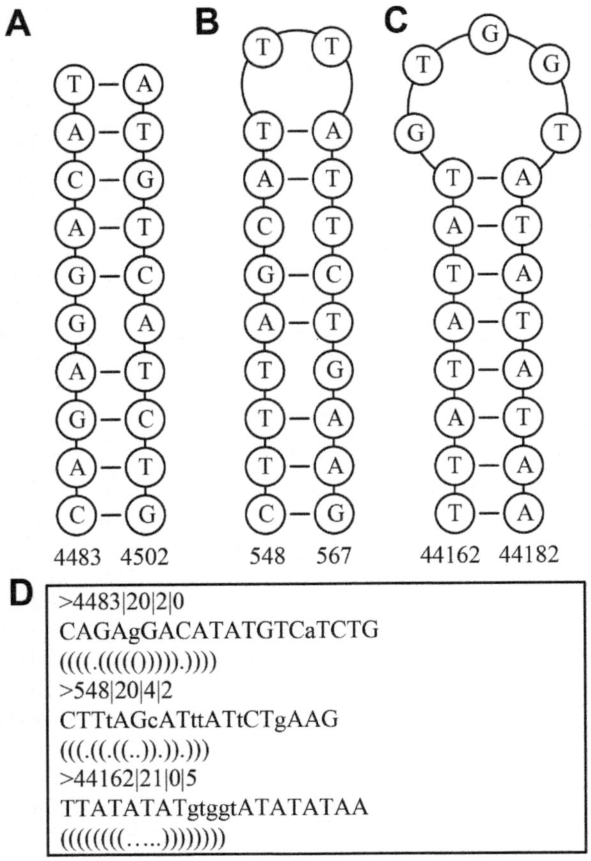

Figure 1. Examples of imperfect inverted repeats detected in the chromosome 1 *of Arabidopsis thaliana* by *detectIR.* Circles highlight the nucleotide bases and numbers represent the start and end genomic coordinates of the imperfect inverted repeats. (A) An imperfect inverted repeat containing only mismatches (un-pairing pair). (B) An imperfect inverted repeat containing both mismatches and a spacer (gaps). (C) An imperfect inverted repeat containing only a spacer (gaps) in the middle. (D) The *detectIR* output for the aforementioned 3 imperfect inverted repeats in the combined format of dot-bracket notation and FASTA. The dots represent the spacer or mismatch nucleotides while brackets indicate the pairing relations. The FASTA description line (*e.g.*, >4483|20|2|0) has the following explanation: > GenomicStartPosition|InvertedRepeatLength|MismatchNumber|GapNumber.

Within the prime number scoring system (also called cumulative scoring system) implemented in *findIR* [24], a subsequence between two bases whose cumulative scores are identical will be recognized as a perfect inverted repeat candidate. This conclusion is based on the assumption that only the scores between reversely complementary bases can completely eliminate each other in the system. If two bases have identical score, the numbers of reversely complementary bases should be equal in the corresponding subsequence [24]. Unfortunately, this assumption is not correct for some cases, because scores also can be partly eliminated between non-complementary bases. For instance, when using the prime number mapping schema: $A \rightarrow 3, T \rightarrow -3, G \rightarrow 7, C \rightarrow -7$, the scores of seven nucleotides A can be eliminated out by that of three nucleotides C (same to T and G). Therefore, if two bases have an identical accumulative score, the numbers of complementary bases in the corresponding subsequence between them are not always equal. In *findIR*, such a case would be still recognized as a perfect inverted repeat candidate. Although these cases could be filtered out later by the downstream process, it clearly increases the computational workload. On the other hand, these cases can be avoided by using large prime numbers (*e.g.*, 10007, 10009), which was exactly adopted by the *findIR* [24].

Different from prime numbers, complex numbers can effectively represent both perfect and imperfect inverted repeats that contain non-complementary pairs in the stem and a central non-palindromic spacer. The complex numbers have been utilized in detecting symmetric palindromes (*e.g.*, ACGGCA, the palindromes without reverse complementary) by Gupta et al. [26], using the following mapping schema:

$$A \rightarrow 1+j, T \rightarrow -1-j, C \rightarrow 1-j, G \rightarrow -1+j$$

Firstly, they divided an input nucleotide sequence into subsequences with the length of a desired palindrome, and then utilized this mapping method to convert each subsequence into numerical series and rearranged the subsequence. Secondly, they use periodicity transformation to calculate a periodic sequence that is closest to the rearranged subsequence. Lastly, through calculating a coefficient between the rearranged subsequence and the periodic sequence to determine and verify each subsequence to be a valid symmetric palindrome [26]. Therefore, their method was not designed for both perfect and imperfect inverted repeat detection that requires nucleotide reverse complementary. In contrast, our usage of complex numbers is different from their approach by deploying a novel mapping schema:

$$A \rightarrow 1, T \rightarrow -1, C \rightarrow j, G \rightarrow -j$$

Using this mapping method, only the scores between reversely complementary bases can really cancel each other out within the numeric scoring system. This method makes sure that the numbers of reversely complementary nucleotides A and T (also C and G) are equal within the sequence candidates of perfect inverted repeat. Furthermore, we can precisely define the upper bound of the score of the imperfect inverted repeats using this complex number mapping schema - the sum of the absolute values of the real part and the imaginary part of C is less than or equal to m, $|real(C)|+|image(C)| \leq m$ (C denotes the score of the subsequence, m represents the maximal number of mismatches allowed – the sum of all nucleotides within the central non-palindromic spacer and the non-complementary pairs in the pairing stem).

Algorithm for perfect inverted repeat detection

The algorithm for perfect inverted repeat detection is based on the principle that a perfect inverted repeat of length h (h>4) must contain a nested perfect inverted repeat of length h-2, which shares the same center. So if we have obtained all the perfect inverted repeats of length h-2, extension of one base at both ends will derive inverted repeat candidates with length h. Among all these inverted repeat candidates, we then filter out those whose terminal bases are not reversely complementary.

The details of our algorithm are shown in Figures 2 and 3. Here, l is the minimal length, L is the maximal length of perfect inverted repeats to be detected, and N is the length of the input sequence S ($l \leq L \leq N$, l and L should be even number).

(1). Mapping sequence to vector. The input sequence S is mapped to a complex number vector M. For example, if input sequence S is 'ATCGAACGAATTCGTTAACC', M = [1,-1, j, -j,1,

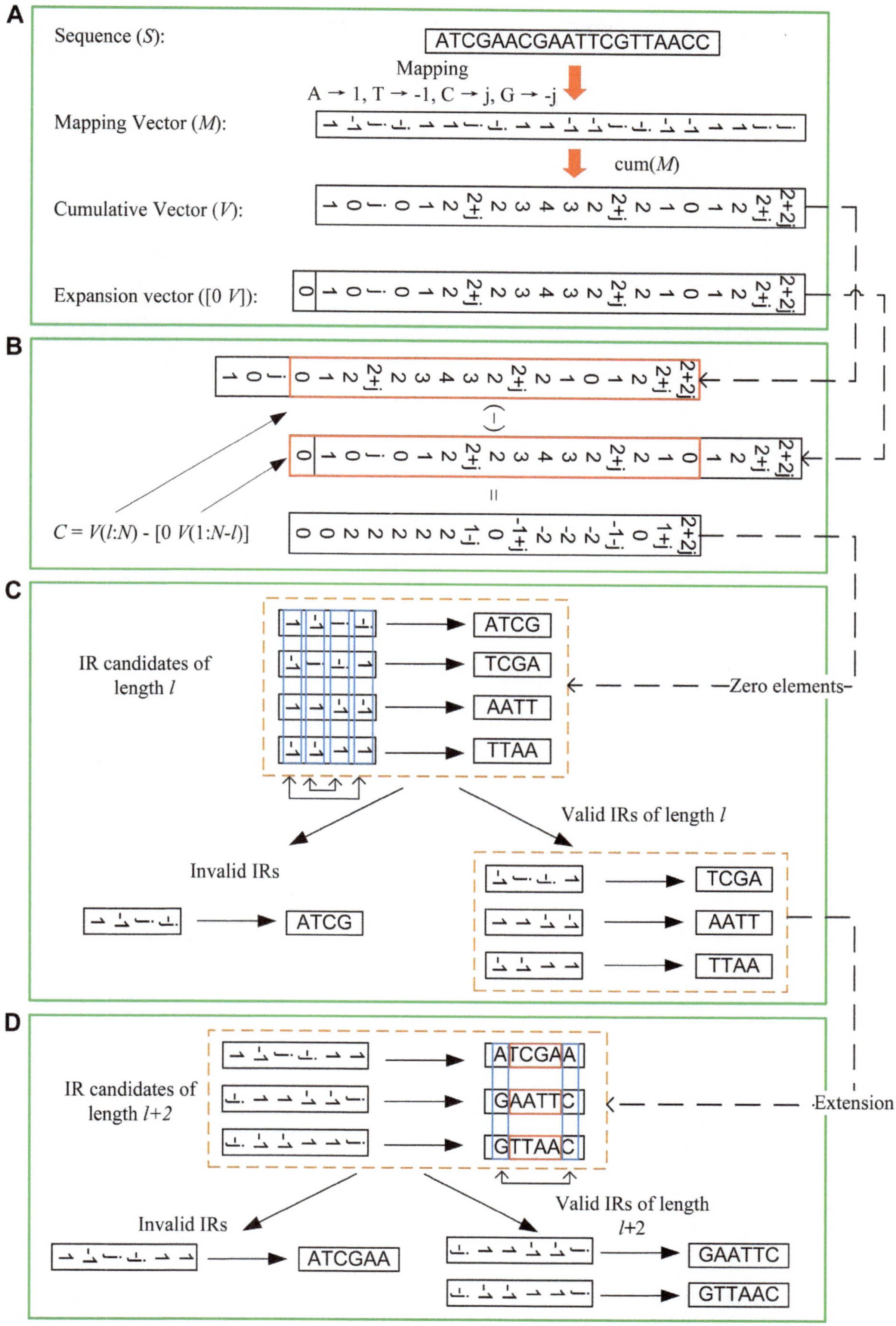
A
Sequence (S):
ATCGAACGAATTCGTTAACC
Mapping
A → 1, T → -1, C → j, G → -j
Mapping Vector (M):
cum(M)
Cumulative Vector (V):
Expansion vector ([0 V]):
B
(−)
C = V(l:N) - [0 V(1:N-l)]
C
IR candidates of length l
ATCG
TCGA
AATT
TTAA
Zero elements
Invalid IRs
ATCG
Valid IRs of length l
TCGA
AATT
TTAA
D
IR candidates of length l+2
ATCGAA
GAATTC
GTTAAC
Extension
Invalid IRs
ATCGAA
Valid IRs of length l+2
GAATTC
GTTAAC

Figure 2. Major steps of the core algorithm for perfect inverted repeat detection. (A) Map a nucleotide sequence to a complex number vector and calculate its cumulative score value. (B) Calculate the scores of all the subsequences of length l (here $l=4$, N is the length of input sequence). (C) Select out perfect inverted repeat candidates and determine valid perfect inverted repeats. (D) Extend one base at both ends of subsequences to obtain longer perfect inverted repeats.

1, j, -j, 1, 1, -1, -1, j, -j, -1, -1, 1, 1, j, j]. Then the cumulative value V of M is calculated (Figure 2A).

(2). Calculation of subsequence score. The scores of all the subsequences of length l are calculated, a subsequence score is defined as the sum of the subsequence's corresponding vector. The scores of all the subsequences of length l can be obtained by the following formula,

$$C = V(l:N) - [0V(1:N-l)]$$

The i-th element $C(i)$ represent the score of the subsequence $S(i{:}i{+}l{-}1) = s_i s_{i+1} \ldots s_{i+l-2} s_{i+l-1}$ (Figure 2B).

(3). Identification of candidates. A subsequence whose score is equal to 0 will be recognized as a candidate of perfect inverted repeat. In this step we will identify all the candidates of length l by finding the zero elements of C,

$$P = \text{find}(C == 0)$$

P represents the indices of the zero elements in vector C.

(4). Validation of candidates. For each perfect inverted repeat candidate, perfect pairing needs to be found between the front half and rear half of bases. We will keep valid perfect inverted repeat candidates, while filter out invalid cases (Figure 2C).

(5). Extension of inverted repeats. Base on the aforementioned principle, extend one base at both ends of inverted repeats identified in the previous step, and select out cases whose new terminal bases are reversely complementary (Figure 2D). For instance, if subsequence $S(i{:}i{+}h{-}3)$ is a perfect inverted repeat of length h-2 identified in previous step, the extended subsequence $S(i{-}1{:}i{+}h{-}2)$ will be a potential inverted repeat of length h. If its terminal bases are either G/C or A/T,

$$M(i-1) + M(i+h-2) = 0$$

Then, $S(i{-}1{:}i{+}h{-}2)$ is a perfect inverted repeat of length h.

(6). Repetition. Repeat the step 5 until $h = L$, then all the perfect inverted repeats of length ranged between l and L have been identified.

Algorithm for imperfect inverted repeat detection

Different from the aforementioned algorithm for perfect inverted repeat detection, to find imperfect inverted repeats of length h, allowing maximal mismatch number m, which is defined as the sum of all nucleotides within the central non-palindromic spacer and the non-complementary pairs in the pairing stem, we will firstly find all subsequences of length h-2 with mismatch number $\leq m$, with the assumption that the nested subsequence of an imperfect inverted repeat with mismatch number $\leq m$ must be a sequence with mismatch number $\leq m$ which share the same center. The major difference between the nested subsequence and the imperfect inverted repeat is that the terminal bases of imperfect inverted repeat must be reversely complementary ('AAAAATTTCT'), while the former does not require meeting this condition ('AAAATTTC').

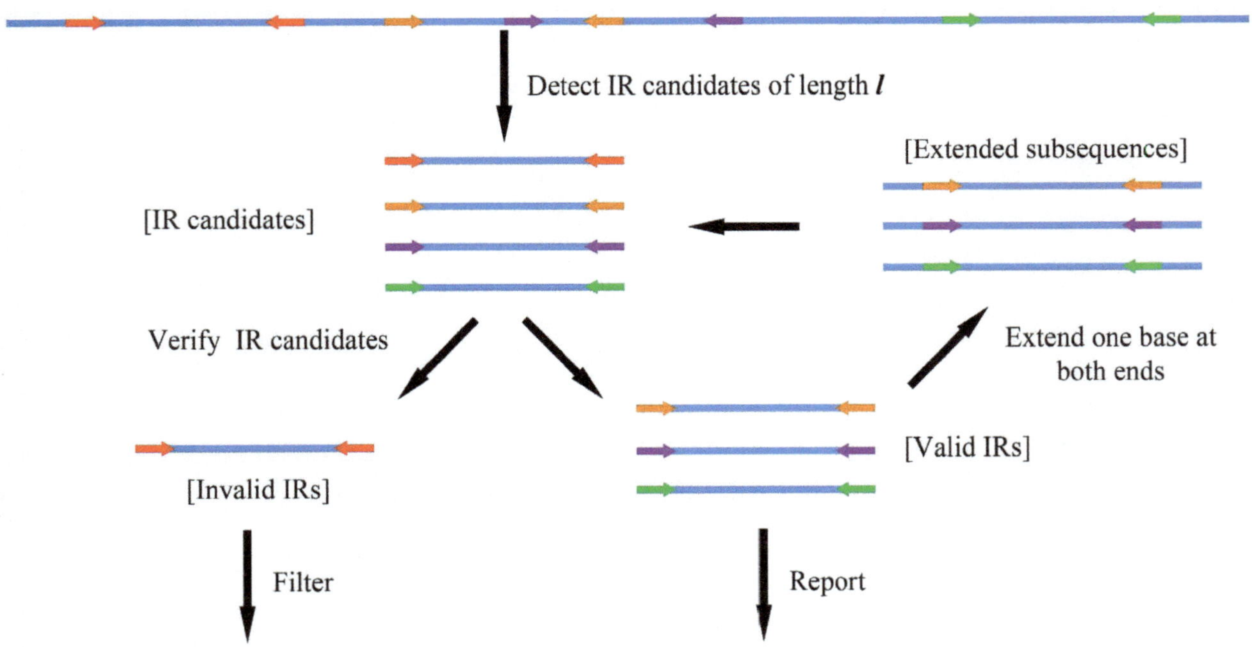

Figure 3. The flowchart of the core algorithm for perfect inverted repeat detection. Arrows in the same color represent the borders of inverted repeats.

Figure 4 shows the core algorithm for imperfect inverted repeat detection. l is the minimal length and L is the maximal length of imperfect inverted repeats to be detected, and N is the length of the input sequence ($l \leq L \leq N$), m is the maximal number of mismatches allowing in each imperfect inverted repeat. The first two steps 1 and 2 are same to the detection of perfect inverted repeats.

(1). Mapping sequence to vector

(2). Calculation of subsequence score

(3). Identification of candidates. If the sum of the absolute values of the real part and the imaginary part of a subsequence's score is less than or equal to m, the subsequence is recognized as an imperfect inverted repeat candidate of length l.

$$|real(C(i))| + |image(C(i))| \leq m$$

(4). Validation of candidates. In this step, the mismatch numbers of all the imperfect inverted repeat candidates of *length l* are calculated. Subsequences that satisfy the following three conditions: (1) the mismatch number is less than or equal to m; (2) the first and last base of the subsequence are reversely complementary; (3) mismatch number is not zero, will be reported as the detected imperfect inverted repeats. While, all the subsequences meeting (1) with/without (2) and (3) will be picked up for the process in the next step (see Figure 4A).

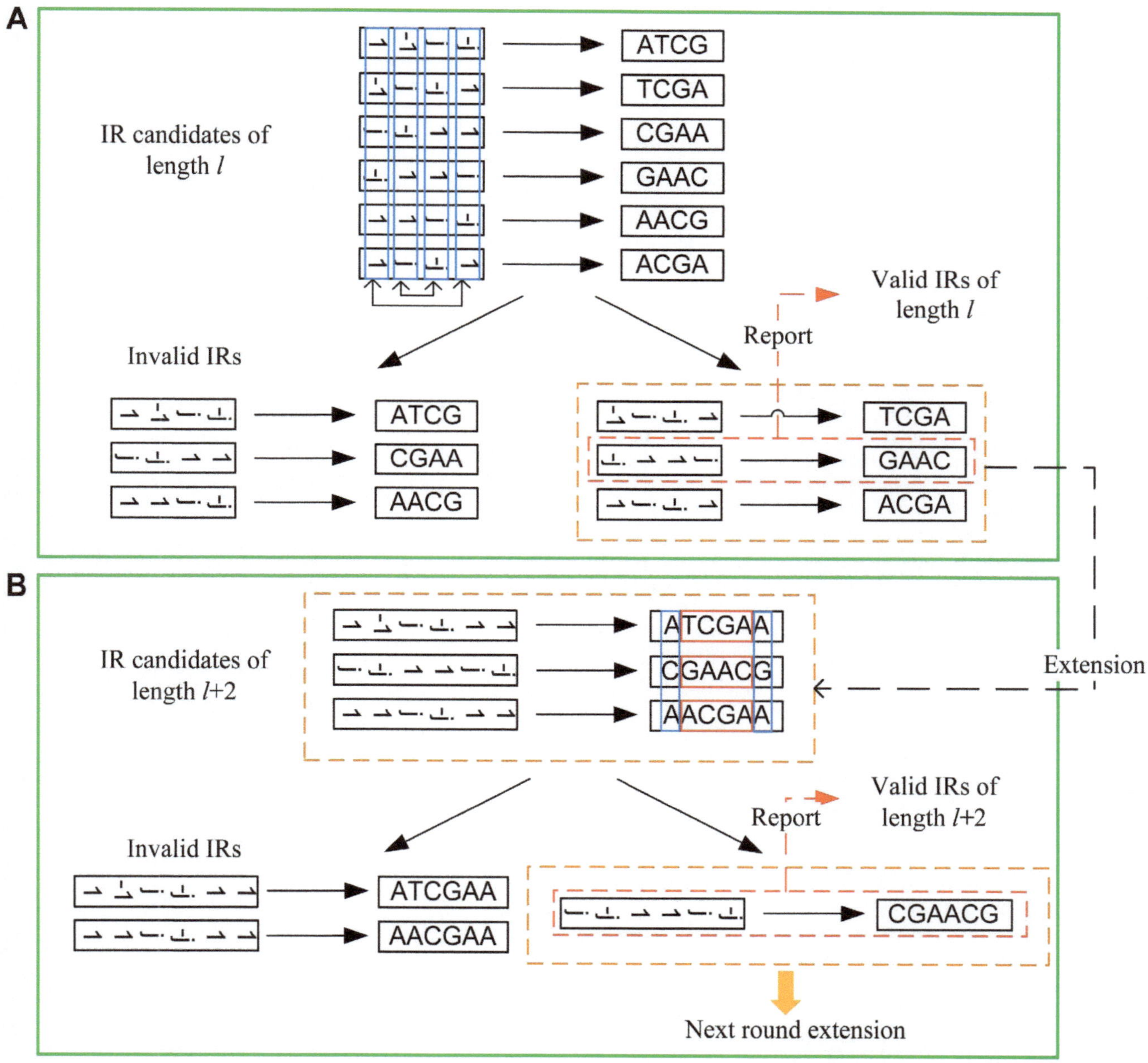

Figure 4. Major steps of the core algorithm for imperfect inverted repeat detection. (A) Select out imperfect inverted repeat candidates (here, we just show part of candidates), report valid imperfect inverted repeats and pick up valid subsequences for the downstream process described in the next step (here $l=4$, $m=2$). (B) Extend one base at both ends of subsequences to obtain longer imperfect inverted repeats. The subsequences locating at both ends of a sequence (*i.e.*, 'ATCGAA') should not be selected for the next round extension.

(5). Extension of subsequences. We will extend one nucleotide at both ends of subsequences generated in the previous step. If the two extended bases are reversely complementary, the corresponding mismatch number of the subsequence keep unchanged, otherwise the mismatch number increases by 2. Then subsequences meeting all three conditions described in step 4 are valid imperfect inverted repeats. Subsequences meeting (1) with/without (2) and (3) will be picked up for the next round extension (see Figure 4B).

For example, when subsequence $S(i{:}i{+}h{-}3)$ of length h-2 has a mismatch number α less than or equal to m, the subsequence $S(i{-}1{:}i{+}h{-}2)$ is a potential imperfect inverted repeats of length h. If,

$$M(i-1)+M(i+h-2)=0, \alpha>0$$

Subsequence $S(i{-}1{:}i{+}h{-}2)$ is an imperfect inverted repeat that meets all given conditions.

(6). Repetition. Repeat the step 5 until $h=L$ (or $h=L$-1), then all imperfect inverted repeats of odd-length (or even-length) ranged between l and L with a mismatch number $\leq m$ have been identified.

(7). Detection of even/odd length inverted repeats. Repeat steps 2–6, starting with calculating the score of subsequences of length l+1. Finally, all imperfect inverted repeats of even-length (or odd-length) ranged between l and L will been identified.

Results

The aforementioned algorithms have been implemented into *detectIR*, which was composed of two MATLAB functions *detectPerfectIR* and *detectImperfectIR* respectively. To evaluate the performance of these two functions, they were compared with four inverted repeat detection tools BioPHP (A PHP program obtained from http://www.biophp.org/minitools/find_palindromes), EMBOSS *palindrome* tool (Stable version 6.3.1), MATLAB built-in *palindromes* function (Matlab R2013b) and MATLAB-based *findIR*. HIV-1 genome and chromosome 1 from *Arabidopsis thaliana*, *Homo sapiens* and *Zea mays* were used as the test data. The detailed step-by-step guide for testing and comparison is available on our sourceforge project website (https://sourceforge.net/projects/detectir). Our source codes and relevant documents are also available as in File S1. The result comparison of perfect inverted repeat detection and imperfect inverted repeat detection is presented below separately. For smaller genomes like *Arabidopsis thaliana* and HIV-1, a standard workstation with 8G RAM should be enough for testing, while large genomes like *Homo sapiens* and *Zea mays* will require at least 32G RAM. For the test results described below, all the tests were performed using Ubuntu 12.04 (precise) 64-bit platform with Intel Xeon (2.00 GHz) processer and 125.9 GB RAM.

Perfect inverted repeat detection

Here, we used each program to search perfect inverted repeats with length between 10 and 1000 *nt*. The detection results are summarized in Table 1. The length distributions of the perfect inverted repeats detected by *detectIR* are shown in Figure S1. It is clear that the numbers of perfect inverted repeats decrease with the increase of inverted repeat length, shorter inverted repeats are much more abundant in genomes (see Figure S1).

To determine the accuracy of *detectPerfectIR*, the outputs from different programs using the same input data were compared against *detectPerfectIR* respectively. The differences discovered between them can be classified into two categories (1) entries only

Table 1. The comparison of *detectPerfectIR* with BioPHP, EMBOSS, MATLAB and *findIR* for perfect inverted repeat detection.

	HIV-1		Arabidopsis thaliana		Homo sapiens		Zea mays	
	IR count	runtime	IR count	runtime	IR count	runtime	IR count	runtime
BioPHP	7	5.56 m	*	*	*	*	*	*
EMBOSS(*palindrome*)	5	<1 s	61,705	34.53 m	347,688	38.74 h	448,928	4.28 h
MATLAB(*palindromes*)	13	0.06 s	266,187	3.27 m	*	*	*	*
findIR	7	0.23 s	142,249	8.80 m	746,925	1.16 h	1,147,428	1.51 h
detectPerfectIR	7	0.05 s	142,249	11.85 s	746,925	1.72 m	1,147,428	2.00 m

*Program crashed in execution or output nothing after 10-day execution.

present in the output of *detectPerfectIR*, (2) entries only present in the output of BioPHP, EMBOSS (*palindrome*), MATLAB (*palindromes*) or *findIR*. As shown in Table 1, consequently, the outputs of *detectPerfectIR* and *findIR* are identical, while *detectPerfectIR* performs much more efficiently.

Entries only present in the output of detectPerfectIR and findIR. The entries only detected by *detectPerfectIR* and *findIR* were found to be valid perfect inverted repeats by human validation. In other words, these cases are missed by the other compared tools. For HIV-1 genome, both EMBOSS and MATLAB missed 2 perfect inverted repeats (see File S2 and S3). For chromosome 1 of *Arabidopsis thaliana*, EMBOSS missed 80,548 perfect inverted repeats (see File S4) and MATLAB missed 86,759 perfect inverted repeats (see File S5). For chromosome 1 of *Homo sapiens*, EMBOSS missed 399,237 perfect inverted repeats (see File S6). For chromosome 1 of *Zea mays*, EMBOSS missed 703,018 perfect inverted repeats (see File S7).

Entries only present in the output of the other compared tools. The entries only found by the other tools prove to be invalid perfect inverted repeats by human validation, which mean the outputs of these tools contain false positives. For the HIV-1 genome, the output of MATLAB contains 8 cases with a gap in the center, like 'CAAAAATTTTG' (see File S3). For chromosome 1 of *Arabidopsis thaliana*, the output of EMBOSS contains 4 invalid cases like 'A-N(60)-T' etc (see File S4). And the output of MATLAB contains 210,697 invalid cases, 46915 of them are subsequences like 'ATTTTTTAAAAAT' with a gap in the center and 163,782 of them are subsequences like 'NNNNNNNNNN' or 'A-N(27)-T' (see File S5). For chromosome 1 of *Zea mays*, the output of EMBOSS contains 4,518 invalid cases (see File S7).

Imperfect inverted repeat detection

In imperfect inverted repeat detection, some tools define continuous mismatches in the center of inverted repeat as gaps; mismatches in other locations are still considered as mismatches, while our algorithm does not differentiate these two types of mismatch. For example, EMBOSS *palindrome* tool will recognize sequence 'AACAACTTTCTT' as an inverted repeat with 1 mismatch and 2 gaps, our tool will recognize it as an inverted repeat with 4 mismatches. MATLAB *palindromes* function can only deal with imperfect inverted repeats containing gaps. So, here we let our function *detectImperfectIR* and MATLAB *palindromes* function detect imperfect inverted repeats of length between 20 and 1000 *nt*, mismatch number (or gap number) ≤6, and let EMBOSS palindrome tool search imperfect inverted repeats of length between 20 and 1000 *nt*, gap number ≤2, and mismatch number ≤2 (Using the definition of EMBOSS). BioPHP and *findIR* are not used here, because they are designed to detect only the perfect inverted repeats. Summaries of the detection results are shown in Table 2. The length distributions of the imperfect inverted repeats detected by *detectIR* are shown in Figure S2. Obviously, the length distribution of imperfect inverted repeats is similar to that of perfect inverted repeats. The number of imperfect inverted repeats of even length is more than those of odd length, and the underlying reason may be that the odd-length inverted repeats must contain a spacer in the middle, which means that the mismatches in the stem should be less. To test this assumption, we run detectIR with an odd maximum mismatch number ($m = 7$). As shown in Figure S3, the numbers of odd-length imperfect inverted repeats are approximate to the numbers of even-length imperfect inverted repeats.

In order to make an unbiased comparison, we will filter out entries with a mismatch number larger than 2 or a gap number larger than 2 (Using the definition of EMBOSS) in the output of

Table 2. The comparison of *detectImperfectIR* with EMBOSS and MATLAB for imperfect inverted repeat detection.

	HIV-1		Arabidopsis thaliana		Homo sapiens		Zea mays	
	IR count	runtime	IR count	runtime	IR count	runtime	IR count	runtime
EMBOSS(*palindrome*)	8	<1 s	65,596	43.48 m	429,662	39.96 h	619,889	5.91 h
MATLAB(*palindromes*)	1	0.07 s	173,659	11.00 m	*	*	*	*
detectImperfectIR	37	0.09 s	311,369	1.48 m	2,166,638	11.83 m	2,878,686	16.63 m

*Program crashed in execution or output nothing after 10-day execution.

detectImperfectIR before comparing it with the output of EMBOSS.

Entries only present in the output of detectImperfectIR. All these entries are validated by human to be imperfect inverted repeats that meet the defined criteria. For HIV-1, EMBOSS missed 9 cases (see File S8), and MATLAB missed 36 cases (see File S9). For instance, both EMBOSS and MATLAB missed case 'ATCAGATGCTAAAGCATATGAT'. For chromosome 1 of *Arabidopsis thaliana*, EMBOSS missed 78,293 cases (see File S10) and MATLAB missed 304,394 cases (see File S11). Both EMBOSS and MATLAB missed cases like 'CTTTAGCATTTATTCTGAAG' and 'ATAATTTAAAA-TAAAATTAT'. For chromosome 1 of *Homo sapiens*, EMBOSS missed 618,357 cases (see File S12). For chromosome 1 of *Zea mays*, EMBOSS missed 825,455 cases (see File S13).

Entries only present in the output of the other compared tools. The entries only present in the output of the other compared tools prove to be false positives again. For chromosome 1 of *Arabidopsis thaliana*, the output of EMBOSS contains 1,765 perfect inverted repeats and 23 entries like 'A-N(27)-TT' (see File S10). The output of MATLAB contains 3,091 perfect inverted repeats and 163,593 entries like 'N(20)' or 'A-N(27)-T' (see File S11). For chromosome 1 of *Homo sapiens*, the output of EMBOSS contains 6,771 perfect inverted repeats (see File S12). For chromosome 1 of *Zea mays*, the output of EMBOSS contains 17,926 perfect inverted repeats and 27,761 entries like 'A-N(100)-T' (see File S13).

Random nucleotide sequence test

To evaluate the efficiency of *detectIR*, we generated several random nucleotide sequences of varied lengths, use function *detectPerfectIR* to detect perfect inverted repeats of length between 4 and 1000, and use function *detectImperfectIR* to detect imperfect inverted repeats of length between 10 and 1000 with mismatches less than or equal to 6. The average runtimes are shown below in Figure 5.

As shown in Figure 5, average runtime of the *detectIR* increases with the increase of the sequence length. The execution time of *detectImperfectIR* is ~6 fold of that of *detectPerfectIR* with same input data, because the perfect inverted repeats has more strict requirements than imperfect inverted repeats which reduce the search space. So it is clear that *detectIR* shows good scalability dealing with large genome sequence inputs.

Availability and Future Directions

detectIR is platform independent and can be used in Windows or Linux as long as MATLAB can be run. The source codes, test and comparison scripts, and documents are freely available at: https://sourceforge.net/projects/detectir.

Clearly, inverted repeats are not randomly distributed in both prokaryotic and eukaryotic genomes. Without a doubt, more wet-lab experiments for important genes are needed to clearly understand their biological functions. However, *in silico* genome-wide scan of inverted repeats can effectively help us to determine their overall distributions and characteristics and discover the groups of inverted repeats that are more likely to have important biological functions. As shown in Information S1, we used *detectIR* to conduct comparative study of perfect and imperfect inverted repeats in *Arabidopsis* genome. We found that both perfect and imperfect inverted repeats are not randomly distributed along the genome, and imperfect inverted repeats are much more abundant than perfect inverted repeats. In particular, imperfect inverted repeats are significantly enriched in near intergenic regions than far intergenic regions, while both perfect and imperfect inverted repeats are significantly more abundant in introns than exons. Our results are in line with the findings in human and yeast genomes [3] [22] [23]. Obviously, the inverted repeats in introns and promoter regions are worthy of closer examination in the future.

In conclusion, we developed an accurate and efficient program *detectIR* for detecting both perfect and imperfect inverted repeats in a given nucleotide sequence. *detectIR* is capable of processing large genome sequences, given enough memory in computation. Compared to BioPHP, EMBOSS *palindrome* tool, MATLAB built-in *palindromes* function and MATLAB-based *findIR*, the test

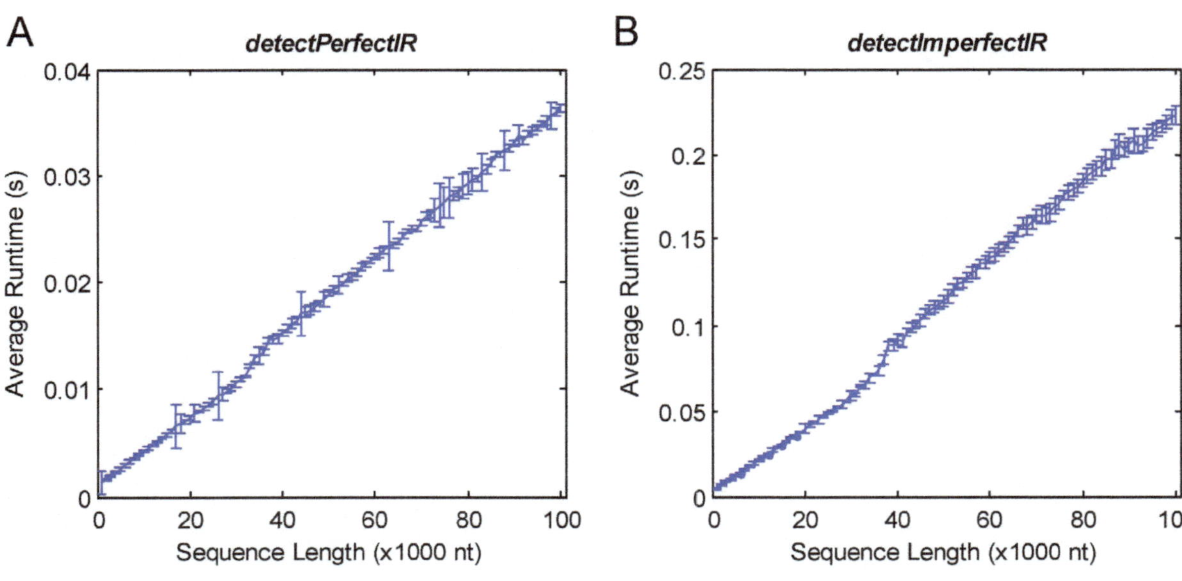

Figure 5. Average runtimes of *detectPerfectIR* and *detectImperfectIR* using random nucleotide sequence inputs of varied lengths. (A) The average runtimes of *detectPerfectIR* using random nucleotide sequence inputs of varied lengths. (B) The average runtimes of *detectImperfectIR* using random nucleotide sequence inputs of varied lengths.

results show that our program can more efficiently detect inverted repeats without sacrificing accuracy. Future directions will focus on improving the program to detect imperfect inverted repeats with indels within the paring stem, and reducing the memory consumption of program.

Supporting Information

Figure S1 Length distributions of perfect inverted repeats in different species detected by *detectIR*.

Figure S2 Length distributions of imperfect inverted repeats in different species detected by *detectIR* with the maximum mismatch number of 6 ($m = 6$).

Figure S3 Length distributions of imperfect inverted repeats in different species detected by *detectIR* with the maximum mismatch number of 7 ($m = 7$).

File S1 Source codes, test and comparison scripts, and user documents of *detectIR*.

File S2 The output files of the perfect inverted repeats detected differentially by *detectIR* and EMBOSS *palindrome* tool (Using the parameters described in the manuscript and HIV-1 genome as input data).

File S3 The output files of the perfect inverted repeats detected differentially by *detectIR* and MATLAB *palindromes* function (Using the parameters described in the manuscript and HIV-1 genome as input data).

File S4 The output files of the perfect inverted repeats detected differentially by *detectIR* and EMBOSS *palindrome* tool (Using the parameters described in the manuscript and chromosome 1 of *Arabidopsis thaliana* as input data).

File S5 The output files of the perfect inverted repeats detected differentially by *detectIR* and MATLAB *palindromes* function (Using the parameters described in the manuscript and chromosome 1 of *Arabidopsis thaliana* as input data).

File S6 The output files of the perfect inverted repeats detected differentially by *detectIR* and EMBOSS *palindrome* tool (Using the parameters described in the manuscript and chromosome 1 of *Homo sapiens* as input data).

File S7 The output files of the perfect inverted repeats detected differentially by *detectIR* and EMBOSS *palindrome* tool (Using the parameters described in the manuscript and chromosome 1 of *Zea mays* as input data).

File S8 The output files of the imperfect inverted repeats detected differentially by *detectIR* and EMBOSS *palindrome* tool (Using the parameters described in the manuscript and HIV-1 genome as input data).

File S9 The output files of the imperfect inverted repeats detected differentially by *detectIR* and MATLAB *palindromes* function (Using the parameters described in the manuscript and HIV-1 genome as input data).

File S10 The output files of the imperfect inverted repeats detected differentially by *detectIR* and EMBOSS *palindrome* tool (Using the parameters described in the manuscript and chromosome 1 of *Arabidopsis thaliana* as input data).

File S11 The output files of the imperfect inverted repeats detected differentially by *detectIR* and MATLAB *palindromes* function (Using the parameters described in the manuscript and chromosome 1 of *Arabidopsis thaliana* as input data).

File S12 The output files of the imperfect inverted repeats detected differentially by *detectIR* and EMBOSS *palindrome* tool (Using the parameters described in the manuscript and chromosome 1 of *Homo sapiens* as input data).

File S13 The output files of the imperfect inverted repeats detected differentially by *detectIR* and EMBOSS *palindrome* tool (Using the parameters described in the manuscript and chromosome 1 of *Zea mays* as input data).

Information S1 The genome-wide distribution of perfect and imperfect inverted repeats in *Arabidopsis thaliana*.

Acknowledgments

We thank Sutharzan Sreeskandarajan for helpful comments on the manuscript. We also want to thank the anonymous reviewers for their valuable comments and suggestions to improve the manuscript.

Author Contributions

Conceived and designed the experiments: CL GJ CY. Performed the experiments: CY. Analyzed the data: CY LL. Contributed reagents/materials/analysis tools: CY. Contributed to the writing of the manuscript: CY LL GJ CL.

References

1. Lilley DM (1980) The inverted repeat as a recognizable structural feature in supercoiled DNA molecules. Proc Natl Acad Sci 77: 6468–6472.
2. Smith GR (2008) Meeting DNA palindromes head-to-head. Genes Dev 22: 2612–2620. doi:10.1101/gad.1724708.
3. Strawbridge EM, Benson G, Gelfand Y, Benham CJ (2010) The distribution of inverted repeat sequences in the Saccharomyces cerevisiae genome. Curr Genet 56: 321–340. doi:10.1007/s00294-010-0302-6.
4. Pearson CE, Zorbas H, Price GB, Zannis-Hadjopoulos M (1996) Inverted Repeats, Stem-Loops, and Cruciforms: Significance for Initiation of DNA Replication. J Cell Biochem 63: 1–20.

5. Chasovskikh S, Dimtchev A, Smulson M, Dritschilo A (2005) DNA transitions induced by binding of PARP-1 to cruciform structures in supercoiled plasmids. Cytometry A 68A: 21–27. doi:10.1002/cyto.a.20187.
6. Allers T, Leach DR (1995) DNA Palindromes Adopt a Methylation-resistant Conformation that is Consistent with DNA Cruciform or Hairpin Formation in Vivo. J Mol Biol 252: 70–85.
7. Gordenin DA, Lobachev KS, Degtyareva NP, Malkova AL, Perkins E, et al. (1993) Inverted DNA repeats: a source of eukaryotic genomic instability. Mol Cell Biol 13: 5315–5322.
8. Hu L, Kim TM, Son MY, Kim S-A, Holland CL, et al. (2013) Two replication fork maintenance pathways fuse inverted repeats to rearrange chromosomes. Nature 501: 569–572. doi:10.1038/nature12500.
9. Brázda V, Laister RC, Jagelská EB, Arrowsmith C (2011) Cruciform structures are a common DNA feature important for regulating biological processes. BMC Mol Biol 12: 33.
10. Bhattacharya M, Das AK (2011) Inverted repeats in the promoter as an autoregulatory sequence for TcrX in Mycobacterium tuberculosis. Biochem Biophys Res Commun 415: 17–23. doi:10.1016/j.bbrc.2011.09.143.
11. Tulin A, Chinenov Y, Spradling A (2003) Regulation of Chromatin Structure and Gene Activity by Poly(ADP-Ribose) Polymerases. Curr Top Dev Biol Volume 56: 55–83.
12. Pelham C, Jimenez T, Rodova M, Rudolph A, Chipps E, et al. (2013) Regulation of HFE expression by poly(ADP-ribose) polymerase-1 (PARP1) through an inverted repeat DNA sequence in the distal promoter. Biochim Biophys Acta BBA - Gene Regul Mech 1829: 1257–1265. doi:10.1016/j.bbagrm.2013.10.002.
13. Voineagu I, Narayanan V, Lobachev KS, Mirkin SM (2008) Replication stalling at unstable inverted repeats: interplay between DNA hairpins and fork stabilizing proteins. Proc Natl Acad Sci 105: 9936–9941.
14. Martinez-Contreras R, Fisette J-F, Nasim FH, Madden R, Cordeau M, et al. (2006) Intronic Binding Sites for hnRNP A/B and hnRNP F/H Proteins Stimulate Pre-mRNA Splicing. PLoS Biol 4: e21. doi:10.1371/journal.pbio.0040021.
15. Nasim F-UH, Hutchison S, Cordeau M, Chabot B (2002) High-affinity hnRNP A1 binding sites and duplex-forming inverted repeats have similar effects on 5′splice site selection in support of a common looping out and repression mechanism. Rna 8: 1078–1089.
16. Howe KJ, Ares M (1997) Intron self-complementarity enforces exon inclusion in a yeast pre-mRNA. Proc Natl Acad Sci 94: 12467–12472.
17. Nakade K, Watanabe H, Sakamoto Y, Sato T (2011) Gene silencing of the Lentinula edodes lcc1 gene by expression of a homologous inverted repeat sequence. Microbiol Res 166: 484–493. doi:10.1016/j.micres.2010.09.004.
18. Hily J-M, Ravelonandro M, Damsteegt V, Bassett C, Petri C, et al. (2007) Plum pox virus coat protein gene Intron-hairpin-RNA (ihpRNA) constructs provide resistance to plum pox virus in Nicotiana benthamiana and Prunus domestica. J Am Soc Hortic Sci 132: 850–858.
19. Wesley SV, Helliwell CA, Smith NA, Wang M, Rouse DT, et al. (2001) Construct design for efficient, effective and high-throughput gene silencing in plants. Plant J 27: 581–590.
20. Yang G (2013) MITE Digger, an efficient and accurate algorithm for genome wide discovery of miniature inverted repeat transposable elements. BMC Bioinformatics 14: 186.
21. Lu C, Chen J, Zhang Y, Hu Q, Su W, et al. (2011) Miniature Inverted-Repeat Transposable Elements (MITEs) Have Been Accumulated through Amplification Bursts and Play Important Roles in Gene Expression and Species Diversity in Oryza sativa. Mol Biol Evol 29: 1005–1017. doi:10.1093/molbev/msr282.
22. Lu L, Jia H, Dröge P, Li J (2007) The human genome-wide distribution of DNA palindromes. Funct Integr Genomics 7: 221–227. doi:10.1007/s10142-007-0047-6.
23. Humphrey-Dixon EL, Sharp R, Schuckers M, Lock R, Gulick P (2011) Comparative genome analysis suggests characteristics of yeast inverted repeats that are important for transcriptional activity. Genome 54: 934–942. doi:10.1139/g11-058.
24. Sreeskandarajan S, Flowers MM, Karro JE, Liang C (2013) A MATLAB-based tool for accurate detection of perfect overlapping and nested inverted repeats in DNA sequences. Bioinformatics. doi:10.1093/bioinformatics/btt651.
25. Rice P, Longden I, Bleasby A (2000) EMBOSS: the European molecular biology open software suite. Trends Genet 16: 276–277.
26. Gupta R, Mittal A, Gupta S (2006) An efficient algorithm to detect palindromes in DNA sequences using periodicity transform. Signal Process 86: 2067–2073. doi:10.1016/j.sigpro.2005.10.008.

$CD161^+$ MAIT Cells Are Severely Reduced in Peripheral Blood and Lymph Nodes of HIV-Infected Individuals Independently of Disease Progression

Johanna Maria Eberhard[1,4⁹], Philip Hartjen[1,2,4⁹], Silke Kummer[1,4], Reinhold E. Schmidt[5,8], Maximilian Bockhorn[3], Clara Lehmann[6], Ashwin Balagopal[7], Joachim Hauber[4,8], Jan van Lunzen[1,4,8*⁹], Julian Schulze zur Wiesch[1,4,8⁹]

1 Infectious Diseases Unit, Department of Medicine, University Medical Center Hamburg-Eppendorf, Hamburg, Germany, **2** Department of Oral and Maxillofacial Surgery, University Medical Center Hamburg-Eppendorf, Hamburg, Germany, **3** Department of General Surgery, University Medical Center Hamburg-Eppendorf, Hamburg, Germany, **4** Heinrich Pette Institute - Leibniz Institute for Experimental Virology, Hamburg, Germany, **5** Department of Immunology and Rheumatology, Hannover Medical School, Hanover, Germany, **6** Department of Internal Medicine I, University Hospital of Cologne, Cologne, Germany, **7** School of Medicine, Johns Hopkins University, Baltimore, Maryland, United States of America, **8** German Center for Infection Research (DZIF), partner site Hamburg and Hannover, Hamburg and Hannover, Germany

Abstract

Mucosal-associated invariant T (MAIT) cells are characterized by the combined expression of the semi-invariant T cell receptor (TCR) Vα7.2, the lectin receptor CD161, as well as IL-18R, and play an important role in antibacterial host defense of the gut. The current study characterized $CD161^+$ MAIT and $CD161^-TCRV\alpha 7.2^+$ T cell subsets within a large cohort of HIV patients with emphasis on patients with slow disease progression and elite controllers. Mononuclear cells from blood and lymph node samples as well as plasma from 63 patients and 26 healthy donors were analyzed by multicolor flow cytometry and ELISA for IL-18, sCD14 and sCD163. Additionally, MAIT cells were analyzed after *in vitro* stimulation with different cytokines and/or fixed *E.coli*. Reduced numbers of $CD161^+$ MAIT cells during HIV infection were detectable in the blood and lymph nodes of all patient groups, including elite controllers. $CD161^+$ MAIT cell numbers did not recover even after successful antiretroviral treatment. The loss of $CD161^+$ MAIT cells was correlated with higher levels of MAIT cell activation; an increased frequency of the $CD161^-TCRV\alpha 7.2^+$T cell subset in HIV infection was observed. *In vitro* stimulation of MAIT cells with IL-18 and IL-12, IL-7 and fixed *E.coli* also resulted in a rapid and additive reduction of the MAIT cell frequency defined by CD161, IL-18R and CCR6. In summary, the irreversible reduction of the $CD161^+$ MAIT cell subset seems to be an early event in HIV infection that is independent of later stages of the disease. This loss appears to be at least partially due to the distinctive vulnerability of MAIT cells to the pronounced stimulation by microbial products and cytokines during HIV-infection.

Editor: R. Keith Reeves, Beth Israel Deaconess Medical Center, Harvard Medical School, United States of America

Funding: This work was supported by the Werner Otto Stiftung, the German Research Agency (SFB841 project A6; JSzW), the DZIF (German Center for Infection Research; RES, JH, JvL, JSzW) and the ECHAM (European Cohort HIV Ageing and Metabolic liver disease; JvL, JME). The funders had no role in study design, data collection and analysis, decision to publish, or preparation of the manuscript.

Competing Interests: The authors have declared that no competing interests exist.

* Email: v.lunzen@uke.de

⁹ These authors contributed equally to this work.

Introduction

Chronic untreated HIV infection is characterized by general immune activation, immune dysregulation, high T cell turnover and a gradual decline of $CD4^+$ T cells through infection and bystander activation induced apoptotic death [1]. The translocation of microbial products from the gastrointestinal (GI) tract to portal and systemic circulation has been proposed as a major driver of the generalized chronic immune activation that is associated with HIV disease progression [2].

A recently described T cell subset with limited receptor diversity and high abundance in mucosal tissues has been shown to recognize microbial products. These cells, termed mucosal-associated invariant T (MAIT) cells, can be identified by the surface expression of CD161 and the invariant TCRVα7.2 segment [1]. In general, MAIT cell responses are restricted by the conserved MHC-related-molecule-1 (MR1) that presents riboflavin precursors derived from bacteria and yeasts predominantly in the gut [3]. The MAIT cell defining surface marker CD161 is a C-type lectin-like membrane receptor that can bind its ligand, the lectin-like transcript 1 (LLT1), with yet unclear function [4,5]. MAIT cells exhibit a tissue-targeting memory phenotype and express high levels of cytokine receptors for IL-18, IL-12 and IL-23 [4,6–8]. Moreover, MAIT cells exhibit specific effector activities such as TNF-α, IFN-γ, IL-17 production as well as granzyme B secretion [4,6,7].

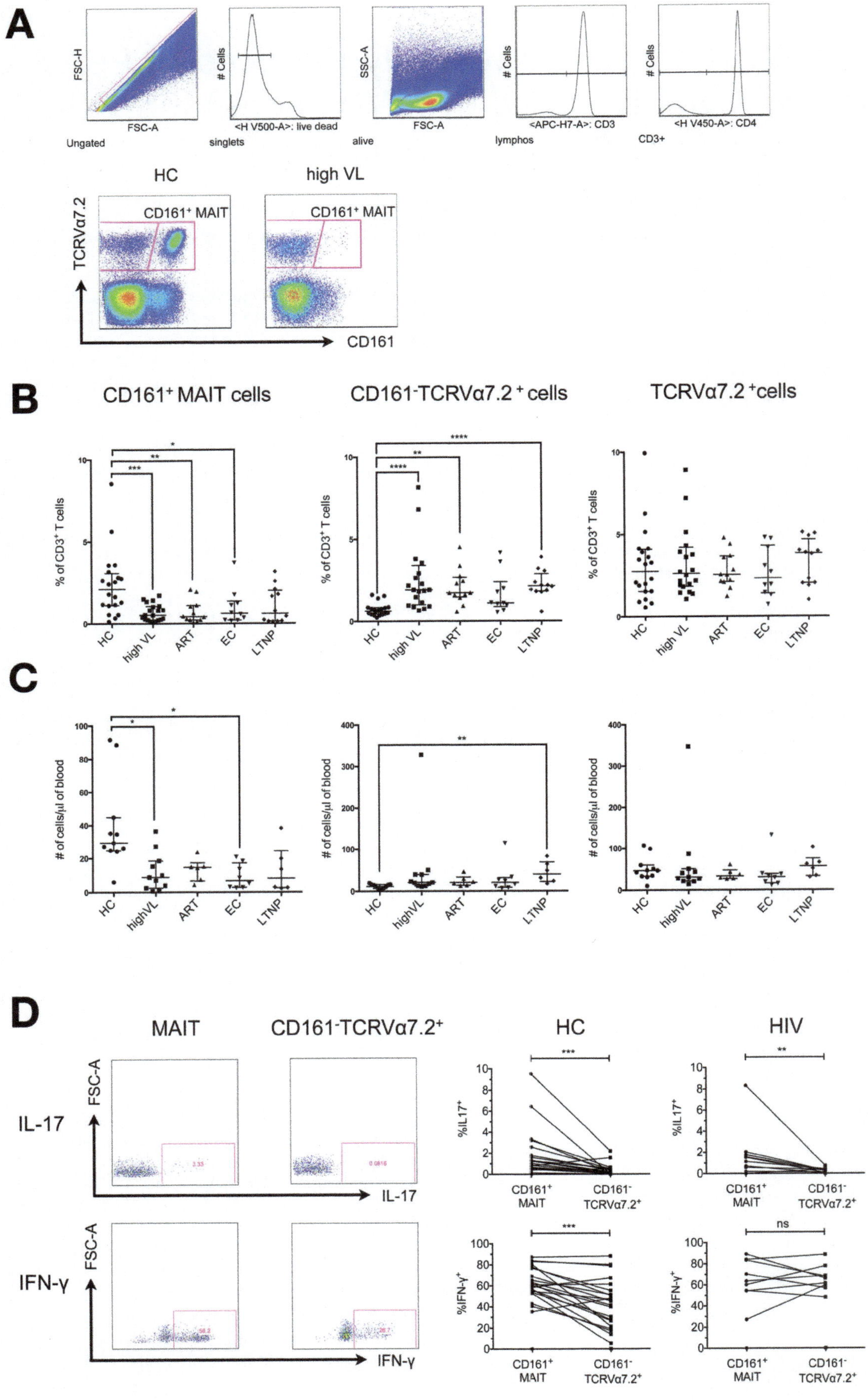
A
FSC-H
FSC-A
Ungated
Cells
<H V500-A>: live dead
singlets
SSC-A
FSC-A
alive
Cells
<APC-H7-A>: CD3
lymphos
Cells
<H V450-A>: CD4
CD3+
HC
high VL
CD161+ MAIT
CD161+ MAIT
TCRVα7.2
CD161
B
CD161+ MAIT cells
CD161-TCRVα7.2+ cells
TCRVα7.2+cells
% of CD3+ T cells
HC
high VL
ART
EC
LTNP
C
# of cells/µl of blood
HC
highVL
ART
EC
LTNP
D
MAIT
CD161-TCRVα7.2+
HC
HIV
IL-17
FSC-A
IL-17
IFN-γ
FSC-A
IFN-γ
%IL17+
%IFN-γ+
CD161+ MAIT
CD161- TCRVα7.2+
ns

Figure 1. CD161$^+$TCRVα7.2$^+$ MAIT cells are severely reduced in the blood of HIV-infected patients. A) Gating Strategy for CD161 and TCRVα7.2 based MAIT cell characterization in the CD4$^-$CD3$^+$T cell subset. All FACS analyses were performed on frozen PBMC samples. Depicted are representative plots from healthy control PBMCs (upper panel). Gating of the MAIT cell subsets comparing a healthy donor (HC) and an HIV patient (lower panel). **B)** Cumulative display of CD161$^+$TCRVα7.2$^+$ MAIT cell frequencies, CD161$^-$TCRVα7.2$^+$ and total TCRVα7.2$^+$ cells in % of CD3$^+$ T cells comparing PBMC samples derived from healthy controls (HC n = 20), untreated patients with high viral loads (high VL n = 20), patients receiving antiretroviral treatment for a at least one year (ART n = 12), elite controller (EC n = 10) and patients with very low viremia and slow progression (< 5000 copies/ml; LTNP n = 12). **C)** Absolute MAIT cell counts, CD161$^-$TCRVα7.2$^+$ and total TCRVα7.2$^+$ cells per µl peripheral blood, calculated based on absolute CD3$^+$ T cell counts (available for 12 HC, 11 high VL, 6 ART, 8 EC and 6 LTNP). All groups were tested for normal distribution with the Kolmogorov-Smirnov test and were compared by the adequate test, ANOVA followed by Tukey's multiple comparisons test or Kruskal-Wallis followed by multiple comparison test, respectively. P-values smaller than 0.05 were considered significant, where *, ** and *** indicate p-values between 0.01 to 0.05, 0.001 to 0.01 and 0.0001 to 0.001, respectively. Bars and lines indicate median, 25% and 75% quartiles. **D)** Representative FACS plots and the percentages of cells that produce the cytokines IL-17 and INF-γ upon stimulation with PMA/ionomycin among MAIT cells and CD161$^-$TCRVα7.2$^+$ cells are shown. PBMC samples derived from healthy donors (n = 22) and HIV-infected patients (ART treated and untreated with high viral loads, n = 10) were analyzed. Asterisks indicate the results of Wilcoxon matched-pairs signed-rank tests.

Recent reports describe a significant loss of CD161$^+$ MAIT cells from the circulation of HIV- infected patients [9–12]. It is thought that the decrease of these cells not only weakens the defense against bacterial pathogens like *Escherichia coli*, *Candida albicans* and *Mycobacterium tuberculosis* (MTB) [1–4], but could also further enhance the intestinal translocation of microbial products, which is related to the chronic activation and exhaustion of the immune system associated with HIV-infection [2,6,9,11,12]. However, the timing, kinetics and mechanisms behind the reduction of peripheral CD161$^+$ MAIT cells in patients with HIV-infection and different disease course has not been fully elucidated. On the one hand, activation induced cell death and accumulation in tissues could explain the severe reduction of MAIT cells. On the other hand a change of phenotype in terms of down-regulation of marker molecules such as CD161 following activation and exhaustion have been suggested as alternative explanation [5–7]. Limited data on the tissue distribution of MAIT cells are available so far, especially with regard to secondary lymphoid tissues. Furthermore, there are extant questions about the early kinetics of MAIT cells during acute infection, and whether patients who exhibit natural control of HIV have spared MAIT cells [8] [11]. In particular, the loss and exhaustion of MAIT cells could have important implications for the mucosal defense against bacterial pathogens in the gut of HIV-infected patients. Latest studies contradict earlier assumptions [9] and show that HIV elite controllers (EC) show activated innate immune responses in comparison to healthy controls despite controlling plasma HIV viremia [13–15]; therefore, these results are consistent with an impaired mucosal barrier.

In the current study, MAIT cells, defined as CD161$^+$ TCR Vα7.2$^+$ CD4$^-$ T cells as well as CD161$^-$TCR Vα7.2$^+$ CD4$^-$ T cells are characterized *ex vivo* and after *in vitro* stimulation in a large cohort of HIV patients with emphasis on patients with slow disease progression and elite controllers (EC). This study aimed to gain further insight into the kinetics as well as possible mechanisms of MAIT cell decline during HIV-infection including the important compartment of lymphoid tissue.

Results

CD161$^+$ MAIT cells are severely reduced in the blood and lymph nodes of HIV-infected patients independently of their disease status

The aim of this study was to comprehensively analyze MAIT cell subsets in the peripheral blood as well as in the lymph node compartment of a large cohort of patients with different HIV disease status.

We first determined the frequency of CD161$^+$ MAIT cells in the peripheral blood in a cohort of healthy, HIV-negative donors (Fig. 1). The vast majority of the CD3$^+$CD161$^+$TCRVα7.2$^+$ MAIT cell population (>90%) either expresses CD8$\alpha\alpha$ or CD8$\alpha\beta$, whereas a smaller subset (<10%) is CD8$^-$CD4$^-$ and only a negligible fraction of these cells expresses the CD4 molecule [10]. For simplicity and for better comparability with previous studies we defined MAIT cells as CD161$^+$TCRVα7.2$^+$CD4$^-$CD3$^+$ T cell population. This gating strategy allowed us to exclude the effect of general CD4$^+$ T cell depletion from the analysis. Our gating strategy is depicted in Fig. 1A. Healthy controls displayed a broad range of MAIT cell frequencies, quantified in two ways: i) as percentage of CD3$^+$ T cells (median = 2.1%, IQR = 1.12–3.06%) and ii) as percentage of CD4$^-$ T cells (mean = 8.12%, IQR = 5.6–12.25%; data not shown) (Fig. 1B). This was reflected in a pattern of similar variation of the absolute number of CD161$^+$ MAIT cells per µl of blood (Fig. 1C) and thus is not merely a consequence of varying parent population sizes. Our results are consistent with previous results from studies that determined MAIT cell frequencies in healthy subjects [5,11,12].

In accordance with previous studies [5–7,13] we observed a severe reduction of the peripheral CD161$^+$ MAIT cell subset of untreated and treated HIV-infected patients (median HC = 2.1%, IQR = 1.12–3.06% vs. median high VL = 0.52%, IQR = 0.22–1.06% and median ART = 0.42%, IQR = 0.22–1.1%, ANOVA followed by Tukey's multiple comparison test: $p<0.001$ and $p<0.01$, respectively) (Fig. 1B, C).

Importantly, we extended the results of the aforementioned studies by characterizing the frequency and function of MAIT cells in a group of elite controllers (n = 10) and long-term nonprogressors (n = 12) (Table 1) to answer the question whether spontaneous viral control or slower disease progression are associated with the preservation of peripheral MAIT cells. Throughout this study LTNPs were defined as: HIV Patients with low viremia (<5000 copies/ml) that maintain a favourable course of infection (CD4 counts>350 cells/µl) over 5 years in the absence of therapy.

Interestingly, we observed a reduction of the CD161$^+$ MAIT cell subset in both groups of patients (LTNP as well as EC) compared to healthy controls (median HC = 2.1%, IQR = 1.12–3.06% vs. median EC = 0.62%, IQR = 0.21–1.37% and median LTNP = 0.61, IQR = 0.14–2.0%) (Fig. 1B). This reduction was slightly less pronounced in EC and not statistically significant for LTNP (ANOVA followed by Tukey's multiple comparison test: $p<0.05$ for EC).

In previously published studies, it has been hypothesized that the disappearance of MAIT cells from the peripheral blood in chronic HIV infection might be best explained by a combination of activation induced cell death and/or homing of MAIT cells to different tissues and the gut [7]. Thus, in order to advance the understanding of possible tissue redistributions of MAIT cells in the course of the HIV infection, we extended our analysis by

Table 1. Cohort (PBMC samples).

	Healthy	high VL	ART	EC	LTNP
number of donors	20	21	12	10	12
% female	53.3	29.4	36.4	57.1	40
age [years]	39.2(±11.2)	39.9(±11.7)	48.9(±16)	46(±11.6)	43.92(±15.3)
time since first diagnosis [month]	-	51.2(±71.6)	101.2(±58.5)	150.5(±69.9)	106.8(±67.1)
viral load [copies/ml]	-	1580000(±3080000)	10 of 12: below detection limit; 2 of 12: <200	below detection limit	986.1 (±1655)
CD4 [c/µl]	798.2(±308.8)	243.6(±289.1)	627.5(±363.1)	780.7(±284.7)	591.8(±176.8)
CD8 [c/µl]	439(±154.1)	951.4(±980.8)	844.3(±266.7)	686.4(±305.9)	1217(±480.9)
CD3 [c/µl]	1323(±418.8)	1594(±1471)	1475(±536.2)	1487(±588.1)	2140(±722.5)
lymphocytes [c/µl]	1785(±527.7)	1613(±1325)	1997(±627.5)	2014(±712.5)	2386(±770)

Shown are means and standard deviation.

inclusion of lymph nodal MAIT cells. As natural killer T cells MAIT cells might have an important role in B cell help [14–16]. Previously, high expression of CCR6 and low expression of CCR7 have been observed on MAIT cells, indicating that these cells are mainly tissue circulating T cells [17].

We also found that lymph node samples of healthy controls and HIV patients (Table 2) generally showed a significantly lower frequency of MAIT cells compared to PBMC of unpaired samples of the same groups ($p<0.01$ in HC and $p<0.0001$ in HIV patients, Mann-Whitney tests), while the frequencies of $CD161^-TCRV\alpha7.2^+$ T cells were not significantly different between the two compartments (Fig. 2A, B). However, analogous to the results obtained for the peripheral blood we observed a further reduction of the lymph nodal $CD161^+$ MAIT cell frequency in HIV-infected patients to a significantly lower median of 0.06% (IQR = 0.04–0.2%, $p = 0.03$) in comparison to healthy controls (Fig. 2). A similar reduction of the $CD161^+$ MAIT frequency was detectable in all LNMC samples of HIV-infected patients regardless of their treatment status (LNMC from 5 untreated and 6 ART-treated patients were included in our analysis). However, it has to be noted that our analysis was limited by the fact that no paired blood - lymph node samples from the same donors were available.

The frequency of the $CD161^-CD4^-$ T cell subset that expressed $TCRV\alpha7.2^+$ but no other MAIT cell-defining markers (e.g. CD161, hence termed: $CD161^-TCRV\alpha7.2^+$ subset), was increased in viremic HIV patients, patients receiving ART and in LTNP (median HC = 0.62%, IQR = 0.44–0.83% vs. median high VL = 1.9%, IQR = 1.0–3.4%, median ART = 1.72%, IQR = 1.46–2.65% and median LTNP = 1.14% IQR = 0.31–4.6%; Kruskal-Wallis test followed by Dunn's multiple comparisons test: $p<0.0001$, $p<0.01$ and $p<0.0001$, respectively) (Fig. 1B middle panel). In the resting state this cell population consists most likely of regular T cells using this Vα chain but their increase in HIV-infected patients might reflect an activation-induced down-regulation of CD161 on the MAIT cell population [13], which was supported by the stable frequency of $TCRV\alpha7.2^+$ T cells within the $CD3^+$ T cell pool (Fig. 1B, right panel). However, only few untreated highly viremic patients showed very high levels of $CD161^-TCRV\alpha7.2^+CD4^-$ T cells. A closer analysis revealed that five of these patients were recently diagnosed as HIV positive and at least three of these patients had a documented primary infection with definite seroconversion (<1 month) (Fig. S1A). For these patients, we used the time since HIV diagnosis as a crude measure for the time of infection (Fig. S1B) as previously described [6]. Therefore, it is intriguing to speculate whether this expansion of the $CD161^-TCRV\alpha7.2^+CD4^-$ T cell subset might be an effect of CD161 down-regulation on former $CD161^+$ MAIT cells, taking place during early stages of infection. While in general, there was a great variation between individual subjects in the frequency of MAIT cells and $CD161^-$ cells in healthy donors as well as in HIV patients, in HIV patients the MAIT/$CD161^-TCRV\alpha7.2^+$ cell ratio was shifted towards the (expanded) $CD161^-TCRV\alpha7.2^+$ portion (Fig. S1). Of note, in lymph nodes we detected a similar shift of this $CD161^+$ MAIT/$CD161^-TCRV\alpha7.2^+$ cell ratio in HIV-infected patients (Fig. 2).

Functional characterization of $CD161^+$ MAIT cells versus $CD161^-TCRV\alpha7.2^+$ cells

MAIT cells are believed to operate by secreting effector cytokines such as TNF-α, IFN-γ as well as IL-17 and IL-22 [1]. In order to assess possible functional impairments of MAIT cells in HIV-infection, we next wanted to explore, whether $CD161^+$ MAIT cells and $CD161^-TCRV\alpha7.2^+CD4^-$ T cells of HIV-infected patients differ in their cytokine secretion profile after unspecific stimulation. Thus, we carried out intracellular cytokine staining assays with PMA/ionomycin-stimulated PBMCs of both groups. Upon PMA/ionomycin-stimulation $CD161^+$ MAIT cells produced slightly more IL-17 ($p<0.001$ and <0.01, for HC and HIV patients respectively) and IFN-γ ($p<0.001$ for HC, no significant difference in HIV patients) as compared to their $CD161^-TCRV\alpha7.2^+$ counterparts (Fig. 1D). This finding is in line with previous results [8] and suggests that both T cell subsets are functionally different, and that $CD161^-TCRV\alpha7.2^+$ cells are less capable to fulfill Tc17 functionality than $CD161^+$ MAIT cells in HIV-infected patients.

Frequencies of activated $CD161^+$ MAIT cells and $CD161^-TCRV\alpha7.2^+$ cells are elevated in the blood of highly viremic HIV patients

In accordance with previous reports [18,19] we observed elevated levels of the soluble activation marker sCD163, a monocyte- and macrophage-specific scavenger receptor, shed during activation, in the plasma of untreated patients (Fig. 3A). A similar trend was observed for levels of sCD14, a marker of monocyte response to LPS [20]. However, this trend did not reach

Table 2. Cohort (LNMC samples).

	Healthy	HIV+(high VL and ART)
number of donors	6	11
age [years]	55 (±16)	44 (±15)
viral load [copies/ml]	-	42516 (±58152)

Shown are means and standard deviation.

statistical significance and was not directly correlated to MAIT cell frequencies (Fig. 3A and data not shown).

In addition to the expression of CD161, MAIT cells are defined by the expression of IL-18R [1]. Therefore, we hypothesized that circulating IL-18 in HIV-infected patients might lead to down-regulation of this receptor as well as to a strong stimulation of these cells. Indeed, IL-18, which is produced by macrophages, dendritic cells and enterocytes, was slightly elevated - though not statistically significant - in the plasma of untreated HIV patients of our cohort when measured in a standard ELISA assay (median high VL = 683.4 pg/ml, IQR = 445.4–1087 pg/ml vs. median HC = 523.4 pg/ml, IQR = 134.2–631 pg/ml) (Fig. 3A). Our results are in line with previous studies that showed that IL-18 is elevated during primary and chronic HIV-infection [21,22].

We next tested the hypothesis whether potent activation of the CD161$^+$ MAIT cell subset could indeed be a possible driving force

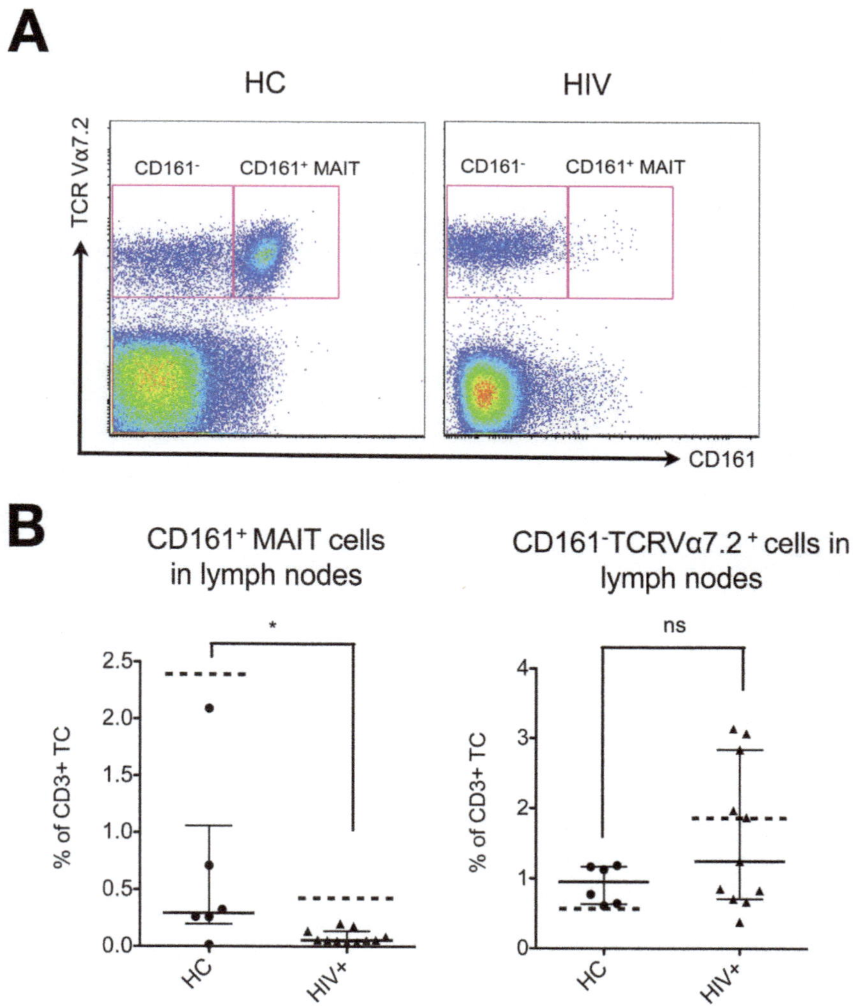

Figure 2. The frequency of CD161$^+$ MAIT cells is severely reduced in lymph nodes of HIV-infected patients. A) Gating strategy for the characterization of MAIT cells and CD161$^-$TCRVα7.2$^+$ cells within the CD4$^-$ T cell subset of lymph node mononuclear cells (LNMC). Representative FACS plots for LNMC from a healthy control and an HIV-infected patient are shown. **B**) Frequencies of CD161$^+$ MAIT cells and CD161$^-$TCRVα7.2$^+$ cells as percentages among CD3$^+$ lymphocytes for LNMC samples derived from healthy controls (healthy, n = 6) and HIV-infected patients (HIV, n = 11). Bars and lines indicate median and interquartile range. Dotted lines indicate the frequencies in the PBMC compartment of unmatched but similar groups for comparison. P-values are results of unpaired Mann-Whitney tests.

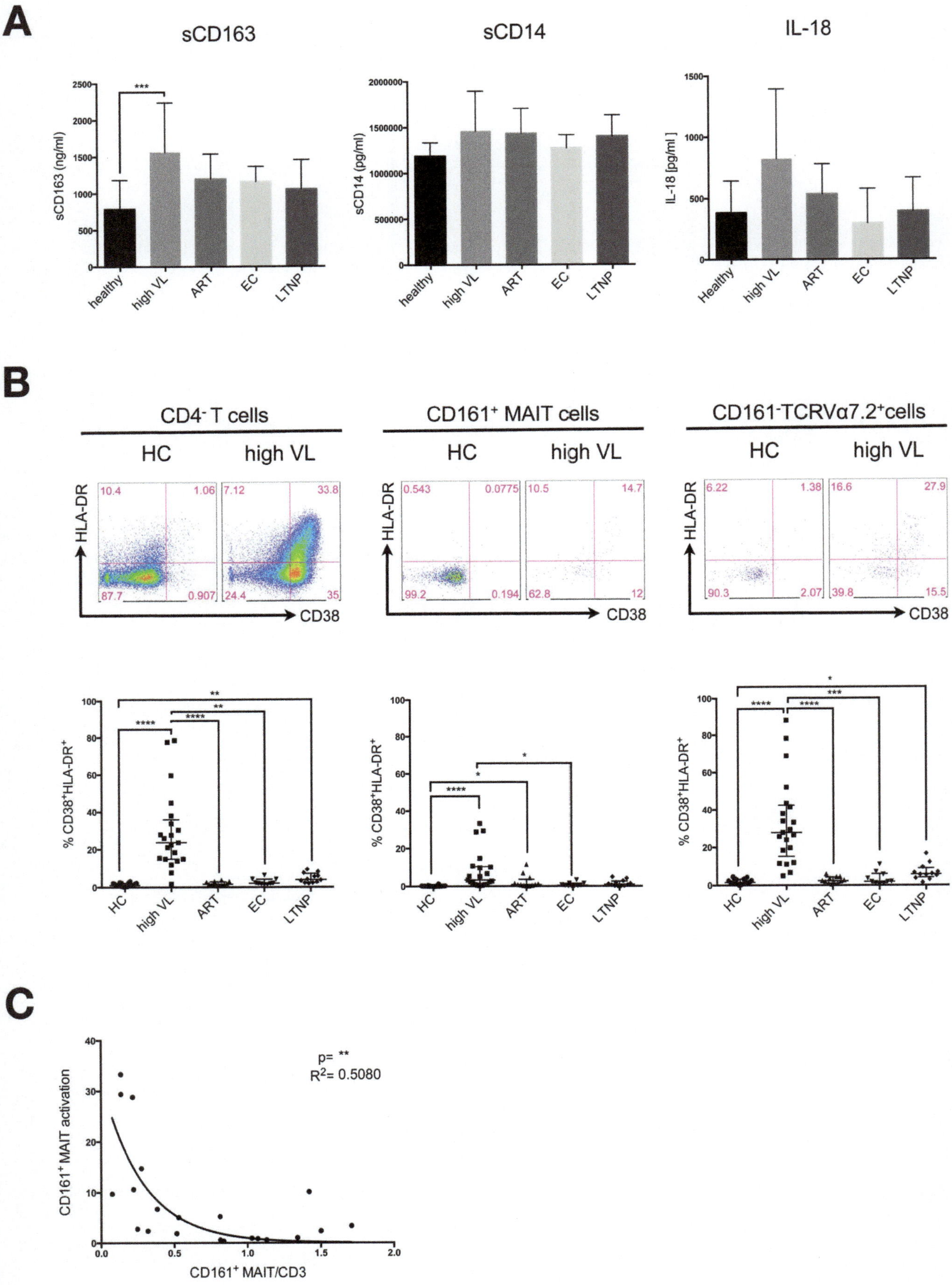
A
sCD163
sCD14
IL-18
sCD163 (ng/ml)
sCD14 (pg/ml)
IL-18 [pg/ml]
healthy
high VL
ART
EC
LTNP
Healthy
B
CD4- T cells
CD161+ MAIT cells
CD161-TCRVα7.2+cells
HC
high VL
HLA-DR
CD38
10.4
1.06
7.12
33.8
87.7
0.907
24.4
35
0.543
0.0775
10.5
14.7
99.2
0.194
62.8
12
6.22
1.38
16.6
27.9
90.3
2.07
39.8
15.5
% CD38+HLA-DR+
C
CD161+ MAIT activation
CD161+ MAIT/CD3
p= **
R2= 0.5080

Figure 3. Frequencies of activated CD161$^+$ and CD161$^-$ TCR Vα7.2$^+$ cells are elevated in the blood of highly viremic HIV patients. A) Plasma levels of sCD163, sCD14 and IL-18 were measured by ELISA in mostly corresponding samples of healthy controls (HC n = 13), highly viremic HIV-infected patients (high VL n = 18), patients receiving ART (ART n = 17), elite controllers (EC n = 6) and long-term nonprogressors (LTNP n = 6). B) Activated cells were defined as CD38$^+$ and HLA-DR$^+$ double positive cells and their frequency was assessed within the CD4$^-$, MAIT and CD161$^-$TCRVα7.2$^+$ populations. PBMC samples were derived from healthy controls (HC), highly viremic HIV-infected patients (high VL), patients receiving ART (ART), elite controllers (EC) and long-term nonprogressors (LTNP). Groups were compared by Kruskal-Wallis test followed by Dunn's multiple comparison test. P-values smaller than 0.05 were considered significant, where *, ** and *** indicate p-values between 0.01 to 0.05, 0.001 to 0.01 and 0.0001 to 0.001 respectively. Bars and lines indicate mean and standard deviation. C) Pearson correlation analysis of CD161$^+$ MAIT cell activation and CD161$^+$ MAIT cell frequency of CD3$^+$ T cells from the untreated high VL patient group. R^2 quantifies goodness of fit to the non-linear regression (exponential grow equation). R^2 is a fraction between 0.0 and 1.0, with 1.0 indicating the best fit.

for MAIT cell depletion. We therefore determined expression of the activation markers HLA-DR and CD38 on the CD161$^+$ MAIT cell subset and their parent population (CD4$^-$CD3$^+$T cells) as well as on the CD161$^-$TCRVα7.2$^+$ cells (Fig. 3B). The frequency of activated cells within the CD161$^+$ MAIT cell subset was significantly elevated in patients with untreated HIV infection and high viral load and slightly in patients receiving ART (median HC = 0.15%, IQR = 0.06–0.28% vs. median high VL = 3.31%, IQR = 0.94–10.35% and median ART = 0.83%, IQR = 0.33–3.63%, Kruskal-Wallis test followed by Dunn's multiple comparisons test: $p<0.0001$ and $p<0.05$, respectively). In fact, the activation level of MAIT cells from elite controllers was also significantly lower compared to highly viremic patients (median EC = 0.39%, IQR = 0.12–1.45%; $p<0.05$).

The CD4$^-$ parent population also showed a very high level of activation in viremic patients in comparison to all other patient groups, which indicates that this activation is part of the general immune activation observed in HIV infection and is not specific for the CD161$^+$ MAIT cell population (Fig. 3B). However, co-expression of CD38 and HLA-DR on the CD161$^+$ MAIT cell subset itself was inversely correlated to the CD161$^+$ MAIT cell frequency (Fig. 3C), indicating that at least an indirect effect of activation (for example at early stages of infection) is likely to be associated with the reduction of the CD161$^+$ MAIT cell subset.

In vitro stimulation of MAIT cells leads to activation and a reduced CD161$^+$ MAIT cell frequency

To determine possible factors that might contribute to the reduction of the CD161$^+$ MAIT cell population in HIV-infection on the one hand or possibly could lead to proliferation on the other hand, we tested the effect of cytokines (i.e. cytokines for which MAIT cells highly express the respective receptor) on CD161$^+$ MAIT cells. Moreover, the hypothesis of microbial translocation as a driving force for MAIT cell reduction in HIV was tested by adding fixed *E.coli* in a bacteria per cell ratio of 100:1 to the *in vitro* culture. In an *in vitro* experiment, PBMCs from healthy donors were stimulated with IL-12, IL-18, IL-7, fixed *E.coli* alone or in combination to elucidate the effect on MAIT cell activation (Fig. 4A, B). No significant alteration in the level of activation or frequency of the CD161$^+$ MAIT cell population was observed with addition of IL-12 or IL-18 alone (Fig. 4A, B). Combined stimulation with IL-12 and IL-18 in contrast led to potent activation of the MAIT cell subset as measured by CD69 expression (unstimulated cells mean = 2.98±1.16% vs. IL-12+IL-18 mean = 53.88±27.04%) accompanied by a slight reduction of the MAIT cell frequency among CD3$^+$ T cells, reflecting synergistic effects of IL-18 and IL-12 (Fig. 4A, B). The reduction of the MAIT cell frequency was confirmed using IL18R or CCR6 expression in addition to CD161 expression as alternative MAIT cell characterization (Fig. S4).

Since IL-7 has been described to be significantly elevated in untreated HIV-Infection [22] and a previous report described IL-7 to be an important cytokine to license MAIT cell effector function [23], the effect of exogenous IL-7 for MAIT cell activation was also tested. In our hands, *in vitro* addition of this cytokine indeed led to the activation of almost the entire CD161$^+$ MAIT cell subset. However, this activation was accompanied by a sharp drop of the CD161$^+$ MAIT cell frequency (Fig. 4A, B).

Addition of fixed *E. coli* also resulted in pronounced CD161$^+$ MAIT cell activation (blank mean = 2.98±1.16% vs. *E. coli* mean = 75.95±14.50%), TCRVα7.2 down-regulation and significant reduction of this cell subset (blank normalized to 1 vs. *E.coli* mean = 0.17±0.15) (Fig. 4A, B).

These results support the hypothesis that the translocation of bacteria and their products as well as consecutively produced pro-inflammatory cytokines (e.g. IL-12, IL-18) contribute to CD161$^+$ MAIT cell over-activation and, in turn to their quantitative reduction in HIV-infected patients [7]. Our results are also in line with a recent report that demonstrated that CD161$^+$ MAIT cells can be stimulated in an TCR independent manner by the cytokines IL-12 and IL-18 [24].

Material and Methods

Study subjects and samples

PBMC as well as lymph node mononuclear cells (derived from hilar and axillary lymph nodes) of in total 63 HIV patients were collected at the University Medical Center Hamburg-Eppendorf and Hannover Medical School, Germany. Healthy individuals (PBMC n = 20, LNMC n = 6) served as controls and for validation of the immunological tests. Written informed consent was obtained from all patients enrolled in this study, which was approved by the Ethics Committee of the Medical Association of Hamburg. The HIV long-term nonprogressor and elite controller cohorts consisted of HIV-infected subjects selected according to viral load, CD4 count, time and duration of HIV infection. The definition of the different stages of the disease were extracted from the electronic databases of the participating centers and confirmed by the treating physicians according to standard classifications and by criteria commonly used in the literature [25,26]. HIV-1 viral load was determined using COBAS amplicor assays with a detection limit of 50 RNA copies/ml. HIV CDC status, antiretroviral treatment, and CD4$^+$ T cell counts were determined via chart review.

Immunophenotypic analysis

For immunophenotypic staining, cryopreserved PBMC or LNMC were thawed using standardized techniques. For exclusion of dead cells PBMCs were stained with the LIVE/DEAD Fixable Aqua Dead Cell Stain Kit (life technologies, Darmstadt, Germany) according to the manufacturer's protocol. To characterize T cell populations, at least 5×10^5 cells were stained with appropriate fluorochrome-conjugated surface antibodies, including anti-CD3 (SK7), anti-CD4 (RPAT4), anti-CD8α (HIT8a), anti-TCRVα7.2 (3C10), anti-CD161 (HP-3G10), anti-HLA-DR (G46-6), anti-CD38 (HIT2, Biolegend), anti-IL-18R (H44), anti-CD69 (FN50),

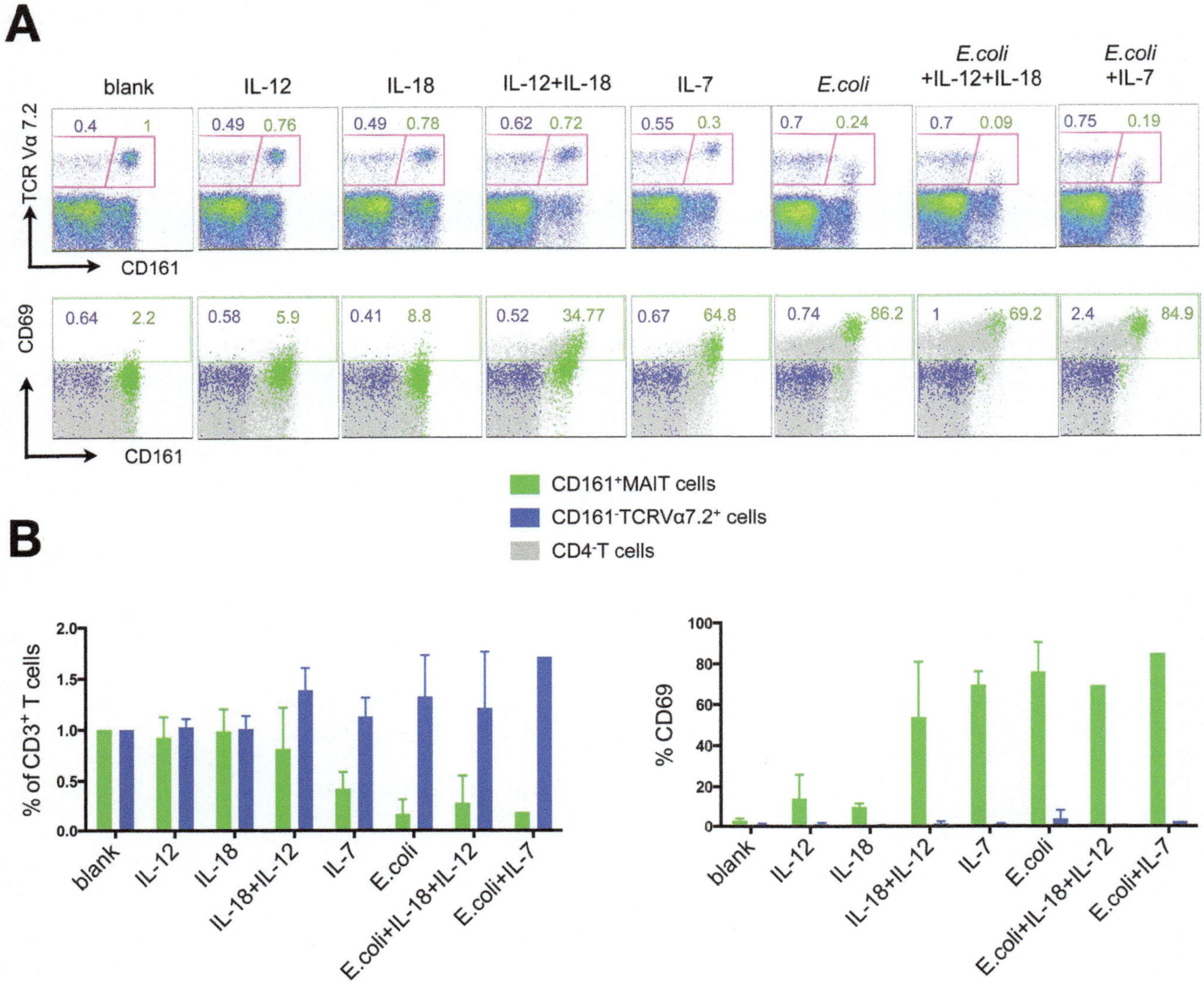

Figure 4. Frequencies of CD161$^+$ MAIT cells are reduced upon *in vitro* stimulation with PFA fixed *E.coli*, IL-7 and combined IL-12 and IL-18. A) Representative FACS plots depicting frequencies of CD161$^-$TCRVα7.2$^+$ cells, CD161$^+$ MAIT cells and all TCRVα7.2$^+$ cells as frequencies of CD3$^+$ T cells after 28 hours of stimulation with IL-12 (100 µg/ml), IL-18 (100 µg/ml) and their combination, IL-7 (100 µg/ml) and PFA fixed *E. coli* (bacteria per cell ratio of 100:1 PBMC). PBMCs were healthy donor-derived and seeded in 1×10^6 cells/well. **B**) Cumulative display of normalized frequencies of CD161$^+$ MAIT cells and CD161$^-$TCRVα7.2$^+$ cells from 3 healthy donors in duplicate measurements for each stimulation setting (apart from *E.coli* in combination with cytokines, which was tested once) measured after 28 hours of stimulation (left panel). Activation levels were assessed by determining the percentage of CD69$^+$ cells within the CD161$^+$ MAIT cell and the CD161$^-$TCRVα7.2$^+$ population.

anti-CCR6 (G034E3) (from Biolegend or BD Biosciences, Heidelberg, Germany) for 20 min at RT in the dark. After surface staining, cells were washed once with PBS and were then resuspended in 0.5% paraformaldehyde. For intracellular cytokine staining, the cells were stimulated with PMA (50 ng/ml) and ionomycin (0.67 µM) for 5 h at 37°C and 5% CO_2 prior to immunophenotypic staining. Brefeldin A (10 g/ml) was added for the last 4 h of the stimulation. Data were collected on a BD LSRII machine using FACS Diva version 5 (BD Biosciences, Heidelberg, Germany).

ELISA of plasma sCD163, sCD14 and IL-18

sCD163 levels in plasma were measured using the Macro163 ELISA kit (Trillium Diagnostics, Bangos, ME). sCD14 levels in plasma were measured using the Human sCD14 Quantikine ELISA kit (R&D Systems, Minneapolis, MN). Plasma levels of IL-18 were measured using the Human IL-18 Platinum ELISA kit (eBioscience, Germany).

Stimulation of PBMCs with cytokines and fixed *E. coli*

PBMCs from healthy donors were freshly isolated and seeded into a 48 well plate (1×10^6 cells/well). IL-12, IL-18 and IL-7 were added with an end concentration of 100 ng/ml. Prior to an experiment, aliquots of 1×10^9 *E.coli* (DH5α)/ml were fixed for 5 min in 1% paraformaldehyde and stored at −80°C. After thawing and washing, *E. coli* was added in a bacteria/cell ratio of 100:1. The PBMCs were stimulated for either 14 or 28 h before surface staining and FACS analysis.

Statistical analysis

All flow cytometric data were analyzed using FlowJo version 9.2 software (Treestar). Statistical analysis was carried out using Prism

5.0 software (GraphPad Software, San Diego, CA). All groups were tested for normal distribution with the Kolmogorov-Smirnov test and were compared by the adequate test. For normally distributed data, parametric tests were applied: for two groups t-tests, for more than two groups ANOVA followed by Tukey's multiple comparisons test. Data that was not normally distributed was tested by the Mann-Whitney test for two unpaired groups, by the Wilcoxon test for paired groups, or Kruskal-Wallis test followed by Dunn's multiple comparisons test for more then two groups, respectively. P-values smaller than 0.05 were considered significant, where *, ** and *** indicate p-values between 0.01 to 0.05, 0.001 to 0.01 and 0.0001 to 0.001, respectively. Pearson's correlation was applied for bivariate correlation analyses. Data are expressed as median, 25% and 75% quartiles or means with standard deviation, respectively (as indicated in the figure legend). $CD161^+$ MAIT cell frequencies were normalized for the *in vitro* stimulation data.

Discussion

Only in the last couple of years the important role of $CD161^+TCRV\alpha7.2^+CD4^-CD3^+$ MAIT cells in the defense of different bacterial (and indirectly in viral) infections has become clear [1,2,6,12,24,27–29]. While great progress has been made in characterizing the phenotypic and functional properties of MAIT cells [1,4,23,24,30–33], many details of MAIT cell function still have to be elucidated.

The current study adds further detail to the recent body of data suggesting diminishing function and decreasing numbers of MAIT cells in HIV infection [5–7]. In particular, frequency and phenotype of MAIT cells during HIV infection with regards to disease status, including HIV LTNP and elite controllers, were analyzed in detail. In accordance with data from a recent study [6] we confirm an irreversible reduction of the $CD161^+$ MAIT cell population in peripheral and lymph nodal tissue of patients with treated and untreated chronic HIV infection. However, while the preliminary results of the study by Leeansyah and coworkers [6] suggests that elite controllers maintain a similar size of their MAIT cell population as healthy controls, we found a significantly reduced MAIT cell frequency, as well as reduced MAIT cell numbers in the ten elite controller patients and a similar trend in twelve long-term nonprogressors included in the present study. These data are potentially of clinical importance and further studies have to elucidate whether the higher general immune activation detected in elite controllers in comparison to healthy controls is in parts due to a lower level of MAIT cells in these patients [34–36].

In functional *in vitro* experiments (Fig. 4) we were able to replicate the proposed model of a constitutive down-regulation of functional MAIT cell markers (i.e. CD161, IL-18R, CCR6) and eventual loss of $TCRV\alpha7.2^+CD4^-CD3^+$ T cells by stimulation with bacterial antigens and pro-inflammatory cytokines in HIV infection [7]. Importantly, we and others found that inflammatory cytokines like IL-12 or IL-18 can activate MAIT cells in a TCR independent manner [24,37]. It is not quite clear in how far the *in vitro* conditions replicate the *in vivo* milieu, but significant shifts towards inflammatory cytokines have been described and it has been proposed that these cytokines add to the pathogenesis of HIV infection [21,22].

Clearly, the current study is limited by the fact that no mucosal tissue was available for any of the patients studied and homing of the MAIT cell population to the gut might be in part responsible for the decrease of the peripheral MAIT cell frequencies. However, two independent studies previously showed a loss of mucosal gut resident MAIT cells in HIV-infected patients [5,6]. In preliminary experiments, we also see high expression of the gut-homing markers CCR9 and beta7 integrin [38] on MAIT cells in the jejunum of healthy controls (data not shown) and up-regulation of CCR9 and beta7 integrin was detected in peripheral MAIT cells in HIV patients (Fig. S3). The frequency of $CCR9^+\beta7^+$ integrin on MAIT cells was inversely correlated with the frequency of MAIT cells supporting the model of partial homing of MAIT cells to the gut in HIV infection [5]. In future prospective efforts it is planned to analyze the gut resident MAIT cell frequencies in HIV patients with different disease course, including HIV elite controllers obtained during routine screening colonoscopies.

In the present study, we also looked at a small number of patients with a recent history of acute retroviral syndrome, early primary HIV infection and/or confirmed recent seroconversion. In line with the results of the recently published studies [5–7], our data indicate that the decrease of peripheral $CD161^+$ MAIT cell numbers seems to be an early event in HIV infection. However, very early in the course of the primary infection we find a relative increase of the $CD161^-$ $TCRV\alpha7.2^+CD4^-CD3^+$ T cell subset suggestive of a down-regulation of CD161 on these cells. This elevation can still be detected at later stages and in different patient groups (Fig. 1B, middle panel). These $CD161^-TCRV\alpha7.2^+CD4^-CD3^+$ T cells were also recently described [5] and appear to have a larger proportion of cells with a similar TCRVβ usage as seen in MAIT cells in HIV-infected patients. In our hands, these highly activated $CD161^-TCRV\alpha7.2^+CD4^-CD3^+$ T cells rapidly develop after *in vitro* stimulation of $CD161^+$ MAIT cells and seem to be less functional *ex vivo* than their $CD161^+$ MAIT cell counterparts (Fig. 1D). In one patient who is included in our study and was treated during early primary infection, the MAIT cell frequency indeed recovered (Fig. S2). In a next step, further prospective clinical studies of patients with primary HIV infection have to establish whether very early initiation of ART can indeed "rescue" the MAIT cell population [39,40].

In ongoing experiments we are now characterizing the transcription factor expression profile (RORγt, Tbet, Gata3, PLZF) of $CD161^+$ MAIT cells versus $CD161^-$ $TCRV\alpha7.2^+CD4^-CD3^+$ T cells in uninfected donors as well as HIV-infected patients in order to explain some of the detected results of this study and to further discriminate relevant MAIT cell subpopulations [14,32,41–43]. For example the ability to secrete IL-17 could well be correlated with expression of the transcription factor RORγt [41]. Of importance, recent studies suggest that iNKT cells and MAIT cells exhibit a proapoptotic propensity with elevated expression of activated caspases, which is correlated with expression of transcription factor PLZF/ZBTB-16 [32]. This would make the loss of MAIT cells due to activation-induced cell death in HIV even more plausible. Also, the manipulation of these transcription factors represents an intriguing target for future therapeutic approaches [44]. The proof of "successful genetic manipulation and reprogramming to pluripotency and re-differentiation of functional MAIT cells" opens at least theoretically further therapeutic options [44,45]. In our hands, it was difficult to culture and expand primary MAIT cells *in vitro* and novel *in vitro* MAIT cell expansion protocols should be developed.

For the time being, it will be important to prospectively examine patients at the first stages of acute HIV infection to understand the exact kinetics of the MAIT cell loss and whether very early initiation of ART during primary HIV infection can indeed rescue the MAIT cell population and thereby possibly minimize subsequent microbial translocation [40]. Other theoretical therapeutic options include the immunomodulatory blockade of circulating cytokines (eg. IL-18) or the use of probiotics to stimulate MAIT cell regeneration and proliferation by activation of the commensal bacterial flora [2,46]. In a next step, the MAIT cell frequency and function have to be comprehensively examined in different tissues, e.g. lung tissue (via BAL) [28,47] or the liver [23] of HIV-infected patients (including elite controllers) in comparison to uninfected controls and, importantly, in HIV/TB or HIV/HCV coinfection [47]. Further studies should also comprehensively look at the different immune cell populations with antibacterial activity (e.g. $\gamma\delta$ T cells, NKT cells or innate lymphoid cells [48,49]) as other cells might compensate the loss of the MAIT cell population. For example, we find a relative expansion of $\gamma\delta$ T cell subsets in HIV infection ([49] and data not shown). Further analysis of MAIT cells might be assisted by the use of MAIT cell tetramer technology [31]. It will also be interesting to see whether the riboflavin metabolites are in itself more reliable and stable markers for bacterial translocation than LPS [30].

In summary, the current study confirms and extends previous studies and suggests that an irreversible reduction of the peripheral $CD161^+$ MAIT as well as an expansion of the $CD161^-TCR V\alpha7.2^+$ subset are early events in HIV infection [5–7,24,47]. The loss is most likely caused by a combination of increased homing to the gut as well as a lacking resistance towards stimulation by microbial products and cytokines leading to a) a change of phenotype, b) loss of function and c) possibly cell death, which takes place in all patients including HIV long-term nonprogressors and elite controllers independently of disease progression.

Supporting Information

Figure S1 The $CD161^+$ MAIT/$CD161^-TCRV\alpha^+$ ratio is shifted in HIV infection. A) Bars indicate each individual's frequency of $CD161^+$ MAIT cells (light grey) and $CD161^-TCRV\alpha^+$ cells (dark grey). Patients with confirmed or suspected acute HIV-infection ($n = 5$) below 1 month post first diagnosis are marked in red. **B**) Comparison of $CD4^+T$ cell frequencies (grey), $CD161^-TCRV\alpha7.2^+$ cell frequencies (blue), $CD161^+$ MAIT cell frequencies (green) of high VL patients below 1 month vs. above 1 month of known HIV-infection. The indicated p-value results from a Mann Whitney test. P-values smaller than 0.05 were considered significant.

Figure S2 Longitudinal $CD161^+$ MAIT cell increase in a patient after early treatment initiation. FACS plots depicting frequencies of $CD161^+$ MAIT (upper right number in green) and $CD161^-TCRV\alpha^+$ cells of the $CD4^-$ T cell population (upper left number in blue) of a patient during acute HIV-infection (Fiebig stage III: ELISA +, Immunoblot -) and 28 month later after immediate initiation of ART.

Figure S3 Migration to the gut is specifically elevated in the $CD161^+$ MAIT cell population. Migrating cells are measured by frequencies of $CCR9^+\beta7integrin^+$ double positive cells of $CD161^+$ MAIT cells and $CD161^-TCRV\alpha7.2^+$ cells, respectively. PBMC samples were derived from healthy controls, highly viremic HIV-infected patients and patients under ART. **A**) Groups were tested for normal distribution by Kolmogorov-Smirnov test and compared by Kruskal-Wallis test followed by Dunn's multiple comparisons test. P-values smaller than 0.05 were considered significant, where *, ** and *** indicate p-values between 0.01 to 0.05, 0.001 to 0.01 and 0.0001 to 0.001 respectively. Bars and lines indicate median and interquartile ranges. **B**) Correlation analysis of $CD161^+$ MAIT cell frequency or $CD161^-TCRV\alpha7.2^+$ cell frequency with the corresponding frequency of $CCR9^+/\beta7^+$ $CD161^+$MAIT cells. R^2 is a fraction between 0.0 and 1.0, with 1.0 indicating the best fit to the linear regression.

Figure S4 The MAIT cell defining markers CD161, IL18R and CCR6 are reduced within the $TCRV\alpha7.2^+$ subset upon stimulation with IL-12 and IL-18, IL-7 and *E.coli*. A) Representative FACS plots depicting frequencies of $CD161^-TCRV\alpha7.2^+$ cells, $CD161^+$ MAIT cells and all $TCRV\alpha7.2^+$ cells as frequencies of $CD3^+$ T cells after 28 hours of stimulation with IL-12 (100 µg/ml), IL-18 (100 µg/ml) and their combination, IL-7 (100 µg/ml) and PFA fixed *E. coli* (bacteria per cell ratio of 100:1 PBMC). PBMCs were healthy donor-derived and seeded in 1×10^6 cells/well.

Acknowledgments

We thank the patients who participated in this study. Furthermore we want to thank Benjamin Otto, from the Department of Clinical Chemistry/Central Laboratories, UKE for providing statistical advice.

Author Contributions

Conceived and designed the experiments: JSzW PH JME JvL. Performed the experiments: JME PH SK. Analyzed the data: JME PH JSzW. Contributed reagents/materials/analysis tools: JvL RES MB CL. Wrote the paper: JME PH JSzW JH JvL. Provided clinical samples: JvL RES MB CL. Carried out the soluble activation marker assays: AB.

References

1. Le Bourhis L, Mburu YK, Lantz O (2013) MAIT cells, surveyors of a new class of antigen: development and functions. Curr Opin Immunol 25: 174–180.
2. Le Bourhis L, Dusseaux M, Bohineust A, Bessoles S, Martin E, et al. (2013) MAIT cells detect and efficiently lyse bacterially-infected epithelial cells. PLoS pathogens 9: e1003681.
3. Le Bourhis L, Martin E, Peguillet I, Guihot A, Froux N, et al. (2010) Antimicrobial activity of mucosal-associated invariant T cells. Nat Immunol 11: 701–708.
4. Patel O, Kjer-Nielsen L, Le Nours J, Eckle SB, Birkinshaw R, et al. (2013) Recognition of vitamin B metabolites by mucosal-associated invariant T cells. Nature communications 4.
5. Cosgrove C, Ussher JE, Rauch A, Gartner K, Kurioka A, et al. (2013) Early and nonreversible decrease of CD161++/MAIT cells in HIV infection. Blood 121: 951–961.
6. Leeansyah E, Ganesh A, Quigley MF, Sonnerborg A, Andersson J, et al. (2013) Activation, exhaustion, and persistent decline of the antimicrobial MR1-restricted MAIT-cell population in chronic HIV-1 infection. Blood 121: 1124–1135.
7. Sandberg JK, Dias J, Shacklett BL, Leeansyah E (2013) Will loss of your MAITs weaken your HAART [corrected]? AIDS 27: 2501–2504.
8. Walker BD (2007) Elite control of HIV Infection: implications for vaccines and treatment. Top HIV Med 15: 134–136.
9. Bello G, Velasco-de-Castro CA, Bongertz V, Rodrigues CA, Giacoia-Gripp CB, et al. (2009) Immune activation and antibody responses in non-progressing elite controller individuals infected with HIV-1. J Med Virol 81: 1681–1690.
10. Walker LJ, Kang Y-H, Smith MO, Tharmalingham H, Ramamurthy N, et al. (2012) Human MAIT and CD8αα cells develop from a pool of type-17 precommitted CD8+ T cells. Blood 119: 422–433.
11. Dusseaux M, Martin E, Serriari N, Peguillet I, Premel V, et al. (2011) Human MAIT cells are xenobiotic-resistant, tissue-targeted, CD161hi IL-17-secreting T cells. Blood 117: 1250–1259.
12. Billerbeck E, Kang YH, Walker L, Lockstone H, Grafmueller S, et al. (2010) Analysis of CD161 expression on human CD8+ T cells defines a distinct functional subset with tissue-homing properties. Proc Natl Acad Sci U S A 107: 3006–3011.

13. Wong EB, Akilimali NA, Govender P, Sullivan ZA, Cosgrove C, et al. (2013) Low levels of peripheral CD161++CD8+ mucosal associated invariant T (MAIT) cells are found in HIV and HIV/TB co-infection. PLoS One 8: e83474.
14. Chang PP, Barral P, Fitch J, Pratama A, Ma CS, et al. (2012) Identification of Bcl-6-dependent follicular helper NKT cells that provide cognate help for B cell responses. Nat Immunol 13: 35–43.
15. King IL, Fortier A, Tighe M, Dibble J, Watts GF, et al. (2012) Invariant natural killer T cells direct B cell responses to cognate lipid antigen in an IL-21-dependent manner. Nat Immunol 13: 44–50.
16. Martin E, Treiner E, Duban L, Guerri L, Laude H, et al. (2009) Stepwise development of MAIT cells in mouse and human. PLoS Biol 7: e54.
17. Le Bourhis L, Guerri L, Dusseaux M, Martin E, Soudais C, et al. (2011) Mucosal-associated invariant T cells: unconventional development and function. Trends Immunol 32: 212–218.
18. Burdo TH, Lo J, Abbara S, Wei J, DeLelys ME, et al. (2011) Soluble CD163, a novel marker of activated macrophages, is elevated and associated with noncalcified coronary plaque in HIV-infected patients. J Infect Dis 204: 1227–1236.
19. Burdo TH, Lentz MR, Autissier P, Krishnan A, Halpern E, et al. (2011) Soluble CD163 made by monocyte/macrophages is a novel marker of HIV activity in early and chronic infection prior to and after anti-retroviral therapy. J Infect Dis 204: 154–163.
20. Sandler NG, Wand H, Roque A, Law M, Nason MC, et al. (2011) Plasma levels of soluble CD14 independently predict mortality in HIV infection. J Infect Dis 203: 780–790.
21. Ahmad R, Sindhu ST, Toma E, Morisset R, Ahmad A (2002) Elevated levels of circulating interleukin-18 in human immunodeficiency virus-infected individuals: role of peripheral blood mononuclear cells and implications for AIDS pathogenesis. J Virol 76: 12448–12456.
22. Napolitano LA, Grant RM, Deeks SG, Schmidt D, De Rosa SC, et al. (2001) Increased production of IL-7 accompanies HIV-1-mediated T-cell depletion: implications for T-cell homeostasis. Nat Med 7: 73–79.
23. Tang XZ, Jo J, Tan AT, Sandalova E, Chia A, et al. (2013) IL-7 licenses activation of human liver intrasinusoidal mucosal-associated invariant T cells. J Immunol 190: 3142–3152.
24. Ussher JE, Bilton M, Attwod E, Shadwell J, Richardson R, et al. (2014) CD161++ CD8+ T cells, including the MAIT cell subset, are specifically activated by IL-12+ IL-18 in a TCR-independent manner. European journal of immunology 44: 195–203.
25. Deeks SG, Walker BD (2007) Human immunodeficiency virus controllers: mechanisms of durable virus control in the absence of antiretroviral therapy. Immunity 27: 406–416.
26. Pereyra F, Addo MM, Kaufmann DE, Liu Y, Miura T, et al. (2008) Genetic and immunologic heterogeneity among persons who control HIV infection in the absence of therapy. J Infect Dis 197: 563–571.
27. Northfield JW, Kasprowicz V, Lucas M, Kersting N, Bengsch B, et al. (2008) CD161 expression on hepatitis C virus-specific CD8+ T cells suggests a distinct pathway of T cell differentiation. Hepatology 47: 396–406.
28. Meierovics A, Yankelevich WJ, Cowley SC (2013) MAIT cells are critical for optimal mucosal immune responses during in vivo pulmonary bacterial infection. Proc Natl Acad Sci U S A 110: E3119–3128.
29. Grimaldi D, Le Bourhis L, Sauneuf B, Dechartres A, Rousseau C, et al. (2014) Specific MAIT cell behaviour among innate-like T lymphocytes in critically ill patients with severe infections. Intensive Care Med 40: 192–201.
30. Birkinshaw RW, Kjer-Nielsen L, Eckle SB, McCluskey J, Rossjohn J (2014) MAITs, MR1 and vitamin B metabolites. Curr Opin Immunol 26: 7–13.
31. Reantragoon R, Corbett AJ, Sakala IG, Gherardin NA, Furness JB, et al. (2013) Antigen-loaded MR1 tetramers define T cell receptor heterogeneity in mucosal-associated invariant T cells. J Exp Med 210: 2305–2320.
32. Gérart S, Sibéril S, Martin E, Lenoir C, Aguilar C, et al. (2013) Human iNKT and MAIT cells exhibit a PLZF-dependent proapoptotic propensity that is counterbalanced by XIAP. Blood 121: 614–623.
33. Lee OJ, Cho YN, Kee SJ, Kim MJ, Jin HM, et al. (2014) Circulating mucosal-associated invariant T cell levels and their cytokine levels in healthy adults. Exp Gerontol 49: 47–54.
34. Krishnan S, Wilson EM, Sheikh V, Rupert A, Mendoza D, et al. (2014) Evidence for Innate Immune System Activation in HIV Type 1-Infected Elite Controllers. J Infect Dis 209: 931–939.
35. Chun T-W, Shawn Justement J, Murray D, Kim CJ, Blazkova J, et al. (2013) Effect of Antiretroviral Therapy on HIV Reservoirs in Elite Controllers. Journal of Infectious Diseases 208: 1443–1447.
36. Pereyra F, Lo J, Triant VA, Wei J, Buzon MJ, et al. (2012) Increased coronary atherosclerosis and immune activation in HIV-1 elite controllers. AIDS 26: 2409–2412.
37. Turtle CJ, Delrow J, Joslyn RC, Swanson HM, Basom R, et al. (2011) Innate signals overcome acquired TCR signaling pathway regulation and govern the fate of human CD161hi CD8α+ semi-invariant T cells. Blood 118: 2752–2762.
38. Mavigner M, Cazabat M, Dubois M, L'Faqihi FE, Requena M, et al. (2012) Altered CD4+ T cell homing to the gut impairs mucosal immune reconstitution in treated HIV-infected individuals. J Clin Invest 122: 62–69.
39. Chen J, Han X, An M, Liu J, Xu J, et al. (2013) Immunological and virological benefits resulted from short-course treatment during primary HIV infection: a meta-analysis. PLoS One 8: e82461.
40. Investigators ST, Fidler S, Porter K, Ewings F, Frater J, et al. (2013) Short-course antiretroviral therapy in primary HIV infection. N Engl J Med 368: 207–217.
41. Constantinides MG, Bendelac A (2013) Transcriptional regulation of the NKT cell lineage. Curr Opin Immunol 25: 161–167.
42. Gordon SM, Carty SA, Kim JS, Zou T, Smith-Garvin J, et al. (2011) Requirements for eomesodermin and promyelocytic leukemia zinc finger in the development of innate-like CD8+ T cells. J Immunol 186: 4573–4578.
43. Alonzo ES, Sant'Angelo DB (2011) Development of PLZF-expressing innate T cells. Curr Opin Immunol 23: 220–227.
44. Wakao H, Fujita H (2013) Toward the realization of cell therapy: the advent of MAIT cells from iPSCs. Cell Cycle 12: 2341–2342.
45. Wakao H, Yoshikiyo K, Koshimizu U, Furukawa T, Enomoto K, et al. (2013) Expansion of functional human mucosal-associated invariant T cells via reprogramming to pluripotency and redifferentiation. Cell Stem Cell 12: 546–558.
46. Wilson NL, Moneyham LD, Alexandrov AW (2013) A systematic review of probiotics as a potential intervention to restore gut health in HIV infection. J Assoc Nurses AIDS Care 24: 98–111.
47. Wong EB, Akilimali NA, Govender P, Sullivan ZA, Cosgrove C, et al. (2013) Low Levels of Peripheral CD161++ CD8+ Mucosal Associated Invariant T (MAIT) Cells Are Found in HIV and HIV/TB Co-Infection. PloS one 8: e83474.
48. Sutton CE, Mielke LA, Mills KHG (2012) IL-17-producing γδ T cells and innate lymphoid cells. European Journal of Immunology 42: 2221–2231.
49. Hartjen P, Meyer-Olson D, Lehmann C, Stellbrink HJ, van Lunzen J, et al. (2013) Vgamma2Vdelta2 T cells are skewed toward a terminal differentiation phenotype in untreated HIV infection. J Infect Dis 208: 180–182.

CD8 and CD4 Epitope Predictions in RV144: No Strong Evidence of a T-Cell Driven Sieve Effect in HIV-1 Breakthrough Sequences from Trial Participants

Kalpana Dommaraju[1,2], Gustavo Kijak[1,2], Jonathan M. Carlson[3], Brendan B. Larsen[4], Sodsai Tovanabutra[1,2], Dan E. Geraghty[5], Wenjie Deng[4], Brandon S. Maust[4], Paul T. Edlefsen[5], Eric Sanders-Buell[1,2], Silvia Ratto-Kim[1,2], Mark S. deSouza[6], Supachai Rerks-Ngarm[7], Sorachai Nitayaphan[8], Punnee Pitisuttihum[9], Jaranit Kaewkungwal[9], Robert J. O'Connell[6], Merlin L. Robb[1,2], Nelson L. Michael[1], James I. Mullins[4], Jerome H. Kim[1], Morgane Rolland[1,2]*

1 US Military HIV Research Program, Walter Reed Army Institute of Research, Silver Spring, Maryland, United States of America, **2** Henry Jackson Foundation, Bethesda, Maryland, United States of America, **3** Microsoft Research, Los Angeles, California, United States of America, **4** Department of Microbiology, University of Washington, Seattle, Washington, United States of America, **5** Vaccine and Infectious Disease Division, Fred Hutchinson Cancer Research Center, Seattle, Washington, United States of America, **6** Armed Forces Research Institute of Medical Sciences, Bangkok, Thailand, **7** Thai Ministry of Public Health, Nonthaburi, Thailand, **8** Royal Thai Army Component, Armed Forces Research Institute of Medical Sciences, Bangkok, Thailand, **9** Faculty of Tropical Medicine, Mahidol University, Bangkok, Thailand

Abstract

The modest protection afforded by the RV144 vaccine offers an opportunity to evaluate its mechanisms of protection. Differences between HIV-1 breakthrough viruses from vaccine and placebo recipients can be attributed to the RV144 vaccine as this was a randomized and double-blinded trial. CD8 and CD4 T cell epitope repertoires were predicted in HIV-1 proteomes from 110 RV144 participants. Predicted Gag epitope repertoires were smaller in vaccine than in placebo recipients ($p = 0.019$). After comparing participant-derived epitopes to corresponding epitopes in the RV144 vaccine, the proportion of epitopes that could be matched differed depending on the protein conservation (only 36% of epitopes in Env vs 84–91% in Gag/Pol/Nef for CD8 predicted epitopes) or on vaccine insert subtype (55% against CRF01_AE vs 7% against subtype B). To compare predicted epitopes to the vaccine, we analyzed predicted binding affinity and evolutionary distance measurements. Comparisons between the vaccine and placebo arm did not reveal robust evidence for a T cell driven sieve effect, although some differences were noted in Env-V2 ($0.022 \leq$ p-value ≤ 0.231). The paucity of CD8 T cell responses identified following RV144 vaccination, with no evidence for V2 specificity, considered together both with the association of decreased infection risk in RV 144 participants with V-specific antibody responses and a V2 sieve effect, lead us to hypothesize that this sieve effect was not T cell specific. Overall, our results did not reveal a strong differential impact of vaccine-induced T cell responses among breakthrough infections in RV144 participants.

Editor: Paul A. Goepfert, University of Alabama, United States of America

Funding: This work was supported in part by an Interagency Agreement Y1-AI-2642-12 between the U.S. Army Medical Research and Material Command and the National Institutes of Allergy and Infectious Diseases and by a cooperative agreement (W81XWH-07-2-0067) between the Henry M. Jackson Foundation for the Advancement of Military Medicine, Inc., and the U.S. Department of Defense. The funders had no role in study design, data collection and analysis, decision to publish, or preparation of the manuscript.

Competing Interests: The authors have declared that no competing interests exist. KD, GK, ST, ESB, SRK, MLR, NLM, JHK, and MR are employees of the US Military HIV Research Program (MHRP). The opinions expressed herein are those of the authors and should not be construed as official or representing the views of the US Department of Defense or the Department of the Army. JMC is an employee of Microsoft Research. This does not alter the authors' adherence to PLOS ONE policies on sharing data and materials.

* Email: mrolland@hivresearch.org

Introduction

The RV144 trial showed modest efficacy in preventing HIV-1 infection with an estimated 31% reduction in HIV-1 infections in the vaccine arm (modified intent to treat population, $p = 0.04$) [1]. Among the 16,402 adult Thai participants, 125 HIV-1 infections were diagnosed following enrollment. We sequenced HIV-1 near full-length genomes from plasma samples collected at the time of HIV-1 diagnosis in 121 subjects [2]. Phylogenetic analyses showed that 110 of these infections were caused by CRF01_AE viruses.

A genetic analysis spurred by the identification of a correlate of risk of infection linked to Env-V2, focused on this Env segment and identified two signatures that distinguished viruses from vaccine and placebo recipients [2]. Viruses derived from vaccine recipients could be differentiated from those from placebo recipients at Env positions 169 and 181, which are contact sites for V2-specific antibodies including some derived from RV144 participants [3]. Genetic signatures in V2, together with the identification of binding antibodies directed against V2 as a correlate of risk of HIV-1 infection [4], suggest that anti-V2 antibodies may have played a role in the protection conferred by the RV144 vaccine.

It is plausible that Env-V2 was not the sole viral determinant impacted by vaccine-induced immune responses. One possible path to explore is the potential role of T-cell mediated immune responses. Analyses performed on samples collected 6 months after the final immunization showed Gag or Env IFN-γ ELISpot responses in 20% of vaccinees vs 7% of placebo recipients [1]. Intracellular cytokine staining assays showed no difference between vaccine and placebo recipients for CD8 responses (Gag CD8: 7% of responders; Env CD8: 11% and 14% of responders among vaccine and placebo recipients, respectively) or for Gag CD4 responses (1% vs 0% of responders), while Env CD4 responses were significantly more frequent in vaccine than in placebo recipients (34% vs 4%, respectively) [1].

To obtain insights on the impact of T cell immunity on founder HIV-1 sequences, potential CD8 and CD4 epitopes can be predicted *in silico* based on sequence motifs matched by class I and II HLA alleles [5,6]. In this study, we performed CD8 and CD4 epitope predictions based on each subject's HLA genotype and HIV-1 proteome sequence(s) using the same methods as in the analysis of breakthrough infections in the Step/HVTN502 trial [5,6], which we have expanded to include comparisons of epitope predictions based on evolutionary distances and predicted affinity binding. We analyzed subject-derived epitope predictions as a function of the epitopes predicted in the RV144 vaccine inserts to investigate whether we could identify features distinguishing the vaccine and placebo group.

Materials and Methods

Ethics Statement

The RV144 clinical vaccine trial was registered with ClinicalTrials.gov and assigned the registration number NCT00223080 (Supporting File S1). The protocol was approved by the ethics committees of the Ministry of Public Health, the Royal Thai Army, Mahidol University, and the Human Subjects Research Review Board of the U.S. Army Medical Research and Materiel Command. It was also independently approved by the World Health Organization and the Joint United Nations Program on HIV/AIDS and by the AIDS Vaccine Research Working Group of the National Institute of Allergy and Infectious Diseases at the National Institutes of Health.

Written informed consent was obtained from all volunteers, who were required to pass a written test of understanding. The consent procedure was approved by the Ethics committees and IRBs listed above.

The RV144 trial was double-blinded and randomized, enrolled 16,402 participants and took place in Thailand between October 2003 and September 2009; the results of the trial were reported by Rerks-Ngarm and colleagues [1], and further details on immune correlates of risk of infection were reported by Haynes and colleagues [4].

HIV-1 sequence data

For RV144 participants who became HIV-1-infected during the RV144 trial (diagnosed between 14 June 2004 and 12 February 2009), HIV-1 near full-length genomes were sequenced from single RNA templates corresponding to plasma samples collected at the time of HIV-1 diagnosis (GenBank accession numbers JX446645–JX448316). Sequences from the 110 subjects who were infected with CRF01_AE viruses were translated to amino acid (AA) sequences, using only sequences with open reading frames.

Vaccine insert sequences corresponded to two lab strains of HIV-1 subtype B and two CRF01_AE viruses isolated in Thailand in 1990 and 1992. The ALVAC-HIV canarypox prime [vCP1521] is a chimeric construct that concatenates *gag* and *pro* of HIV-1 subtype B (strain LAI) with gp120 of CRF01_AE (strain 92TH023) fused to a 28-AA-long segment of the transmembrane-anchoring portion of gp41 HIV-1-B strain LAI (HXB2 position AA 684:711 of HXB2 gp160). The AIDSVAX B/E boost was composed of two gp120 proteins with N-terminal truncations (HIV-1 protein started at AA42 of HXB2 gp160): one protein was HIV-1 subtype B (strain MN) and one was HIV-1 CRF01_AE (strain CM244).

HLA genotyping

High-resolution typing of class I and II HLA was performed by DNA sequence-based typing (SBT) and by the sequence-specific oligonucleotide probe (SSOP) method, with concordant results. Class I SBT was carried out by PCR amplification and subsequent dye terminator nucleotide sequencing of exons 2 and 3, with ambiguous types being resolved to four digits using the dbMHC SBT interpretation interface [7] (http://www.ncbi.nlm.nih.gov/projects/gv/mhc/). Class II SBT were genotyped in the CLIA/ASHI accredited lab of William Hildebrand at the University of Oklahoma Health Sciences Center using in-house PCR and sequencing methodologies. The entirety of exon 2 was DNA sequenced for all class II loci with additional exons DNA sequenced for DQB1 (exon 3), DQA1 (exon 3), and DPB1 (exons 3 & 4). DNA sequence analysis and HLA allele assignment were performed with Assign-SBT v3.5.1 software (Conexio Genomics). The HLA database for allele assignment was updated with IMGT release 3.0.0 May 5th 2010. Any ambiguous types that remained following DNA Sequence Based Typing were resolved to 4-digits using the PEL-FREEZ UNITRAY SSP, Life Technologies. SSOP was conducted using the LABType SSO Class I HD system (One Lambda, Canoga Park, CA), which is based on Luminex xMAP technology, and results were interpreted using the accompanying HLA Fusion 2.0.0 software. HLA types are reported according to the IMGT/HLA nomenclature (version 3.7.0, http://www.ebi.ac.uk/imgt/hla/ambig.html).

$CD4^{+}$ and $CD8^{+}$ T cell epitope predictions

CTL epitope predictions were done with the NetMHCpan 2.4 Server, which predicts binding of peptides to each subject's HLA genotype using artificial neural networks [8] (http://www.cbs.dtu.dk/services/NetMHCpan/). Predictions were done for 9-mers, because it is the favored length for binding (predictions for other lengths are made from approximations based on 9-mers, and are thus less accurate). CD4 epitope predictions were done with the NetMHCIIpan 2.1 Server, which predicts binding of peptides to each subject's MHC class II HLA-DR alleles using artificial neural networks [9] (http://www.cbs.dtu.dk/services/NetMHCIIpan/). Predicted epitopes were 15-mers, and unique epitopes were retained based on the core 8-mer peptide sequence: between several overlapping peptides with an identical core peptide, the peptide that had the strongest predicted binding affinity was retained.

Predictions are given with IC50 values (in nM), with a threshold of 50 nM for an epitope to be considered a strong binder (SB); weak binders (WB) have a predicted IC50 between 50 and 500 nM.

Epitopes were predicted on the translated AA sequences corresponding to Gag, Pol, Env and Nef based on each subject's class I and II HLA alleles. In parallel, epitopes were predicted in the vaccine insert sequences using all the HLA/HLA-DR alleles in the cohort of 110 RV144 subjects. For each subject, all unique HLA-peptide binding pairs were retained, leading to some peptides being counted multiple times for each HLA to which it was predicted to bind.

Subject-specific epitopes were matched to the vaccine-derived epitopes – epitopes were matched when the subject- and vaccine-derived peptides (with the same HXB2 positions) had at least 67% AA identity, or a maximum of 3 mismatches for a 9-mer; we consider that 9-mers with 4 or more mismatches cannot be aligned with confidence and our rationale for not aligning such 9-mers is that the sequences are too distant for the peptide to be recognized by a vaccine-elicited response [10]. Matched epitope predictions were analyzed based on the respective binding affinity values of the matched epitopes, and on the evolutionary distance calculated between the matched epitopes. For each matched subject-derived and vaccine-derived epitope pair, the binding affinity value was calculated as the ratio of the binding affinity for the subject-derived epitope to the binding affinity of the vaccine-derived epitope. The evolutionary distance was calculated between the subject-derived and vaccine-derived epitope based on the HIV-specific matrix (HIV-between-10%) developed by Nickle and colleagues [11].

For each subject, summary distances were computed based on matched pairs of predicted epitopes (if there were no predicted epitope or no matched pair, then the distance could not be defined and the subject's information was not used). Wilcoxon rank sum tests (equivalently, the Mann-Whitney test) with exact 2-sided p-values were used to test for a different distribution in summary measures between the vaccine and placebo groups.

Phylogenetic dependency networks

We used phylogenetic dependency networks, a statistical model of evolution that simultaneously takes into account HIV-1 AA co-variation, linkage disequilibrium among HLA alleles, and shared ancestry in the HIV-1 phylogeny to identify the primary source of selection pressure acting on each HIV codon [12]. For each gene, a maximum likelihood phylogenetic tree was constructed and a model of conditional adaptation was created for the vaccine status and for every HLA gene, amino acid position and state. The null hypothesis is that the observations depend on the phylogenetic tree structure; then, adaptation due to each variable is modeled along the tree by an additive process. Results were adjusted for multiple comparisons, using q values of ≤ 0.2 with an associated p-value threshold of ≤ 0.05 (implying a false-positive proportion of 20% among identified associations).

Association between viral loads and HLA alleles

We analyzed the effect of the HLA (2 digit) genotype on viral loads measured at the time of HIV-1 diagnosis (VL corresponding to the plasma sample sequenced).

L1-regularized linear regression analyses were used to test which features predict VL for each sample. A bootstrap procedure (sample with replacement 1,000 times) was used to estimate a bootstrap support frequency for a given predictor and its effect size on viral loads.

Results

Gag epitope repertoires from vaccine recipients were smaller than those of placebo recipients

We performed CD8 and CD4 epitope predictions based on each subject's genotype and HIV-1 genomic sequences derived at the time of HIV-1 diagnosis. To avoid the misidentification of effects that would be due to a phylogenetic difference, we only included the 110 subjects infected with CRF01_AE viruses – see Flowchart on Figure 1. For these 44 vaccine and 66 placebo recipients, the vaccine efficacy was estimated at 34% (95% C.I. = 7.8%, 54.7%) (compared to 31% in the full mITT cohort [1]), thus allowing vaccine/placebo investigations of the impact of the vaccine. Epitope predictions from two subjects in a linked HIV-1 transmission were included since, despite being infected with nearly identical viruses, both subjects had different HLA genotypes and thus non-overlapping predicted epitope repertoires (Figure 2A).

The number of predicted epitopes for each subject depends on both the genotype of the individual and the HIV-1 sequence they were infected with. There was no difference in the distribution of HLA types between the vaccine and placebo groups; then we looked at the epitopes predicted for these HLA alleles. When the vaccine and placebo groups were compared, there was no difference in the number of predicted CD8 epitopes in Pol, Env and Nef: Median number of epitopes in Pro: $n = 5$ (vaccine) and $n = 6$ (placebo), $p = 0.464$; in RT-IN: $n = 116$ (vaccine) and $n = 117.5$ (placebo), $p = 0.707$; in Env: $n = 64$ (vaccine) and $n = 66$ (placebo), $p = 0.238$; in Nef: $n = 25$ (vaccine) and $n = 26.5$ (placebo), $p = 0.408$ (Table 1). In contrast, there were significantly fewer Gag epitopes predicted in sequences from vaccine recipients ($n = 45$) than in those from placebo recipients ($n = 51.5$), $p = 0.019$ (Table 1).

Env epitopes from RV144 participants poorly matched vaccine-derived epitopes

We can hypothesize that, due to vaccine-engendered escape mutations, fewer epitopes may have a corresponding matched epitope in the vaccine insert sequence in sequences from vaccine recipients than in those from placebo recipients. For each subject, the list of predicted autologous class I and class II epitopes was compared to corresponding epitopes predicted in the vaccine insert strain to identify pairs of matched subject+vaccine epitopes (Schematic representation for class I epitopes in Figure 2B). Considering each vaccine insert sequence separately, we found no difference between vaccine and placebo recipients in the ratio of subject-derived epitopes that could be matched to vaccine-derived epitopes for any of the HIV-1 proteins: $p \geq 0.314$ vs CM244, $p \geq 0.214$ vs LAI (MN for Env), $p \geq 0.540$ vs 92TH023. Since the RV144 vaccine was composed of proteins of different subtype (Subtype B and CRF01_AE; while all subjects evaluated were infected with CRF01_AE) and of proteins that are relatively variable (Env-gp120) or conserved (Gag/Pro), we tested if these factors affected the ability to match predicted autologous epitopes to the predicted epitopes in the inserts. We found that the ratio of matched epitopes differed depending on the protein and on the vaccine reference considered but not on the vaccine/placebo status. The proportion of matched epitopes is much higher in Pol, Gag, or Nef (73 to 91%) than in Env, for which only about a third (36%) of predicted epitopes in subject-derived sequences could be matched to epitopes identified in the vaccine inserts (Table 2). In addition, there were subtype-specific differences, with significantly more subject-derived epitopes matched against the CM244 (also CRF01) than against the MN (or LAI; both subtype B) vaccine insert. For example, an average of 55% of Env predicted epitopes were matched against CM244 compared to 7% matched against MN ($p < 0.0001$) whether vaccine or placebo recipients are considered. The limited number of matched epitopes is due to the high diversity between Env sequences, hence the large distance between specific strains, which is amplified when attempting cross-subtype epitope matching.

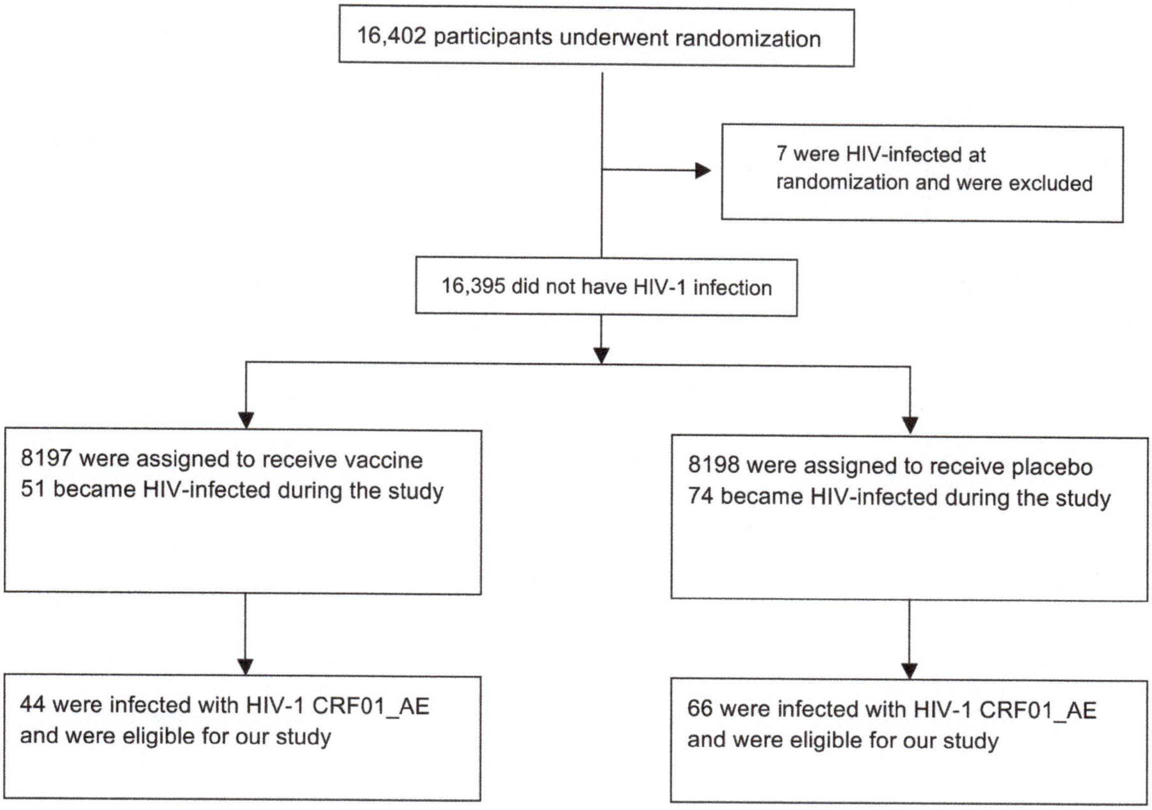

Figure 1. Flowchart diagram of HIV-1 breakthrough infections in RV144.

No vaccine/placebo distinction in Gag, Pro, Gp120 epitope comparisons against the vaccine inserts

Under the hypothesis that vaccine-induced immune responses could lead to escape mutations in sequences from vaccinees, we used epitopes predicted based on each subject's genotype to test whether epitope changes relative to the vaccine inserts differed between the vaccine and placebo groups. Because the vaccine was multivalent, we compared the epitopes predicted in RV144

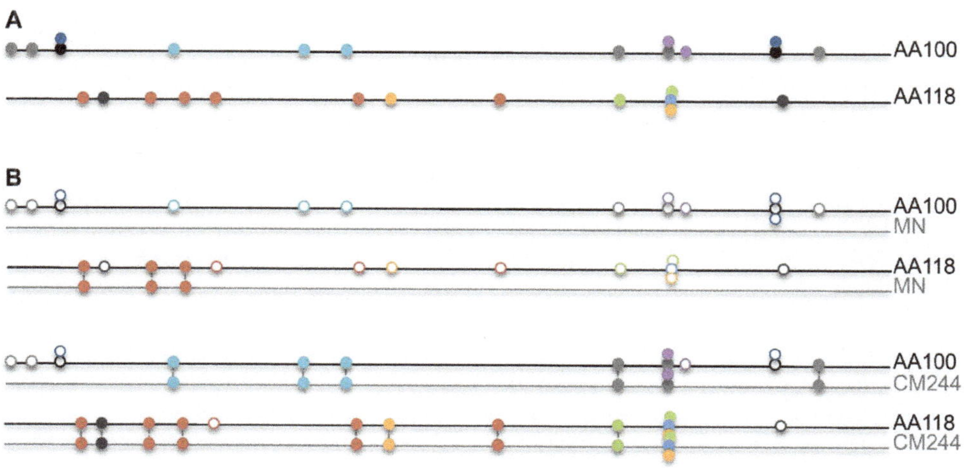

Figure 2. Schematic representation of epitope predictions in RV144 HIV-1 breakthrough sequences, and their comparison to RV144 vaccine inserts. A. Each line represents the Env-gp120 sequence from a subject and each circle a CD8 epitope prediction (different colors for different HLA alleles). The figure represents epitopes predicted based on each subject's HLA class I genotype for two subjects who were infected with a nearly identical virus (AA100: HLA-A*02:03, HLA-A*24:10, HLA-B*18:01, HLA-B*18:02, HLA-C*07:04; AA118: HLA-A*11:01, HLA-A*24:07, HLA-B*44:03, HLA-C*01:02, HLA-C*07:01). B. Epitope repertoires from a given subject are compared to the epitope predictions for the vaccine insert sequences (CM244 and MN) based on that subject's HLA class I genotype. Empty circles represent epitopes predicted in the sequence from a subject that could not be matched to a corresponding epitope prediction based on the vaccine insert sequence and the subject's HLA class I genotype. More subject-derived epitopes were matched against the vaccine insert CM244 than against MN; both subjects were infected by a CRF01-AE virus like CM244, while MN is a subtype B virus.

Table 1. Number of CD8 epitopes predicted for each subject depending on his HLA type.

	Gag		Pro		Env	
	Placebo	Vaccine	Placebo	Vaccine	Placebo	Vaccine
Nr of subjects	66	44	65	43	66	44
Median	51.5	45	6	5	66	64
Mean	52.71	46.11	6.39	6.21	69.68	64.75
p-value	0.019		0.464		0.238	
	RT-IN		**Nef**			
	Placebo	**Vaccine**	**Placebo**	**Vaccine**		
Nr of subjects	66	44	66	44		
Median	117.5	116	26.5	25		
Mean	116.30	113.80	26.42	25.30		
p-value	0.707		0.408			

Predictions are given for proteins that corresponded to the vaccine inserts (Gag, Pro, Env), and for proteins that were not part of the vaccine (RT-IN, and Nef).

participants' sequences to the subtype B and CRF01_AE reference strains included in the vaccine (CRF01_AE: CM244 and 92TH023; subtype B: LAI and MN). We tested both differences in binding affinities (by comparing predicted IC50 for the epitopes in the vaccinee's sequence and in the vaccine insert) and in evolutionary distances (i.e., protein distances between RV144 participants' epitopes and vaccine-derived epitopes were calculated using an HIV-specific substitution model). We looked for evidence of a difference between vaccine and placebo group by analyzing predictions in proteins that were part of the vaccine (Gag, Pro, Gp120) and used as control the epitope predictions derived from RT-IN and Nef (to test the hypothesis that there would be no difference between the vaccine and placebo group outside of the vaccine insert).

We first looked at predicted CD8 and CD4 epitopes defined as both weak and strong binders. We found no difference between the vaccine and placebo group either when we focused on binding affinities or evolutionary distances for the different proteins and references considered (data not shown). Second, we focused on the subset of epitopes identified as strong binders (i.e., with a predicted IC50≤50 nM). Again, there was no concordant evidence of a difference between the vaccine and placebo group, although, for CD8 epitope predictions, there was a trend suggesting a difference between the vaccine and placebo groups in Pro ($p = 0.080$) and gp120 ($p = 0.065$) when binding affinities of predicted epitopes were considered (Table 3). In addition, when the analysis was limited to V2, some results were significant (0.022≤p-value≤0.231; see below). Comparisons of epitope predictions in RT-IN and Nef verified that there was also no distinction between the vaccine and placebo group for proteins not included in the vaccine (p-values≥0.16 for both CD4 and CD8 predictions).

Env-V2 and Env-V3-specific comparisons of epitope predictions

Given the results of the RV144 correlates of risk study [4], a V2-specifc analysis was performed. While analyses of CD8 epitope predictions that included both strong and weak binders showed that only the comparison of V2-binding affinity measures against CM244 was significant ($p = 0.017$), the results were more consistent when we focused on the subset of epitopes identified as strong binders (i.e., with a predicted IC50≤50 nM) (Table 3). Data were not available against the subtype B vaccine boost (MN) because subject-derived epitopes were too divergent to be matched to the vaccine strain. For predicted strong CD8 binders, there was a significant difference between the vaccine and placebo group in the V2 region of Env when binding affinities were considered. Comparisons were significant against the CRF01_AE strains (CM244 $p = 0.022$; 92TH023 $p = 0.047$). When evolutionary distances were considered for CD8 epitopes, there was only a trend suggesting a difference between the vaccine and placebo group against the CRF01_AE strains (CM244 $p = 0.058$; 92TH023 $p = 0.231$).

When CD4 epitope predictions were considered, there were weak trends suggesting a greater number of strong binders in the

Table 2. Subject-specific epitopes matched to vaccine-derived epitopes.

Matched epitopes	Gag	Pol	Env	Nef
CD8	4,629/5,509	12,198/13,368	5,545/15,520	2,389/2,860
CD8 (%)	84%	91%	36%	84%
CD4	11,177/13,419	25,273/29,921	13,109/36,738	3,006/4,119
CD4 (%)	83%	84%	36%	73%

Epitopes were considered matched when the subject- and vaccine-derived peptides had at least 67% AA identity. Number and percentages of matched epitopes are given for all of the 110 subjects in the cohort; there was no difference between the vaccine and placebo groups.

Table 3. CD8 and CD4 epitopes predicted to be strong binders matched against different vaccine inserts.

CD8 epitope predictions - Binding affinity						
Gag	**P CM244 (66)**	**V CM244 (44)**	**P LAI (66)**	**V LAI (44)**		
Mean	0.996	0.965	0.979	0.979		
p-value	0.266		0.813			
Pro	**P CM244 (31)**	**V CM244 (20)**	**P LAI (31)**	**V LAI (20)**		
Mean	0.24	0.338	0.426	0.354		
p-value	0.08		0.333			
gp120	**P CM244 (66)**	**V CM244 (44)**	**P MN (66)**	**V MN (44)**	**P 92TH (66)**	**V 92TH (44)**
Mean	0.95	0.997	0.623	0.676	0.826	0.864
p-value	0.065		0.468		0.448	
V2	**P CM244 (58)**	**V CM244 (35)**	**P MN (0)**	**V MN (0)**	**P 92TH (58)**	**V 92TH (35)**
Mean	0.957	1.123	n.a.	n.a.	0.017	0.114
p-value	0.022		n.a.		0.047	
V3	**P CM244 (13)**	**V CM244 (9)**	**P MN (0)**	**V MN (0)**	**P 92TH (0)**	**V 92TH (0)**
Mean	0.903	0.548	n.a.	n.a.	n.a.	n.a.
p-value	0.108		n.a.		n.a.	
RT-In	**P CM244 (66)**	**V CM244 (44)**	**P LAI (66)**	**V LAI (44)**		
Mean	1	1	0.439	0.641		
p-value	n.a.		0.378			
Nef	**P CM244 (66)**	**V CM244 (44)**	**P LAI (66)**	**V LAI (44)**		
Mean	0.98	0.9	0.669	0.635		
p-value	0.162		0.958			
CD8 epitope predictions - Evolutionary distance						
Gag	**P CM244 (66)**	**V CM244 (44)**	**P LAI (66)**	**V LAI (44)**		
Mean	0.033	0.051	0.142	0.139		
p-value	0.351		0.998			
Pro	**P CM244 (31)**	**V CM244 (20)**	**P LAI (31)**	**V LAI (20)**		
Mean	0.124	0.14	0.152	0.113		
p-value	0.851		0.361			
gp120	**P CM244 (66)**	**V CM244 (44)**	**P MN (66)**	**V MN (44)**	**P 92TH (66)**	**V 92TH (44)**
Mean	0.056	0.064	0.005	0.005	0.014	0.016
p-value	0.403		0.356		0.859	
V2	**P CM244 (58)**	**V CM244 (35)**	**P MN (0)**	**V MN (0)**	**P 92TH (58)**	**V 92TH (35)**
Mean	0.095	0.101	n.a.	n.a.	0.049	0.025
p-value	0.058		n.a.		0.231	
V3	**P CM244 (13)**	**V CM244 (9)**	**P MN (0)**	**V MN (0)**	**P 92TH (0)**	**V 92TH (0)**
Mean	0.21	0.148	n.a.	n.a.	n.a.	n.a.
p-value	0.227		n.a.		n.a.	
RT-In	**P CM244 (66)**	**V CM244 (44)**	**P LAI (66)**	**V LAI (44)**		
Mean	0.002	0.002	0.038	0.03		
p-value	0.792		0.616			
Nef	**P CM244 (64)**	**V CM244 (44)**	**P LAI (64)**	**V LAI (44)**		
Mean	0.081	0.087	0.281	0.247		
p-value	0.803		0.458			
CD4 epitope predictions - Binding affinity						
Gag	**P CM244 (62)**	**V CM244 (43)**	**P LAI (62)**	**V LAI (43)**		
Mean	0.991	0.985	1.002	0.948		
p-value	0.688		0.296			

Table 3. Cont.

CD8 epitope predictions - Binding affinity						
Pro	**P CM244 (40)**	**V CM244 (22)**	**P LAI (40)**	**V LAI (22)**		
Mean	0.816	0.804	0.897	0.971		
p-value	0.794		0.662			
gp120	**P CM244 (59)**	**V CM244 (43)**	**P MN (59)**	**V MN (43)**	**P 92TH (59)**	**V 92TH (43)**
Mean	0.86	0.847	0.548	0.374	0.528	0.4
p-value	0.989		0.127		0.336	
V2	**P CM244 (45)**	**V CM244 (22)**	**P MN (45)**	**V MN (22)**	**P 92TH (45)**	**V 92TH (22)**
Mean	1.001	1.14	n.a.	n.a.	0	0.045
p-value	0.177		n.a.		0.162	
V3	**P CM244 (15)**	**V CM244 (4)**	**P MN (15)**	**V MN (4)**	**P 92TH (15)**	**V 92TH (4)**
Mean	0.314	0.259	n.a.	n.a.	n.a.	n.a.
p-value	0.881		n.a.		n.a.	
RT-In	**P CM244 (62)**	**V CM244 (43)**	**P LAI (62)**	**V LAI (43)**		
Mean	0.999	1	0.689	0.6		
p-value	0.416		0.403			
Nef	**P CM244 (54)**	**V CM244 (35)**	**P LAI (54)**	**V LAI (35)**		
Mean	1.001	1.044	0.28	0.201		
p-value	0.202		0.186			
CD4 epitope predictions - Evolutionary distance						
Gag	**P CM244 (61)**	**V CM244 (43)**	**P LAI (61)**	**V LAI (43)**		
Mean	0.021	0.025	0.112	0.089		
p-value	0.806		0.04			
Pro	**P CM244 (40)**	**V CM244 (22)**	**P LAI (40)**	**V LAI (22)**		
Mean	0.111	0.076	0.121	0.095		
p-value	0.299		0.732			
gp120	**P CM244 (59)**	**V CM244 (43)**	**P MN (59)**	**V MN (43)**	**P 92TH (59)**	**V 92TH (43)**
Mean	0.097	0.083	0.025	0.015	0.046	0.035
p-value	0.108		0.12		0.195	
V2	**P CM244 (45)**	**V CM244 (22)**	**P MN (0)**	**V MN (0)**	**P 92TH (45)**	**V 92TH (22)**
Mean	0.168	0.089	n.a.	n.a.	0.041	0.047
p-value	0.01		n.a.		0.602	
V3	**P CM244 (15)**	**V CM244 (4)**	**P MN (0)**	**V MN (0)**	**P 92TH (15)**	**V 92TH (4)**
Mean	0.235	0.2	n.a.	n.a.	0.043	0.176
p-value	0.96		n.a.		0.272	
RT-In	**P CM244 (62)**	**V CM244 (43)**	**P LAI (62)**	**V LAI (43)**		
Mean	0.006	0.002	0.035	0.035		
p-value	0.332		0.65			
Nef	**P CM244 (54)**	**V CM244 (35)**	**P LAI (54)**	**V LAI (35)**		
Mean	0.107	0.105	0.347	0.405		
p-value	0.956		0.296			

Epitopes were predicted in all HIV-1 proteome sequences derived from RV144 breakthrough infections. The epitopes were matched against epitopes derived from the RV144 vaccine inserts of subtype B (MN, LAI) or CRF01_AE (CM244, 92TH023); two epitope characteristics were used to compare epitopes from the breakthrough to the vaccine: the predicted binding affinity for each epitope and the protein distance between the epitope sequences. One summary measure was computed for each protein and each subject, and comparisons were done between the vaccine (V) and placebo (P) groups (the number of vaccine and placebo recipients included in each group is in parenthesis) with Mann-Whitney tests for proteins corresponding to those included in the RV144 vaccine insert (Gag, Pro, gp120 (including V2)) and those not part of the RV144 vaccine (RT-IN, Nef).

V2 of vaccinees compared to the placebo group (CM244 $p = 0.177$; 92TH023 $p = 0.162$), and significantly greater evolutionary distances in placebo recipients against CM244 ($p = 0.010$), but not against 92TH023 ($p = 0.602$).

Given that high responses to V3 have been associated with a lower risk of HIV-1 infection among vaccinees who had low gp120-specific plasma IgA: (OR = 0.49, p = 0.007), we also performed a V3-specific analysis for CD8 and CD4 epitopes. There was no significant distinction found between the vaccine and placebo groups using the tests described above ($p>0.108$), noting that there were no epitopes in V3 that had enough similarity with MN for the corresponding epitopes to be matched (i.e., less than 2/3 of the residues of a peptide matched).

Parallels between V2 and V3 were notable: i) both V2 and V3 were a hotspot of RV144-induced antibody responses [13]; ii) V2- and V3-specific binding antibodies were identified as correlates of risk of infection in RV144; and iii) they harbored signature sites of RV144 vaccination. Statistical analyses that interrogated individual sites in Env from RV144 participants identified two sites in V2 (sites 169 and 181, [2]) and one in V3 (site 317). Thus, we looked specifically at predicted epitopes in V2 and V3 that spanned the signature sites. Figure 3 shows the overlap between CD8 and CD4 predicted epitopes in V2 and V3: we note that because multiple alleles can restrict the same peptide the number of epitope predictions starting at a specific location can surpass the number of subjects in the cohort. In addition, there are epitopes spanning the signature sites in both V2 and V3; however, no distinction was detected between the vaccine and placebo group (Table S1 in File S2).

No allele-specific effect in vaccine/placebo epitope comparisons against the vaccine inserts

By analyzing Env sequence data as a function of each subject's genotype on a site-by-site basis with a phylogenetically-corrected method, five DRB1 and one class I HLA alleles (DRB1*03, DRB1*04, DRB1*07, DRB1*11, DRB1*15, A*68) were associated with specific AA polymorphisms in Env. However, the limited number of subjects with a given allele (ranging from four with DRB1*11 to 33 with DRB1*15) did not allow us to perform meaningful vaccine/placebo comparisons restricted to carriers of these specific alleles.

Next, when $\log_{10}$ viral loads (measured at the time of sampling for viral genome sequencing, corresponding to early infection as the last negative visit happened six months prior diagnosis) were analyzed as a function of Env sequence together with each subject's genotype, HLA alleles HLA-A*11 and HLA-B*46 were associated with higher viral loads, although the effect sizes were small (HLA-A*11: weight = 0.23, bootstrap support = 0.87; HLA-B*46: weight = 0.12, bootstrap support = 0.70). We therefore examined epitope metrics for carriers of HLA-A*11 (n = 59), HLA-B*46 (n = 40), as well as for carriers of HLA-A*02 as this is another frequent allele in the RV144 cohort (n = 53). We repeated the analysis described above by taking into account separately the predicted epitopes restricted by HLA-A*02, HLA-A*11, and HLA-B*46; including strong and weak binders (focusing only on strong binders reduced the subset of predicted epitopes to a number too small for adequate comparisons).

For these allele-specific comparisons, there was no difference between the vaccine and placebo groups whether evolutionary distances or binding affinity were considered – the smallest p-values were p = 0.206 for evolutionary distances (gp120 vs CM244 for HLA-A*02), and p = 0.123 for binding affinity measures (V2 vs CM244 for HLA-B*46) (Table S2 in file S2). There was a p-value = 0.045 for Nef epitope predictions restricted by HLA-A*11; this result should probably not be viewed as a significant vaccine/placebo distinction given the high number of tests performed, that Nef was not part of the vaccine, and that it is a comparison against the cross-subtype reference (subtype B) while all subjects analyzed here were infected with CRF01_AE viruses.

No relationship between epitopic distances and the duration of HIV-1 infection

We looked at the relationship between the evolutionary distance (defined above) and the mean diversity in each subject, the latter of which can be used as a measure of the age of the infection. The hypothesis is that if the epitope distances track intra-host diversity it could be interpreted as a sign of intra-host evolution, i.e., a post-infection effect. We found no relationship between the epitopic evolutionary distance and the mean diversity in each subject: For V2 CD8 predictions: Spearman correlation coefficient $\rho = -0.113$ (p = 0.283); for V2 CD4 predictions: Spearman correlation coefficient $\rho = 0.011$ (p = 0.929). There was also no relationship between the epitopic evolutionary distance and the number of days since the last negative visit in each subject (V2 CD8 predictions: Spearman correlation coefficient $\rho = -0.188$ (p = 0.071); V2 CD4 predictions: Spearman correlation coefficient $\rho = -0.075$ (p = 0.544)).

Discussion

Here we analyzed epitope predictions derived from HIV-1 genome sequences corresponding to 110 CRF01_AE breakthrough infections in the RV144 trial, including 44 vaccine and 66 placebo recipients. We tested for evidence of a distinction between the vaccine and placebo groups and found evidence potentially suggestive of a weak T cell driven sieve effect among breakthrough viruses as vaccine/placebo comparisons showed a) some evidence of a signal converging on the Env-V2 segment, and b) smaller Gag epitope repertoires in vaccine recipients compared to placebo recipients.

One indication that the V2 signal, although weak, may be genuine is the fact that differences between the vaccine and placebo group were only seen when comparisons were made against CRF01_AE strains (CM244, 92TH023). No difference was seen when subject-derived sequences were compared to epitopes derived from the subtype B MN strain; this appears logical as the MN boost protein would seem unlikely to have elicited a substantial number of cross-reactive T cell responses toward infecting CRF01_AE viruses, which at the epitope level often differed from MN by 4–5 residues out of nine in a CTL epitope. The lack of V2 signal against MN as a reference could be expected as cross-reactivity decreases drastically with more than 2 mutations out of 9 residues in a CTL epitope [10] - a typical instance when epitopes are compared between subtype B and CRF01_AE. An additional factor that may explain the identification of a vaccine/placebo distinction in V2 is the fact that 60% of the CD4 responses detected in a subset of RV144 vaccine recipients were directed against V2 [14], although, paradoxically, these responses were not identified post-infection, suggesting that antigen-specific T cells could possibly have been preferentially infected and deleted [15]. Importantly, it is possible that the signal detected in V2 was the consequence of an antibody-mediated effect, as binding antibodies targeting V2 were associated with a decreased risk of HIV-1 infection in the RV144 trial. As such, two vaccine-associated signatures in V2 [2] that were linked to vaccine-derived binding antibodies [3] were located within predicted CD8/4 epitopes. Overall, it is difficult to hypothesize that T cell driven immune responses played an important role in the protection associated with the RV144 vaccine because few RV144 subjects mounted CD8/CD4 responses following RV144 vaccination [1]. However, we cannot discount that T cell responses may have played a role in

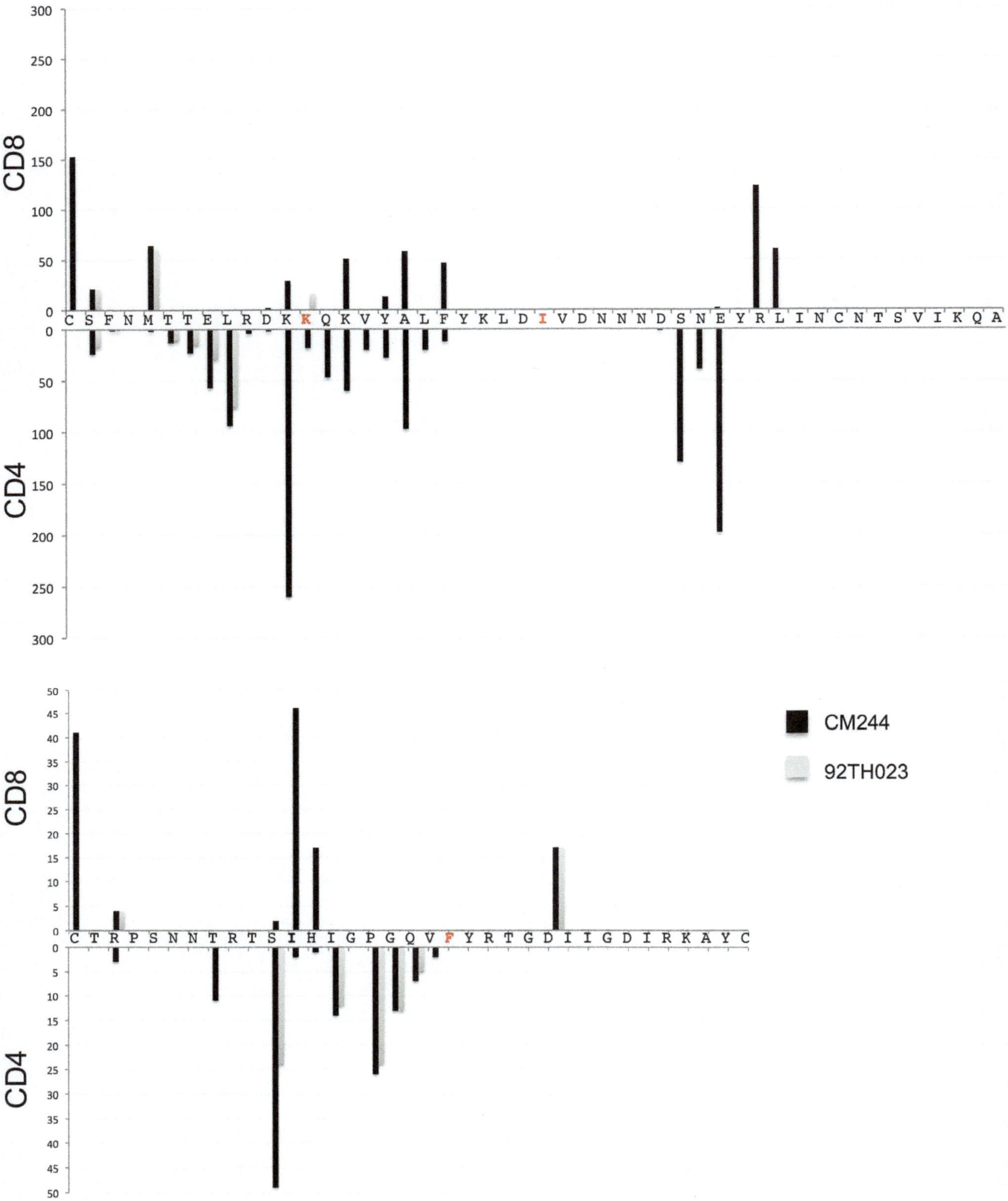

Figure 3. Overlap between predicted CD8 and CD4 epitopes in Env-V2 and -V3 in sequences from HIV-1-infected RV144 participants. The x-axis corresponds to the V2 and V3 sequence, and the y-axis corresponds to the number of predicted epitopes starting at each position. The epitope predictions correspond to all unique HLA/peptide combinations, hence the number of epitope predictions starting at a specific location can surpass the number of subjects in the cohort because a given peptide can be predicted as an epitope for multiple HLA alleles. The amino acids in red correspond to sites that were identified as genetic signatures that distinguished breakthrough sequences from vaccine and placebo recipients.

a more restricted way as the limited sensitivity of the T cell assays employed in the RV144 trial means that some responses may not have been detected.

Our results were generally, but not necessarily, in agreement between the CD8 and CD4 epitope predictions. It has to be noted that CD4 epitopes are less well defined than CD8 epitopes in the context of HIV-1 natural infection, hence *in silico* predictions of CD4 epitopes are less accurate than those for CD8 epitopes. It is possible that the absence of information and algorithms for the prediction of epitopes in HLA class II alleles common in Thailand may underestimate epitope enumeration and bias this analysis. To overcome the uncertainty in epitope predictions, additional analyses were focused on a few V2 epitopes that had been precisely characterized in some RV144 participants ([16]; and personal communication from Mark deSouza and Silvia Ratto-Kim). For example, we specifically looked at predicted epitopes corresponding to the peptide that showed the highest recognition in a study of responses from 25 RV144 vaccine recipients following vaccination: peptide VHALFYKLDIVPIED (AA 172–186) [16]. However, these epitope comparisons focused on the experimental data showed no distinction between vaccine and placebo groups, while this may be due in part to the small number of subjects, it also illustrates the limited congruence between *in silico* predictions and mapped CTL responses, as previously noted [6].

The second signal we identified was the significantly ($p = 0.019$) smaller size of Gag epitope repertoires among vaccine recipients compared to placebo recipients. One interpretation is that there could be more escape mutations in Gag sequences from vaccinees (due to vaccine-induced responses), and that these mutations prevented certain sequence motifs from being recognized as epitopes. Another interpretation is that vaccine efficacy might depend on the number of Gag epitopes in the circulating viruses, implying that viruses with canonical epitopes were more likely to be blocked from establishing infection. Some evidence of a vaccine/placebo distinction in Gag is interesting as Gag is typically a preferential target of T cell responses compared to the V2 region of Env. Indeed, a T cell driven sieve effect may have been expected to be uncovered in an immunodominant region of the proteome, as was shown in a study of the Step trial [6]. Analyses of epitope repertoires from breakthrough infections in the Step trial showed a distinction between the vaccine and placebo group that was largely driven by an effect in Gag. Several factors allowed for the detection of a T cell based signal in Gag in the Step trial: i) most subjects mounted T cell responses following vaccination; ii) there are immunodominant responses in Gag; iii) a Gag immunodominant response (SL9) was restricted by a common allele in the Step cohort (HLA-A*02); iv) Gag is a relatively conserved protein allowing for an easier identification of genetic signals than a more variable protein (such as Env); v) there was no env immunogen to potentially shift immunodominance patterns in vaccinees.

Lastly, our results differ from those of Gartland and colleagues [17], who reported evidence of greater predicted HLA binding escape for an HLA A*02 peptide in vaccine versus placebo recipients, and greater vaccine efficacy in A*02-positive participants than in A*02-negative participants (VE = 54% versus 3%, P = 0.05). We note that a comprehensive test of all HLA alleles in the RV144 cohort failed to show that A*02 modified vaccine efficacy. The differences between our studies could also be due to the fact that the MN-derived V2 peptide linked to the findings by Gartland and colleagues was not included as a predicted epitope in our analysis, because we only considered as a predicted epitope the peptides that had a predicted binding affinity <500 nm (different methods can be used to analyze sequences without conditioning on the presence of potential epitopes [18]). Besides, few MN-derived epitopes were included in our cross-proteome analysis since subtype B- (MN vaccine insert) and CRF01_AE- (breakthrough viruses) derived epitopes were poorly matched; the MN peptide highlighted in [17] showed three to six AA differences with corresponding breakthrough-derived peptides, suggesting a limited probability of cross-reactive CTL responses with the breakthrough peptides (knowing that the MN component of the RV144 vaccine was a protein boost, which would not typically be expected to elicit CTL responses).

In conclusion, while there is some evidence that T cell driven immune responses may have been associated with genetic changes in HIV-1 breakthrough viruses from vaccinees, the fact that most results are not strongly corroborated across our proteome-wide epitope comparisons is consistent with weak CD8-driven cytotoxic T cell responses in RV144. Hence, in the absence of evidence for strong CD8+ T cell epitopic signals across the RV144 vaccine inserts, the most conservative interpretation of our findings for V2 epitope predictions would suggest a relationship to V2-specific binding antibody responses previously identified as a correlate of risk in RV144 [4].

Acknowledgments

Disclaimer: Data correspond to some breakthrough infections in the RV144 vaccine efficacy trial (ClinicalTrials.gov registration number NCT00223080); results of the RV144 trial were published by Rerks-Ngarm and colleagues [1].

We thank Drs. Peter B. Gilbert, Alexandra Schuetz, Rasmi Thomas for helpful discussions and comments on the manuscript.

Author Contributions

Conceived and designed the experiments: MR. Performed the experiments: KD JMC. Analyzed the data: KD MR JMC. Contributed reagents/materials/analysis tools: GK JMC BBL ST ESB DEG WD BSM PTE SRK MdS SRN SN PP JK. Contributed to the writing of the manuscript: MR KD JMC BBL ROC MLR NLM JIM JHK.

References

1. Rerks-Ngarm S, Pitisuttithum P, Nitayaphan S, Kaewkungwal J, Chiu J, et al. (2009) Vaccination with ALVAC and AIDSVAX to prevent HIV-1 infection in Thailand. N Engl J Med 361: 2209–2220.
2. Rolland M, Edlefsen PT, Larsen BB, Tovanabutra S, Sanders-Buell E, et al. (2012) Increased HIV-1 vaccine efficacy against viruses with genetic signatures in Env V2. Nature.
3. Liao HX, Bonsignori M, Alam SM, McLellan JS, Tomaras GD, et al. (2013) Vaccine induction of antibodies against a structurally heterogeneous site of immune pressure within HIV-1 envelope protein variable regions 1 and 2. Immunity 38: 176–186.
4. Haynes BF, Gilbert PB, McElrath MJ, Zolla-Pazner S, Tomaras GD, et al. (2012) Immune-correlates analysis of an HIV-1 vaccine efficacy trial. N Engl J Med 366: 1275–1286.

5. Rolland M, Heckerman D, Deng W, Rousseau C, Coovadia H, et al. (2008) Broad and Gag-biased HIV-1 epitope repertoires are associated with lower viral loads. PLoS ONE 3: e1424.
6. Rolland M, Tovanabutra S, deCamp AC, Frahm N, Gilbert PB, et al. (2011) Genetic impact of vaccination on breakthrough HIV-1 sequences from the STEP trial. Nat Med 17: 366–371.
7. Hurley CK, Mack SJ, Mickelson E, Marsh S, Tilanus MGJ, et al. (2006) HLA typing and informatics. in immunobiology of the human MHC, in J A Hansen (ed), 13th International Histocompatibility Workshop protocols IHWG Press, Seattle, WA: 179–352.
8. Nielsen M, Lundegaard C, Blicher T, Lamberth K, Harndahl M, et al. (2007) NetMHCpan, a method for quantitative predictions of peptide binding to any HLA-A and -B locus protein of known sequence. PLoS ONE 2: e796.
9. Nielsen M, Justesen S, Lund O, Lundegaard C, Buus S (2010) NetMHCIIpan-2.0 - Improved pan-specific HLA-DR predictions using a novel concurrent alignment and weight optimization training procedure. Immunome Res 6: 9.
10. Rolland M, Frahm N, Nickle DC, Jojic N, Deng W, et al. (2011) Increased breadth and depth of cytotoxic T lymphocytes responses against HIV-1-B Nef by inclusion of epitope variant sequences. PLoS ONE 6: e17969.
11. Nickle DC, Heath L, Jensen MA, Gilbert PB, Mullins JI, et al. (2007) HIV-specific probabilistic models of protein evolution. PLoS One 2: e503.
12. Carlson JM, Brumme ZL, Rousseau CM, Brumme CJ, Matthews P, et al. (2008) Phylogenetic dependency networks: inferring patterns of CTL escape and codon covariation in HIV-1 Gag. PLoS Comput Biol 4: e1000225.
13. Karasavvas N, Billings E, Rao M, Williams C, Zolla-Pazner S, et al. (2012) The Thai Phase III HIV Type 1 Vaccine trial (RV144) regimen induces antibodies that target conserved regions within the V2 loop of gp120. AIDS Res Hum Retroviruses 28: 1444–1457.
14. de Souza MS, Ratto-Kim S, Chuenarom W, Schuetz A, Chantakulkij S, et al. (2012) The Thai phase III trial (RV144) vaccine regimen induces T cell responses that preferentially target epitopes within the V2 region of HIV-1 envelope. J Immunol 188: 5166–5176.
15. Douek DC, Betts MR, Hill BJ, Little SJ, Lempicki R, et al. (2001) Evidence for increased T cell turnover and decreased thymic output in HIV infection. J Immunol 167: 6663–6668.
16. de Souza MS, Ratto-Kim S, Chuenarom W, Schuetz A, Chantakulkij S, et al. (2012) The Thai phase III trial (RV144) vaccine regimen induces T cell responses that preferentially target epitopes within the V2 region of HIV-1 envelope. Journal of immunology 188: 5166–5176.
17. Gartland AJ, Li S, McNevin J, Tomaras GD, Gottardo R, et al. (2014) Analysis of HLA A*02 Association with Vaccine Efficacy in the RV144 HIV-1 Vaccine Trial. Journal of virology 88: 8242–8255.
18. Edlefsen PT, Gilbert PB, Rolland M (2013) Sieve analysis in HIV-1 vaccine efficacy trials. Curr Opin HIV AIDS 8: 432–436.

Methodological Challenges in Collecting Social and Behavioural Data Regarding the HIV Epidemic among Gay and Other Men Who Have Sex with Men in Australia

Iryna B. Zablotska[1*], Andrew Frankland[1,2], Martin Holt[3], John de Wit[3], Graham Brown[4,5], Bruce Maycock[5], Christopher Fairley[6,7], Garrett Prestage[1,4]

1 The Kirby Institute, The University of NSW Australia, Sydney, NSW, Australia, **2** School of Psychiatry, The University of NSW Australia, Sydney, NSW, Australia, **3** Centre for Social Research in Health, The University of NSW Australia, Sydney, NSW, Australia, **4** The Australian Research Centre in Sex, Health and Society, La Trobe University, Melbourne, VIC, Australia, **5** Curtin University, Perth, WA, Australia, **6** Central Clinical School, Monash University, Melbourne, VIC, Australia, **7** Melbourne Sexual Health Centre, Melbourne, VIC, Australia

Abstract

Background: Behavioural surveillance and research among gay and other men who have sex with men (GMSM) commonly relies on non-random recruitment approaches. Methodological challenges limit their ability to accurately represent the population of adult GMSM. We compared the social and behavioural profiles of GMSM recruited via venue-based, online, and respondent-driven sampling (RDS) and discussed their utility for behavioural surveillance.

Methods: Data from four studies were selected to reflect each recruitment method. We compared demographic characteristics and the prevalence of key indicators including sexual and HIV testing practices obtained from samples recruited through different methods, and population estimates from respondent-driven sampling partition analysis.

Results: Overall, the socio-demographic profile of GMSM was similar across samples, with some differences observed in age and sexual identification. Men recruited through time-location sampling appeared more connected to the gay community, reported a greater number of sexual partners, but engaged in less unprotected anal intercourse with regular (UAIR) or casual partners (UAIC). The RDS sample overestimated the proportion of HIV-positive men and appeared to recruit men with an overall higher number of sexual partners. A single-website survey recruited a sample with characteristics which differed considerably from the population estimates with regards to age, ethnically diversity and behaviour. Data acquired through time-location sampling underestimated the rates of UAIR and UAIC, while RDS and online sampling both generated samples that underestimated UAIR. Simulated composite samples combining recruits from time-location and multi-website online sampling may produce characteristics more consistent with the population estimates, particularly with regards to sexual practices.

Conclusion: Respondent-driven sampling produced the sample that was most consistent to population estimates, but this methodology is complex and logistically demanding. Time-location and online recruitment are more cost-effective and easier to implement; using these approaches in combination may offer the potential to recruit a more representative sample of GMSM.

Editor: Koustuv Dalal, Örebro University, Sweden

Funding: Gay Community Periodic Survey and PASH study in New South Wales (NSW), Australia, were funded by the NSW Ministry of Health, in Victoria by Victoria Department of Health, and in Queensland by Queensland Health. The CONNECT study was funded by the Project Grant from the National Health and Medical Research Council, Australia (NHMRC 630547). The Kirby Institute and the Centre for Social Research in Health receive funding from the Australian Government Department of Health and Ageing. The funders had no role in study design, data collection and analysis, decision to publish, or preparation of the manuscript.

Competing Interests: The authors have declared that no competing interests exist.

* Email: izablotska@nchecr.unsw.edu.au

These authors contributed equally to this work.

Introduction

In recent decades, a substantial body of research amongst gay men who have sex with men (GMSM) has accumulated, with a particular focus on mapping the trends in a range of social and behavioural factors. An emphasis on behavioural surveillance has been driven by the importance of monitoring behaviours relevant to the transmission of HIV and other sexually transmitted infections (STIs), providing data for targeted HIV and STI prevention policy, and for evaluating health-promotion efforts. [1] In countries with concentrated HIV epidemics among GMSM, there has been a strategic value in focusing on gay and bisexual men living in metropolitan areas [2,3], given the concentration of new HIV infections within this group. [4] Also, accessing a broader, more representative sample of GMSM is challenging, and social-behavioural research and behavioural surveillance have been reliant on a limited number of recruitment methods such as convenience, time-location and online sampling. [5–8] A number of methodological issues persist in the field, including limited generalizability and a lack of certainty over how the samples generated by each recruitment approach differ from one another. [9,10] The absence of a validated sampling frame limits the ability to evaluate these different recruitment approaches, and identify the methodology most likely to produce a representative sample. [11] These issues are critical, given that the utility of behavioural surveillance efforts rest on the identification of representative subgroups that allow researchers to gather reliable data. The importance of these data in guiding health policy and community-based education highlights the potential risk of incomplete or inaccurate surveillance data [12].

In recent years, peer-referral approaches such as Respondent-Driven Sampling (RDS) have become more widespread [13], offering both a methodology for accessing hard-to-reach populations as well as the potential to produce population estimates of key behavioural indicators. [14] Although not free from bias [15], these estimates provide novel social and behavioural data within the GMSM population, as well as an opportunity to explore differences in the behavioural profiles of GMSM accessed via different recruitment approaches. The current study aimed to assess and compare multiple recruitment strategies for studying social and behavioural factors relevant to HIV transmission among GMSM. Additionally, we sought to determine if each sample described the same population, to document the differences in the samples produced by each method, and to explore which method provided the optimal balance between reliability, representativeness, and cost.

Methods

Population and samples

The following data sources were selected to represent different recruitment methods:

1) *Gay Community Periodic Surveys (GCPS), funded by the State Departments of Health* in six Australian jurisdictions, are part of the national HIV behavioural surveillance system and have been used to collected data on HIV related behaviours among gay men annually since 1996. The methodology of data collection has been described previously. [16] Briefly, these repeated surveys employ convenience time-location sampling and recruit gay men at gay community venues, events and clinics. They collect information about socio-demographic characteristics of participants, their sexual partnerships and practices, illicit drug use and testing for HIV and STI. The core socio-demographic and behavioural questions have remained stable since the start of the surveys in 1996.
2) The study of Contemporary Norms in Networks and Communities of GMSM (CONNECT) was funded by the Australian National Health and Medical Research Council. This cross-sectional multi-site survey was specifically focused on: 1) investigating the patterns of connections between individuals in GMSM communities and assess how they shape HIV-related behaviours; 2) assessing the relationship between social norms and sexual practices, and 3) comparing the norms and patterns of behaviour in geographically and epidemiologically distinct GMSM populations in the capital cities of three Australian states New South Wales (NSW), Victoria and Western Australia, in order to identify local community norms and barriers to effective HIV prevention. This quantitative study recruited participants using two recruitment methods: RDS in stage I (CONNECT-I, February 2011- April 2012) and Internet-based recruitment in stage II (CONNECT-II, June - August 2012). The methods of CONNECT-I have been described previously. [17] The online recruitment for CONNECT-II was conducted using online advertisement and e-blast emails about the study to the membership of the Squirt website. This website offers its members the opportunity to meet other men for online connections and finding partners. The same data collection tool was used in both stages, and questions collecting information about socio-demographic characteristics, sexual practices and testing for HIV/STI were adopted from the GCPS. In this analysis, the sample recruited by CONNECT-I was used to examine the characteristics of an RDS sample.
3) As the source of sample(s) recruited online, we considered studies that satisfied the following criteria: 1) participants included men living in the same cities as the participants of the CONNECT-I and GCPS, 2) enrolment was conducted during approximately the same time-frame as in the latter two studies, 3) comparable data collection tools, particularly with respect to socio-demographic, behavioural and testing indicators, and 4) recruitment of GMSM online. The CONNECT-II sample was used as an example of a sample recruited specifically through a single website, and the Pleasure and Sexual Health (PASH) study provided a sample recruited through multiple websites. The PASH study was commissioned and funded by the Departments of Health in the states of NSW, Victoria, South Australia and Western Australia. Its design and methods have been described previously. [18] The study participants were recruited online, and quantitative socio-demographic and behavioural information was collected using tools developed by GCPS.

In all studies included in this analysis behavioural information was collected anonymously; clinical records were not used; personal identifying information was not collected, and participants were not asked to provide written informed consent. For each of the studies included in this analysis, approvals have been obtained from the appropriate Human Research Ethics Committees: for CONNECT – from the University of NSW Australia (HREC 09381) and Curtin University, Perth (SPH-04-2010)); for PASH – from the University of NSW Australia (HREC 07207), and for GCPS - from the University of NSW Australia (HREC 09209).

Data analyses

We used the data from the selected datasets to compare the characteristics of the samples and the prevalence of sexual and testing practices among the participants. The variables of interest included the following socio-demographic factors: age in years (under 25 (reference group), 25–34, 35–44, 45–54 and 55 or more), ethnic background (Anglo-Australian versus Other), level of education (up to three years of high school (reference category), completed high school, tertiary diploma and university degree), having been tested for HIV in the past (Yes versus No), HIV serostatus (positive (reference group), negative or unknown/not sure). We also explored sexual identity of the participants (gay/bisexual (reference group), bisexual, heterosexual and other), indicators of gay social engagement including number of friends who are gay (a few (reference group), some, most or all) and time

Table 1. Estimated population prevalence of socio-demographic and behavioural factors among gay men: CONNECT I study (estimates derived using respondent-driven sampling).

Variables	Crude proportion (n) N=937 [1]%	Point estimate of the population adjusted proportion (%)	95% bootstrapped confidence interval for the population adjusted proportion (%)
Age group (years)			
<25	15.8% (146)	14.9%	9.2%–21.9%
25–34	37.0% (341)	38.8%	30.7%–46.5%
35–44	25.0% (230)	26.3%	19.7%–31.7%
45–54	15.4% (142)	13.7%	8.9%–20.2%
55+	6.8% (63)	6.4%	3.2%–10.9%
Ethnic background			
Anglo-Australian	61.6% (570)	62.9%	56.7%–68.8%
Other	38.4% (356)	37.1%	31.2%–43.3%
Education			
Up to 3 years HS	6.7% (62)	5.7%	3.0%–8.0%
Year 12/HSC/TEE	16.7% (155)	20.5%	15.7%–25.4%
Tertiary diploma	24.2% (224)	24.9%	20.5%–30.7%
University level	52.4% (486)	48.9%	42.5%–55.0%
Ever tested for HIV			
No	9.4% (86)	10.7%	6.2%–16.6%
Yes	90.6% (832)	89.3%	83.4%–93.8%
HIV serostatus			
positive	**11.7%** (110)	7.7%	4.1%–11.3%
negative	75.5% (707)	78.0%	72.3%–83.8%
Don't know/nor sure	12.8% (120)	14.3%	9.5%–19.9%
Sexual identity			
Gay/homosexual	94.2% (855)	96.0%	94.0%–98.1%
Bisexual	3.0% (27)	1.9%	0.5%–3.4%
Heterosexual	0.1% (1)	0.2%	0%–0.4%
Other	2.8% (25)	2.0%	0.5%–3.7%
Gay friends			
A few	0.6% (5)	0.2%	0%–0.8%
Some	**17.3%** (158)	26.2%	20.7%–33.0%
Most	31.7% (290)	34.5%	29.2%–40.4%
All	**50.6%** (463)	39.1%	31.6%–45.3%
Time spent with gay friends			
A little	**0.5%** (5)	0.0%	–
Some	**13.7%** (126)	20.2%	15.0%–27.5%
Most	39.1% (359)	39.1%	33.0%–44.8%
All	46.6% (428)	40.7%	32.7%–47.7%
No sex partners (last 6 months)			
One	24.7% (217)	31.5%	24.7%–38.0%
2–5	7.3% (64)	8.3%	5.2%–12.0%
6–10	28.6% (252)	32.1%	26.6%–38.5%
11–20	15.1% (133)	12.5%	8.8%–17.1%
21–50	**21.0%** (185)	13.6%	9.4%–17.4%
>50	3.3% (29)	2.0%	0.7%–3.7%
Anal sex with regular partners			
No partners	45.8% (360)	41.2%	33.1%–47.2%

Table 1. Cont.

Variables	Crude proportion (n) N = 937 [1]%	Point estimate of the population adjusted proportion (%)	95% bootstrapped confidence interval for the population adjusted proportion (%)
No anal sex	5.0% (39)	5.1%	2.1%–8.5%
All anal sex with condoms	11.1% (87)	8.4%	5.5%–13.2%
Some anal sex without condoms	**38.2%** (300)	45.3%	38.5%–52.9%
Anal sex with casual partners			
No partners	30.9% (281)	37.2%	30.5%–44.1%
No anal sex	4.3% (39)	4.6%	2.0%–7.3%
All anal sex with condoms	29.6% (269)	28.2%	22.7%–33.8%
Some anal sex without condoms	35.3% (321)	30.1%	24.5%–36.3%

[1]Denominators for individual variables may differ from the grand total due to some missing responses.
Note; Highlighted in bold are variable categories where the crude estimates fall outside the asymptotically unbiased estimates of the 95% bootstrapped confidence intervals.

spent with gay friends (a little (reference group), some, most and all), and sexual practices in the preceding six months including number of sex partners (one (reference group), 2–5, 6–10, 11–20, 21–50 or more than 50), and unprotected anal intercourse, separately for regular and casual partners (UAIR and UAIC respectively, both coded as no partners, no anal sex, all sex with condoms or some sex without condoms).

We also used the RDS sample from the CONNECT-I study and RDS partition analysis to produce population estimates of the indicators considered in this analysis. Table 1 presents crude proportions and the asymptotically unbiased prevalence. The RDSII estimator was used to derive sampling weights for each variable for further calculation of asymptotically unbiased estimates. Bootstrapping with 1,000 replicates was used to calculate the population prevalence confidence intervals. Although these estimates are unlikely to be free from bias, they are more likely to be less biased than estimates from the selected samples due to the use of weighting for the probability of selection of recruits. [10] We compared the sample proportions across the studies that used different recruitment methods, specifically convenience time-location sampling, RDS and convenience online sampling, and also compared the sample estimates with the population level estimates produced by RDS partition analysis. The only other data source that previously produced population estimates of interest was the telephone-based survey used by the Australian Study of Health and Relationships (ASHM). [19,20] Because it was conducted almost a decade prior to the selected studies (in 2003) and had limited number of indicators of interest, it had limited value for our comparison.

As the CONNECT–I study was conducted in NSW, Victoria and Western Australia, and population estimates of interest could be obtained for only these three jurisdictions, we limited the samples from all studies to only those participants who reported living in these three states.

We used Pearson's $\chi 2$ test for independence and logistic regression with Type I error of 5% to compare the proportions. All analyses were executed in STATA 12.0 (StataCorp, College Station, TX, USA).

Results

The crude and estimated population proportions of socio-demographic and behavioural characteristics of gay men in three major Australian states of New South Wales, Victoria and Western Australia are presented in Table 1. The majority of Australian GMSM was estimated to identify as gay or homosexual, and to report high levels of gay social engagement. Estimated HIV testing rates were high, with 89.3% (83.4–93.8%) having ever been tested. Population levels of unprotected anal intercourse were estimated to be at 45.3% (38.5%–52.9%) with regular partners and 30.1% (24.5%–36.3%) with casual partners. The comparison of crude and population-adjusted proportions shows that crude proportions for most variable categories fall within the confidence limits of the asymptotically unbiased estimates of the population-adjusted proportions, indicating little relative bias.

The distributions of the same socio-demographic and behavioural factors in the samples recruited using different recruitment approaches are presented in Table 2. GCPS includes 10,842 men, who were recruited using convenience time-location sampling. CONNECT-I recruited 937 men using RDS, CONNECT-II recruited 667 men online through a single website and PASH recruited 2,306 GMSM online through various websites. GCPS was a behavioural surveillance sample and was used as a reference group in comparisons of the socio-demographic and behavioural characteristics across the samples. CONNECT-I was generally similar to the GCPS with respect to age (except that it had a significantly higher proportion of men aged 25–34 as compared to the rest of the sample). Both online-recruited samples had more age differences compared to the GCPS than CONNECT-I. The proportion of Anglo-Australian men was significantly lower in CONNECT-I and PASH than in the GCPS. As to level of education and having ever being tested for HIV, men in the CONNECT-I were largely similar to those in the GCPS sample; the online samples were less similar. CONECT-I and PASH were similar to the GCPS with respect to HIV serostatus. Significant differences were observed across the samples with respect to sexual identity, particularly the online samples recruited significantly higher proportions of bisexual men and, respectively, lower proportions of men who identified themselves as gay or homosexual. Significant differences were observed across all

Table 2. Comparison of sample proportions of socio-demographic and behavioural factors among gay men recruited using different sampling methods.

Study name (Sampling method)	GCPS (Time-location)	CONNECT I (Respondent-driven)		CONNECT II (Internet-based, a single website)		PASH (Internet-based, multiple websites)	
Variables	**Sample propor tion**	**Sample propor tion**	**Chi2 test p-value for the comparison with GCPS sample**	**Sample propor tion**	**Chi2 test p-value for the comparison with GCPS sample**	**Sample propor tion**	**Chi2 test p-value for the comparison with GCPS sample**
	N = 10,842	**N = 937**		**N = 667**		**N = 2,306**	
Age group (years)							
<25	15.1	15.8	0.557	12.33	0.065	21.3	**0.000**
25–34	32.6	37.0	**0.007**	21.11	**0.000**	30.1	**0.043**
35–44	27.1	25.0	0.161	24.66	0.197	27.1	0.978
45–54	16.8	15.4	0.269	26.52	**0.000**	15.1	0.078
55+	8.4	6.8	0.101	15.37	**0.000**	6.5	**0.008**
Ethnic background							
Anglo-Australian	65.9	61.6	**0.008**	69.4	0.074	62.9	**0.007**
Other	34.2	38.4	**0.008**	30.6	0.074	37.1	**0.007**
Education							
Up to 3 years HS	7.3	6.7	0.515	10.2	**0.008**	12.1	**0.000**
Year 12/HSC/TEE	18.0	16.7	0.326	15.0	0.061	13.9	**0.000**
Tertiary diploma	20.6	24.2	**0.011**	26.7	**0.000**	20.4	0.831
University level	54.1	52.4	0.326	48.1	**0.005**	53.6	0.688
Ever tested for HIV							
No	10.6	9.4	0.233	20.9	**0.000**	15.2	**0.000**
Yes	89.4	90.6	0.233	79.1	**0.000**	84.8	**0.000**
HIV serostatus							
positive	10.3	11.7	0.17	8.1	0.067	9.4	0.193
negative	75.7	75.5	0.848	60.0	**0.000**	75.4	0.711
Don't know/nor sure	14.0	12.8	0.329	31.9	**0.000**	15.2	0.114
Sexual identity							
Gay/homosexual	88.5	94.2	**0.000**	69.7	**0.000**	87.4	0.138
Bisexual	6.3	3.0	**0.000**	27.7	**0.000**	10.3	**0.000**
Heterosexual	2.8	0.1	**0.001**	0.5	**0.004**	0.4	**0.000**
Other	2.4	2.8	0.507	2.1	0.649	2.0	0.228
Gay friends							
A few	1.4	0.6	**0.035**	12.1	**0.000**	4.9	**0.000**
Some	16.6	17.3	0.603	34.7	**0.000**	35.6	**0.000**

Table 2. Cont.

Study name (Sampling method)	GCPS (Time-location)	CONNECT I (Respondent-driven)		CONNECT II (Internet-based, a single website)		PASH (Internet-based, multiple websites)	
Variables	**Sample propor tion**	**Sample propor tion**	**Chi2 test p-value for the comparison with GCPS sample**	**Sample propor tion**	**Chi2 test p-value for the comparison with GCPS sample**	**Sample propor tion**	**Chi2 test p-value for the comparison with GCPS sample**
	N = 10,842	**N = 937**		**N = 667**		**N = 2,306**	
Most	36.7	31.7	**0.003**	31.1	**0.008**	27.9	**0.000**
All	45.4	50.6	**0.002**	22.1	**0.000**	31.6	**0.000**
Time spent with gay friends							
A little	1.7	0.5	**0.012**	8.0	**0.000**	7.9	**0.000**
Some	17.1	13.7	**0.008**	36.3	**0.000**	31.6	**0.000**
Most	40.8	39.1	0.318	34.7	**0.004**	39.6	0.269
All	40.4	46.6	**0.000**	21.0	**0.000**	21.0	**0.000**
No sex partners (last 6 months)							
One	13.9	24.7	**0.000**	12.7	0.524	14.3	0.621
2–5	22.2	7.3	**0.000**	7.9	**0.000**	21.7	0.622
6–10	26.2	28.6	0.111	32.0	**0.022**	25.9	0.815
11–20	14.7	15.1	0.708	19.6	**0.015**	14.3	0.677
20–50	19.0	21.0	0.134	22.5	0.118	20.5	0.095
>50	4.1	3.3	0.237	5.4	0.269	3.3	0.055
Anal sex with regular partners							
No partners	42.0	45.8	**0.038**	76.6	**0.000**	44.7	**0.019**
No anal sex	6.4	5.0	0.108	2.4	**0.000**	7.2	0.189
All anal sex with condoms	17.5	11.1	**0.000**	5.9	**0.000**	10.5	**0.000**
Some anal sex without condoms	34.1	38.2	**0.02**	15.1	**0.000**	37.6	**0.001**
Anal sex with casual partners							
No partners	38.4	30.9	**0.000**	58.2	**0.000**	31.1	**0.000**
No anal sex	12.9	4.3	**0.000**	5.4	**0.000**	11.1	**0.022**
All anal sex with condoms	28.3	29.6	0.403	15.1	**0.000**	29.2	0.372
Some anal sex without condoms	20.4	35.3	**0.000**	21.3	0.593	28.6	**0.000**

Table 3. Comparison of the sample and population estimates of prevalence of socio-demographic and behavioural factors among gay men.

Study name (Sampling method)		GCPS (Time-location)		CONNECT I (Respondent-driven)		CONNECT II (Internet-based, a single website)		PASH (Internet-based, multiple websites)	
Variables	**95% CI for the population estimate**	**Sample propor tion**	**Compared with Population estimate**	**Sample propor tion**	**Compared with population estimate**	**Sample propor tion**	**Compared with population estimate**	**Sample propor tion**	**Compared with population estimate**
		N = 10,842		**N = 937**		**N = 667**		**N = 2,306**	
Age group (years)									
<25	9.2%–21.9%	15.1%		15.8%		12.33%		21.3%	
25–34	30.7%–46.5%	32.6%		37.0%		21.11%	↓	30.1%	↓
35–44	19.7%–31.7%	27.1%		25.0%		24.66%		27.1%	
45–54	8.9%–20.2%	16.8%		15.4%		26.52%	↑	15.1%	
55+	3.2%–10.9%	8.4%		6.8%		15.37%	↑	6.5%	
Ethnic background									
Anglo-Australian	56.7%–68.8%	65.9%		61.6%		69.4%	↑	62.9%	
Other	31.2%–43.3%	34.2%		38.4%		30.6%	↓	37.1%	
Education									
Up to 3 years HS	3.0%–8.0%	7.3%		6.7%		10.2%	↑	12.1%	↑
Year 12/HSC/TEE	15.7%–25.4%	18.0%		16.7%		15.0%	↓	13.9%	↓
Tertiary diploma	20.5%–30.7%	20.6%		24.2%		26.7%		20.4%	↓
University level	42.5%–55.0%	54.1%		52.4%		48.1%		53.6%	
Ever tested for HIV									
No	6.2%–16.6%	10.6%		9.4%		20.9%	↑	15.2%	
Yes	83.4%–93.8%	89.4%		90.6%		79.1%	↓	84.8%	
HIV serostatus									
positive	4.1%–11.3%	10.3%		11.7	↑	8.1%		9.4%	
negative	72.3%–83.8%	75.7%		75.5%		60.0%	↓	75.4	
DK/nor sure	9.5%–19.9%	14.0%		12.8%		31.9%	↑	15.2	
Sexual identity									
Gay/homosexual	94.0%–98.1%	88.5%	↑	94.2%		69.7%	↓	87.4	↓
Bisexual	0.5%–3.4%	6.3%		3.0%		27.7%	↑	10.3	↑
Heterosexual	0%–0.4%	2.8%	↑	0.1%		0.5%	↑	0.4	
Other	0.5%–3.7%	2.4%	↓	2.8%		2.1%		2.0	
Gay friends									
A few	0%–0.8%	1.4%	↑	0.6%		12.1%	↑	4.9	↑
Some	20.7%–33.0%	16.6%	↓	17.3%	↓	34.7%	↑	35.6	↑
Most	29.2%–40.4%	36.7%		31.7%		31.1%		27.9	↓

Table 3. Cont.

Study name (Sampling method)		GCPS (Time-location)		CONNECT I (Respondent-driven)		CONNECT II (Internet-based, a single website)		PASH (Internet-based, multiple websites)	
Variables	**95% CI for the population estimate**	**Sample propor tion**	**Compared with Population estimate**	**Sample propor tion**	**Compared with population estimate**	**Sample propor tion**	**Compared with population estimate**	**Sample propor tion**	**Compared with population estimate**
		N = 10,842		**N = 937**		**N = 667**		**N = 2,306**	
All	31.6%–45.3%	45.4%	↑	50.6%	↑	22.1%	↓	31.6	
Time spent with gay friends									
A little	–	1.7%		0.5%		8.0%		7.9	
Some	15.0%–27.5%	17.1%		13.7%	↓	36.3%	↑	31.6	↑
Most	33.0%–44.8%	40.8%		39.1%		34.7%		39.6	
All	32.7%–47.7%	40.4%		46.6%		21.0%	↓	21.0	↓
No sex partners (last 6 months)									
One	24.7%–38.0%	13.9%	↓	24.7%		12.7%	↓	14.3	↓
2–5	5.2%–12.0%	22.2%	↑	7.3%		7.9%		21.7	↑
6–10	26.6%–38.5%	26.2%		28.6%		32.0%		25.9	↓
11–20	8.8%–17.1%	14.7%		15.1%		19.6%	↑	14.3	
20–50	9.4%–17.4%	19.0%	↑	21.0%	↑	22.5%	↑	20.5	↑
>50	0.7%–3.7%	4.1%	↑	3.3%		5.4%	↑	3.3	
Anal sex with regular partners									
No partners	33.1%–47.2%	42.0%		45.8		76.6%	↑	44.7	
No anal sex	2.1%–8.5%	6.4%		5.0		2.4%		7.2	
All anal sex with condoms	5.5%–13.2%	17.5%	↑	11.1		5.9%		10.5	
Some anal sex without condoms	38.5%–52.9%	34.1%	↓	38.2	↓	15.1%	↓	37.6	↓
Anal sex with casual partners									
No partners	30.5%–44.1%	38.4		30.9		58.2	↑	31.1	
No anal sex	2.0%–7.3%	12.9	↑	4.3		5.4		11.1	↑
All anal sex with condoms	22.7%–33.8%	28.3		29.6		15.1	↓	29.2	
Some anal sex without condoms	24.5%–36.3%	20.4	↓	35.3		21.3		28.6	

↑ significantly higher than the population estimate (p-value<0.05).
↓ significantly lower than the population estimate (p-value<0.05).

studies with respect to gay social engagement (number of gay friends and time spent with gay friends). Participants in both CONNECT studies were different from men in the GCPS in terms of the number of sex partners, while men in PASH were similar to the GCPS participants in this regard. All studies found different prevalence rates of UAIC and UAIR.

We then compared the sample proportions for the same set of variables obtained from each of the four studies with the estimated population proportions (see Table 3). In the GCPS, the distributions of variables measuring age, ethnic background, education, ever being tested for HIV and time spent with gay friends fell within confidence limits estimated for population proportions. The proportion of HIV positive men was overestimated as was the proportion of men identifying themselves as gay/homosexual and heterosexual. Importantly, GCPS overestimated the proportion of men who had 2–5 and more than 20 partners in preceding six months, the proportion of men who always used condoms in anal sex with regular partners and the proportion of men who did not have anal sex with causal partners. CONNECT-I sample proportions were the closest to the population estimates, with only a few differences, most important of which were overestimated proportion of men with 20–50 partners within six months and underestimated proportion of men engaging in UAIR. CONNECT-II sample had significant differences from the population estimates on all variables. PASH fell outside of confidence limits for population estimates of men in the 25 to 34 age group, education, most categories of variables describing gay social engagement and the number of sex partners. Regarding two key indicators of anal sex, all studies underestimated the proportion of men who had UAIR within a six month period and the GCPS samples underestimated the proportion of men having UAIC within a six month period.

A secondary analysis was conducted using the GCPS and PASH samples, based on the observation that these samples tended to differ from the population estimates in the opposite direction from one another. We carried out simulations using a composite of both samples, with different recruitment ratios of participants recruited in physical venues versus online (1:1, 1:2, 1:3, 1:4, 1:5), in order to identify which sample composition was most consistent with population estimates (data not presented; available on request). These simulations demonstrated that as the sample ratio reached 1:5, the observed sample characteristics became more consistent with the population estimates, particularly with regards to UAIC. Regardless of the recruitment ratio, we still observed differences between the composite sample and the population estimates with regards to UAIR, number of sexual partners, and sexual identification.

Discussion

In the current study, we identified differences in the social and behavioural profile of adult GMSM based on how they were recruited, using a number of sampling approaches commonly employed in behavioural surveillance research. Additionally, we presented the population estimates for a number of socio-demographic and behavioural characteristics of GMSM in three major Australia states. Three primary sampling methodologies were utilized: time-location, RDS, and online recruitment. For the latter, two separate samples were recruited via either a single or multiple websites. All samples were recruited from the same source population and collected the same information, which allowed assessing the scope of comparability between the samples recruited using different recruitment methods. Each sample was compared against RDS-derived population estimates with regards to demographic, social and behavioural indicators commonly measured in behavioural surveillance research amongst GMSM.

Men recruited through time-location sampling (GCPS) shared a similar socio-demographic profile as the population estimated by RDS, and no differences were noted in HIV testing or serostatus. These men appeared more connected to the gay community, spending a greater amount of time with a larger number of gay friends then the overall population, which is unsurprising given sample ascertainment. These men also reported a greater number of sexual partners, although they engaged in less unprotected anal intercourse (with either regular or casual partners). Men recruited through RDS were the most consistent with the population estimates, with no socio-demographic differences noted. The RDS sample slightly overestimated the proportion of HIV-positive men, and also appeared to recruit men with an overall higher number of sexual partners. Few behavioural differences were noted, aside from the RDS sample underestimating the proportion of men engaging in UAIR.

GMSM who were recruited through a single-website survey differed considerably from the population estimates. This sample contained a higher proportion of men aged over 45, was less ethnically diverse, and included a greater proportion of men with high-school only education. These men were less likely to have ever undergone HIV testing, and were more likely to be unaware of their HIV status. This method produced a sample of men who appeared to be less connected to the gay community, and who were more likely to report no sexual contact with either a causal or regular partner in the past six months. In comparison, the online sample recruited through multiple websites was more consistent with population estimates. Overall, few socio-demographic differences were noted, although this sample contained more variation in sexual identification. These men tended towards spending less time with gay friends than the overall population, and had fewer gay friends. These findings are consistent with the profiles described in two previous Australian studies the Private Lives-2 [21] and e-Male [22,23], which both reported similar patterns of socio-demographic characteristics, sexual identification and HIV testing history. Few behavioural differences were noted in the PASH sample compared to population estimates, although this sample underestimated the proportion of UAIR as well as the proportion of men who did not engage in any anal intercourse with a casual partner.

The socio-demographic profile of GMSM appeared relatively stable across different sampling methods, with greater differences observed amongst the sample recruited through a single website. This approach seems vulnerable to a self-selection bias, given its reliance on recruiting men who have subscribed to a specific website. When men were recruited through a range of websites, the resulting sample was more consistent with the overall population estimates. The social characteristics that varied the most between samples related to gay social engagement patterns. Unsurprisingly, men recruited through time-location sampling appeared to have greater connections to other gay men, likely driven by the use of established gay social venues as recruitment sites and the explicit focus on recruiting community-attached men in the study.

Of particular interest was the stability of key behavioural indicators, such as sexual practices, which are one of the primary outputs of behavioural surveillance amongst GMSM. Each of the separate recruitment methods produced samples that differed from the RDS-derived population estimates with regards to key behavioural indicators such as unprotected anal intercourse with either casual or regular partners. Data acquired through time-location sampling underestimated the rates of both UAIR and

UAIC, while RDS and online sampling both generated samples that underestimated UAIR. Given that time-location sampling remains the gold-standard recruitment approach for GMSM behavioural research, the finding that a sample recruited using this methodology underestimated the prevalence of sexual practices strongly related to the transmission of HIV is an important one, particularly in the context of reports of increased rates of UAIC and HIV diagnoses. [24] The lower rates of UAIC in the GCPS sample may reflect the reality that GMSM who utilize the venues that serve as recruitment sites are more likely to be exposed to health-promotion messages than men with fewer connections to the gay community, such as those accessed through online recruitment. In addition, these community-attached men are also more likely to be the target audience for many HIV prevention strategies, such as those emphasizing the risk posed by UAIC in the transmission of HIV.

Of the four recruitment approaches, RDS produced the sample with proportions closest to the RDS-derived population estimates. However, several other factors require consideration when comparing sampling methodologies. Each recruitment approach differed in the level of input required, as well as the value or utility of the data it provided. Time-location sampling, as used in the GPCS, is currently a gold-standard method for recruitment GMSM for behavioural surveillance studies, and is capable of producing samples representative of the overall sampling frame as long as the selection of venues is adequate. Additionally, the GCPS in Australia allows for measuring trends over time, with consistent data collection protocols established from 1996. However, this need for consistency limits the flexibility of the content in the GPCS although there has been some scope for collecting one-off data about specific issues. [25] Further, the use of the same venues over time makes the GCPS sensitive to changes in venue clientele. The growing prominence of online social networks as a way to locate sexual partners may limit the potential for the GCPS to capture GMSM who have shifted away from physical venues, particularly young gay men who are underrepresented in typical GCPS samples. [26] The funding and staffing demands of the GCPS are slightly greater than online data collection, although the study's profile in the community limits the amount of advertising required.

Online recruitment offers a clear alternative to time-location sampling, particularly given the prominence of the Internet in gay men's social and sexual networks. [27] It also offers the potential of recruiting a broader sample of GMSM, by including men who are not accessed via traditional location-based recruitment which focus on community-attached gay men. Both the Connect-II and PASH studies had lower costs and logistic demands relative to the GCPS, although advertising requirements were greater. The importance of selecting the websites through which men are recruited appeared critical; the Connect-II study was based on men accessed through a single website, and this sample was perhaps the most divergent from population estimates. The PASH study recruited men through a range of websites and also differed from population estimates with regards to both social and behavioural factors. Intriguingly, the direction of these differences was often in the opposite direction as the differences between the GCPS and the population estimates. Based on our secondary analysis, we observed that combining both venue-based and online recruitment generated a sample with characteristics more consistent to the population estimates than any of the individual recruitment methods. This suggests that online recruitment and time-location sampling tap into overlapping but distinct subgroups with important qualitative differences, and combining the two approaches might offer the potential for recruiting a more inclusive and representative sample of GMSM. Similarly, Guo et al. reported different behavioural and demographic profile amongst Chinese MSM based on sampling methodology, and encouraged the careful selection of multiple recruitment approaches in improving the representativeness of MSM samples [9].

Finally, despite the consistency between population estimates and the group recruited via RDS, this methodology is perhaps too complex and logistically demanding to be easily incorporated into routine behavioural surveillance among GMSM in Australia. This methodology may be more appropriate for investigation of population issues, as well as exploring specific empirical questions rather than ongoing surveillance. It has some value in offering the potential to produce population estimates, as well as utility as a reference for evaluating the reliability of other sampling approaches. Although this methodology can be considered as a potentially superior form of convenience sampling, the results produced by it are still prone to some residual bias and should be interpreted with caution [10].

The current data clearly indicate the potential for different recruitment approaches to produce samples of GMSM with differing social and behavioural profiles. To our knowledge, this is the first study to evaluate the statistical significance of the differences between the samples recruited from the same source population using differing recruitment approaches. The findings suggest the need for careful consideration of the changing nature of social and sexual networks, and the influence this shift has had on data derived from traditional venue-based recruitment methodologies. The current data emphasize the importance of a clear understanding of the relative strengths of each recruitment approach, and the need for a clearly articulated rationale for the selection of a particular method. Rather than a methodological limitation, this highlights an important opportunity for accessing a broader, more representative sample of GSMM by combining traditional time-location sampling with online recruitment. Further investigation of this is necessary, in order to ascertain the most effective and reliable way of gathering the data necessary for providing an empirically sound basis for health-promotion and intervention efforts.

Acknowledgments

The authors would like to acknowledge the key community partners - the state-based AIDS Councils and PLWHA organizations in New South Wales, Victoria and Western Australia for being instrumental in the conduct of the Gay Community Periodic Surveys and the CONNECT study. Many thanks go to all study participants for sharing their life experiences with the research team.

Author Contributions

Conceived and designed the experiments: IZ JDW GB BM CF GP MH. Performed the experiments: IZ JDW GB BM CF GP MH. Analyzed the data: IZ AF. Contributed to the writing of the manuscript: IZ AF. Further contributed to writing the manuscript and preparing it for publication: MH JDW GB BM CF GP.

References

1. World Health Organization (2013) Guidelines for Second Generation HIV Surveillance: An Update: Know Your Epidemic. Available: http://www.ncbi.nlm.nih.gov/books/NBK158982/. Accessed 2014 Oct 14.
2. Rehle T, Lazzari S, Dallabetta G, Samoah-Odei E (2004) Second-generation HIV surveillance: better data for decision-making. BullWorld Health Organ 82: 121–127.

3. Garnett GP, Garcia-Calleja JM, Rehle T, Gregson S (2006) Behavioural data as an adjunct to HIV surveillance data. Sex TransmInfect 82 Suppl 1: i57–i62.
4. The Kirby Institute, The University of New South Wales. (2013) *HIV, viral hepatitis and sexually transmissible infections in Australia:* Annual Surveillance Report 2013. Available: http://kirby.unsw.edu.au/publications. Accessed 2014 Oct 14.
5. McFarland W, Caceres CF (2001) HIV surveillance among men who have sex with men. AIDS 15 Suppl 3: S23–S32.
6. Elford J, Jeannin A, Spencer B, Gervasoni JP, van de Laar MJ, et al. (2009) HIV and STI behavioural surveillance among men who have sex with men in Europe. EuroSurveill 14(47) pii: 19414.
7. Paquette D, Kropp R, Cule S, Wylie J, Husbands W, et al. (2008) HIV prevalence and associated risk behaviours among men who have sex with men (MSM) in Canada.; 2008 7/10/2008; Mexico City, Mexico.
8. Paquette D, De Wit J (2010) Sampling Methods Used in Developed Countries for Behavioural Surveillance Among Men who have Sex with Men. Aids and Behavior 14: 1252–1264.
9. Guo Y, Li XM, Fang XY, Lin XY, Song Y, et al. (2011) A comparison of four sampling methods among men having sex with men in China: implications for HIV/STD surveillance and prevention. Aids Care-Psychological and Socio-Medical Aspects of Aids/Hiv 23: 1400–1409.
10. McCreesh N, Frost SDW, Seeley J, Katongole J, Tarsh MN, et al. (2012) Evaluation of Respondent-driven Sampling. Epidemiology 23: 138–147.
11. Johnston LG, Malekinejad M, Kendall C, Iuppa IM, Rutherford GW (2008) Implementation challenges to using respondent-driven sampling methodology for HIV biological and behavioral surveillance: field experiences in international settings. AIDS Behav 12: S131–S141.
12. Grulich A, O'Donnell D, de Wit JB (2010) Surveillance, epidemiology and behavioural research to guide HIV prevention policy. N S W Public Health Bull. 21(3–4):96.
13. Malekinejad M, Johnston LG, Kendall C, Kerr LR, Rifkin MR, et al. (2008) Using respondent-driven sampling methodology for HIV biological and behavioral surveillance in international settings: a systematic review. AIDS Behav 12: S105–S130.
14. Magnani R, Sabin K, Saidel T, Heckathorn D (2005) Review of sampling hard-to-reach and hidden populations for HIV surveillance. AIDS 19 Suppl 2: S67–S72.
15. McCreesh N, Copas A, Seeley J, Johnston LG, Sonnenberg P, et al. (2013) Respondent Driven Sampling: Determinants of Recruitment and a Method to Improve Point Estimation. Plos One 8(10)
16. Zablotska IB, Kippax S, Grulich A, Holt M, Prestage G (2011) Behavioural surveillance among gay men in Australia: methods, findings and policy implications for the prevention of HIV and other sexually transmissible infections. Sex Health 8: 272–279.
17. Zablotska I, De Wit J, Brown G, Maycock B, Fairley CK, et al. (2013) Protocol for a Respondent-Driven Sampling Study Exploring the Roles of Peer Norms in HIV-Related Practices of Gay Men. World Journal of AIDS 3: 320–326.
18. Prestage G, Down IA, Bradley J, McCann PD, Brown G, et al. (2012) Is Optimism Enough? Gay Men's Beliefs About HIV and Their Perspectives on Risk and Pleasure. Sexually Transmitted Diseases 39: 167–172.
19. Smith AMA, Rissel CE, Richters J, Grulich AE, de Visser RO (2003) Sex in australia: The rationale and methods of the Australian study of health and relationships. Australian and New Zealand Journal of Public Health 27: 106–117.
20. Grulich AE, de Visser RO, Smith AMA, Rissel CE, Richters J (2003) Sex in Australia: Homosexual experience and recent homosexual encounters. Australian and New Zealand Journal of Public Health 27: 155–163.
21. Lyons A, Pitts M, Grierson J, Smith A, McNally S, et al. (2012) Sexual Behavior and HIV Testing Among Bisexual Men: A Nationwide Comparison of Australian Bisexual-Identifying and Gay-Identifying Men. Aids and Behavior 16: 1934–1943.
22. Holt M, Rawstorne P, Wilkinson J, Worth H, Bittman M, et al. (2012) HIV testing, gay community involvement and internet use: social and behavioural correlates of HIV testing among Australian men who have sex with men. AIDS Behav 16: 13–22.
23. Holt M, Rawstorne P, Worth H, Bittman M, Wilkinson J, et al. (2011) Predictors of HIV Disclosure Among Untested, HIV-Negative and HIV-Positive Australian Men Who had Anal Intercourse with Their Most Recent Casual Male Sex Partner. Aids and Behavior 15: 1128–1139.
24. Zablotska IB, Prestage G, Middleton M, Wilson D, Grulich AE (2010) Contemporary HIV diagnoses trends in Australia can be predicted by trends in unprotected anal intercourse among gay men. AIDS 24: 1955–1958.
25. Zablotska IB, Grulich AE, De Wit J, Prestage G (2011) Casual sexual encounters among gay men: familiarity, trust and unprotected anal intercourse. AIDS Behav 15: 607–612.
26. Zablotska IB, Holt M, Prestage G (2012) Changes in gay men's participation in gay community life: implications for HIV surveillance and research. AIDS Behav 16: 669–675.
27. Elford J (2006) Changing patterns of sexual behaviour in the era of highly active antiretroviral therapy. CurrOpinInfectDis 19: 26–32.

Cardiac Health Risk Stratification System (CHRiSS): A Bayesian-Based Decision Support System for Left Ventricular Assist Device (LVAD) Therapy

Natasha A. Loghmanpour[1], Marek J. Druzdzel[2,3], James F. Antaki[1]*

1 Department of Biomedical Engineering, Carnegie Mellon University, Pittsburgh, Pennsylvania, United States of America, **2** Decision Systems Laboratory, School of Information Sciences, University of Pittsburgh, Pittsburgh, Pennsylvania, United States of America, **3** Faculty of Computer Science, Bialystok University of Technology, Bialystok, Poland

Abstract

This study investigated the use of Bayesian Networks (BNs) for left ventricular assist device (LVAD) therapy; a treatment for end-stage heart failure that has been steadily growing in popularity over the past decade. Despite this growth, the number of LVAD implants performed annually remains a small fraction of the estimated population of patients who might benefit from this treatment. We believe that this demonstrates a need for an accurate stratification tool that can help identify LVAD candidates at the most appropriate point in the course of their disease. We derived BNs to predict mortality at five endpoints utilizing the Interagency Registry for Mechanically Assisted Circulatory Support (INTERMACS) database: containing over 12,000 total enrolled patients from 153 hospital sites, collected since 2006 to the present day, and consisting of approximately 230 pre-implant clinical variables. Synthetic minority oversampling technique (SMOTE) was employed to address the uneven proportion of patients with negative outcomes and to improve the performance of the models. The resulting accuracy and area under the ROC curve (%) for predicted mortality were 30 day: 94.9 and 92.5; 90 day: 84.2 and 73.9; 6 month: 78.2 and 70.6; 1 year: 73.1 and 70.6; and 2 years: 71.4 and 70.8. To foster the translation of these models to clinical practice, they have been incorporated into a web-based application, the Cardiac Health Risk Stratification System (CHRiSS). As clinical experience with LVAD therapy continues to grow, and additional data is collected, we aim to continually update these BN models to improve their accuracy and maintain their relevance. Ongoing work also aims to extend the BN models to predict the risk of adverse events post-LVAD implant as additional factors for consideration in decision making.

Editor: Yiru Guo, University of Louisville, United States of America

Funding: Funding was provided by the 1R41 HL120428-01, 1R01HL086918, and U01HL101066-01 National Institutes of Health grants. The funders had no role in study design, data collection and analysis, decision to publish, or preparation of the manuscript.

Competing Interests: The authors have declared that no competing interests exist.

* Email: antaki@cmu.edu

Introduction

Cardiac transplantation currently represents the most definitive treatment for end-stage heart failure (ESHF) with 90% 1-year survival and a 70% 5-year survival. However, there is a need for alternate therapies due to the limited supply of donor organs. For those ineligible for a heart transplant, or unable to wait, an alternative life-sparing therapy is to implant a left ventricular assist devices (LVAD). These devices have been used for nearly 25 years to support ESHF patients while awaiting transplant and have been consistently shown to improve mortality. The technology has now progressed to the point where they are offered as permanent or so-called Destination Therapy (DT). According to current estimates, the number of ESHF patients who may benefit from LVAD therapy is between 80,000 and 200,000 annually. [1]

LVAD Risk Scores

Optimal and responsible use of LVAD therapy requires a procedure for selecting patients who are most likely to benefit, and less likely to suffer adverse complications. In general, as a patient's disease progresses, the probability of poor outcomes increases. It is therefore important to identify candidates early in the progression of their disease so as not to miss the optimal window of opportunity [2,3]. The window is considered between INTERMACS level 7 and 3, where 7 is clinically stable but history of previous decompensation and 3 is stable but Inotrope dependent [4]. This has motivated the development of risk scores to stratify patients based on the factors that have historically been associated with outcomes, such as patient characteristics, advances in mechanical circulatory support technology and surgical experience.

The most commonly cited score is the Lietz-Miller Destination Therapy Risk Score (DTRS), which was derived from a patient cohort with first generation pumps [5]. The first generation LVADs were pulsatile flow pumps, which attempted to mimic the physiological conditions. One-year survival in subjects undergoing the first generation pulsatile flow HeartMate XVE implantation for DT in the Randomized Evaluation of Mechanical Assistance for the Treatment of Congestive Heart failure (REMATCH) trial was 52% [6]. Enrollment criteria of initial studies emphasized hemodynamic variables. The DTRS analyzed 45 baseline parameters and outcomes in 280 DT patients in the post-REMATCH era. The most important determinants of in-hospital mortality were poor nutrition, hematological abnormalities, markers of end-organ and RV dysfunction and lack of inotropic support. Patients were stratified into low, medium, high and very high risk based on a score calculated from these predictors to correspond with 1-year survival [5]. The DTRS, however, has many limitations. The majority of patients in the derivation cohort were ambulatory, older men with large body surface area. Co-morbidities such as diabetes, cardiac cachexia or obesity were under-represented, while psychosocial factors or echocardiographic parameters were not considered.

Since the DTRS was derived, there has been major advances in the technology. In particular, second generation (continuous flow) pumps have become available that are smaller in size, have simpler technique for implantation, longer durability and present reduced risk of thromboembolism, infection and malfunction. Consequently, the frequency of adverse events has diminished, which has further expanded the candidacy pool for LVAD therapy. This has rendered the DTRS less accurate [7]. Other risk scores have been introduced, but are limited for a variety of reasons, such as limited independent variables or limited training data (e.g. from a single center.) For example, a recently introduced HeartMate II Risk Score (HMRS) relies on only five preoperative variables for predicting 90 day survival; the long-term (1 year) model only contained two: age and implant center experience [8].

Clinical Decision Support Systems

The transition from paper to electronic medical records provides both a challenge and great opportunity for clinical decision making. On the one hand, the ever increasing quantity of information collected on a typical LVAD patient can overwhelm a clinical team, and arguably may introduce more uncertainty due to data incompleteness and noisiness. On the other hand, the wealth of information embedded in these data are ideal for computer-based Clinical Decision Support Systems (CDSS) [9,10]. This is the motivation for developing the Cardiac Health Risk Stratification System (CHRiSS). CHRiSS is a web-enabled decision support tool that provides patient-specific predictions of mortality at 5 endpoints post-implant: 30 day, 90 day, 6 month, 1 year and 2 year. It offers several advantages over traditional LVAD risk scores. Since it is based on a Bayesian machine learning algorithm, it can better represent the influence of large sets of interrelated variables as compared to traditional Cox model multivariate predictors [11,12]. Unlike most risk scores which compute survival at one time point, CHRiSS provides predictions of both short-term and long-term mortality. Since CHRiSS is implemented as an interactive software application, it also permits the user to explore various "what if" scenarios.

The purpose of this study is to evaluate the accuracy and sensitivity of the Bayesian Networks (BNs) in the CHRiSS tool. Accuracy is evaluated both in terms of True Negative (ability to predict survival) and True Positive (ability to predict mortality), which is also depicted by the receiver operating characteristics (ROC) curve. Sensitivity analysis was performed to identify the strongest predictive variables that are associated with either increased or decreased chance of survival post-LVAD.

Methods

This study was conducted with a comprehensive dataset, known as the Interagency Registry for Mechanically Assisted Circulatory Support (INTERMACS). This is the largest national registry for U.S. Food and Drug Administration (FDA) approved mechanical circulatory support devices that is jointly sponsored by the National Heart, Lung, and Blood Institute (NHLBI), Centers for Medicare and Medicaid Services (CMS), FDA and industry. The registry has over 12,000 total enrolled patients (over 8,000 continuous flow LVADs) from 153 hospital sitesand has been collecting data since 2006 to the present day. The dataset consists of over 300 pre-implant clinical variables, subdivided into six main categories: demographics, co-morbidities and limitations from transplant listing, laboratory values, hemodynamics, medications and quality of life questionnaires and surveys. A co-morbidity in this context is defined as a medical condition or disease that exists simultaneously with another condition or disease. They can either be independent or related conditions or diseases.

Patient Cohort

Institutional Review Board approval was obtained through hospitals participating within INTERMACS. The study described in this submission was approved by the INTERMACS Data, Access, Analysis, and Publication Committee (DAAP). Written informed consent was acquired from participants before being enrolled in INTERMACS. The Data Coordinating Center at University of Alabama at Birmingham provided us the data once it was de-identified. The data used in the present study was anonymized and de-identified prior to analysis. Inclusion criteria for this study was: use of a continuous flow LVAD as the primary implant and age>19, thus excluding pediatric patients. Patients who ultimately received an Right Ventricular Assist Device (RVAD) were included as long as the initial implant was an LVAD and an RVAD was placed thereafter. The specific type of RVAD was not considered. Total Artificial Heart recipients were excluded from this study. This translated to 8,050 patients from year 2006 to 2013 in the initial dataset. Data from patients whose LVAD was electively removed (e.g., due to transplantation or recovery) were censored at the time of event (See Table 1).

Pre-processing

The raw data from the registry was pre-processed to transform continuous data into discrete bins (required by the Bayesian algorithm) and to fill in missing data, described below.

Discretization. Discretization was done based on a balance of equal frequency binning and published upper and lower limits of clinically normal values [13,14]. Table S1 provides the list of variables with their respective formats and input values. Clinical scenarios and outcomes, such as events during hospitalization, adverse events prior to implant and interventions within 48 hours of implant, were defined using the INTERMACS definitions.

Missing data. The patient records provided by the INTERMACS data set were found to be routinely incomplete (see Table S1 for percentages missing). Missing data was separated into two categories: *missing at random* (MAR), and *missing not at random* (MNAR) [15]. Missing demographics and lab values, for example, were considered to be either MAR, in which case we assumed the most probable values (i.e. BMI between 24–27 since it is considered normal). The method of using normal values has been cited in previous studies to produce superior results compared to

Table 1. Mortality statistics, censored for explant and transplant.

Endpoint	Survival No. (%)	Death No. (%)	Total	Survival SMOTE No. (%)	Death SMOTE No. (%)	Total SMOTE No. (%)
30 Day	7620 (95.2)	387 (4.8)	8007	7620 (90.8)	774 (9.2)	8394
90 Day	7024 (90.5)	737 (9.5)	7761	7024 (82.6)	1474 (17.3)	8498
6 Month	6245 (86.1)	1007 (13.9)	7252	6245 (75.6)	2014 (24.4)	8259
1 Year	5241 (79.7)	1334 (20.3)	6575	5241 (66.2)	2668 (33.7)	7909
2 Year	4432 (72.7)	1667 (27.3)	6099	4432 (57.1)	3334 (42.9)	7766

SMOTE: synthetic minority oversampling technique.

listwise deletion and other methods [16]. Missing co-morbidities, on the other hand were considered MNAR, in which case we assumed that it was not a concern for that patient. This is standard procedure for handling MNAR data in medical datasets. For example, if a patient has no record of a chest x-ray then the doctor probably did not feel the need to order one. In these cases, it is common to assume a "normal" value, which in the case of the x-ray would be *not ordered* as opposed to *unknown*, or simply *missing*. Additional data in the MAR category were missing laboratory and hemodynamic values were designated as *not ordered*. Missing medication data was considered MNAR, in which we assumed that no such medication was prescribed. Finally, missing quality of life metrics were considered MNAR, and designated as *unknown*. This was justified based on voluntary and sporadic participation in the two quality of life surveys, the EuroQoL [17] (offered since the beginning of the registry)and the Kansas City Cardiomyopathy Questionnaire (KCCQ) [18] implemented after 2012.

Synthetic Minority Oversampling Technique (SMOTE)

A common challenge in data mining that inhibits the predictive ability of the model, is an uneven distribution of the outcome (survival post-LVAD). In medicine, there is often a larger portion of the cohort that are free of death or adverse event as compared to the number of events. The 30-day mortality rate in INTERMACS is 4.8%, compared to a 95.2% survival rate. With such a discrepancy, the model will always predict the majority class (survival) if uncertain how to classify a new patient. This will pose a setback clinically, as it is most important to identify the high-risk patients (early mortality).

One of the most frequently cited methods for addressing this bias is SMOTE [19], which is used when the minority class is increased by creating synthetic examples rather than by over-sampling with replacement. The minority class (mortality) is over-sampled by taking each minority class sample and introducing synthetic examples along the line segments joining any or all of the k minority class nearest neighbors. For this study we increased the minority class by 100%, which would essentially double the mortality number at each endpoint, while the survival number remained unchanged. The 100% was identified by incrementally increasing the percentage from 0% to 100% and identifying the best performing percentage. We set the cut off at 100% to ensure there would be at least an even number of actual and synthetic cases, as opposed to more synthetic compared to actual cases. Synthetic samples are generated by taking the difference between the instance (or patient) under consideration and its nearest neighbor. This difference was multiplied by a random number between 0 and 1, and added to the feature vector under consideration. (This causes the selection of a random point along the line segment between two specific features.) SMOTE effectively forces the decision region of the minority class to become more general. Table 1 juxtaposes the dataset before and after application of SMOTE.

Bayesian Networks

The machine learning methods used for the present study were built upon Bayesian techniques used previously by our group for multiple decision support studies, including: optimal VAD weaning [20], the need for right ventricular support due to right ventricular failure [21–23] and a two-center study to predict 90-day survival for continuous flow LVADs [24,25]. Bayesian networks (BNs) [26] are acyclic directed graphs in which nodes represent random variables and directed arcs (represented as arrows) between pairs of variables represent influences between them. In addition to the graph structure, a BN is equipped with conditional probability tables (CPT), associated with each node, and describes the probability distribution over the variable's values conditional on all combinations of values of its immediate predecessors (parents) in the graph. A BN is a representation of a factorization of the joint probability distribution over its variables. Independence between a pair of variables is represented by absence of a directed arrow between these variables. Explicit representation of independences results in significant savings in the number of parameters necessary to represent the complete joint probability distribution, making BNs highly practical even in very complex domains.

The joint probability distribution represented by a BN can be updated in the light of new evidence by means of Bayes theorem. Efficient algorithms exist that given observed values of some of the variables, produce the new joint (conditional) probability distribution over the remaining variables. While the quality of the results rests on the quality of the underlying representation of the joint probability distribution, BNs have been shown to be very robust to precision of their parameters [27] and there are indications that possible errors in structure (i.e., incorrect independences) have also limited influence on the quality of the results [28].

To illustrate, one may consider a simple BN model in Figure S1, modeling risk factors related to LVAD survival. The network models the joint probability distribution over the four factors and the survival variable. Not all variables need to be known. For example, we could derive from the network the average survival probability for a center with limited LVAD experience.

For this study, we evaluated four BNs: *Näive Bayes*, *Tree-Augmented Näive Bayes*, *Bayesian Search* and the *Greedy Thick Thinning Algorithm* [29]. We ultimately chose the *Greedy Thick Thinning Algorithm* as the final model based on a tradeoff between complexity and accuracy. The model starts with an empty graph and iteratively adds and removes arcs as it builds the

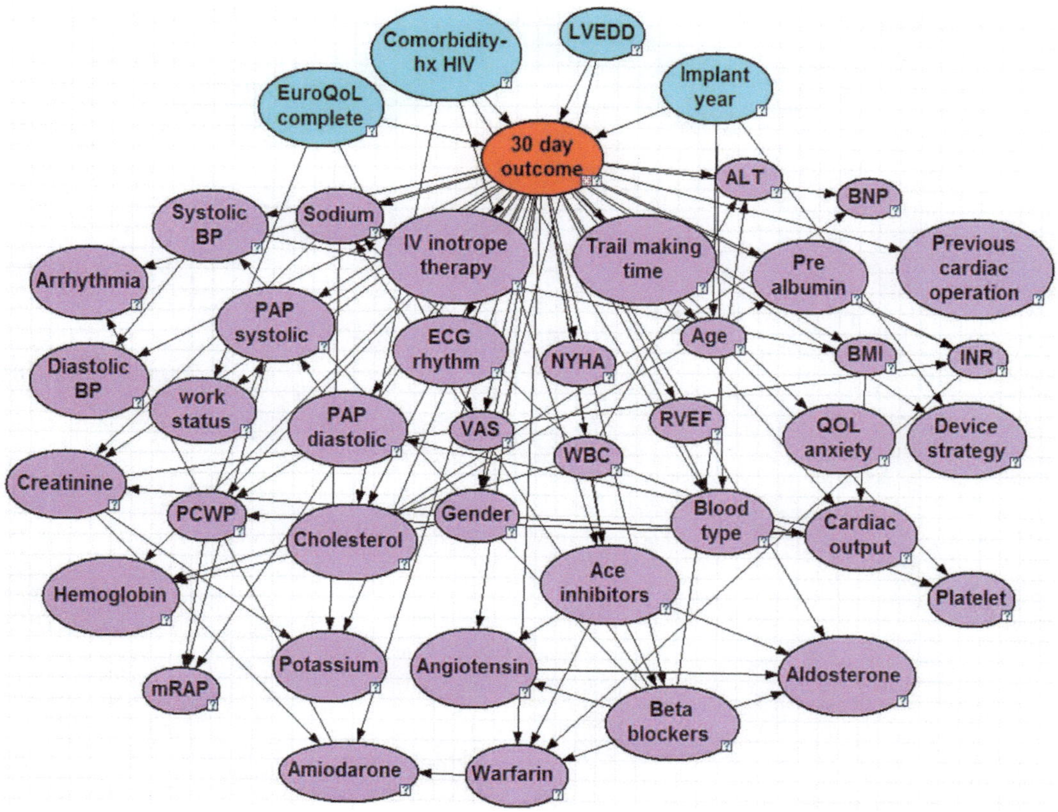

Figure 1. 30 Day Bayesian Model. Node colors: red = class, blue = parent, purple = child. Question marks identify nodes that do not have specific evidence set and use the population distribution as the prior distribution. LVEDD = left ventricle end diastolic diameter, ALT = alanine transaminase, BP = blood pressure, mRAP = mean right atrial pressure, PCWP = pulmonary capillary wedge pressure, VAS = visual analog scale, BNP = B-type natriuretic peptide, WBC = white blood cell, NYHA = New York Heart Association functional class, RVEF = right ventricle ejection fraction, INR = international normalized ratio, BMI = body mass index, ECG = Electrocardiography, QOL = quality of life, hx HIV = history of human immunodeficiency virus.

network, incrementally increasing the Bayesian scoring metric: in this case, the K2 prior distribution over the parameters [30].

Markov Blanket

We applied the Markov Blanket to simplify the network and reduce the likelihood of over-fitting the model to the dataset (i.e. performs well only on the training data, but unable to generalize to other datasets). It has been shown in previous studies that using the Markov Blanket is one of the most effective and efficient methods of feature selection [31]. The Markov Blanket for each of the BN models was comprised of the class node and the family of nodes that make it conditionally independent of all other nodes in the network. This includes the parents, the children and the parents of the children, or spouses [26].

Evaluation

Ten-fold cross validation was the vehicle for model derivation and optimization. The BN classifiers were evaluated on an independent testing/holdout dataset comprised of a training set of approximately 90% of the data records and a testing set from the remaining approximate 10%. The models were derived, built and implemented using two open-source machine learning software libraries: The GeNIe modeling environment developed by the Decision Systems Laboratory of the University of Pittsburgh [32] and the machine learning library WEKA (Waikato Environment for Knowledge Analysis) [33]. Performance metrics included: Accuracy, True Positive, True Negative and area under the ROC curve (AUC). A sensitivity analysis was also performed, where all variables are kept constant and a single parameter is changed to observe the direct affects. This is then expanded to change additional parameters to visualize their additive affects.

Results

The optimized BNs can be seen in Figures 1–5, and a summary of their performance can be found in Table 2. Accuracy was greatest for the 30 day model with 95% and lowest for the 2 year model with 71%. The True Positive (proportion of patients who were correctly predicted to not survive) was greatest for the 2 year at 65% and lowest for the 90 day model at 23%. The True Negative (proportion of patients who were correctly predicted to survive past the endpoint) was greatest for the 30 day model at nearly 100% and lowest for the 2 year model at 76%. The ROC % was greatest for the 30 day model at 93% and lowest for the 6 month, 1 year and 2 year models (all 71%).

30 Day Model

The 30-day mortality model consisted of 44 nodes and 93 arcs. There are four parent nodes for 30 day mortality: whether or not a patient completed the EuroQoL survey, a history of HIV, implant year, and left ventricular end diastolic dimension (LVEDD), an indicator of dilated cardiomyopathy. Positive HIV was the strongest predictive node, followed by the implant year. When a

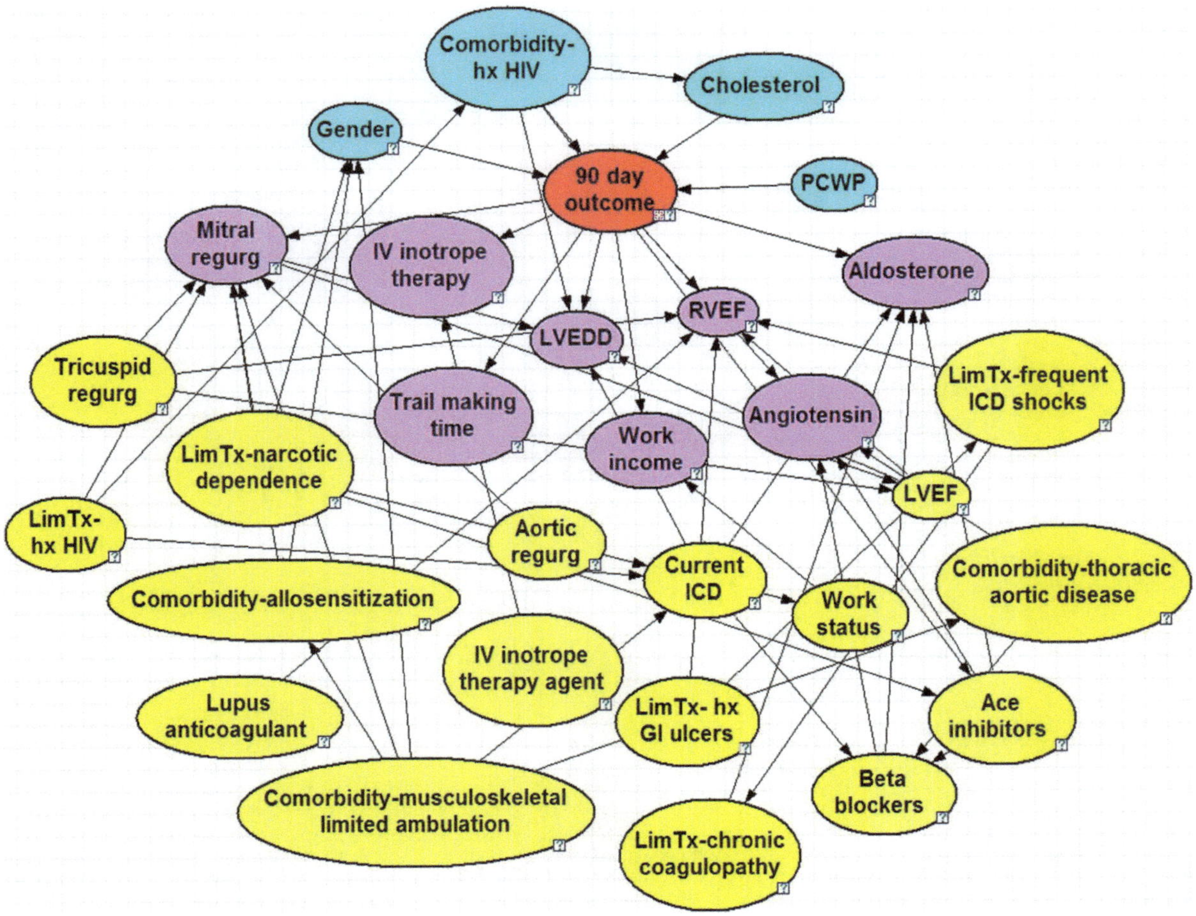

Figure 2. 90 Day Bayesian Model. Node colors: red = class, blue = parent, purple = child, yellow = spouse. Question marks identify nodes that do not have specific evidence set and use the population distribution as the prior distribution. LVEDD = left ventricle end diastolic diameter, PCWP = pulmonary capillary wedge pressure, RVEF = right ventricle ejection fraction, LVEF = left ventricle ejection fraction, hx HIV = history of human immunodeficiency virus, ICD = implantable cardioverter defibrillator, Lim tx = limitation for transplant listing, GI = gastrointestinal, IV = intravenous.

patient is indicated to have a history of HIV, then the baseline likelihood of survival drops from 95% (when no patient-specific evidence is specified) to 53% and drops further to 43% chance of survival when the LVEDD is above 75 mm. The children nodes includes a combination of laboratory values (sodium, BNP and platelets), hemodynamics (mean right arterial pressure, diastolic blood pressure and ECG rhythm), demographics (age and gender) and pre-implant medication (beta blockers, aldosterone and amiodarone). This model was the one exception to using the Markov Blanket, as it would approach nearly 150 nodes with the inclusion of the spousal nodes and would be more prone to over-fitting the dataset. For the model, we simply used the parents and children nodes, which put it at a comparable size as the other endpoint Bayesian models.

90 Day Model

The 90-day model consisted of 30 nodes and 56 arcs. There are four parent nodes: gender, co-morbidity of HIV, cholesterol and pulmonary capillary wedge pressure. History of HIV decreased 90-day chance of survival from 87% to 52% and, when combined with elevated cholesterol (above 150 mg/dL), further decreases to 47%. The chance of survival increases (as compared to the baseline) to 91% if a patient's cholesterol is below 110 mg/dL and they do not have HIV. The children nodes include variables such as mitral regurgitation, right ventricular ejection fraction and work income. Spouse nodes include tricuspid and aortic regurgitation, pre-implant beta blockers, pre-implant ace inhibitors, and left ventricular ejection fraction.

6 Month Model

The 6-month model consisted of 34 nodes and 70 arcs. There are five parent nodes: limitation for transplant due to thoracic aortic disease, creatinine, number of cardiac hospitalizations within the 12 months prior to LVAD implant, cholesterol and HIV. Compared to the baseline chance of survival at 6 months of 76%, the limitation for transplant reduces to 48%, and when combined with creatinine levels below 1.1 mg/dL further reduces to 37%. The children nodes include variables such as BMI, work income and angiotensin. Spouse nodes include presence of an implantable cardioverter defibrillator (ICD), admission reason before implant, history of gastrointestinal bleeding, limitation for transplant listing due to advanced age, and the INTERMACS profile (from level 1 critical cardiogenic shock to level 7 resting heart failure symptoms but stable).

1 Year Model

The 1-year model consisted of 39 nodes and 76 arcs. There are six parent nodes: co-morbidity of HIV, limitation for transplant

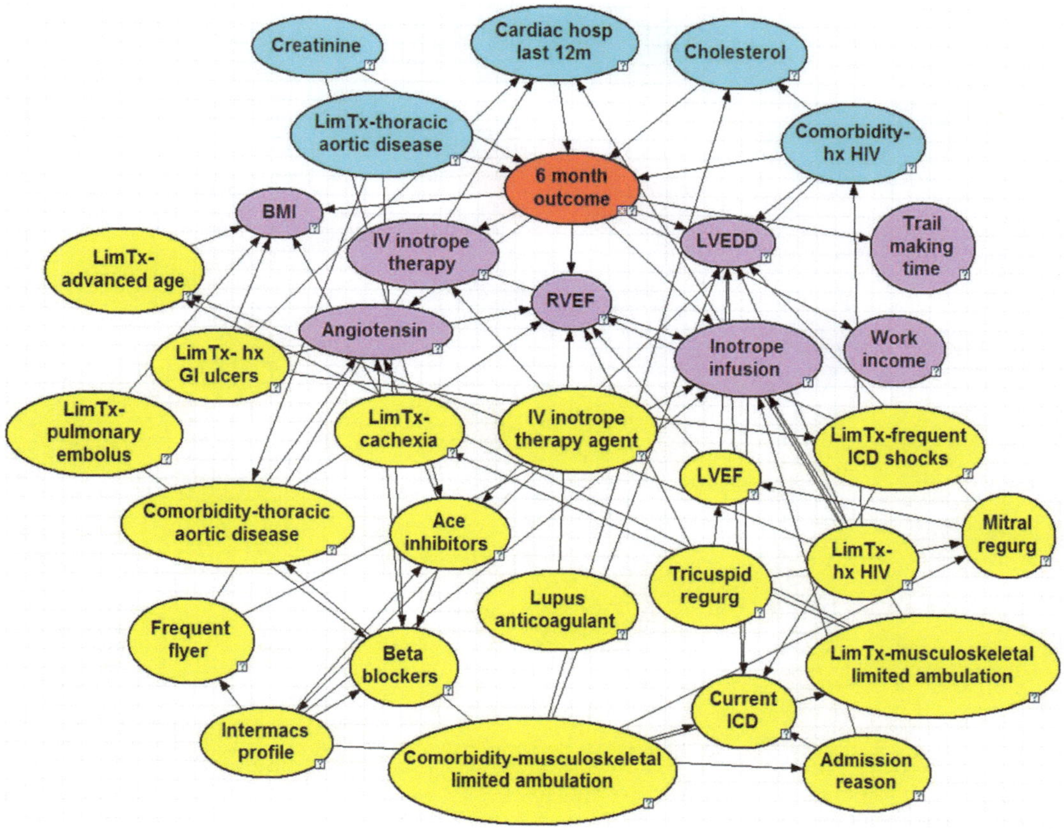

Figure 3. 6 Month Bayesian Model. Node colors: red = class, blue = parent, purple = child, yellow = spouse. Question marks identify nodes that do not have specific evidence set and use the population distribution as the prior distribution. LVEDD = left ventricle end diastolic diameter, RVEF = right ventricle ejection fraction, LVEF = left ventricle ejection fraction, hx HIV = history of human immunodeficiency virus, BMI = body mass index, ICD = implantable cardioverter defibrillator, Lim tx = limitation for transplant listing, GI = gastrointestinal, IV = intravenous.

listing due to thoracic aortic disease, gender, implant year, limitation for transplant listing due to pulmonary hypertension and cholesterol. The baseline chance of survival at 1 year post-implant is 75%, and more recent implants (2013) have higher chances of survival (86%) compared to implants done between 2008–2010 (64–66%). Although this is likely due to shorter follow up times for the more recent implants, it may also reflect advances in implant techniques and changes in the patient post-VAD management. Similar to the other models, both a history of HIV and thoracic aortic disease have major impacts on the chance of 1 year survival. The children nodes include age, right ventricular ejection fraction, BMI, ace inhibitors and diastolic blood pressure. Spouse nodes include admission reason, systolic blood pressure, the INTERMACS profile, temporary mechanical circulatory device, current ICD and co-morbidity due to cachexia (malnutrition).

2 Year Model

The model for 2-year mortality consisted of 45 nodes and 78 arcs. There are eight parent nodes: pro-BNP, BNP, co-morbidity of solid organ cancer, implant year, gender, limitation for transplant listing due to limited social support, patient refusal for transplant listing, and limitation for transplant listing due to large BMI. The baseline 2-year chance of survival is 69%, which increases by 5% if the patient's BNP levels are below 540 pg/dL and increases further to 84% if the implant was done more recently. The chance of survival falls below the baseline (to 62%) if BNP is elevated above 1200 pg/dL, drops further to 58% if the patient declines transplant listing and drops even further to 50% if the patient also has limited social support. The children nodes included age, trail making time (a neuro-psychological test of visual attention and task switching), co-morbidity due to a history of illicit drug use and blood type. Spousal nodes included limitation for transplant listing due to peripheral vascular disease, the INTERMACS profile, being a so-called *frequent flyer* (patients who are repeatedly in and out of the hospital emergency room), the IV inotrope therapy agent and age.

HMRS

The HMRS was derived and validated for 90-day and 1-year mortality and identifies patients as either low risk (4–8% mortality), medium risk (11–16% mortality) or high risk (25–29% mortality). When applied to the INTERMACS database, 93.1% of patients were predicted as low risk with a 9% morality rate, 4.4% were predicted as medium risk with a 16% mortality rate, and 2.3% were predicted as high risk with a 14.6% mortality rate. The ROC for the 90-day HMRS score was 60.3% compared to 73.9% for the 90-day CHRiSS model and the 1-year HMRS score 57.4% compred to 70.9% for the 1-year CHRiSS model.

Discussion

The decision to refer a patient for LVAD therapy entails processing numerous, dynamically evolving and inter-related

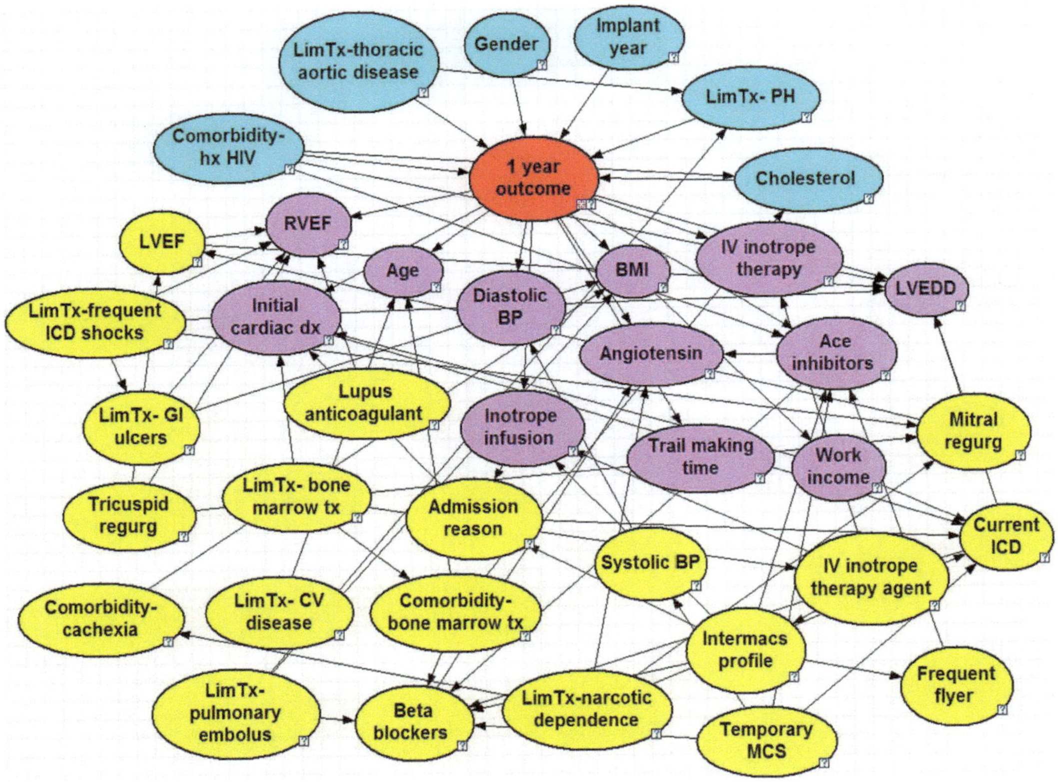

Figure 4. 1 Year Bayesian Model. Node colors: red = class, blue = parent, purple = child, yellow = spouse. Question marks identify nodes that do not have specific evidence set and use the population distribution as the prior distribution. LVEDD = left ventricle end diastolic diameter, RVEF = right ventricle ejection fraction, BMI = body mass index, lim tx PH = limitation for transplant listing due to pulmonary hypertension, IV = intravenous, ICD = implantable cardioverter defibrillator, CV = cardiovascular, GI = gastrointestinal, BP = blood pressure, hx HIV = history of human immunodeficiency virus, MCS = mechanical circulatory support.

clinical variables, which is a complex task filled with uncertainty. The trajectory by which a patient may be offered the option to receive a LVAD involves multiple specialties and decision points. The extensive volume of information and data that must be considered (demographics, labs, history, family support, insurance, etc.) is at odds with the rapidity with which some decisions must be made. Deferring a decision to implant an LVAD, may allow the severity of ESHF to progress thereby increasing the likelihood of an adverse event. Lietz and Miller describe an "optimal window" for LVAD implantation, beyond which the operative risk may deem the intervention futile. However, the key to successful and timely implementation of LVAD therapy is the proper identification of the patient who will benefit from this type of therapy: before clinical instability occurs, which has a major impact on the downstream morbidity and mortality with this intervention.

The advanced heart failure team must evaluate risk in terms of both immediate complications as well as likelihood of repeated readmissions due to longer-term complications. Hence there is a need for a CDSS to aid the physicians in pre-LVAD candidate assessment, by providing personalized risk predictions to ultimately encourage earlier intervention in the appropriate patients. We envision two steps (with iteration) when using CHRiSS: the clinician would first input the variables available for that patient and calculate their initial risk and then adjust actionable variables to perform the "what if" scenarios. For example, a clinician assessing a patient who is initially malnourished (has lower levels of albumin), could then adjust the albumin to the normal range and see if the prognosis improves and by how much.

Such a dynamic CDSS does not exist for advanced HF patients and the BNs offer several advantages over the traditional statistical methods used to derive risk scores such as the HMRS or DTRS. Current risk scores are limited by their: (1) simplistic four to nine variable summed scoring system; (2) inability to co-evolve with the changing HF risk factors and emerging treatment options; and (3) requirement to know a fixed set of variables and inability to be computed when any are missing. BNs address these limitations, as they are able to: (1) account for hundreds of inter-related variables in a single model; (2) dynamically update as risk factors change and different drugs are created; and (3) compute predictions with missing values by using the prior probabilities encoded within each variable node. The current study demonstrated the potential for developing advanced CDSS based on these models in the domain of HF, as well as other medical applications.

For example, in the absence of any decision tool, expert judgment resulted in the correct prognosis of survival at 1 year 79.7% (n = 5241 patients) of the time (true survival rate, see Table 1). This translates to 20.3% (n = 1334 patients) frequency of incorrect judgment of survival. (Presuming that the decision to implant an LVAD in these patients was predicated on positive 1-year survival prognosis.) With the added contribution of CHRiSS in decision-making, 85.3% (see True Negative in Table 2) of these 79.7% (actual survival from Table 1) would be corroborated by the prognostic model. Thereby denying an LVAD from 14.7% of these patients who would have survived, had the physician followed CHRiSS recommendation. On the other hand, the expert incorrectly predicted survival in 20.3% (n = 1334, mortality

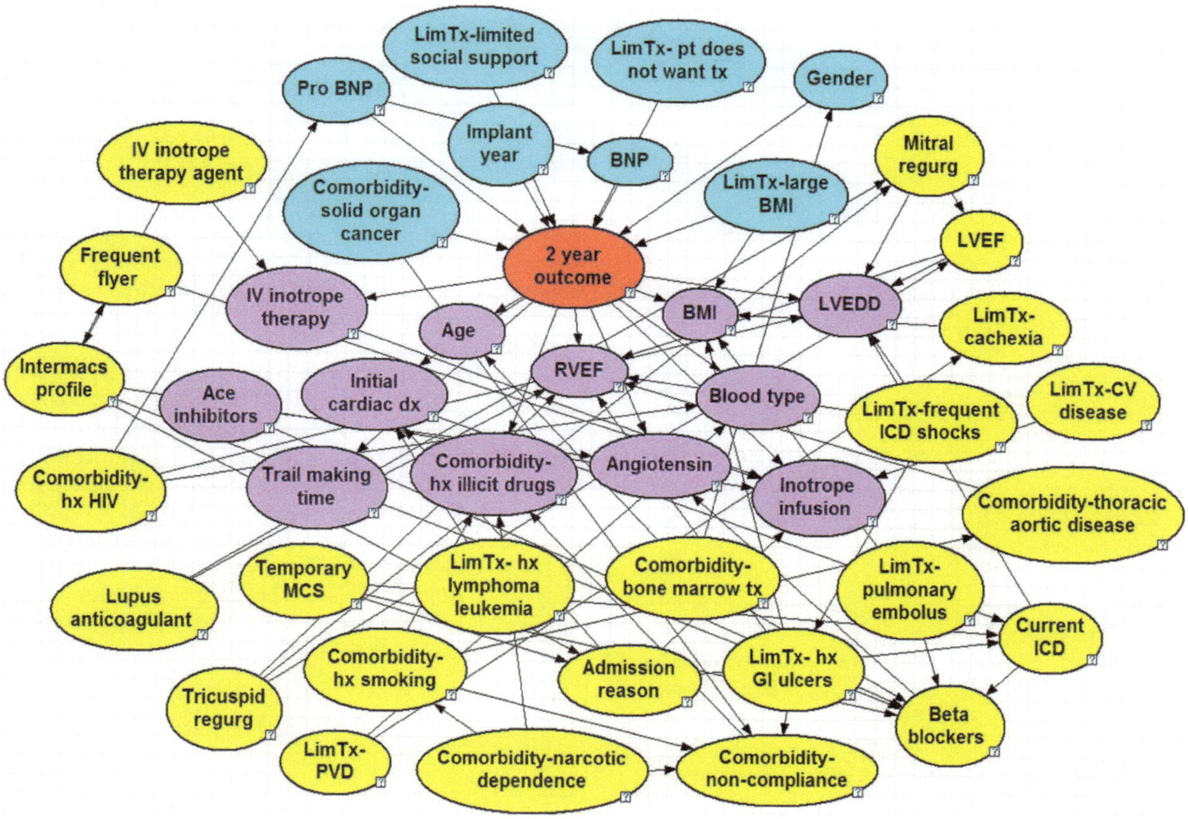

Figure 5. 2 Year Bayesian Model. Node colors: red = class, blue = parent, purple = child, yellow = spouse. Question marks identify nodes that do not have specific evidence set and use the population distribution as the prior distribution. LVEDD = left ventricle end diastolic diameter, BNP = B-type natriuretic peptide, LVEF = left ventricle ejection fraction, GI = gastrointestinal, IV = intravenous, ICD = implantable cardioverter defibrillator, PVD = peripheral vascular disease, hx HIV = history of human immunodeficiency virus, BMI = body mass index, MCS = mechanical circulatory support, CV = cardiovascular.

% from Table 1). CHRiSS would have predicted almost half of these patients, hence sparing 667 patients from a suboptimal outcome. Although there is no way of knowing, retrospectively, how long these LVAD patients would have survived if they did not receive a LVAD, the additional insight provided by CHRiSS would assist the patient and physician in weighing the risks and benefits of the various courses of treatment. For example, these patients may be prioritized for cardiac transplantation, thereby making better use of limited organ supply for those who would not otherwise survive on a LVAD (in exchange for a transplant patient who would have done just as well on a LVAD.)

The 2-year CHRiSS model correctly identified 65% of patients who would not survive past the endpoint, which would be very important to know for DT patients to decide if they wish to accept this risk considering chance of surviving (and thriving) for many years with this end of life treatment. Following the same logic for predicting short-term outcomes, CHRiSS would spare half of the 387 patients from undergoing a major surgery who would do very poorly during the recovery post-implant. The 30-day model could aid in vetting potential high risk DT and bridge to transplant (BTT) candidates. Paradoxically, the performance of the 90-day and 6-month models were not as good as the 30-day, 1-year, and 2-year models. This may be attributable to the heterogeneity in causes of death, which may confound the Bayesian Network to identify specific predictive variables.

Table 2. Summary of Bayesian Model Performance.

Endpoint	Accuracy (%)	True Positive (Dead) (%)	True Negative (Alive) (%)	ROC (%)
30 Day	94.9	51.0	99.4	92.5
90 Day	84.2	22.9	97.1	73.9
6 Month	78.2	30.3	93.7	70.6
1 Year	73.1	49.1	85.3	70.6
2 Year	71.4	65.0	76.2	70.8

ROC = receiver operating characteristic curve.

We had also conducted a sensitivity analysis to observe the direct effects of each variable on the outcome, as well as the additive effects of several variables. The variables that created the greatest effect on the outcome were presented in the results section for each model. For the short-term outcome, positive HIV increased likelihood of mortality by 42% at 30-days and 35% at 90-days. Each of these percentages were further increase by 5–10% when adding an enlarged LVEDD (dilated cardiomyopathy) or elevated cholesterol, respectively. When considering long-term predictors (2-year model), one of the parent nodes was BNP, which had bi-modal effects: normal levels lead to reduced chance of mortality by 5% and elevated levels increased mortality by 7%.

The use and acceptance of Bayesian methodology are becoming increasingly prevalent in the medical community (see, for example [34–42]). For example, in 2010, the FDA released a guidance for the use of Bayesian statistics in medical device clinical trials [43]. In 2013, the United Network for Organ Sharing (UNOS) proposed the adoption of a new Bayesian methodology to better identify those transplant programs that may be underperforming in the area of patient and graft survival.

Although the methods described in this study are more advanced than the current risk scores used in HF prognosis, the results are far from perfect. There are several limitations that may adversely affect performance, including inherent retrospective bias, imbalance of the outcome variable, and extensive missing data. We aim to address these limitations in our ongoing prospective studies. It is also important to clarify that the CHRiSS models are able to discern likelihood of mortality for patients receiving an LVAD and does not allude to any predictions for patients not receiving the device. We plan to perform a follow up study that will derive BN models based on both INTERMACS data, as well as a HF cohort for those who do not receive an LVAD. Nevertheless, the current models are able to provide decision support to the HF clinicians regarding potential future LVAD recipients.

This study was the first application of the Bayesian Network algorithm to a cohort of LVAD recipients. Although the current models outperform the current LVAD risk scores, there is an opportunity to improve them yet further as additional prospective data is collected, and additional risk factors are added to the model. Most certainly, the Bayesian models better represent the complex inter-variable relationships between clinical variables, better emulating human logic, which in turn makes them more appealing to end users.

Supporting Information

Figure S1 A simple Bayesian network model modeling risk factors related to LVAD survival.

Table S1 Many = not all format options listed, DT = destination therapy, BTT = bridge to transplant, BTR = bridge to recovery, CPB = cardiopulmonary bypass, MI = myocardial infarction, ECMO = extracorporeal membrane oxygenator, CABG = coronary artery bypass graft, IABP = intra-aortic balloon pump, INR = international normalized ratio, ICD = implantable cardioverter defibrillator, BNP = B-type natriuretic peptide, WBC = white blood cell, ALT = alanine transaminase, AST = aspartate aminotransferase, CRP = C-Reactive Protein, LVEF = left ventricle ejection fraction, LVEDD = left ventricle end diastolic diameter, RVEF = right ventricle ejection fraction, PCWP = pulmonary capillary wedge pressure, NYHA = New York Heart Association functional class, HF = heart failure, GI = gastrointestinal, HIV = human immunodeficiency virus.

Acknowledgments

We would like to thank Dr. Manreet Kanwar, Dr. Srinivas Murali and Dr. Raymond Benza at Allegheny General Hospital for their clinical insight and expertise. We thank Dr. James Kirklin, Dr. Francis Pagani and Dr. David Naftel of INTERMACS for allowing us to use their registry for the study. We would lastly like to thank Susan Meyers and Grant Studdard for their administrative, database, and statistical assistance with INTERMACS. Models described in this paper have been constructed using GeNIe, a modeling environment for graphical probabilistic models available at http://genie.sis.pitt.edu/.

Author Contributions

Conceived and designed the experiments: NAL JFA MJD. Performed the experiments: NAL. Analyzed the data: NAL. Contributed reagents/materials/analysis tools: MJD. Wrote the paper: NAL JFA. Created the software used in analysis: MJD. Provided technical insight: MJD. Provided funding: JFA.

References

1. Lietz K, Miller LW (2008) Destination therapy: current results and future promise. In: Seminars in thoracic and cardiovascular surgery. Elsevier, volume 20, pp. 225–233.
2. Miller LW (2011) Left ventricular assist devices are underutilized. Circulation 123: 1552–1558.
3. Stewart GC, Stevenson LW, Miller LW (2011) Keeping left ventricular assist device acceleration on track. Circulation 123: 1559–1568.
4. Peura JL, Colvin-Adams M, Francis GS, Grady KL, Hoffman TM, et al. (2012) Recommendations for the use of mechanical circulatory support: Device strategies and patient selection a scientific statement from the american heart association. Circulation 126: 2648–2667.
5. Lietz K, Long JW, Kfoury AG, Slaughter MS, Silver MA, et al. (2007) Outcomes of left ventricular assist device implantation as destination therapy in the post-rematch era implications for patient selection. Circulation 116: 497–505.
6. Rose EA, Moskowitz AJ, Packer M, Sollano JA, Williams DL, et al. (1999) The rematch trial: rationale, design, and end points. The Annals of thoracic surgery 67: 723–730.
7. Teuteberg JJ, Ewald GA, Adamson RM, Lietz K, Miller LW, et al. (2012) Risk assessment for continuous flow left ventricular assist devices: does the destination therapy risk score work? an analysis of over 1,000 patients. Journal of the American College of Cardiology 60: 44–51.
8. Cowger J, Sundareswaran K, Rogers JG, Park SJ, Pagani FD, et al. (2013) Predicting survival in patients receiving continuous flow left ventricular assist devicesthe heartmate ii risk score. Journal of the American College of Cardiology 61: 313–321.
9. Brahnam S, Jain LC (2011) Intelligent Decision Support Systems in Healthcare. Springer.
10. Musen MA, Middleton B, Greenes RA (2014) Clinical decision-support systems. In: Biomedical informatics, Springer. pp. 643–674.
11. Berry DA (2006) Bayesian clinical trials. Nature Reviews Drug Discovery 5: 27–36.
12. Ibrahim JG, Chen MH, Sinha D (2005) Bayesian survival analysis. Wiley Online Library.
13. Kratz A, Ferraro M, Sluss PM, Lewandrowski KB (2004) Laboratory reference values. New England Journal of Medicine 351: 1548–1564.
14. Parameters NH (2009) Laboratory values. Edwards Lifesciences website: www edwards com.
15. Lin JH, Haug PJ (2008) Exploiting missing clinical data in bayesian network modeling for predicting medical problems. Journal of biomedical informatics 41: 1–14.
16. Oniœko A, Druzdzel MJ, Wasyluk H (2002) An experimental comparison of methods for handling incomplete data in learning parameters of bayesian networks. In: Intelligent Information Systems 2002, Springer. pp. 351–360.
17. EuroQol G (1990) Euroqol–a new facility for the measurement of health-related quality of life. Health policy (Amsterdam, Netherlands) 16: 199.
18. Faller H, Steinbüchel T, Schowalter M, Spertus JA, Störk S, et al. (2004) [the kansas city cardiomyopathy questionnaire (kccq)–a new disease-specific quality

of life measure for patients with chronic heart failure]. Psychotherapie, Psychosomatik, medizinische Psychologie 55: 200–208.
19. Chawla NV, Bowyer KW, Hall LO, Kegelmeyer WP (2011) Smote: synthetic minority over-sampling technique. arXiv preprint arXiv:11061813.
20. Santelices LC, Wang Y, Severyn D, Druzdzel MJ, Kormos RL, et al. (2010) Development of a hybrid decision support model for optimal ventricular assist device weaning. The Annals of thoracic surgery 90: 713–720.
21. Wang Y, Simon MA, Bonde P, Harris BU, Teuteberg JJ, et al. (2012) Decision tree for adjuvant right ventricular support in patients receiving a left ventricular assist device. The Journal of Heart and Lung Transplantation 31: 140–149.
22. Wang Y, Simon M, Bonde P, Harris BU, Teuteberg JJ, et al. (2012) Prognosis of right ventricular failure in patients with left ventricular assist device based on decision tree with smote. Information Technology in Biomedicine, IEEE Transactions on 16: 383–390.
23. Wang Y, Rosé CP, Ferreira A, McNamara DM, Kormos RL, et al. (2010) A classification approach for risk prognosis of patients on mechanical ventricular assistance. In: Machine Learning and Applications (ICMLA), 2010 Ninth International Conference on. IEEE, pp. 293–298.
24. Loghmanpour N, Kanwar M, Wang Y, Snyder T, Horstmanshof D, et al. (2013) A novel, risk stratification model using bayesian networks for continuous flow left ventricular assist device 90-day survival. The Journal of Heart and Lung Transplantation 32: S232.
25. Kanwar M, Loghmanpour N, Wang Y, Snyder T, Horstmanshof D, et al. (2013) A novel, risk stratification model using bayesian networks for continuous-flow left ventricular assist device 90-day survival. Journal of the American College of Cardiology 61.
26. Pearl J (1988) Probabilistic reasoning in intelligent systems: networks of plausible inference. Morgan Kaufmann.
27. Oniœko A, Druzdzel MJ (2013) Impact of precision of bayesian network parameters on accuracy of medical diagnostic systems. Artificial intelligence in medicine 57: 197–206.
28. Oniœko ADM (2014) Impact of bayesian network model structure on the accuracy of medical diagnostic systems. 13th International Conference on Artificial Intelligence and Soft Computing (ICAISC-2014).
29. Heckerman D (1998) A tutorial on learning with Bayesian networks. Springer.
30. Cooper GF, Herskovits E (1991) A bayesian method for constructing bayesian belief networks from databases. In: Proceedings of the Seventh conference on Uncertainty in Artificial Intelligence. Morgan Kaufmann Publishers Inc., pp. 86–94.
31. Koller D, Sahami M (1996) Toward optimal feature selection.
32. Druzdzel MJ (1999) Genie: A development environment for graphical decision-analytic models. In: Proceedings of the AMIA Symposium. American Medical Informatics Association, p. 1206.
33. Witten IH, Frank E (2005) Data Mining: Practical machine learning tools and techniques. Morgan Kaufmann.
34. Hoot N, Aronsky D (2005) Using bayesian networks to predict survival of liver transplant patients. In: AMIA annual symposium proceedings. American Medical Informatics Association, volume 2005, p. 345.
35. Lucas P (2001) Bayesian networks in medicine: a model-based approach to medical decision making. In: Proceedings of the EUNITE workshop on Intelligent Systems in patient Care. pp. 73–97.
36. Eom JH, Kim SC, Zhang BT (2008) Aptacdss-e: A classifier ensemble-based clinical decision support system for cardiovascular disease level prediction. Expert Systems with Applications 34: 2465–2479.
37. Sadeghi S, Barzi A, Sadeghi N, King B (2006) A bayesian model for triage decision support. International Journal of Medical Informatics 75: 403–411.
38. Gevaert O, De Smet F, Timmerman D, Moreau Y, De Moor B (2006) Predicting the prognosis of breast cancer by integrating clinical and microarray data with bayesian networks. Bioinformatics 22: e184–e190.
39. Charitos T, Van Der Gaag LC, Visscher S, Schurink KA, Lucas PJ (2009) A dynamic bayesian network for diagnosing ventilator-associated pneumonia in icu patients. Expert Systems with Applications 36: 1249–1258.
40. Austin RM, Onisko A, Druzdzel MJ (2010) The pittsburgh cervical cancer screening model: a risk assessment tool. Archives of pathology & laboratory medicine 134: 744–750.
41. Cao C, Leong TY, Leong AP, Seow FC (1998) Dynamic decision analysis in medicine: a data-driven approach. International journal of medical informatics 51: 13–28.
42. Diez FJ, Mira J, Iturralde E, Zubillaga S (1997) Diaval, a bayesian expert system for echocardiography. Artificial Intelligence in Medicine 10: 59–73.
43. FDA (2010). Guidance for the use of bayesian statistics in medical device clinical trials.

Permissions

All chapters in this book were first published in PLOS ONE, by The Public Library of Science; hereby published with permission under the Creative Commons Attribution License or equivalent. Every chapter published in this book has been scrutinized by our experts. Their significance has been extensively debated. The topics covered herein carry significant findings which will fuel the growth of the discipline. They may even be implemented as practical applications or may be referred to as a beginning point for another development.

The contributors of this book come from diverse backgrounds, making this book a truly international effort. This book will bring forth new frontiers with its revolutionizing research information and detailed analysis of the nascent developments around the world.

We would like to thank all the contributing authors for lending their expertise to make the book truly unique. They have played a crucial role in the development of this book. Without their invaluable contributions this book wouldn't have been possible. They have made vital efforts to compile up to date information on the varied aspects of this subject to make this book a valuable addition to the collection of many professionals and students.

This book was conceptualized with the vision of imparting up-to-date information and advanced data in this field. To ensure the same, a matchless editorial board was set up. Every individual on the board went through rigorous rounds of assessment to prove their worth. After which they invested a large part of their time researching and compiling the most relevant data for our readers.

The editorial board has been involved in producing this book since its inception. They have spent rigorous hours researching and exploring the diverse topics which have resulted in the successful publishing of this book. They have passed on their knowledge of decades through this book. To expedite this challenging task, the publisher supported the team at every step. A small team of assistant editors was also appointed to further simplify the editing procedure and attain best results for the readers.

Apart from the editorial board, the designing team has also invested a significant amount of their time in understanding the subject and creating the most relevant covers. They scrutinized every image to scout for the most suitable representation of the subject and create an appropriate cover for the book.

The publishing team has been an ardent support to the editorial, designing and production team. Their endless efforts to recruit the best for this project, has resulted in the accomplishment of this book. They are a veteran in the field of academics and their pool of knowledge is as vast as their experience in printing. Their expertise and guidance has proved useful at every step. Their uncompromising quality standards have made this book an exceptional effort. Their encouragement from time to time has been an inspiration for everyone.

The publisher and the editorial board hope that this book will prove to be a valuable piece of knowledge for researchers, students, practitioners and scholars across the globe.

List of Contributors

Chia-Jui Yang
Department of Internal Medicine, Far East Memorial Hospital, New Taipei City, Taiwan

Nan-Yao Lee
Department of Internal Medicine, Far East Memorial Hospital, New Taipei City, Taiwan

Tun-Chieh Chen
Department of Internal Medicine, Kaohsiung Medical University Hospital and College of Medicine, Kaohsiung Medical University, Kaohsiung, Taiwan
Department of Internal Medicine, Kaohsiung Municipal Ta-Tung Hospital, Kaohsiung Medical University, Kaohsiung, Taiwan

Yu-Hui Lin
Department of Internal Medicine, Taichung Veterans General Hospital, Taichung, Taiwan

Shiou-Haur Liang
Department of Internal Medicine, E-Da Hospital/I-Shou University, Kaohsiung, Taiwan,

Po-Liang Lu
Department of Internal Medicine, Kaohsiung Medical University Hospital and College of Medicine, Kaohsiung Medical University, Kaohsiung, Taiwan

Wen-Chi Huang
Department of Internal Medicine, Kaohsiung Chang Gung Memorial Hospital, Chang Gung University College of Medicine, Kaohsiung, Taiwan

Hung-Jen Tang
Department of Internal Medicine, Chi-Mei Medical Center, Tainan, Taiwan

Chen-Hsiang Lee
Department of Internal Medicine, Kaohsiung Chang Gung Memorial Hospital, Chang Gung University College of Medicine, Kaohsiung, Taiwan

Hsi-Hsun Lin
Department of Internal Medicine, E-Da Hospital/I-Shou University, Kaohsiung, Taiwan,

Yen-Hsu Chen
Department of Internal Medicine, Kaohsiung Medical University Hospital and College of Medicine, Kaohsiung Medical University, Kaohsiung, Taiwan

Wen-Chien Ko
Department of Internal Medicine, Far East Memorial Hospital, New Taipei City, Taiwan

Chien-Ching Hung
Department of Internal Medicine, National Taiwan University Hospital and National Taiwan University College of Medicine, Taipei, Taiwan
Department of Medical Research, China Medical University Hospital, Taichung, Taiwan
China Medical University, Taichung, Taiwan

Shan Qiao and Xiaoming Li
Prevention Research Center, Carman and Ann Adams Department of Pediatrics, School of Medicine, Wayne State University, Detroit, Michigan, United States of America

Bonita Stanton Zhang
Institute of Global Health, Vanderbilt University, Nashville, Tennessee, United States of America

Chen Yuejiao Zhou, Zhiyong Shen and Zhenzhu Tang
Guangxi Center of Disease Control and Prevention, Guangxi, China

Sten H. Vermund
Vanderbilt Institute for Global Health, Vanderbilt University School of Medicine, Nashville, Tennessee, United States of America
Department of Pediatrics, Vanderbilt University School of Medicine, Nashville, Tennessee, United States of America

Meridith Blevins
Vanderbilt Institute for Global Health, Vanderbilt University School of Medicine, Nashville, Tennessee, United States of America
Department of Biostatistics, Vanderbilt University School of Medicine, Nashville, Tennessee, United States of America

Troy D. Moon
Vanderbilt Institute for Global Health, Vanderbilt University School of Medicine, Nashville, Tennessee, United States of America
Department of Pediatrics, Vanderbilt University School of Medicine, Nashville, Tennessee, United States of America

Eurico José
Friends in Global Health, Quelimane and Maputo, Mozambique

Linda Moiane
Friends in Global Health, Quelimane and Maputo, Mozambique

José A. Tique
Vanderbilt Institute for Global Health, Vanderbilt University School of Medicine, Nashville, Tennessee, United States of America
Friends in Global Health, Quelimane and Maputo, Mozambique

Mohsin Sidat
School of Medicine, Universidade Eduardo Mondlane, Maputo, Mozambique

Philip J. Ciampa
Vanderbilt Institute for Global Health, Vanderbilt University School of Medicine, Nashville, Tennessee, United States of America
Department of Medicine, Vanderbilt University School of Medicine, Nashville, Tennessee, United States of America

Bryan E. Shepherd
Vanderbilt Institute for Global Health, Vanderbilt University School of Medicine, Nashville, Tennessee, United States of America
Department of Biostatistics, Vanderbilt University School of Medicine, Nashville, Tennessee, United States of America

Lara M. E. Vaz
Vanderbilt Institute for Global Health, Vanderbilt University School of Medicine, Nashville, Tennessee, United States of America
Department of Preventive Medicine, Vanderbilt University School of Medicine, Nashville, Tennessee, United States of America
Friends in Global Health, Quelimane and Maputo, Mozambique

Anna Vassall
London School of Hygiene and Tropical Medicine, London, United Kingdom

Sudhashree Chandrashekar
London School of Hygiene and Tropical Medicine, London, United Kingdom
St John's Research Institute, Bangalore, India

Michael Pickles
London School of Hygiene and Tropical Medicine, London, United Kingdom
Kingdom Imperial College, London, United Kingdom

Tara S. Beattie
London School of Hygiene and Tropical Medicine, London, United Kingdom

Govindraj Shetty
Karnataka Health Promotion Trust, Bangalore, India

Parinita Bhattacharjee
St John's Research Institute, Bangalore, India

Marie-Claude Boily
Imperial College, London, United Kingdom

Peter Vickerman
London School of Hygiene and Tropical Medicine, London, United Kingdom

Janet Bradley
URESP, Centre de recherche du CHU de Québec, Québec, Canada

Michel Alary
URESP, Centre de recherche du CHU de Québec, Québec, Canada
Département de médecine sociale et préventive, Université Laval, Québec, Canada

Stephen Moses
Karnataka Health Promotion Trust, Bangalore, India

Charlotte Watts
London School of Hygiene and Tropical Medicine, London, United

Xingguang Li
State Key Laboratory for Infectious Disease Prevention and Control, National Center for AIDS/STD Control and Prevention, Chinese Center for Disease Control and Prevention, Beijing, China, and Collaborative Innovation Center for Diagnosis and Treatment of Infectious Diseases, Hangzhou, Zhejiang, China
HIV Molecular Epidemiology and Virology Research Group, The State Key Laboratory of Virology, Wuhan Institute of Virology, University of Chinese Academy of Sciences, Wuhan, Hubei, China

Xihui Zang
Jilin Provincial Center for Disease Control and Prevention, Changchun, Jilin, China

Chuanyi Ning
State Key Laboratory for Infectious Disease Prevention and Control, National Center for AIDS/STD Control and Prevention, Chinese Center for Disease Control and Prevention, Beijing, China, and Collaborative Innovation Center for Diagnosis and Treatment of Infectious Diseases, Hangzhou, Zhejiang, China
Guangxi Key Laboratory of AIDS Prevention and Treatment & School of Public Health, Guangxi Medical University, Nanning, Guangxi, China

Yi Feng, Cunxin Xie, Xiang He, Hui Xing and Yiming Shao
State Key Laboratory for Infectious Disease Prevention and Control, National Center for AIDS/STD Control and Prevention, Chinese Center for Disease Control and Prevention, Beijing, China, and Collaborative Innovation Center for Diagnosis and Treatment of Infectious Diseases, Hangzhou, Zhejiang, China

Yutaka Takebe
State Key Laboratory for Infectious Disease Prevention and Control, National Center for AIDS/STD Control and Prevention, Chinese Center for Disease Control and Prevention, Beijing, China, and Collaborative Innovation Center for Diagnosis and Treatment of Infectious Diseases, Hangzhou, Zhejiang, China
AIDS Research Center, National Institute of Infectious Diseases, Tokyo, Japan

Liuyan Sun, Qi Guo
Jilin Provincial Center for Disease Control and Prevention, Changchun, Jilin, China

Marcia L. Kalish
Vanderbilt Institute for Global Health, Vanderbilt University School of Medicine, Nashville, Tennessee, United States of America

Tamil Kendall
Women and Health Initiative and Takemi Program in International Health, Department of Global Health and Population, Harvard School of Public Health, Boston, Massachusetts, United States of America

Tim Lane, Thomas Osmand, Alexander Marr, Starley B. Shade and Susan Kegeles
Center for AIDS Prevention Studies, University of California San Francisco, San Francisco, California, United States of America

Kristin Dunkle
Rollins School of Public Health, Emory University, Atlanta, Georgia, United States of America

Theodorus Sandfort
HIV Center for Clinical and Behavioral Studies, Columbia University, New York, New York, United States of America

Helen Struthers
Anova Health Institute, Johannesburg, South Africa
Division of Infectious Diseases & HIV Medicine, Department of Medicine, University of Cape Town, Cape Town, South Africa

James A. McIntyre
Anova Health Institute, Johannesburg, South Africa
School of Public Health & Family Medicine, University of Cape Town, Cape Town, South Africa

Benjamin Trinité, Chi N. Chan, Caroline S. Lee, Saurabh Mahajan and David N. Levy
Department of Basic Science, New York University College of Dentistry, New York, New York, United States of America

Yang Luo and Mark A. Muesing
Aaron Diamond AIDS Research Center, New York, New York, United States of America

Joy M. Folkvord, Michael Pham and Elizabeth Connick
Department of Medicine, University of Colorado Denver, Aurora, Colorado, United States of America

Viraj Kulkarni and Barbara K. Felber
Human Retrovirus Pathogenesis Section, Vaccine Branch, Center for Cancer Research, National Cancer Institute at Frederick, Frederick, Maryland, United States of America

Antonio Valentin, George N. Pavlakis and Margherita Rosati
Human Retrovirus Section, Vaccine Branch, Center for Cancer Research, National Cancer Institute at Frederick, Frederick, Maryland, United States of America

Morgane Rolland and James I. Mullins
Departments of Microbiology, Medicine and Laboratory Medicine, University of Washington, Seattle, Washington, United States of America

Matthew P. Fox
Center for Global Health & Development, Boston University, Boston, Massachusetts, United States of America
Health Economics and Epidemiology Research Office, Department of Internal Medicine, School of Clinical Medicine, Faculty of Health Sciences, University of the Witwatersrand, Johannesburg, South Africa
Department of Epidemiology, Boston University School of Public Health, Boston, Massachusetts, United States of America

Kate Shearer
Health Economics and Epidemiology Research Office, Department of Internal Medicine, School of Clinical Medicine, Faculty of Health Sciences, University of the Witwatersrand, Johannesburg, South Africa

Mhairi Maskew
Health Economics and Epidemiology Research Office, Department of Internal Medicine, School of Clinical Medicine, Faculty of Health Sciences, University of the Witwatersrand, Johannesburg, South Africa

Gesine Meyer-Rath
Center for Global Health & Development, Boston University, Boston, Massachusetts, United States of America
Health Economics and Epidemiology Research Office, Department of Internal Medicine, School of Clinical Medicine, Faculty of Health Sciences, University of the Witwatersrand, Johannesburg, South Africa

Kate Clouse
Health Economics and Epidemiology Research Office, Department of Internal Medicine, School of Clinical Medicine, Faculty of Health Sciences, University of the Witwatersrand, Johannesburg, South Africa
Vanderbilt Institute for Global Health, Vanderbilt University, Nashville, Tennessee, United States of America

Ian Sanne
Health Economics and Epidemiology Research Office, Department of Internal Medicine, School of Clinical Medicine, Faculty of Health Sciences, University of the Witwatersrand, Johannesburg, South Africa
Clinical HIV Research Unit, Department of Internal Medicine, School of Clinical Medicine, Faculty of Health Sciences, University of the Witwatersrand, Johannesburg, South Africa

Thijs Booiman, Viviana Cobos Jimé nez, Karel A. van Dort, Angé lique B. van 't Wout and Neeltje A. Kootstra
Department of Experimental Immunology, Sanquin Research, Landsteiner Laboratory and Center for Infection and Immunity (CINIMA) at the Academic Medical Center of the University of Amsterdam, Amsterdam, The Netherlands

Denny McLaughlin
Department of Biochemistry, Microbiology and Immunology, Faculty of Medicine, University of Ottawa, Ottawa, Ontario, Canada

Elliott Faller
Department of Biochemistry, Microbiology and Immunology, Faculty of Medicine, University of Ottawa, Ottawa, Ontario, Canada
Ottawa Hospital Research Institute, Ottawa, Ontario, Canada

Scott Sugden
Department of Biochemistry, Microbiology and Immunology, Faculty of Medicine, University of Ottawa, Ottawa, Ontario, Canada

Paul MacPherson
Department of Biochemistry, Microbiology and Immunology, Faculty of Medicine, University of Ottawa, Ottawa, Ontario, Canada
Department of Medicine, Faculty of Medicine, University of Ottawa, Ottawa, Ontario, Canada
Division of Infectious Diseases, Ottawa Hospital General Campus, Ottawa, Ontario, Canada
Ottawa Hospital Research Institute, Ottawa, Ontario, Canada

Camilla Tincati and Matteo Basilissi
Department of Health Sciences, Clinic of Infectious Diseases and Tropical Medicine, "San Paolo" Hospital, University of Milan, Milan, Italy

Elisabetta Sinigaglia
Blood Transfusion Unit, "San Paolo" Hospital, Milan, Italy

Esther Merlini
Department of Health Sciences, Clinic of Infectious Diseases and Tropical Medicine, "San Paolo" Hospital, University of Milan, Milan, Italy

Giovanni Carpani
Blood Transfusion Unit, "San Paolo" Hospital, Milan, Italy

Antonella d'Arminio Monforte
Department of Health Sciences, Clinic of Infectious Diseases and Tropical Medicine, "San Paolo" Hospital, University of Milan, Milan, Italy

Giulia Marchetti
Department of Health Sciences, Clinic of Infectious Diseases and Tropical Medicine, "San Paolo" Hospital, University of Milan, Milan, Italy

Camden J. Hallmark
Houston Department of Health and Human Services, Houston, Texas, United States of America

Jennifer Skillicorn
Department of Epidemiology and Biostatistics, School of Public Health and Health Services, George Washington University, Washington, DC, United States of America

Thomas P. Giordano
Center for Innovations in Quality, Effectiveness and Safety, Michael E. DeBakey VA Medical Center, Houston, Texas, United States of America
Department of Medicine, Baylor College of Medicine, Houston, Texas, United States of America

Jessica A. Davila
Center for Innovations in Quality, Effectiveness and Safety, Michael E. DeBakey VA Medical Center, Houston, Texas, United States of America
Department of Medicine, Baylor College of Medicine, Houston, Texas, United States of America

Marlene McNeese
Houston Department of Health and Human Services, Houston, Texas, United States of America

Nestor Rocha, Avemaria Smith and Stacey Cooper
HIV/AIDS, Hepatitis, STD, and TB Administration, District of Columbia Department of Health, Washington, DC, United States of America

Amanda D. Castel
Department of Epidemiology and Biostatistics, School of Public Health and Health Services, George Washington University, Washington, DC, United States of America

Walter R. Lopes de Campos, Nthato Chirwa, Grace London and Lia S. Rotherham
Emerging Health Technologies Competency Area, Biosciences Unit, Council for Scientific and Industrial Research, Pretoria, South Africa

Lynn Morris
National Institute for Communicable Diseases, Sandringham, South Africa

Bongani M. Mayosi
Department of Medicine, Groote Schuur Hospital and University of Cape Town, Cape Town, South Africa

Makobetsa Khati
Emerging Health Technologies Competency Area, Biosciences Unit, Council for Scientific and Industrial Research, Pretoria, South Africa
Department of Medicine, Groote Schuur Hospital and University of Cape Town, Cape Town, South Africa

Tendesayi Kufa
The Aurum Institute, Johannesburg, South Africa
The School of Public Health, University of the Witwatersrand, Johannesburg, South Africa

Tonderai Mabuto and Evans Muchiri
The Aurum Institute, Johannesburg, South Africa,

Salome Charalambous
The Aurum Institute, Johannesburg, South Africa
The School of Public Health, University of the Witwatersrand, Johannesburg, South Africa

Dominique Rosillon
GlaxoSmithKline Vaccines, Wavre, Belgium

Gavin Churchyard
The Aurum Institute, Johannesburg, South Africa
The School of Public Health, University of the Witwatersrand, Johannesburg, South Africa

Rebecca C. Harris
CROMSOURCE on behalf of GlaxoSmithKline Vaccines, Wavre, Belgium

Congting Ye
Department of Automation, Xiamen University, Xiamen, Fujian 361005, China
Department of Biology, Miami University, Oxford, Ohio 45056, United States of America

Guoli Ji
Department of Automation, Xiamen University, Xiamen, Fujian 361005, China
Innovation Center for Cell Biology, Xiamen University, Xiamen, Fujian 361005, China

Lei Li
Department of Automation, Xiamen University, Xiamen, Fujian 361005, China
Department of Biology, Miami University, Oxford, Ohio 45056, United States of America

Chun Liang
Department of Biology, Miami University, Oxford, Ohio 45056, United States of America
State Key Laboratory for Biology of Plant Diseases and Insect Pests, Institute of Plant Protection, Chinese Academy of Agricultural Sciences, Beijing 100193, China

Johanna Maria Eberhard
Infectious Diseases Unit, Department of Medicine, University Medical Center Hamburg-Eppendorf, Hamburg, Germany
Heinrich Pette Institute - Leibniz Institute for Experimental Virology, Hamburg, Germany

Philip Hartjen
Infectious Diseases Unit, Department of Medicine, University Medical Center Hamburg-Eppendorf, Hamburg, Germany
Department of Oral and Maxillofacial Surgery, University Medical Center Hamburg-Eppendorf, Hamburg, Germany

Silke Kummer
Infectious Diseases Unit, Department of Medicine, University Medical Center Hamburg-Eppendorf, Hamburg, Germany
Heinrich Pette Institute - Leibniz Institute for Experimental Virology, Hamburg, Germany

Reinhold E. Schmidt
Department of Immunology and Rheumatology, Hannover Medical School, Hanover, Germany
German Center for Infection Research (DZIF), partner site Hamburg and Hannover, Hamburg and Hannover, Germany

Maximilian Bockhorn
Department of General Surgery, University Medical Center Hamburg-Eppendorf, Hamburg, Germany

Clara Lehmann
Department of Internal Medicine I, University Hospital of Cologne, Cologne, Germany, 7 School of Medicine, Johns Hopkins University

Ashwin Balagopal
Baltimore, Maryland, United States of America

Joachim Hauber
Heinrich Pette Institute - Leibniz Institute for Experimental Virology, Hamburg, Germany
German Center for Infection Research (DZIF), partner site Hamburg and Hannover, Hamburg and Hannover, Germany

Jan van Lunzen
Infectious Diseases Unit, Department of Medicine, University Medical Center Hamburg-Eppendorf, Hamburg, Germany
Heinrich Pette Institute - Leibniz Institute for Experimental Virology, Hamburg, Germany
German Center for Infection Research (DZIF), partner site Hamburg and Hannover, Hamburg and Hannover, Germany

Julian Schulze zur Wiesch
Infectious Diseases Unit, wDepartment of Medicine, University Medical Center Hamburg-Eppendorf, Hamburg, Germany
Heinrich Pette Institute - Leibniz Institute for Experimental Virology, Hamburg, Germany

German Center for Infection Research (DZIF), partner site Hamburg and Hannover, Hamburg and Hannover, Germany

Iryna B. Zablotska
The Kirby Institute, The University of NSW Australia, Sydney, NSW, Australia

Andrew Frankland
The Kirby Institute, The University of NSW Australia, Sydney, NSW, Australia,
School of Psychiatry, The University of NSW Australia, Sydney, NSW, Australia

Martin Holt and John de Wit
Centre for Social Research in Health, The University of NSW Australia, Sydney, NSW, Australia,

Graham Brown
The Australian Research Centre in Sex, Health and Society, La Trobe University, Melbourne, VIC, Australia
Curtin University, Perth, WA, Australia

Bruce Maycock
Curtin University, Perth, WA, Australia

Christopher Fairley
Central Clinical School, Monash University, Melbourne, VIC, Australia
Melbourne Sexual Health Centre, Melbourne, VIC, Australia

Garrett Prestage
The Kirby Institute, The University of NSW Australia, Sydney, NSW, Australia
The Australian Research Centre in Sex, Health and Society, La Trobe University, Melbourne, VIC, Australia

Natasha A. Loghmanpour
Department of Biomedical Engineering, Carnegie Mellon University, Pittsburgh, Pennsylvania, United States of America

Marek J. Druzdzel
Decision Systems Laboratory, School of Information Sciences, University of Pittsburgh, Pittsburgh, Pennsylvania, United States of America
Faculty of Computer Science, Bialystok University of Technology, Bialystok, Poland

James F. Antaki
Department of Biomedical Engineering, Carnegie Mellon University, Pittsburgh, Pennsylvania, United States of America

Index

A

Aids-related Complications, 49-56

Antenatal Care (anc), 49, 52, 155

Anti-gp120 Aptamer, 146

Antibodies, 79, 84-87, 91, 93-94, 112, 115-119, 124, 147, 152, 193, 198-199, 205, 207-208

Antibody Assays, 87

Antiretroviral Therapy, 2-3, 5, 9, 20-23, 25-28, 33, 56, 58, 82, 96, 98, 104-106, 113, 120, 126, 129, 134-135, 146, 156, 164-165, 167, 169, 171, 173-175, 197, 219

Antiretroviral Therapy (art), 27, 33, 96

Art Initiation, 20-23, 67, 96-98, 100-101, 103

B

Bayesian Networks, 220-222, 229

Behavioural Surveillance, 209-210, 212, 217-219

Benzathine Penicillin G (bpg), 1

Bone Impairment, 131, 133

Broad Epitope Recognition, 84

C

Cardiac Health Risk Stratification System (chriss), 220-221, 223, 225, 227, 229

Cardiovascular Impairment, 127-129, 133-134

Cd4 T-cells, 115-125

Cd62l (l-selectin), 69, 71, 73, 75, 77, 79, 81, 83

Cd161+ Mait Cells, 187, 189-191, 193-197

Cell Viability Assays, 116

Centers for Disease Control And Prevention (cdc), 156

Chronic Untreated Hiv Infection, 187

Combination Antiretroviral Therapy, 2-3, 5, 20, 22-23, 26-27, 165, 167, 169, 171, 173, 175

Commercial Sex, 10-13, 15, 18, 38

Community Mobilisation, 29-31, 33-38

Community-based Evaluation, 155, 157, 159, 161, 163

D

Detectir, 176-179, 181-185

Down-modulation, 69-73, 75, 77-79, 81, 83

F

Female Sex Workers, 10-11, 13, 15, 17-19, 29, 31, 33, 35, 37-38

Flow Cytometry, 73, 78-80, 116-124, 127-128, 130, 153, 187

Former Plasma Donors (fpds), 39

Foxo1 Activity, 69-71, 73, 75, 77-79, 81, 83

G

Gmsm, 209-210, 212, 217-218

H

Heterosexual Transmission, 10, 44, 46

Hiv Care Continuum, 136

Hiv Epidemic, 25, 35, 38, 47-49, 56, 66-67, 104, 209, 211, 213, 215, 217, 219

Hiv Impact, 33-34

Hiv Infected Children, 20-21, 23, 25, 27

Hiv Prevention, 10-12, 15-18, 27, 29-31, 33-35, 37-38, 58-59, 67-68, 104, 137-138, 144, 161, 163-164, 210, 218-219

Hiv Testing, 11-12, 15-17, 19, 30, 49-61, 63-68, 96-98, 101, 104, 136-145, 155-164, 209, 212, 217, 219

Hiv-1 Genotype, 42, 44, 46-47

Hiv-1 Infected Macrophages, 106, 149

Hiv-1 Molecular

Epidemiologic Investigation, 40

Hiv-1 Replication, 69-70, 73, 81-83, 106-107, 109-113

Hiv-1 Subtype C, 146-149, 151-153

Hiv-1 Tat Protein, 75, 82, 115-122, 124-126

Hiv-associated Cardiomyopathy (hivcm), 146

Hiv-associated Tuberculosis, 165, 167, 169, 171, 173, 175

Hiv-infected Individuals, 120, 125, 165, 173, 187, 197

Hiv-infected Patients, 1-3, 6-9, 115-116, 125-127, 131, 134, 147, 174-175, 189-191, 193, 195-197

Hiv-positive Msm, 58-59, 65

Hla Genotyping, 199

Hmrs, 221, 225-226

Houston, Texas, 136, 138

Human Cardiomyocytes, 146-147, 149-153

Human Immune Deficiency Virus (hiv), 165

Humoral Immune Responses, 84-89, 91, 93, 95

I

Il-7 Receptor Alpha-chain, 115, 117, 119, 121, 123, 125-126

Imperfect Inverted Repeats, 176-185

Incremental Impact Estimation, 32

Interagency Registry For Mechanically Assisted Circulatory Support (intermacs), 220
Invariant Natural Killer T (inkt), 127, 129, 131, 133-135

L

Left Ventricular Assist Device (lvad) Therapy, 220
Lymph Nodes, 77, 82, 126, 187, 189-191, 193, 195, 197

M

Macrophages, 75, 82, 106-109, 111-114, 125, 146, 149, 151-154, 191, 197
Matlab, 176-177, 182-186
Mexico, 49-50, 55-56, 219
Molecular Epidemiology, 39, 41, 43, 45, 47
Mozambique, 20-28
Mpumalanga Men's Study (mpms), 58-59, 61, 63, 65, 67
Msm, 1, 3, 5-8, 30, 39-42, 44, 46-48, 58-61, 64-68, 129, 167, 218-219
Mucosal-associated Invariant T (mait) Cells, 187

N

Nyanza Province, 155-161, 163

P

P24ce Dna Vaccine, 84-85, 87, 89, 91, 93, 95
Peripheral Blood, 69-70, 78, 109, 113-114, 116, 125-126,
128-129, 149, 187, 189-191, 193, 195, 197
Phenotyping Human Cardiomyocytes, 147
Phosphodiesterase 8a, 106-107, 109, 111, 113
Phylogenetic Tree, 40, 43, 45, 200
Pmtct Uptake, 155, 157, 159, 161, 163
Pre-art Initiation, 96
Psychological Fears, 10-13, 15, 17-19

R

Random Nucleotide Sequence Test, 184
Rapid Plasma Reagin (rpr), 1-2
Respondent-driven Sampling (rds), 59, 209
Reverse Transcription, 74, 77, 81, 106-107, 109-113, 146
Rv144 Vaccine, 198-201, 204-205, 207

S

Southern India, 29, 38
Synthetic Minority Oversampling Technique
(smote), 220, 222
Syphilis, 1-3, 5-11, 18-19, 32, 48, 68

T

T-cell Driven Sieve Effect, 198-199, 201, 203, 205, 207
Treponema Pallidum, 1
Tuberculosis, 22-26, 134, 144, 165-167, 169, 171, 173-175, 186, 189

U

Unaids Strategic Investment, 29

V

Vector Calculation, 176-177
Vertical (mother-to-child) Transmission, 49
Virologically-suppressive Treatment, 127

W

Women's Hiv Disease Progression, 53
World Health Organization, 26, 28, 55, 58, 96, 105, 155, 164, 199, 218